Lecture Notes in Computer Science 8539

Commenced Publication in 1973
Founding and Former Series Editors:
Gerhard Goos, Juris Hartmanis, and Jan van Leeuwen

T0190068

Hiroshi Fujita   Takeshi Hara
Chisako Muramatsu (Eds.)

Breast Imaging

12th International Workshop, IWDM 2014
Gifu City, Japan, June 29 – July 2, 2014
Proceedings

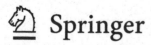

Springer

Volume Editors

Hiroshi Fujita
Takeshi Hara
Chisako Muramatsu
Gifu University Graduate School of Medicine
Department of Intelligent Image Information
1-1 Yanagido, Gifu, Gifu 501-1194, Japan
E-mail: {fujita, chisa}@fjt.info.gifu-u.ac.jp, takeshi.hara@mac.com

ISSN 0302-9743   e-ISSN 1611-3349
ISBN 978-3-319-07886-1   e-ISBN 978-3-319-07887-8
DOI 10.1007/978-3-319-07887-8
Springer Cham Heidelberg New York Dordrecht London

Library of Congress Control Number: 2014940080

LNCS Sublibrary: SL 6 – Image Processing, Computer Vision, Pattern Recognition,
and Graphics

Typesetting: Camera-ready by author, data conversion by Scientific Publishing Services, Chennai, India

Printed on acid-free paper

Springer is part of Springer Science+Business Media (www.springer.com)

Preface

This volume of Springer's *Lecture Notes in Computer Science* series comprises the scientific proceedings of the 12th International Workshop on Breast Imaging (IWDM 2014), which was held June 29-July 2, 2014, in Gifu City, Japan. This workshop was formerly called the International Workshop on Digital Mammography, IWDM for short. Although the term "Digital Mammography" was changed to "Breast Imaging" starting from the last meeting (IWDM 2012), we still kept the familiar abbreviation "IWDM." This new naming is to make clear the recognition of the movement in breast imaging from mammography toward more recent emerging technologies and multimodality imaging solutions. The IWDM meetings traditionally bring together a diverse set of researchers (physicists, mathematicians, computer scientists, and engineers), clinicians (radiologists, surgeons), and representatives of industry, who are jointly committed to developing technology for early detection of and subsequent patient management in breast cancer. The conference series was initiated at a 1993 meeting of the SPIE in San Jose, with subsequent meetings hosted every two years. Previous meetings have been held in York (1994), Chicago (1996), Nijmegen (1998), Toronto (2000), Bremen (2002), Durham (2006), Tucson (2008), Girona (2010), and Philadelphia (2012). This year was the first time the workshop was held in an in Asian region in the history of the workshop over the past 20 years.

A total of 122 paper submissions from around 20 countries were received for IWDM 2014. Each of the abstracts along with the maximum four-page supporting documents was reviewed in a blind process by two members of the Scientific Committee, which led to a final selection of 27 oral presentations and 76 posters during the two and a half days of sequential scientific sessions. Eleven profound talks, including a plenary lecture, eight keynotes, and two luncheon seminars, were given by invited speakers in IWDM 2014. Of these 11 talks, ten short abstracts are included in the front matter of this volume, and six full review papers by these speakers followed by 97 final peer-reviewed papers constitute a comprehensive state of the art in breast imaging today in this proceedings volume (LNCS 8539).

Invited speakers, who are working as breast surgeons, radiologists, medical physicists at hospitals, and researchers in universities or companies, were chosen discreetly. As mentioned above, this workshop was the first meeting held in an Asian area, and thus we selected the themes that are specific to issues of dense breast, screening means, and imaging modalities. Dr. Noriaki Ohuchi of Tohoku University Graduate School of Medicine, Japan, gave a lecture on the efficacy of ultrasonography screening by sharing the updated data from the randomized clinical trial for Japanese women in their 40s. Dr. Woo-Kyung Moon of Seoul National University Hospital, Republic of Korea, presented data on the current breast imaging diagnosis and screening in Korea. Dr. Ruey-Feng Chang of the

National Taiwan University, Taiwan, gave a review on computer-aided diagnosis for B-mode, elastography, and automated ultrasound, and Dr. Kwan-Hoong Ng of the University of Malaya, Malaysia, gave a review on the quantitative measurement and clinical utility of breast density. Dr. Michael K. O'Connor of the Mayo Clinic, USA, presented diagnostic and screening application of molecular breast imaging in women with dense breasts. Dr. Julian Marshall of Hologic Inc., USA, discussed the current situation in mammography CAD with the advent of tomosynthesis, while Dr. Etta D. Pisano of the Medical University of South Carolina, USA, provided a review of tomosynthesis and an overview of the Tomosynthesis Mammographic Imaging Screening Trial (TMIST) design. Dr. Andrew D. A. Maidment of the University of Pennsylvania, USA, presented his work on virtual clinical trials for the assessment of new screening modalities. Dr. Elizabeth Krupinski of the University of Arizona, USA, gave an overview of current breast cancer telemedicine services in Arizona. A special luncheon seminar was given by Dr. Tsuyoshi Shiina of Kyoto University, Japan, with the topic of real-time tissue elastography. Another luncheon seminar was presented by two invited speakers, Dr. Ch. Mueller-Leisse and Dr. Mechthild Schulze-Hagen of Maria Hilf Moenchengladbach, Germany, who talked about the clinical benefit of tomosynthesis.

Finally, a meeting as large and successful as IWDM 2014 is only possible through the tireless work of many people. First, I would like to acknowledge the excellent work of the Scientific Committee in guaranteeing scientific significance by means of providing feedback to the authors for the final papers. Second, special thanks need to go to Takeshi Hara and Chisako Muramatsu for making this meeting a reality, to Norimitsu Shinohara for working many hours to recruit the industrial partners, and to Xiangrong Zhou for making and renewing the workshop web-site daily. Third, thanks go to all the advisory board members and local Organizing Committee members listed herein. Finally, we are grateful to our academic partners, cooperating organizations, and industrial partners for their enthusiastic support for the scientific progress in breast imaging.

June 1, 2014   Hiroshi Fujita

Organization

Workshop Chair

Hiroshi Fujita   Gifu University, Japan

Scientific Committee

Susan M. Astley   University of Manchester, UK
Ulrich Bick   Charité University, Germany
Hilde Bosmans   University Hospitals of KU Leuven, Belgium
Hiroshi Fujita   Gifu University, Japan
Maryellen L. Giger   University of Chicago, USA
Takeshi Hara   Gifu University, Japan
Nico Karssemeijer   Radboud University Nijmegen Medical Centre
                             The Netherlands
Elizabeth A. Krupinski   University of Arizona, USA
Andrew D.A. Maidment   University of Pennsylvania, USA
Joan Martí   University of Girona, Spain
Etta D. Pisano   Medical University of South Carolina, USA
Martin J. Yaffe   University of Toronto, Canada
Reyer Zwiggelaar   Aberystwyth University, UK

Local Organizing Committee Chairs

Chisako Muramatsu   Gifu University, Japan
Xiangrong Zhou   Gifu University, Japan

Local Organizing Committee

Daisuke Fukuoka   Gifu University, Japan
Tomoko Matsubara   Nagoya Bunri University, Japan
Hiroko Nishide   Gifu University of Medical Science, Japan
Norimitsu Shinohara   Gifu University of Medical Science, Japan

Special Advisors

Kunio Doi   University of Chicago, USA,
                             and Gunma Prefectural College of Health
                             Sciences, Japan
Tokiko Endo   National Hospital Organization Higashi Nagoya
                             National Hospital, Japan

Advisory Board

Tetsuro Katafuchi	Gifu University of Medical Science, Japan
Yoshie Kodera	Nagoya University, Japan
Woo-Kyung Moon	Seoul National University Hospital Republic of Korea
Shigeru Nawano	International University of Health and Welfare Mita Hospital, Japan
Shigeru Sanada	Kanazawa University, Japan
Nachiko Uchiyama	National Cancer Center, Japan

Plenary Lecture

Effectiveness of Ultrasonography Screening for Breast Cancer; Up-Dated Data from the RCT of 76,196 Women Aged 40-49 (J-START)

Noriaki Ohuchi, Akihiko Suzuki, and Takanori Ishida

Department of Surgical Oncology, Graduate School of Medicine,
Tohoku University, Sendai, Japan
{noriaki-ohuchi,takanori}@med.tohoku.ac.jp
Akihiko1622@me.com

At present, mammography (MG) is the only method for breast cancer screening that has evidence of decreasing mortality. However, MG does not achieve sufficient screening accuracy in women aged 40 to 49, as the U.S. Preventive Services Task Force (USPSTF) has recently recommended against routine screen MG in women aged 40 to 49 years. Supplemental screening ultrasonography (US) has the potential to depict early breast cancers not seen on MG. However, randomized controlled trials (RCTs), cohort studies, or case-control studies have not been completed to assess the efficacy of screening US to reduce breast cancer mortality, and the effectiveness has not been verified.

In 2007, we planned the RCT to assess effectiveness of US screening for breast cancer in women aged 40-49, with a design to study 50,000 women with MG and US (intervention group), and 50,000 women with MG only (control group). The primary endpoints are sensitivity and specificity, and the secondary endpoint is rate of advanced breast cancers.

The cumulative total number of participants registered is 76,196 (38,313 in the intervention group and 37,883 in the control group). The study was designed so that participants registered at their first examination underwent examinations by the same method for the subsequent two years. The second examinations were completed by end of March 2013. Among the 76,196 participants, 74.5% of women had undertaken second screening, while information including the presence of interval cancer is obtained from a further 22.6% using a questionnaire. As of end of December 2013, only 2.9% of participants are unclear for their follow-up.

This study is the first large-scale RCT carried out to clarify the effectiveness of US screening for breast cancer. It requires objective judgment regarding the advantages and disadvantages of the introduction of US screening, and it is anticipated that J-START project will make a significant contribution to establish a scientific justification for its introduction. RCT is the most appropriate way to make scientific analysis and verification of the effectiveness of new modality in cancer diagnosis and treatment, although such trials are extremely costly, take long time until the final evaluation confirmed.

We believe that J-START, a prospective and challenging trial to evaluate effectiveness of screening modality, would make an important contribution to the world, with leading to the cancer mortality reduction in future generations.

Keynote Talks

Virtual Clinical Trials for the Assessment of Novel Breast Screening Modalities

Andrew D.A. Maidment

University of Pennsylvania, Dept. of Radiology, Philadelphia, PA, USA
Andrew.Maidment@uphs.upenn.edu

Validation of any imaging system is challenging due to the huge number of system parameters that should be evaluated. The ultimate metric of system performance is a clinical trial. However, the use of clinical trials is limited by cost and duration. We are strong proponents of a preclinical alternative, in the form of Virtual Clinical Trials (VCT), which model human anatomy, image acquisition, display and processing, and image analysis and interpretation. A complete VCT pipeline was envisioned by combining the breast anatomy and image acquisition simulation pipeline developed at the University of Pennsylvania, with the MeVIC image display and observation pipeline developed by researchers at Barco. Today an integrated virtual clinical trial design program, *VCTdesigner*, and a virtual clinical trial management program, *VCTmanager*, are freely available (www.VCTworld.org). The pipeline design is flexible and extensible, making it possible to add functionality easily and rapidly. It is our hope that by freely distributing the VCTmanager software, our field can standardize on this platform for running VCT.

Computer-Aided Diagnosis for B-mode, Elastography and Automated Breast Ultrasound

Ruey-Feng Chang[1,2] and Chung-Ming Lo[1]

[1]Department of Computer Science and Information Engineering
National Taiwan University, Taipei, Taiwan
{rfchang,d97001}@csie.ntu.edu.tw
[2]Graduate Institute of Biomedical Electronics and Bioinformatics
National Taiwan University, Taipei, Taiwan

This review paper encapsulates the presentation of the computer-aided diagnosis (CAD) development in the session of US imaging at IWDM 2014. The development includes novel methodologies in conventional B-mode and modern ultrasound modalities such as elastography and automated breast ultrasound. For B-mode images, gray-scale invariant texture features were proposed to solve the changing of echogenicities from various ultrasound systems. Speckle patterns were analyzed to show the properties of tiny scatterers with microstructure contained in breast tissues for tissue characterization. Using quantified sonographic findings in tumor classification can achieve better diagnostic result than combining all features together. Elastography CAD systems use automatic tumor segmentation and clustering method to reduce operator-dependence. Dynamic sequence features were extracted from a sequence of elastograms to provide tumor stiffness without selecting slices. Another approach was selecting slices with quality evaluation methods. Both approaches reduced the overloads of physicians in slice selection. Automated breast ultrasound system is developed to automatically scan the whole breast and build the volumetric breast structure. Three-dimensional morphology, texture, and speckle features were proposed and combined to provide more diagnostic information than two-dimensional features. These CAD systems for B-mode, elastography, and automated breast ultrasound are good at malignancy evaluation and would be helpful in clinic use.

Breast Imaging Diagnosis and Screening in Korea

Woo Kyung Moon, M.D.

Department of Radiology, Seoul National University Hospital,
Seoul, Korea

In Korea, national cancer screening program (NCSP) began in 1999 for five major cancers, including stomach, breast, uterine cervix, liver and colorectal cancers. The NCSP recommends biennial breast cancer screening for females over 40 years of age with mammogram $\pm$ clinical breast examination as the screening tool. The Korean Society of Breast Imaging (KSBI) developed guidelines and standards of quality management for mammography from 1999. On January 14, 2003, the national assembly of Korea approved the Acts including quality management for mammography. Annual inspection includes the facilities to meet minimum quality standards for personnel, equipment, and phantom image. Every three year, on site survey and evaluation of clinical image are added. Mammography accreditation program has been helping facilities improve the image quality by peer review and professional feedback.

The breast cancer screening rate increased from 33.2% in 2004to55.2% in 2009. According to previously published reports in Korea, there were variations in performance indicators across the institutions, but these differences were not extreme; Performance of screening mammography was associated with sensitivity of 85.0-91.5%, specificity of 95.0-99.0%, PPV_1 of 0.8-2.5%, PPV_2 of 18.0-27.7%, recall ratesof 5.1-13.0%, and cancer detection rates of 0.5-2.0/1000. Compared with the ideal goal of ACR in USA, PPV_1 and cancer detection rates are lower than the goal of ACR. It is probably due to lower cancer incidence in Korea than that of USA. In the near future, results of 10 year performance and outcome measurements of NCSP in Korea will be reported.

Although mammography screening is the only method presently considered appropriate for mass screening of asymptomatic women, the success in cancer detection has been limited in women with small and dense breasts, especially in Asian women. Other or new breast imaging technologies having potential role in breast screening are digital mammography, breast ultrasound including automated whole breast US, MRI, digital breast tomosynthesis. The digital mammographic imaging screening trial (DMIST) found that digital mammography performed significantly better than analog mammography in premenopausal and perimenopausal women, those aged $<$ 50 years, and those with dense breasts. Ultrasound is an ideal supplement tomammography. The results of a multicenter trial of supplemental screening breast ultrasound for women at high risk with dense breast tissue have been promising. Several studies found that ultrasound alone caught breast tumors that mammography couldn't see in 0.1-0.5% of patients. Previously Published Data of screening US in Korea show similar cancer detection rate, reported 0.35% - 0.5%. However, the operator dependence of hand held ultrasound is a major concern with respect to the widespread use of whole breast screening ultrasound. Recently developed automated whole breast ultrasound is more readily reproducible, has 3D capability through multi-planar reconstruction, and allows delayed interpretation outside of real time, optimizing the radiologist's reading environment. Magnetic resonance imaging has been used with success in the screening of high-risk women. From 2007, the ACS issued recommendations for screening breast MRI among certain high-risk women. Recently developed digital breast tomosynthesis (DBT) allows cross-sectional visualization of breast tissue that the overlying and underlying anatomical tissue can be effectively removed when viewing individual slices. Thus overcoming the problem of super-positioning that reduces the effectiveness of mammography. It also has a potential role for breast screening. However, there are no large, peer-reviewed studies that support the routine use of other imaging techniques, these are not recommended to be widely used until a clear outcome benefit is established for breast cancer screening.

Measurement and Clinical Use of Breast Density

Kwan-Hoong Ng and Susie Lau

Department of Biomedical Imaging and University of Malaya
Research Imaging Centre,
Faculty of Medicine, University of Malaya, Kuala Lumpur, Malaysia
ngkh@ummc.edu.my

Breast density is loosely defined as the amount of fibroglandular tissue in the breast compared to the total amount of breast tissue. In this review paper we consider the three ways of describing breast density as seen on a mammogram: pattern-based, area-based and volumetric-based and explain the rationale for each along with detailing the various ways of estimating each of them (visual, semi-automated, and fully automated). We also consider the use of other imaging modalities of estimating breast density, including CT. Clinically, breast density has now moved from being a controversial, even derided subject to one which is widely accepted with an expanding number of clinical uses. It is proven that a woman's breast density is a strong predictor of the failure of mammographic screening to detect breast cancer and thus can be used to indicate where alternate modalities might be considered. It is proven that breast density is a strong predictor of the risk of developing breast cancer and thus can be used to start to consider tailored screening programs. We review the current widely known clinical uses along with the lesser known uses, such as assessing the benefits of chemoprevention and generating more accurate radiation dose estimates. Breast density is becoming an increasingly important clinical tool; there is an increasing need for accurate and consistent density measures along with an understanding of how the various measures compare.

Low-Dose Molecular Breast Imaging - Diagnostic and Screening Applications in Women with Dense Breasts

Michael K. O'Connor

Department of Radiology, Mayo Clinic, Rochester, MN
mkoconnor@mayo.edu

Approaches to imaging the breast with nuclear medicine and/or molecular imaging methods have been under investigation since the early 1990s. Nuclear medicine procedures, which detect the preferential uptake of a radiotracer in breast lesions, have the potential to offer valuable functional information that complements conventional anatomical imaging techniques such as mammography and ultrasound.

Despite initial enthusiasm for scintimammography, nuclear medicine techniques in general have struggled to gain mainstream acceptance by the breast imaging community. In the last 5-10 years, older-generation scintillating gamma systems, such breast-specific gamma imaging systems, have been replaced by a new generation of dual detector cadmium zinc telluride [CZT] detectors that perform direct conversion [DC] of gamma ray energy to signal and yield improved spatial and energy resolution. Using CZT-based detectors, DC-Molecular breast Imaging [DC-MBI] has demonstrated the ability to reliably detect breast tumors in a variety of diagnostic and screening settings. Recent improvements in both the detector technology and patient preparation have enabled the associated radiation dose from DC-MBI to be reduced to less than 1.5 mSv. The most robust evidence for the clinical use of DC-MBI is in the screening of women with dense breast tissue. In two large screening studies, the addition of DC-MBI to mammography was significantly more sensitive than mammography alone in detecting cancer (91% vs. 25%, $p < 0.001$). Supplemental screening with DC-MBI detected an additional 8.3 cancers per 1000 women, which compares very favorably to other modalities in screening women with dense breasts.

Will New Technologies Replace Mammography CAD as We Know It?

Julian Marshall, Ashwini Kshirsagar, Sibel Narin, and Nikos Gkanatsios

Hologic, Inc., Santa Clara, CA, USA

Since its commercial introduction in 1998, Mammography computer-aided detection (CAD) has been one of the few CAD technologies widely implemented in clinical practice. The original concept of CAD marks as overlays on images has been broadly accepted, although new paradigms have been proposed and successfully tested that could one day challenge that original approach. But now, as breast imaging evolves further with the advent of digital breast tomosynthesis, new image processing techniques are developing that may cause us to re-evaluate the clinical requirements for Mammography CAD as we know it. What clinical problems in breast imaging are not solved by tomosynthesis, and how can CAD help us with those problems?

Tomosynthesis: What We Know Now and Why TMIST Is Needed

Etta D. Pisano

Department of Radiology and Radiological Science,
Medical University of South Carolina,
Charleston, USA
pisanoe@musc.edu

Digital Breast Tomosynthesis provides pseudo three-dimensional viewing of breast tissue on a technological platform similar to conventional two-dimensional digital mammography. The technology is being incorporated into clinical environments across the world. This presentation provides a review of the current published literature concerning the clinical use of digital breast tomosynthesis and an overview of the design of a proposed North American Tomosynthesis Mammographic Imaging Screening Trial (TMIST).

Advanced Telecommunications in Breast Imaging– Streamlining Telemammography, Telepathology & Teleoncology Services to Improve Patient Care

Elizabeth A. Krupinski

Department of Medical Imaging, University of Arizona,
Tucson, AZ USA
krupinski@radiology.arizona.edu

Teleradiology services are very common worldwide, and Full Field Digital Mammography (FFDM) systems have made it possible to include mammography. This is important because breast cancer is the most common cancer in women in many parts of the world and it is the second leading cause of cancer deaths. In rural and medically underserved areas, mammography rates are lower than in urban areas for a variety of reasons, including lack of dedicated screening facilities and/or personnel, poor compliance, and large distances between patients and clinics (making it difficult to return for follow-up care). Once possible cancers are detected, biopsies are performed but in many cases reports are very slow to get back to the patient and/or local clinician impacting treatment and follow-up. Telepathology can address this situation. Patients may also require oncology services and in rural areas they are often limited or non-existent. Real-time teleoncology services can facilitate treatment and counseling. Finally, breast care support and education can be facilitated by virtual support groups and broadcasting education lectures.

Luncheon Seminar

Real-Time Tissue Elastography:
Theory and Usefulness for Breast Cancer Diagnosis

Tsuyoshi Shiina

Department of Human Health Sciences, Graduate School of Medicine,
Kyoto University, Kyoto, Japan
shiina@hs.med.kyoto-u.ac.jp

Disease tissues, such as breast cancer, become hard as the disease progresses. Therefore, ultrasound tissue elasticity imaging, i.e., elasography has attracted much attention as a modality that provides novel diagnostic information regarding tissue stiffness, and various techniques for elasography have been proposed in the last two decades.

The most widely available commercial elastography method today is strain imaging using external tissue compression and generating images of the resulting tissue strain. The most fundamental external force is manually applying pressure with a probe on the body surface, similar to an ordinary ultrasound examination, which is referred to as strain elastography.

Advantages of ultrasonic examination, such as real-time and simple (freehand) operation, must be preserved in the ultrasound elastography system. In a freehand compression, it is necessary to have a large dynamic range of strain for stable measurement that does not depend on a compression speed and quantity. The Combined Autocorrelation Method (CAM) was developed by our group as an image reconstruction method suited for clinical application. It produces an elasticity image with high-speed processing and accuracy, and achieves a wide dynamic range for strain estimation by combining envelope correlation and phase shift while avoiding aliasing errors. As a result of collaboration of our group and Hitachi Medical Corporation the first practical system of ultrasound elastography based on strain elastography was released in 2003 based on the CAM.

Its efficacy was demonstrated in the diagnosis of breast-cancer tumors together with an elasticity score proposed at the same time, and it is currently being used in various fields of clinical medicine other than breast-cancer diagnosis, such as prostate-cancer, arteriosclerosis, chronic hepatitis.

Strain elastography has the advantages of being easy to use and providing elasticity images in real time and with a high spatial resolution in a manner similar to conventional ultrasonography. Many manufacturers today produce ultrasonographic equipment with a strain elastography function. Recently, another elastography approach (shear wave imaging) that provides stiffness images based upon the shear wave propagation speed has been practically applied. Features and equipment of each method, i.e., their merits and limitations, must be clarified for their appropriate use. Recently, to help users of ultrasound elastography, academic societies of medical ultrasound, such as WFUMB, EFSUMB, and JSUM, have started to prepare guidelines.

Elastography further improves the value of ultrasonography with the ability to provide new diagnostic information related to tissue characterization. On the other hand, it is still an evolving technology with much technical potential for clinical application in the future including expanding its scope of application, quantification, 3D measurement, and treatment support, etc. One might anticipate that it will further evolve in the future and attain a position as a third mode of ultrasound imaging behind B-mode and Doppler method.

Table of Contents

Ultrasound

Breast Density

Imaging Physics I

CAD

Tomosynthesis

Imaging Physics II

ICT and Image Processing

Poster Papers

Virtual Clinical Trials for the Assessment of Novel Breast Screening Modalities

Andrew D.A. Maidment

University of Pennsylvania, Dept. of Radiology, Philadelphia, PA, USA
Andrew.Maidment@uphs.upenn.edu

Abstract. Validation of any imaging system is challenging due to the huge number of system parameters that should be evaluated. The ultimate metric of system performance is a clinical trial. However, the use of clinical trials is limited by cost and duration. We are strong proponents of a preclinical alternative, in the form of Virtual Clinical Trials (VCT), which model human anatomy, image acquisition, display and processing, and image analysis and interpretation. A complete VCT pipeline was envisioned by combining the breast anatomy and image acquisition simulation pipeline developed at the University of Pennsylvania, with the MeVIC image display and observation pipeline developed by researchers at Barco. Today an integrated virtual clinical trial design program, *VCTdesigner*, and a virtual clinical trial management program, *VCTmanager*, are freely available (www.VCTworld.org). The pipeline design is flexible and extensible, making it possible to add functionality easily and rapidly. It is our hope that by freely distributing the VCTmanager software, our field can standardize on this platform for running VCT.

Keywords: Virtual clinical trials, observer models, anatomy models, imaging simulations, breast cancer, imaging.

1   Introduction

Validation of any imaging system is challenging due to the huge number of system parameters that should be evaluated. The ultimate metric of system performance is a clinical trial. However, the use of clinical trials is limited by cost and duration. In addition, trials involving ionizing radiation require repeated irradiation of volunteers, which may be impractical. In particular, breast-screening trials have a low incidence of disease; therefore, radiation must be used judiciously. We are, therefore, strong proponents of a preclinical alternative, in the form of *Virtual Clinical Trials* (VCT), which model human anatomy, image acquisition, display and processing, and image analysis and interpretation.

We coined the phrase "Virtual Clinical Trials" in 2009, in anticipation of the growing abilities of anatomy and imaging system simulations, together with innovations in observer models. A complete VCT pipeline (Fig. 1) was envisioned by combining the breast anatomy and image acquisition simulation pipeline developed at the University of Pennsylvania, with the MeVIC image display and observation pipeline developed

H. Fujita, T. Hara, and C. Muramatsu (Eds.): IWDM 2014, LNCS 8539, pp. 1–8, 2014.

by researchers at Barco, Inc. Today an integrated virtual clinical trial design program, *VCTdesigner*, and a virtual clinical trial management program, *VCTmanager*, are freely available (www.VCTworld.org).

We believe that VCTs have at least two significant roles: quantitative and objective assessment of system performance in the design of novel imaging methods; and, validation of clinical trial designs prior to execution of real clinical trials. Traditionally, novel imaging methods (whether acquisition systems, display systems or image processing solutions) are evaluated with simple test objects (uniform fields, edges, etc.) and limited clinical data sets. Similarly, clinical trials are restricted to volunteers meeting specific entry criteria, such as age or absence of prior disease, to simplify study design and data analysis. These traditional evaluation methods provide tractable results that allow one to grade or rank systems in terms of superiority *vis-a-vis* that specific test or that particular patient group; however, these tests do not necessarily predict clinical performance in the full clinical population.

By contrast, a VCT is cast in terms of close surrogates of real clinical tasks, such as the detection or classification of calcifications or masses in the breast, or the estimation of breast density or parenchymal properties. Thus, it is expected that rankings obtained by a VCT would closely match clinical performance. We also expect that results of a VCT can act as a guide for the design of actual clinical trials, by allowing clinical researchers to simulate various trial designs *a priori* and to calculate the effect and power more accurately when designing clinical trials. VCTs can also extend the results of a clinical trial by simulating patients otherwise excluded (e.g., detection of multifocal disease in women with surgical clips).

While we have concentrated, to date, on VCT for x-ray imaging of the breast, the methods presented here are general and thus are applicable to imaging other body parts with a variety of image modalities. In addition, while we explicitly discuss the use of observer models as surrogates for human observers, it is also relevant to consider VCT for quantitative measurement systems, such as computer-aided diagnosis (CAD) systems and systems designed to estimate breast density or breast cancer risk.

2   VCTworld

The *VCTmanager* simulation pipeline is implemented in an extensible C++ and OpenCL software platform. The structure of the pipeline is illustrated in Fig. 1. Synthetic breast images are generated using the breast anatomy and imaging simulation methods developed at the University of Pennsylvania (UPenn) over the last two decades [1-5]. Normal breast anatomy is simulated with a recursive partitioning algorithm using octrees [5]. Lesions can be included automatically based upon a configurable set of rules [6]. Phantom deformation due to clinical breast positioning and compression is simulated using a finite element (FE) model and rapid post-FE software [7]. DBT image acquisition is currently simulated by ray tracing projections through the phantoms, assuming a polyenergetic x-ray beam without scatter, and an ideal detector model. Processed or reconstructed images are obtained using the Real-Time Tomography, LLC (RTT) image reconstruction and processing software [8]. Other imaging modalities are also supported, although not yet fully integrated, including dedicated breast CT, magnetic resonance imaging, and ultrasound imaging.

The display and virtual observer simulation is based upon MeVIC (Medical Virtual Imaging Chain) [9-11] developed at Barco. Datasets (volumes of interest) of projection images or tomographic image stacks, with and without simulated lesions, are input to the display and virtual observer portion of the simulation pipeline. Each stack is first decomposed into spatiotemporal frequency components using a 3D fast Fourier transform (FFT). Various elements of the human visual system (HVS) are simulated in the Fourier domain. Then, a 3D inverse FFT is applied to the perceived amplitudes to transform the perceived image(s) back into the space-time domain. Finally, the results are input to a multi-slice channelized Hotelling observer (msCHO) developed by Platiša et al [12]. Further details of the simulation have been provided previously [11].

The simulation modules in the pipeline are interconnected using an XML-based dynamic parsimonious data representation, offering a high level of control for the simulations. The data are structured at two levels. At a high-level, the clinical trial is defined in terms of the research arms (e.g., defining the modalities or modality parameters to be tested, and the patient population). At the next level, *virtual patient* or *virtual imaging study* data are defined that parallel the DICOM metadata for an equivalent imaging procedure on the system(s) being simulated together with such demographic data as can be simulated. For example, this information can include a unique name and numerical identifier; study information such as modality, date and time; series and image information including acquisition parameters and desired display state (for presentation/for processing); and demographic data including breast size, breast density, etc. These data both guide the simulation and serve as the source of the DICOM metadata for the image files that are created.

An example of the simulation is shown in Fig. 2. A single slice from the breast anatomy model containing a calcification cluster is shown in Fig. 2A. The actual model consists of a 450 mL breast compressed to 5 cm with isotropic voxels of dimension (200 µm) [3]. The choice of voxel size is modality and task dependent. Each voxel is assigned a unique tissue type (adipose, fibroglandular, calcification, etc.) that is indicated by the grayscale in the figure. A projection mammogram is shown in Fig. 2B, simulating a Selenia Dimensions (Hologic, Bedford MA) 2D acquisition, and processed with Adara™ (RTT, Villanova PA). A magnified region is inset. Finally, a tomosynthesis reconstruction in shown in Fig 2C, simulated with a 3D Selenia Dimensions acquisition geometry, and reconstructed with Briona™ (RTT).

Trial design is performed using the matching *VCTdesigner* software. At the current time, we use simulations of full calcification clusters and complex breast masses for human observer trials; while for the virtual clinical trials, we typically simulate a single calcification or a simple mass. Typical VCT trials can involve 3,000-30,000 image datasets per condition, depending upon the desired statistics. The vast majority of the *VCTworld* software is optimized to run on the GPU allowing us to simulate a single image (breast generation through observer simulation) in less than a minute, and thus simulate complete VCT in less than a day.

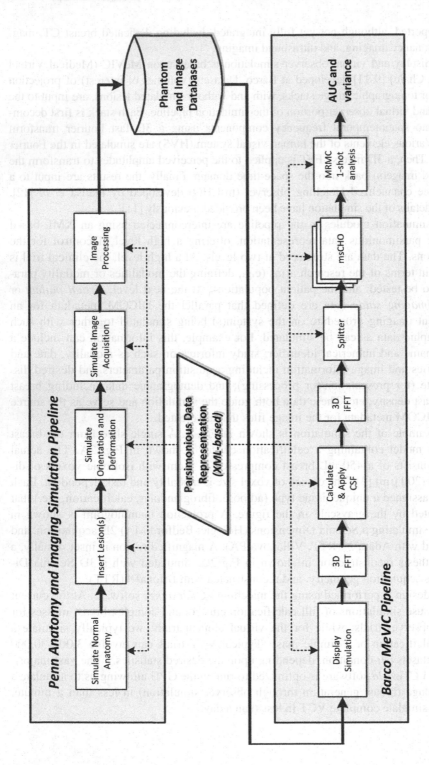

Fig. 1. Flow chart of the VCTmanager pipeline for simulation of breast anatomy, image acquisition, display and observation

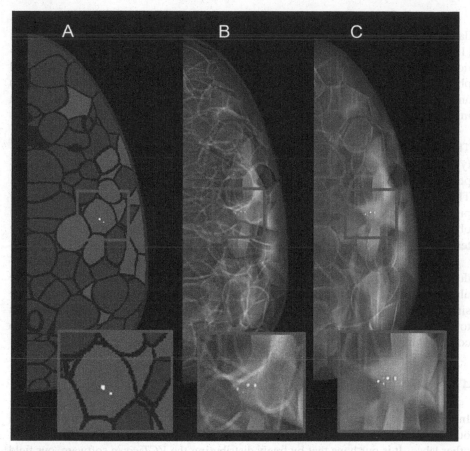

Fig. 2. Example of a breast model with calcifications in cross-section (A), together with the resulting mammogram (B), and DBT slice (C). A magnified image is inset

3   VCT Validation

It is essential that all VCT software be extensively validated. Without such validation, the results are unlikely to have clinical value. The vast majority of our efforts in the last two decades have been on validating our VCT pipeline and constituent software. We have two basic validation approaches. First, we attempt to validate the simulation results against the task being tested. For example, in early testing of our anatomy simulation, we compared texture measures of our simulated images against similar measures of clinical mammograms [1]. In this evaluation, we determined whether the distribution of texture values of an individual simulated breast was consistent with that of a real breast, and whether the distribution of the set of all simulated breasts matched a large set of real breasts. In this way, we concluded that we were able to simulate virtually any breast that might be seen clinically.

The VCT pipeline has been validated for a variety of applications, including the validation and optimization of digital breast tomosynthesis (DBT) reconstruction methods [13-15], DBT image denoising methods [16], ultrasound tomography (UST) reconstruction and segmentation methods [17], analysis of power spectra descriptors in simulated phantom DBT images [18], analysis of texture properties in digital mammography (DM) and DBT images [19, 20], analysis of tumor detectability in DBT [21, 22], and breast imaging dosimetry [23].

Next, once we develop a validation method, we attempt to automate the process. This allows for *regression testing* of future software generations. Given the complexity of the simulation software, regression testing allows us to determine whether prospective changes to the software alter the fundamental operation of the pipeline. These tests are hierarchical, allowing testing from individual components to the entire pipeline. As functionality is added to the pipeline, more extensive testing with human observers or machine observers is periodically necessary; when applicable, these new tests are added to the regression test set.

Finally, physical versions of the 3D anthropomorphic phantom have also been produced and used to validate various applications [24, 25]. This phantom provides the ultimate validation of the acquisition simulation method, as it is possible to compare the simulated and real images of the phantom directly. The addition of simulated lesions to the phantom provide further opportunities for validation, as it is then possible to compare human and machine detection directly.

4   The Future of VCTs

In the last five years, the term "Virtual Clinical Trials" has entered into routine use in our field. There is substantial research on the topic, both by our collaborators and by other labs. It is our hope that by freely distributing the *VCTworld* software, our field can standardize on this platform for running VCT. The pipeline design is flexible and extensible, making it possible to add functionality easily and rapidly.

There is an increasing demand for features, as the use of VCTs increase. We need to create models with increased realism and of all body parts, to extend the use of VCT. Similarly, we need observer models that better match human observers in terms of the tasks that are to be evaluated. Observer models that involve search and models that can detect complex lesions are required; for example, support of calcification clusters having a variety of sizes and numbers of calcifications, or models that can detect masses with a variety of shapes and sizes, or models that can detect lesions with both calcifications and masses. Ultimately, we will need to create general observers; observers that can read medical images of any body part or disease.

Acknowledgements. Research reported in this publication was supported in part by the National Cancer Institute of the National Institutes of Health under award number R01CA154444. The content is solely the responsibility of the author and does not necessarily represent the official views of the National Institutes of Health. The author would like to thank his collaborators Predrag Bakic and Joe Chui from the University of Pennsylvania, David Pokrajac from Delaware State University, and Ali Avanaki, Kathryn Espig, Tom Kimpe, Cedric Marchessoux and Albert Xthona from Barco. The author would like to thank our advisors Bill Ecklund, Miguel Eckstein, Elizabeth Krupinski and Ljiljana Platiša. Finally, the author would like to acknowledge the researchers at more than 50 universities and companies who now use our VCT phantoms, images and software. Andrew Maidment is a member of the Scientific Advisory Board of RTT.

References

1. Bakic, P.R., Albert, M., Brzakovic, D., Maidment, A.D.A.: Mammogram synthesis using a 3D simulation. II. Evaluation of synthetic mammogram texture. Medical Physics 29(9), 2140–2151 (2002)
2. Bakic, P.R., Albert, M., Brzakovic, D., Maidment, A.D.A.: Mammogram synthesis using a 3D simulation. I. Breast tissue model and image acquisition simulation. Medical Physics 29(9), 2131–2139 (2002)
3. Bakic, P.R., Albert, M., Brzakovic, D., Maidment, A.D.A.: Mammogram synthesis using a three-dimensional simulation. III. Modeling and evaluation of the breast ductal network. Medical Physics 30(7), 1914–1925 (2003)
4. Carton, A.K., Bakic, P., Ullberg, C., Derand, H., Maidment, A.D.: Development of a physical 3D anthropomorphic breast phantom. Med. Phys. 38(2), 891–896 (2011)
5. Pokrajac, D.D., Maidment, A.D., Bakic, P.R.: Optimized generation of high resolution breast anthropomorphic software phantoms. Med. Phys. 39(4), 2290–2302 (2012)
6. Shankla, V., Pokrajac, D., Weinstein, S.P., DeLeo, M., Tuite, C., Roth, R., et al.: Automatic insertion of simulated microcalcification clusters in a software breast phantom. In: SPIE Medical Imaging 2014: Physics of Medical Imaging, San Diego, CA. SPIE, vol. 9033 (2014)
7. Maidment, A.D.A., Bakic, P.R., Ruiter, N.V., Richard, F.: Model-based comparison of two breast tissue compression methodologies. Medical Physics 31(6), 1786 (2004)
8. Kuo, J., Ringer, P.A., Fallows, S.G., Bakic, P.R., Maidment, A.D.A., Ng, S.: Dynamic reconstruction and rendering of 3D tomosynthesis images. In: Pelc, N.J., Samei, E., Nishikawa, R.M. (eds.) Medical Imaging 2011:Proceedings of the SPIE, Orlando, FL. Proceedings of the SPIE, vol. 7961 (2011)
9. Marchessoux, C., Kimpe, T., Vansteenkiste, E., Staelens, S., Schelkens, P., Bosmans, H., et al. (eds.): Medical Virtual Imaging Chain (MeVIC). Medical Image Perception Conference XIII, Santa Barbara, CA (2009)
10. Braeckman, G., Marchessoux, C., Besnehard, B., Barbarien, J., Schelkens, P. (eds.): Perceptually optimized compression for heterogenous content in the context of medical networked applications, San Francisco. SPIE Electronic Imaging (2010)
11. Avanaki, A.N., Espig, E.S., Marchessoux, C., Krupinski, E.A., Bakic, P.R., Kimpe, T.R.L., et al.: Integration of spatio-temporal contrast sensitivity with a multi-slice channelized Hotelling observer. In: Medical Imaging 2013: Image Perception, Observer Performance, and Technology Assessment, Orlando, FL. SPIE, vol. 8673, p. 86730H (2013)
12. Platisa, L., Goossens, B., Vansteenkiste, E., Badano, A., Phillips, W. (eds.): Channelized Hotelling observer for detection tasks in multi-slice images. Medical Image Perception Society (MIPS), Santa Barbara (2009)

13. Bakic, P.R., Ng, S., Ringer, P., Carton, A.-K., Conant, E.F., Maidment, A.: Validation and Optimization of Digital Breast Tomosynthesis Reconstruction using an Anthropomorphic Software Breast Phantom. In: Samei, E., Pelc, N. (eds.) SPIE Medical Imaging: Physics of Medical Imaging, San Diego, CA, vol. 7622 (2010)
14. Bakic, P.R., Ringer, P., Kuo, J., Ng, S., Maidment, A.D.A.: Analysis of Geometric Accuracy in Digital Breast Tomosynthesis Reconstruction. In: Martí, J., Oliver, A., Freixenet, J., Martí, R. (eds.) IWDM 2010. LNCS, vol. 6136, pp. 62–69. Springer, Heidelberg (2010)
15. Zeng, R., Park, S., Bakic, P.R., Myers, K.J.: Is the Outcome of Optimizing the System Acquisition Parameters Sensitive to the Reconstruction Algorithm in Digital Breast Tomosynthesis? In: Maidment, A.D.A., Bakic, P.R., Gavenonis, S. (eds.) IWDM 2012. LNCS, vol. 7361, pp. 346–353. Springer, Heidelberg (2012)
16. Vieira, M.A.C., Bakic, P.R., Maidment, A.D.A.: Effect of denoising on the quality of reconstructed images in digital breast tomosynthesis. In: Physics of Medical Imaging, Lake Buena Vista, FL. SPIE (2013)
17. Bakic, P.R., Li, C., West, E., Sak, M., Gavenonis, S.C., Duric, N., et al.: Comparison of 3D and 2D Breast Density Estimation from Synthetic Ultrasound Tomography Images and Digital Mammograms of Anthropomorphic Software Breast Phantoms. In: Pelc, N.J., Samei, E., Nishikawa, R.M. (eds.) SPIE Medical Imaging: Physics of Medical Imaging Lake Buena Vista, FL, vol. 7961 (2011)
18. Lau, A.B., Bakic, P.R., Reiser, I., Carton, A.-K., Maidment, A.D.A., Nishikawa, R.M.: An Anthropomorphic Software Breast Phantom for Tomosynthesis Simulation: Power Spectrum Analysis of Phantom Reconstructions. Medical Physics 37, 3473 (2010)
19. Bakic, P.R., Keller, B., Zheng, Y., Wang, Y., Gee, J.C., Kontos, D., et al.: Testing Realism of Software Breast Phantoms: Texture Analysis of Synthetic Mammograms. In: Physics of Medical Imaging, Lake Buena Vista. SPIE, vol. 8668 (2013)
20. Abbey, C.K., Bakic, P.R., Pokrajac, D.D., Maidment, A.D.A., Eckstein, M.P., Boone, J.: Non-Gaussian Statistical Properties of Virtual Breast Phantoms. In: Kupinski, CM-TaM (eds.) SPIE Image Perception, Observer Performance, and Technology Assessment, San Diego. SPIE, vol. 9037 (2014)
21. Young, S., Park, S., Anderson, K., Badano, A., Myers, K.J., Bakic, P.R.: Estimating DBT performance in detection tasks with variable-background phantoms. In: Samei, E., Hsieh, J. (eds.) SPIE Medical Imaging: Physics of Medical imaging, Lake Buena Vista, FL, vol. 7258 (2009)
22. Young, S., Bakic, P.R., Myers, K.J., Jennings, R.J., Park, S.: A virtual trial framework for quantifying the detectability of masses in breast tomosynthesis projection data. Medical Physics 40(5), 051914 (2013)
23. Dance, D.R., Hunt, R.A., Bakic, P.R., Maidment, A.D.A., Sandborg, M., Ullman, G., et al.: Breast dosimetry using high-resolution voxel phantoms. Radiation Protection Dosimetry 114, 359–363 (2005)
24. Carton, A.-K., Bakic, P.R., Ullberg, C., Maidment, A.D.A.: Development of a 3D high-resolution physical anthropomorphic breast phantom. In: Samei, E., Pelc, N.J. (eds.) SPIE Medical Imaging: Physics of Medical Imaging, San Diego, CA, vol. 7622 (2010)
25. Carton, A.-K., Bakic, P.R., Ullberg, C., Derand, H., Maidment, A.D.A.: Development of a physical 3D anthropomorphic breast phantom. Medical Physics 38(2), 891–896 (2011)

Computer-Aided Diagnosis for B-Mode, Elastography and Automated Breast Ultrasound

Ruey-Feng Chang[1,2] and Chung-Ming Lo[1]

[1] Department of Computer Science and Information Engineering
National Taiwan University, Taipei, Taiwan
{rfchang,d97001}@csie.ntu.edu.tw
[2] Graduate Institute of Biomedical Electronics and Bioinformatics
National Taiwan University, Taipei, Taiwan

Abstract. This review paper encapsulates the presentation of the computer-aided diagnosis (CAD) development in the session of US imaging at IWDM 2014. The development includes novel methodologies in conventional B-mode and modern ultrasound modalities such as elastography and automated breast ultrasound. For B-mode images, gray-scale invariant texture features were proposed to solve the changing of echogenicities from various ultrasound systems. Speckle patterns were analyzed to show the properties of tiny scatterers with microstructure contained in breast tissues for tissue characterization. Using quantified sonographic findings in tumor classification can achieve better diagnostic result than combining all features together. Elastography CAD systems use automatic tumor segmentation and clustering method to reduce operator-dependence. Dynamic sequence features were extracted from a sequence of elastograms to provide tumor stiffness without selecting slices. Another approach was selecting slices with quality evaluation methods. Both approaches reduced the overloads of physicians in slice selection. Automated breast ultrasound system is developed to automatically scan the whole breast and build the volumetric breast structure. Three-dimensional morphology, texture, and speckle features were proposed and combined to provide more diagnostic information than two-dimensional features. These CAD systems for B-mode, elastography, and automated breast ultrasound are good at malignancy evaluation and would be helpful in clinic use.

Keywords: Computer-aided diagnosis, breast cancer, ultrasound.

1 Introduction

Breast cancer has become the most common cancer in women [1]. Early detection and treatment are useful to reduce the mortality [2]. Ultrasound (US), as an imaging tool, is widely used on clinical breast examination. The sonographic appearances of breast tumors are interpreted by radiologists to distinguish between malignant and benign tumors [3]. With the development of imaging technology, more and more US-related modalities are proposed to provide diagnostic information. These modalities either present the underlying tissue composition for characterization or establish the

H. Fujita, T. Hara, and C. Muramatsu (Eds.): IWDM 2014, LNCS 8539, pp. 9–15, 2014.
© Springer International Publishing Switzerland 2014

volumetric breast structure for reviewing. The growing data generated from various modalities is useful for radiologists to make more accurate diagnostic decision. However, it would be a time-consuming task to review various US images. Computer-aided diagnosis (CAD) systems are emerging tools to give assistance in clinical use. The advanced CAD systems integrate interdisciplinary knowledge including digital imaging processing, pattern recognition, artificial intelligence classifier, and statistical analysis to speed up the diagnostic procedure and reduce oversight errors. The quantitative analysis generated by CAD systems also provides more details for malignancy estimation and treatment evaluation. Besides, CAD systems can be installed in common computers and be automatically updated via internet. The state-of-art CAD system technologies for various US modalities were presented in the session of US imaging at IWDM 2014 as addressed in this review paper. Section 2 describes the novel CAD technologies for breast US modalities including B-mode, elastography, and automated breast ultrasound.

2   Novel CAD Technologies

2.1   B-Mode

After transferring the US wave to tissues, the return echo is detected and measured to construct a two-dimensional image known as brightness mode (B-mode) frame. B-mode is the most common US imaging technique used on clinical examination. Developing breast CAD based on B-mode images provides an immediate assistance for diagnosis. American College of Radiology establishes the standard Breast Imaging Reporting and Data System (BI-RADS) Lexicon [4] to describe the dominant sonographic findings of a tumor in B-mode. Including shape, orientation, margins, lesion boundary, echo pattern, and posterior acoustic features are classified into morphology or texture features and are quantified in various CAD systems. Morphology features presenting the shape characteristics of tumors are almost invariant under different US parameter settings. However, texture features based on gray-scale analysis are easily affected by the changing of echogenicities. Yang et al. [5] proposed using ranklet transform to rearrange the pixel values by their intensity rankings in an image. Extracting gray-level co-occurrence matrix (GLCM) texture features from the multi-resolution and orientation-selective transformed images resulted in better diagnostic performance than those from wavelet transform. Three databases from different US systems were used in the experiment including Acuson Sequoia (Acuson Siemens, Mountain View, CA, USA), GE LOGIQ 7 (GE Medical Systems, Milwaukee, WI, USA), and Voluson 730 expert (GE Medical systems, Kretz Ultrasound, Zipf, Austria). Via ranklet transform, the performances of area under receiver operating characteristic curve (AUC) were 0.918, 0.943, and 0.934 while the wavelet transform achieved 0.847, 0.922, and 0.867. For the generalization ability of CAD systems, the texture analysis based on ranklet transform would be more robust.

More quantitative features were extracted from B-mode images to provide extra diagnostic information over conventional features. Moon et al. [6] extracted speckle patterns in B-mode to analyze the scatterers with microstructure contained in breast tissues. Tiny scatterers such as tissue parenchyma generate the constructive and de-structive interference called speckle presented by granular appearance in US images. The AUC of speckle features is significantly better than that of conventional B-mode features (0.93 vs. 0.86, p-value=0.0359).

Different classification method used in CAD systems can also lead to different re-sult in distinguishing malignant from benign tumors. Moon et al. [7] suggested quan-tifying six BI-RADS descriptive categories rather than combing all features together for tumor classification. Multiple quantitative features were used to interpret a BI-RADS descriptive category such as shape. In the classification, if one or more malig-nant findings were shown on a tumor, it was classified to be malignant. Otherwise, it was benign. The CAD based on quantified BI-RADS findings achieved significantly better partial AUC (over 90% sensitivity) than that of the conventional CAD using all features together (0.90 vs. 0.76, p-value<0.05). The performance is promising in eva-luating tumor malignancy to avoid missing carcinomas. Fig. 1 shows a B-mode US image.

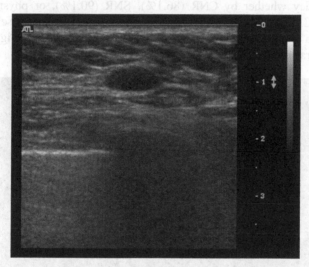

Fig. 1. A B-mode ultrasound image acquired from an ATL HDI 5000 scanner (Philips, Bothell, WA, USA)

2.2   Elastography

Elastography is a dynamic imaging technique using US to estimate tumor stiffness under an external force. In the acquisition, a B-mode image is displayed side by side with the corresponding elastogram to provide anatomical information. A sequence of elastograms containing 50-90 slices is stored during the manual compression. The gray-scale value of elastogram pixels is 0-255. Harder tissues are darker with lower pixel values while softer tissues are closer to 255. Automatic tumor segmentation [8] was proposed to delineate the tumor contour in both B-mode images and elastograms to reduce user-dependence and accurately estimate tumor stiffness. Fuzzy c-means clustering was used in classifying the pixels within a delineated tumor into bright or dark clusters rather than using a fixed intensity threshold.

To extract more complete stain information from the dynamic elastography, tumor boundary tracking mechanism was used in a CAD [9] to calculate stiffness features of the total sequence to reduce the influence of slice selection. The segmentation result of the first slice, as a template, was applied on adjacent slices. The method considered the variation caused by manual compression and save time of physicians in slice selection. The performance of whole sequence analysis achieved significantly better AUC than that of using only a selected slice (0.90 vs. 0.75, p-value=0.002).

Another CAD [10] automatically chooses a slice with the best quality for diagnosis. The quality was determined based on the signal-to-noise (SNR) ratio within the segmented tumor or the contrast-to-noise (CNR) ratio between the segmented tumor and surrounding normal tissues on a elastogram. As a result, both strain features extracted from the SNR and CNR slices can achieve as good performance as those of the physician-selected slice. Combining B-mode and strain features together obtained the best accuracy whether by CNR (86.1%), SNR (90.1%), or physician-selected (89.4%). The CAD approach reduces the overload of physicians in selecting slices and generates a promising diagnostic performance for clinical use. Fig. 2 shows an image slice extracted from an elastogram sequence.

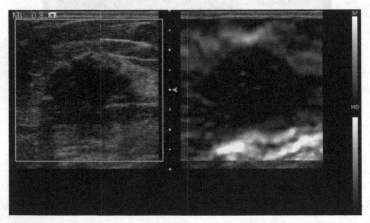

Fig. 2. An elastogram acquired by an ACUSON S2000 ultrasound system (Siemens Medical Solutions, Mountain View, CA)

2.3   Automated Breast Ultrasound

Early detection is helpful to reduce the mortality of breast cancer [2]. However, conventional US equipped with hand-held probe which highly depends on operator experience is not practical to be used in screening. The standardization of scanning and US documentation is necessary to control the examination quality. Performing screening of thousands of patients using manual US is also time-consuming. With the growing of imaging techniques, automated breast ultrasound (ABUS) systems have been developed to make the US screening become acceptable. ABUS systems automatically scan the whole breast and build the volumetric three-dimensional (3-D) breast structure for reviewing. The ABUS systems have been used on clinical examination to improve the detection rate of breast cancers [11]. CAD systems for ABUS systems were also developed to provide more diagnostic information.

Moon et al. [12] extracted quantitative 3-D morphology and texture features after applying 3-D segmentation on ABUS images. The morphology features such as margin and compactness of volume structure were described using the distances between tumor center and boundary voxels. More features were calculated from the difference between the tumor contour and the best-fit ellipse including surface ratio, volume overlapping ratio, and number of non-overlapping regions on the boundary. For texture features, GLCM was used to analyze the correlations between voxels in the segmented tumor volume. The performance of the best combination of 3-D features achieved the AUC of 0.9466. In the further study [13], the statistics and texture of speckle voxels mentioned in the previous B-mode section were extracted from ABUS images to explore more diagnostic information. The performance of the speckle features was comparable to that of the morphological features (AUC=0.91 vs. 0.91, p-value>0.05). Upon the complementary advantage, combining the speckle and morphology features obtained a significantly better AUC than using the morphology features alone (0.96 vs 0.91, p-value=0.0154). Fig. 3 shows the illustration of ABUS images.

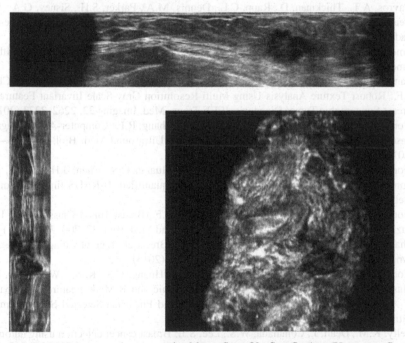

Fig. 3. A 3-DABUS image volume acquired by a SomoVu ScanStation (U-system, San Jose, CA, USA) can be observed from axial (top), sagittal (left), and coronal (right) view

3   Conclusions

Nowadays, more and more modalities are developed to provide novel information about the physical and mechanical properties of breast tissues. The overloads of image examinations need to be reduced to deal with the growing population suffering from breast cancer. CAD systems proposed to accelerate the diagnostic procedure and quantify the likelihood of malignancy are significant tools in future health care. The advances of breast US CAD systems for B-mode, elastography, and ABUS were presented in the session of US imaging at IWDM 2014 as addressed in this review paper.

Acknowledgments. The authors thank the National Science Council (NSC 101-2221-E-002-068-MY3), Ministry of Economic Affairs (102-EC-17-A-19-S1-164), Department of Health (DOH102-TD-C-111-001), and Ministry of Education (AE-00-00-06) of the Republic of China for the financial support.

Reference

1. Jemal, A., Siegel, R., Xu, J., Ward, E.: Cancer Statistics. CA-Cancer J. Clin. 60, 277–300 (2010)
2. Sickles, E.A.: Breast imaging: From 1965 to the present. Radiology 215, 1–16 (2000)
3. Stavros, A.T., Thickman, D., Rapp, C.L., Dennis, M.A., Parker, S.H., Sisney, G.A.: Solid breast nodules: Use of sonography to distinguish between benign and malignant lesions. Radiology 196, 123–134 (1995)
4. American College of Radiology: Breast Imaging Reporting and Data System, 4th ed. American College of Radiology (2003)
5. Yang, M.C., Moon, W.K., Wang, Y.C.F., Bae, M.S., Huang, C.S., Chen, J.H., Chang, R.F.: Robust Texture Analysis Using Multi-Resolution Gray-Scale Invariant Features for Breast Sonographic Tumor Diagnosis. IEEE Trans. Med. Imaging 32, 2262–2273 (2013)
6. Moon, W.K., Lo, C.M., Huang, C.S., Chen, J.H., Chang, R.F.: Computer-Aided Diagnosis Based on Speckle Patterns in Ultrasound Images. Ultrasound Med. Biol. 38, 1251–1261 (2012)
7. Moon, W.K., Lo, C.M., Cho, N., Chang, J.M., Huang, C.S., Chen, J.H., Chang, R.F.: Computer-aided diagnosis of breast masses using quantified BI-RADS findings. Comput. Methods Programs Biomed. 111, 84–92 (2013)
8. Moon, W.M., Chang, S.C., Huang, C.S., Chang, R.F.: Breast Tumor Classification Using Fuzzy Clustering for Breast Elastography. Ultrasound Med. Biol. 37, 700–708 (2011)
9. Chang, S.C., Lai, Y.C., Chou, Y.H., Chang, R.F.: Breast elastography diagnosis based on dynamic sequence features. Med. Phys. 40, 022905 (2013)
10. Moon, W.K., Chang, S.C., Chang, J.M., Cho, N., Huang, C.S., Kuo, J.W., Chang, R.F.: Classification of Breast Tumors Using Elastographic and B-Mode Features: Comparison of Automatic Selection of Representative Slice and Physician-Selected Slice of Images. Ultrasound Med. Biol. 39, 1147–1157 (2013)
11. Kelly, K.M., Dean, J., Comulada, W.S., Lee, S.J.: Breast cancer detection using automated whole breast ultrasound and mammography in radiographically dense breasts. Eur. Radiol. 20, 734–742 (2010)

12. Moon, W.K., Shen, Y.W., Huang, C.S., Chiang, L.R., Chang, R.F.: Computer-Aided Diagnosis for the Classification of Breast Masses in Automated Whole Breast Ultrasound Images. Ultrasound Med. Biol. 37, 539–548 (2011)
13. Moon, W.K., Lo, C.M., Chang, J.M., Huang, C.S., Chen, J.H., Chang, R.F.: Computer-aided classification of breast masses using speckle features of automated breast ultrasound images. Med. Phys. 39, 6465–6473 (2012)

Measurement and Clinical Use of Breast Density

Kwan-Hoong Ng and Susie Lau

Department of Biomedical Imaging and University of Malaya Research Imaging Centre,
Faculty of Medicine, University of Malaya, Kuala Lumpur, Malaysia
ngkh@um.edu.my

Abstract. Breast density is loosely defined as the amount of fibroglandular tissue in the breast compared to the total amount of breast tissue. In this review paper we consider the three ways of describing breast density as seen on a mammogram: pattern-based, area-based and volumetric-based and explain the rationale for each along with detailing the various ways of estimating each of them (visual, semi-automated, and fully automated). We also consider the use of other imaging modalities of estimating breast density, including CT. Clinically, breast density has now moved from being a controversial, even derided subject to one which is widely accepted with an expanding number of clinical uses. It is proven that a woman's breast density is a strong predictor of the failure of mammographic screening to detect breast cancer and thus can be used to indicate where alternate modalities might be considered. It is proven that breast density is a strong predictor of the risk of developing breast cancer and thus can be used to start to consider tailored screening programs. We review the current widely known clinical uses along with the lesser known uses, such as assessing the benefits of chemoprevention and generating more accurate radiation dose estimates. Breast density is becoming an increasingly important clinical tool; there is an increasing need for accurate and consistent density measures along with an understanding of how the various measures compare.

Keywords: BI-RADS, breast cancer, breast density, mammography, volumetric breast density.

1 Introduction

Breast density is loosely defined as the amount of fibroglandular tissue in the breast compared to the total amount of breast tissue. It is a strong predictor of the failure of mammographic screening to detect breast cancer lesions [1]. It is also a strong predictor of the risk of developing breast cancer [2] with increased density tending to be associated with higher breast cancer risk (after adjustments for other parameters) [3, 4]. It is the goal of many researchers and companies to develop a reliable and realistic measure of density, not subject to human interpretation, i.e., objective and reproducible.

H. Fujita, T. Hara, and C. Muramatsu (Eds.): IWDM 2014, LNCS 8539, pp. 16–23, 2014.
© Springer International Publishing Switzerland 2014

2   Measurement of Mammographic Breast Density Today

2.1   Visual Assessments

Radiologists have been assessing breast density visually and subjectively from two dimensional images of breast since the mid-1970s. Wolfe [5] and Tabár [6] are the two best known pattern-based visual assessment methods but have proven hard to implement in practice due to subjectivity whereas the more quantitative BI-RADS breast density category system has proven more popular. The BI-RADS [7] works by dividing density into four gross categories. Initially, those categories were simple descriptive terms ("fatty", "scattered density", "heterogeneously dense", "extremely dense"), but the BI-RADS 4th Ed. [8] included quantitative elements: fatty was "<25%" glandular; scattered density was "25%–50%" glandular; heterogeneous density was "51%–75%" glandular; and extremely dense was ">75%" glandular. However, the 5th Ed. [9] removed the quantitative elements because, the authors argued, it made no difference to US radiologists' judgment of density.

Table 1. Overview of development of pattern-based breast density assessment methods

Year	Method/ References	Brief Description
1976	Wolfe Wolfe [5]	Qualitative classification of mammographic density into four parenchymal-patterns.
1997	Tabár Gram *et al.* [6]	Classification of mammograms in 5 patterns based on a histologic-mammographic correlation with a 3D, thick-slice technique, and on the relative proportion of four "building blocks".
1993	BI-RADS (3rd Ed) ACR [7]	Standardized reporting system by ACR for classifying mammography into four categories.
2013	BI-RADS (5th Ed) ACR [9]	Comprehensive guide by ACR providing standardized breast imaging terminology, report organization, assessment structure, and classification system for mammography (four-category), ultrasound, and MRI of the breast.

2.2   Quantitative Area Assessments

Breast density can be estimated by area assessment, i.e., fraction of 2D breast image that appears dense. Several methods have been developed to quantify the dense areas based upon segmentation [10] and interactive thresholding methods [11].

The quantitative semi-automatic threshold method, as implemented by the Cumulus software has been the mainstay for screen-film mammography. However, this method is observer-dependent, labor-intensive and time-consuming. One challenging question remains: How to delineate the dense area accurately, objectively, and speedily?

Table 2. Overview of development of areal breast density assessment methods

Year	Method/ References	Brief Description
1988	SCC Boyd *et al.* [12]	Based on mammographic density percentage given by radiologists and divided into six categories of unequal intervals.
1994	Cumulus Byng *et al.* [11]	The boundaries of the breast tissue and the threshold for dense tissue are identified, and the software calculates the areas of the breast and dense tissue.
1998	Madena Ursin *et al.* [13]	Identify and quantify radiographic density patterns by measuring the percentage of the mammogram that contains densities in a specified range.
2000	ABDM Heine *et al.* [14]	A statistical method based on a chi-square probability analysis that allows the automated discrimination of fat from fibroglandular tissue.
2003	BI-RADS (4th Ed) ACR [8]	Quantitative classification, modification of Wolfe's classification, and is defined using percentages of density divided into quartiles.
2012	M-Vu Breast Density (VuCOMP) www.vucomp.com/ products/breast-density [15]	Computer algorithms which evaluate breast structures and textures to differentiate between fatty and dense regions. Dense breast area is then converted to one of the four density categories corresponding to BI-RADS.
2012	ImageJ Li *et al.* [16]	Automated analysis of breast density to construct a measure that mimics Cumulus. It includes additional features of mammograms for improving the risk associations of breast density and breast cancer risk.
2012	AutoDensity Nickson *et al.* [17]	Segmentation and classification similar to Cumulus by identifying white tissue as 'dense' (breast density segmentation). The method finds an optimal threshold for each mammogram independently.

2.3   Quantitative Volumetric Assessments

Fully automated methods have been developed to measure the true physical breast density, these methods measure volume of fibroglandular tissue (dense tissue), volume of breast and then compute the ratio, the volumetric breast density (VBD). VBD has the advantage of being independent of equipment, exposure factors and radiographic technique. Results so far suggest that volumetric measures are at least as strongly associated with breast cancer risk as those produced by the area-based approaches.

Table 3. Overview of development of VBD assessment methods

Year	Method/ References	Brief Description
1989	h_{int} Highnam *et al.* [18]	A method to normalize mammograms by calculating anatomical information from it. From the h_{int} image, each pixel represents the thickness of 'interesting' (non-fat) tissue of the compressed breast on that pixel during acquisition.
1999	SMF Highnam *et al.* [18]; Brady *et al.* [19]	SMF provides a representation of the amount of non-fat tissue at each location in a mammogram. From the compressed breast thickness, the SMF representation provides a volumetric estimate of dense tissue in the breast.
2003	Cumulus V Pawluczyk *et al.* [20]	The method is based on initial calibration of the imaging system with a tissue-equivalent device and the subsequent correction for variations through images of a step wedge placed adjacent to the breast during imaging.
2005	BD (SXA) Shepherd *et al.* [21]	The method measures breast composition (Breast Compositional Density) using single X-ray absorptiometry techniques (SXA). Breast density is measured by comparing the opacity to two reference standards imaged with each breast.
2008	Quantra Hartman *et al.* [22]	The method estimates the thickness of fibroglandular breast tissue for each pixel and aggregates these values to compute the total breast volume. The fibroglandular tissue volume is found by referencing each pixel's attenuation to the attenuation of pixels for fat.
2010	Volpara Highnam *et al.* [23]; van Engeland *et al.* [24]	The method is based on a relative physics model, and is an extension of h_{int} and SMF representations. The key differences with SMF are in the robustness and reliability of the results, especially in dense breasts, and not including skin in the dense tissue volume.
2010	Spectral Ding *et al.* [25]	Differences in the energy spectrum are used to differentiate between adipose and fibroglandular tissue to provide objective VBD measurement.

2.4   Breast Density from other Imaging Modalities

Computed Tomography (CT). The most straightforward method of measuring volumetric radiological density is from CT as it enhances visualization of glandular tissue and architecture with its volume data as compared to other breast imaging techniques [26]. It also eliminates the influence of overlapping tissues, and adds to detailed quantitative analysis of breast tissue composition and structural organization [27].

Magnetic Resonance Imaging (MRI). MRI images can be produced that provide signals related to the fat and water composition of the breast. Since the water composition is highly correlated with the amount of fibroglandular tissue, these images are useful for breast density assessment. Several groups are developing approaches to quantify breast density using MRI. As an example, van Engeland et al. [24] reported a method to segment glandular tissue in MRI data.

Ultrasound. Several novel methods for measuring breast density and breast cancer risk have been developed. These depend on the acoustic velocity difference in breast tissue. Ultrasound percent density was determined by segmenting high sound speed areas from each tomogram, integrating over the entire breast, and dividing by total breast area. Their results showed that utilizing sound speed in tissues could be implemented to evaluate breast density [28].

Digital Breast Tomosynthesis (DBT). DBT could provide more accurate measures of the dense breast tissue and ultimately result in more accurate measures of risk. Early work suggests this is more difficult than might seem due to blurring of density across slices. Still, this is projection x-rays, thus, volumetric measurements seem to be very likely. Current research focuses on developing VBD estimation techniques and new approaches to characterize the volumetric complexity of the breast tissue using DBT parenchymal texture analysis [29].

3   Clinical Uses of Breast Density Today

A major problem with screening younger women is that mammographic density is higher than in older women and this would obscure detection of cancers. The obscuring effect is due to the dense fibroglandular tissue and cancers having very similar x-ray attenuation properties. Density measures are being used to determine women who would benefit from adjunctive screening.

Breast density measurements have been used to track changes in density patterns which occur over time or with medical treatment. This is useful to assess the effectiveness of chemoprevention such as the administration of Tamoxifen [30].

In the US, many states now have laws stating that women have to be informed of their breast density so that they understand the risk of their cancer being missed and the risk of cancer developing. As of November 1, 2013, thirteen states have enacted as law, fourteen other states have introduced bills, and a federal law is being proposed. An advocate group, Are You Dense, Inc. (www.areyoudense.org), is spearheading the public awareness about breast density and suggesting to women that they should enquire about an ultrasound or MRI in addition to their mammograms.

4   Clinical Uses of Breast Density Tomorrow

Both global and regional breast density changes over time could be monitored using VBD tools, and this would be very useful for management of the disease, and detection of the early signs of breast cancer.

As risk models are becoming more robust and useful, and since breast density is an independent variable in the equation, the accurately measured density value is important. Risk models including dense fibroglandular volume may more accurately predict breast cancer risk than current risk models [31] and be used to adjust screening intervals.

VBD also enables us to estimate breast specific personalized radiation dose. Globally accepted and validated algorithm along with knowledge of VBD allows for more accurate mean glandular dose comparison and standardization [32].

Information of population-based VBD would also enable us to determine at what age screening should begin [33], and there is some discussion now of base-line scans to determine tailored breast screening programs at an early age. Breast density information should be told to surgeons and it influences patient selection for breast-conserving surgery.

5   Conclusions

Breast density has several clinical uses today, and many more being investigated, but we must be cognizant that other variables such as BMI need to also be factored in for some of the uses, especially related to risk of developing breast cancer. There are various ways of estimating breast density, and ultimately the ways which provide the most useful clinical information for the specific purpose will be used. For many uses, accuracy of assessment is not critical, but for others such as tracking of Tamoxifen effectiveness, greater accuracy might be needed. Researchers and commercial companies are now bringing systems to market which look promising to resolve the clinical needs.

In the quest for the ideal breast density system that should have access to a dataset of breast consisting of a voxel by voxel description of the breast tissue in all its forms (glandular, fibrous, fat, etc.). In reality we need a good measure which is highly correlated to risk of missing cancer to decide who should get adjunctive imaging. Volumetric measures of breast density are more accurate predictors of breast cancer risk than risk factors alone and than percent dense area.

Furthermore, for special cases such as chemo-prevention analysis (hormone replacement therapy) we might need greater accuracy, that might be derived from mammography and better quality control, or from tomosynthesis, or from CT and/or MRI.

Standardization is essential for international comparison studies due to variation in mammographic density assessment arising from different techniques and radiologists. Breast cancer risk assessment and patient education can be combined to empower women with knowledge about their personal risk and provide a fully automated risk assessment tool for physicians. An internationally standardized breast density notification protocol is necessary to rectify the growing diversity [32].

The development of a valid universal standard tool for measuring mammographic density is vital for accurate risk prediction (on a population and individual level) and to tailor preventive measures, including breast screening, according to a woman's risk.

Acknowledgement. This research was supported by the High Impact Research Grant UM.C/HIR/MOHE/06 from the Ministry of Higher Education, Malaysia.

References

1. Pisano, E.D., Gatsonis, C., Hendrick, E., Yaffe, M., Baum, J.K., Acharyya, S., Conant, E.F., Fajardo, L.L., Bassett, L., D'Orsi, C., Jong, R., Rebner, M.: Diagnostic Performance of Digital versus Film Mammography for Breast-Cancer Screening. N. Engl. J. Med. 353, 1773–1783 (2005)
2. Boyd, N.F., Guo, H., Martin, L.J., Sun, L., Stone, J., Fishell, E., Jong, R.A., Hislop, G., Chiarelli, A., Minkin, S., Yaffe, M.J.: Mammographic density and the risk and detection of breast cancer. N. Engl. J. Med. 356, 227–236 (2007)
3. Boyd, N., Martin, L., Yaffe, M., Minkin, S.: Mammographic density and breast cancer risk: current understanding and future prospects. Breast Cancer Res. 13, 223 (2011)
4. Yaffe, M.: Mammographic density. Measurement of mammographic density. Breast Cancer Res. 10, 209 (2008)
5. Wolfe, J.N.: Risk for breast cancer development determined by mammographic parenchymal pattern. Cancer 37, 2486–2492 (1976)
6. Gram, I.T., Funkhouser, E., Tabár, L.: The Tabár classification of mammographic parenchymal patterns. Eur. J. Radiol. 24, 131–136 (1997)
7. ACR: Breast Imaging Reporting and Data System® (BI-RADS®). 3rd edn. American College of Radiology, Reston (1998)
8. ACR: Breast Imaging Reporting and Data System® (BI-RADS®), 4th edn. American College of Radiology, Reston (2003)
9. ACR: Breast Imaging Reporting and Data System® (BI-RADS®) Atlas, 5th edn. American College of Radiology, Reston (2014)
10. Sivaramakrishna, R., Obuchowski, N., Chilcote, W., Powell, K.: Automatic segmentation of mammographic density. Acad. Radiol. 8, 250–256 (2001)
11. Byng, J.W., Boyd, N.F., Fishell, E., Jong, R.A., Yaffe, M.J.: The quantitative analysis of mammographic densities. Phys. Med. Biol. 39, 1629–1638 (1994)
12. Boyd, N., Byng, J., Jong, R., Fishell, E., Little, L., Miller, A., Lockwood, G., Tritchler, D., Yaffe, M.: Quantitative classification of mammographic densities and breast cancer risk: results from the Canadian National Breast Screening Study. J. Natl. Cancer Inst. 87, 670–675 (1995)
13. Ursin, G., Astrahan, M.A., Salane, M., Parisky, Y.R., Pearce, J.G., Daniels, J.R., Pike, M.C., Spicer, D.V.: The detection of changes in mammographic densities. Cancer Epidemiol. Biomarkers Prev. 7, 43–47 (1998)
14. Heine, J.J., Velthuizen, R.P.: A statistical methodology for mammographic density detection. Med. Phys. 27, 2644–2651 (2000)
15. http://www.vucomp.com/products/breast-density
16. Li, J., Szekely, L., Eriksson, L., Heddson, B., Sundbom, A., Czene, K., Hall, P., Humphreys, K.: High-throughput mammographic-density measurement: a tool for risk prediction of breast cancer. Breast Cancer Res. 14, R114 (2012)
17. Nickson, C., Arzhaeva, Y., Aitken, Z., Elgindy, T., Buckley, M., Li, M., English, D., Kavanagh, A.: AutoDensity: an automated method to measure mammographic breast density that predicts breast cancer risk and screening outcomes. Breast Cancer Res. 15, R80 (2013)

18. Highnam, R., Brady, M.: Mammographic Image Analysis. Kluwer Academic Publishers (1999)
19. Brady, M., Gavaghan, D., Simpson, A., Parada, M.M., Highnam, R.: eDiamond: A Grid-Enabled Federated Database of Annotated Mammograms. In: Grid Computing, pp. 923–943. John Wiley & Sons (2003)
20. Pawluczyk, O., Augustine, B., Yaffe, M., Rico, D., Yang, J., Mawdsley, G., Boyd, N.: A volumetric method for estimation of breast density on digitized screen-film mammograms. Med. Phys. 30, 352–364 (2003)
21. Shepherd, J., Herve, L., Landau, J., Fan, B., Kerlikowske, K., Cummings, S.: Novel use of single X-ray absorptiometry for measuring breast density. Technol. Cancer Res. Treat 4, 173–182 (2005)
22. Hartman, K., Highnam, R.P., Warren, R., Jackson, V.: Volumetric Assessment of Breast Tissue Composition from FFDM Images. In: Krupinski, E.A. (ed.) IWDM 2008. LNCS, vol. 5116, pp. 33–39. Springer, Heidelberg (2008)
23. Highnam, R., Brady, S.M., Yaffe, M.J., Karssemeijer, N., Harvey, J.: Robust breast composition measurement - volpara™. In: Martí, J., Oliver, A., Freixenet, J., Martí, R. (eds.) IWDM 2010. LNCS, vol. 6136, pp. 342–349. Springer, Heidelberg (2010)
24. van Engeland, S., Snoeren, P., Huisman, H., Boetes, C., Karssemeijer, N.: Volumetric breast density estimation from full-field digital mammograms. IEEE Trans. Med. Imaging 25, 273–282 (2006)
25. Ding, H., Molloi, S.: Quantification of breast density with spectral mammography based on a scanned multi-slit photon-counting detector: a feasibility study. Phys. Med. Biol. 57, 4719–4738 (2012)
26. Boone, J.M., Kwan, A.L., Yang, K., Burkett, G.W., Lindfors, K.K., Nelson, T.R.: Computed tomography for imaging the breast. J. Mammary Gland Biol. Neoplasia 11, 103–111 (2006)
27. Nelson, T.R., Cervino, L.I., Boone, J.M., Lindfors, K.K.: Classification of breast computed tomography data. Med. Phys. 35, 1078–1086 (2008)
28. Glide, C., Duric, N., Littrup, P.: Novel approach to evaluating breast density utilizing ultrasound tomography. Med. Phys. 34, 744–753 (2007)
29. Dobbins III, J.T., Godfrey, D.J.: Digital x-ray tomosynthesis: current state of the art and clinical potential. Phys. Med. Biol. 48, 65–106 (2003)
30. Li, J., Humphreys, K., Eriksson, L., Edgren, G., Czene, K., Hall, P.: Mammographic density reduction is a prognostic marker of response to adjuvant tamoxifen therapy in postmenopausal patients with breast cancer. J. Clin. Oncol. 31, 2249–2256 (2013)
31. Shepherd, J., Kerlikowske, K., Ma, L., Duewer, F., Fan, B., Wang, J., Malkov, S., Vittinghoff, E., Cummings, S.: Volume of mammographic density and risk of breast cancer. Cancer Epidemiol Biomarkers Prev. 20, 1473–1482 (2011)
32. Ng, K.H., Yip, C.H., Taib, N.A.: Standardisation of clinical breast-density measurement. Lancet Oncol. 13, 334–336 (2012)
33. Lokate, M., Stellato, R.K., Veldhuis, W.B., Peeters, P.H., van Gils, C.H.: Age-related changes in mammographic density and breast cancer risk. Am. J. Epidemiol. 178, 101–109 (2013)

Low-Dose Molecular Breast Imaging - Diagnostic and Screening Applications in Women with Dense Breasts

Michael K. O'Connor

Department of Radiology, Mayo Clinic, Rochester, MN
mkoconnor@mayo.edu

Abstract. Approaches to imaging the breast with nuclear medicine and/or molecular imaging methods have been under investigation since the early 1990s. Nuclear medicine procedures, which detect the preferential uptake of a radiotracer in breast lesions, have the potential to offer valuable functional information that complements conventional anatomical imaging techniques such as mammography and ultrasound.

Despite initial enthusiasm for scintimammography, nuclear medicine techniques in general have struggled to gain mainstream acceptance by the breast imaging community. In the last 5-10 years, older-generation scintillating gamma systems, such breast-specific gamma imaging systems, have been replaced by a new generation of dual detector cadmium zinc telluride [CZT] detectors that perform direct conversion [DC] of gamma ray energy to signal and yield improved spatial and energy resolution. Using CZT-based detectors, DC-Molecular breast Imaging [DC-MBI] has demonstrated the ability to reliably detect breast tumors in a variety of diagnostic and screening settings. Recent improvements in both the detector technology and patient preparation have enabled the associated radiation dose from DC-MBI to be reduced to less than 1.5 mSv. The most robust evidence for the clinical use of DC-MBI is in the screening of women with dense breast tissue. In two large screening studies, the addition of DC-MBI to mammography was significantly more sensitive than mammography alone in detecting cancer (91% vs. 25%, $p < 0.001$). Supplemental screening with DC-MBI detected an additional 8.3 cancers per 1000 women, which compares very favorably to other modalities in screening women with dense breasts.

1   Introduction

Women with mammographic breast density in the upper quartile have an associated three to five time's greater risk of developing breast cancer relative to women with breast density in the lower quartile. Although mammography is the standard tool for breast cancer screening and the only method shown to significantly decrease breast cancer mortality, its sensitivity is strongly inversely related with breast density. In the U.S., recognition of this limitation of mammography has spurred patient advocacy groups for new legislation that would mandate disclosure of breast density information directly to women.

How this disclosure will impact patients is not yet fully understood. However, it is likely to accelerate the development of supplemental screening techniques as patients

H. Fujita, T. Hara, and C. Muramatsu (Eds.): IWDM 2014, LNCS 8539, pp. 24–29, 2014.
© Springer International Publishing Switzerland 2014

look for alternatives to mammography. The most obvious candidates are ultrasound, contrast-enhanced breast MRI and tomosynthesis. An option not generally considered is molecular breast imaging [MBI]. This presentation will review the recent developments in MBI technology. It will also review potential diagnostic applications of MBI, including monitoring response to neoadjuvant chemotherapy and present clinical results from 2 large screening studies.

2   Molecular Breast Imaging – Recent Developments

Molecular breast imaging is a nuclear medicine procedure that employs a dedicated dual-head gamma camera for imaging uptake of a radiopharmaceutical, typically Tc-99m sestamibi, in the breast. In the last 5 years, older-generation scintillating gamma systems, such breast-specific gamma imaging [BSGI] systems, have been replaced by a new generation of dual detector compact gamma cameras. These systems perform a direct conversion [DC] of gamma ray energy to electronic signal (non-scintillating) using solid-state cadmium zinc telluride [CZT] detectors and yield improved spatial and energy resolution compared to BSGI systems. Using CZT-based detectors, DC-MBI has demonstrated the ability to reliably detect breast tumors in a variety of diagnostic settings. Detection of breast cancer with MBI relies on differences in functional uptake of Tc-99m sestamibi, rather than differences in the attenuation coefficients of tissues in the breast as with mammography. DC-MBI has been studied in both the diagnostic and screening settings. A key issue in the use of DC-MBI in both settings is the radiation dose associated with this procedure. Over the last 5 years, significant improvements have been made in the DC-MBI technology which now allow count density and diagnostic accuracy to be maintained at administered doses of ~240 MBq (6.5 mCi) giving an effective (whole-body) radiation dose of 1.9 mSv (1-3). More recent work in patients has shown that improved control over patient metabolic status (e.g. requiring that patients fast for >4 hours prior to injection of the Tc-99m sestamibi) enables further reduction in the administered dose to <190 MBq (<5 mCi) Tc-99m sestamibi giving an effective radiation dose of <1.5 mSv. This is now comparable to the effective dose from mammography and tomosynthesis and is low enough to allow consideration of widespread use of MBI for both diagnostic and screening applications.

3   Diagnostic and Screening Applications of MBI

The potential uses of MBI in the clinical setting are listed below. Best uses include screening, which is discussed in more detail below, evaluation of patients who are unable or unwilling to undergo MRI, and monitoring response to neoadjuvant chemotherapy (NAC).

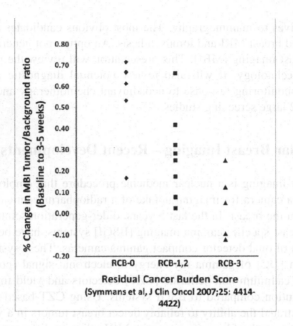

Fig. 1. Percent changes in the MBI T/B ratio from baseline to 3-5 weeks as a function of their final residual cancer burden score. Adapted from Mitchell D, et al (4).

- Best Uses of MBI
  - Screening dense breast (especially if additional risk factors)
  - Qualifies for, but unable / unwilling to undergo, MRI
  - Follow-up neoadjuvant chemotherapy (early evidence supports)
- Acceptable Uses of MBI
  - Problem solving for breast imagers
  - Nipple discharge
  - Persistent clinical concern with negative mammography / ultrasound
  - History of silicone injections

Early prediction of response to NAC offers a potential opportunity to change treatment strategy in cases of inadequate response. Clinical examination, mammography, and ultrasound provide only a modest correlation between tumor size and response to NAC. Contrast enhanced MRI has been used for evaluating response, but further work is needed to establish its value, due to heterogeneity in study design of investigations performed thus far. Several studies using FDG-PET have shown a correlation between standardized uptake value after NAC and final pathological response and to date FDG-PET is the most promising technique for monitoring NAC. MBI may offer an alternative and less expensive method for evaluation of response. Previous studies had shown that breast tumor uptake of sestamibi could accurately assess the response to NAC and may be as useful as FDG-PET in this application. A recent study from

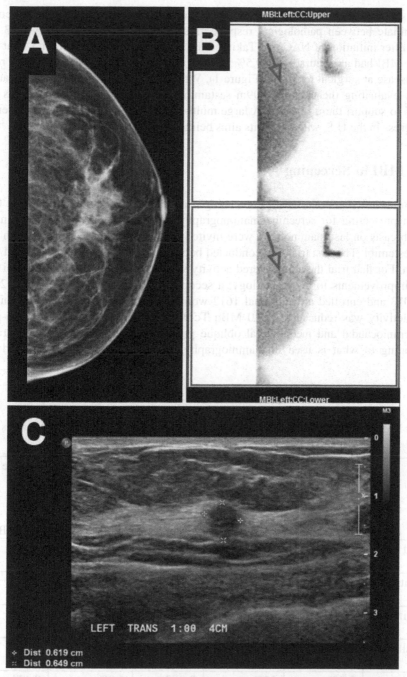

Fig. 2. A) Screening mammogram (Left CC view). No evidence of malignancy. B) Left CC views from upper and lower detector on MBI study performed 1 week after mammogram. Arrows indicate area of focal uptake. C) Ultrasound of area of concern showed a 6 x 7 x 6 mm hypoechoic mass with irregular margins confirmed at biopsy as an invasive tubular carcinoma.

Mayo showed that a simple measurement of tumor / background ratio [T/B] could differentiate between pathological responders and non-responders as early as 3 - 5 weeks after initiation of NAC (4). Taking a threshold of 50% reduction in T/B at 3-5 weeks, MBI had an accuracy of 89.5% for predicting the presence or absence of residual disease at surgical resection (Figure 1). While these results are promising, larger studies evaluating the use of Tc-99m sestamibi and dedicated gamma cameras are needed to support these findings. A large multi-center trial (ContraMIBI) is currently in progress in the U.S. with one of its aims being to confirm these findings.

4   MBI in Screening

Over the last 5 years two separate screening trials have been completed. In each trial women presenting for screening mammography with heterogeneously or extremely dense breasts on last mammogram were invited to undergo MBI, performed with Tc-99m sestamibi. The first trial was conducted between 2008 and 2010 and enrolled 936 women. For that trial the administered activity was ~740 MBq Tc-99m sestamibi (5). After improvements to the technology, a second trial was conducted between 2011 and 2013 and enrolled an additional 1612 women. In this second trial, the administered activity was reduced to ~240 MBq Tc-99m sestamibi. Bilateral, 10 min-per-view craniocaudal and mediolateral oblique projections were acquired (comparable positioning to what is used in mammography). Breast radiologists interpreted the

Table 1. Combined results of Two Screening Trials of MBI

(Abbr: DMX: digital mammography, Yield: # cancers per 1000 screened, PPV1: # cancers per abnormal screen, PPV3: # cancers per biopsy performed)

	DMX alone	DC-MBI alone	p-value (DMX alone vs. DC-MBI alone	Combination of DMX + adjunct DC-MBI	p-value (DMX alone vs. DMX + DC-MBI)
Yield	3.1 (8/2548)	10.2 (26/2548)	<0.001	11.4 (29/2648)	<0.001
Sensitivity	25% (8/32)	81% (26/32)	<0.001	91% (29/32)	<0.001
Specificity	90% (2262/2516)	93% (2345/2516)	<0.001	84% (2115/2516)	<0.001
Recall Rate	10% (264/2548)	7.7% (196/2548)	<0.001	16.8% (427/2548)	<0.001
PPV1	3.0% (8/264)	13% (26/196)	0.003	6.8% (29/427)	0.111
PPV3	21% (8/38)	31% (27/88)	0.451	27% (30/113)	0.643

MBI studies while blinded to mammography findings. Assessments of 1-5 (paralleling BI-RADS) were assigned; 3 or higher was considered positive. Positive MBI studies were then compared with screening mammogram to rule out benign explanation for MBI findings; diagnostic workup was performed if assessment remained positive. Reference standard was determined by pathology findings within 365 days of imaging or negative findings on next annual screen. Both trials yielded essentially identical results in terms of sensitivity and specificity. Between the two trials, a total of 32 patients were diagnosed with breast cancer: 3 were detected by mammography only, 21 by DC-MBI only, 5 by both, and 3 by neither. Performance characteristics of mammography, DC-MBI, and the combination are given in Table 1. Adjunct screening with DC-MBI in women with dense breasts significantly increased yield by 8.3 cancers per 1000 screened; this supplemental yield is higher than that observed for supplemental ultrasound (3.5 – 4.4). Positive predictive value was not reduced with adjunct MBI as has been observed with adjunct ultrasound or MRI.

5   Conclusions

With the improvements in the underlying technology behind DC-MBI and optimization of patient preparation, we believe that MBI has a role to play in both the diagnostic and screening setting and may be of particular value as an adjunct technique to mammography and tomosynthesis in screening women with dense breast tissue.

References

1. Hruska, C.B., Weinmann, A.L., O'Connor, M.K.: Proof of concept for low-dose molecular breast imaging with a dual-head CZT gamma camera. Part I. Evaluation in phantoms. Med. Phys. 39, 3466–3475 (2012)
2. Hruska, C.B., Weinmann, A.L., Tello-Skjerseth, C.M., Wagenaar, E.M., Conners, A.L., Tortorelli, C.L., Maxwell, R.W., Rhodes, D.J., O'Connor, M.K.: Proof of concept for low-dose molecular breast imaging with a dual-head CZT gamma camera. Part II. Evaluation in patients. Med. Phys. 39, 3476–3483 (2012)
3. Swanson, T.N., Troung, D.T., Paulsen, A., Hruska, C.B., O'Connor, M.K.: Adsorption of Tc-99m Sestamibi onto Plastic Syringes: Evaluation of the Factors affecting the Degree of Adsorption and their Impact on Clinical Studies. JNMT 41, 247–252 (2013)
4. Mitchell, D., Hruska, C.B., Boughey, J.C., Wahner-Roedler, D.L., Jones, K.N., Tortorelli, C., Conners, A.L., O'Connor, M.K.: Tc-99m sestamibi molecular breast imaging to assess tumor response to neoadjuvant chemotherapy in women with locally advanced breast cancer. Clin. Nucl. Med. 38, 949–956 (2013)
5. Rhodes, D.J., Hruska, C.B., Phillips, S.W., Whaley, D.H., O'Connor, M.K.: Dedicated Dual-Head Gamma Imaging for Breast Cancer Screening in Women with Mammographically Dense Breasts. Radiology 258, 106–118 (2011)

Will New Technologies
Replace Mammography CAD as We Know It?

Julian Marshall, Ashwini Kshirsagar, Sibel Narin, and Nikos Gkanatsios

Hologic, Inc, Santa Clara, CA, USA

Abstract. Since its commercial introduction in 1998, Mammography computer-aided detection (CAD) has been one of the few CAD technologies widely implemented in clinical practice. The original concept of CAD marks as overlays on images has been broadly accepted, although new paradigms have been proposed and successfully tested that could one day challenge that original approach. But now, as breast imaging evolves further with the advent of digital breast tomosynthesis, new image processing techniques are developing that may cause us to re-evaluate the clinical requirements for Mammography CAD as we know it. What clinical problems in breast imaging are not solved by tomosynthesis, and how can CAD help us with those problems?

Keywords: Mammography, Tomosynthesis, Generated 2D, Computer-aided Detection, CAD.

Authors' Note: This paper is not intended as a scientific paper. Instead, it is intended to be a bit controversial – to foster thought and get the research community thinking about how Mammography CAD should be adapted in a changing Breast Imaging world.

1 Introduction

In the United States, approximately 82% of full-field digital mammography (FFDM) machines (~10,000 of 12,246[1]) feed images to a Mammography CAD system; that 82% number is referred to as the "adoption rate". The adoption rate in other countries is lower, such as in Spain (~46%) and Taiwan (~35%).

The effectiveness of Mammography CAD has long been the subject of debate. Several important studies have demonstrated benefit from the use of CAD[2,3,4,5], while

---

[1] Data from US FDA website for MQSA National Statistics as of January 1, 2014.

[2] Freer TW et al. Screening Mammography with Computer-aided Detection: Prospective Study of 12,860 Patients in a Community Breast Center. Radiology 2001; 220:781–786.

[3] Cupples et al. Impact of computer-aided detection in a regional screening mammography program. AJR. 2005;185: 944-950.

[4] Gromet M. Comparison of Computer-Aided Detection to Double Reading of Screening Mammograms: Review of 231,221 Mammograms. AJR. 2008;190: 854-859.

H. Fujita, T. Hara, and C. Muramatsu (Eds.): IWDM 2014, LNCS 8539, pp. 30–37, 2014.
© Springer International Publishing Switzerland 2014

others have questioned those benefits[6,7]. Even though CAD has been successful in finding cancers at earlier stage[3], using a CAD system as a 2nd reader ensures an increased recall rate; the radiologist has already read the case prior to seeing the CAD marks, so additional cancers can only be found if additional cases are recalled.

1.1 The Very Real Problems Mammography CAD Was To Solve

In Spain, CAD adoption was driven by the cost savings associated with no longer double-reading and the potential for a higher cancer detection rate; in the United States, CAD adoption was driven by a very favorable reimbursement climate and the potential for finding cancers earlier.

Interviews with radiologists reveal:

1. Most clinicians value Mammography CAD because of its very high sensitivity, especially for detecting small and subtle calcification clusters.
2. Most clinicians do not value the mass detection capability because of poor specificity, despite CAD's high sensitivity and the fact that it correctly marks many cancers in prior mammograms[8].

This gives us hope that CAD is addressing the major human failings in mammography reading – observational oversight and satisfaction of search.

Most Mammography CAD systems operate as second-readers. After a first review of the images, the workstation shows the CAD marks. Often, the radiologist has already looked at those locations and can quickly dismiss the false marks (especially for calcifications). Most mass marks can be similarly dismissed, but some areas of superimposed tissue masquerading as potential mass lesions and marked by CAD may cause the radiologist to worry – to second-guess if they are real lesions or not – slowing down reading (especially for readers with less experience).

Mammography CAD users want improved CAD performance and clinical effectiveness. But, to a large extent, CAD algorithms may not improve much further because they share the same limitations as human observers; super-imposed tissue limits sensitivity and specificity because lesions simply cannot be seen, or because normal overlapping tissue looks disturbing.

2   The Introduction of Digital Breast Tomosynthesis

The application of tomosynthesis in breast imaging was proposed by Niklason et al[9] in 1997. By acquiring a number of low-dose X-rays of the breast from different angles

5   Gilbert FJ et al. Single Reading with Computer-Aided Detection for Screening Mammography. N Engl J Med 2008; 359:1675-1684.
6   Gur D et al. Changes in Breast Cancer Detection and Mammography Recall Rates After the Introduction of a Computer-Aided Detection System. J Natl Cancer Inst (2004) 96 (3): 185-190.
7   Fenton JJ et al. Influence of Computer-Aided Detection on Performance of Screening Mammography. N Engl J Med 2007; 356:1399-1409.
8   FDA PMA P970058. Data on file.

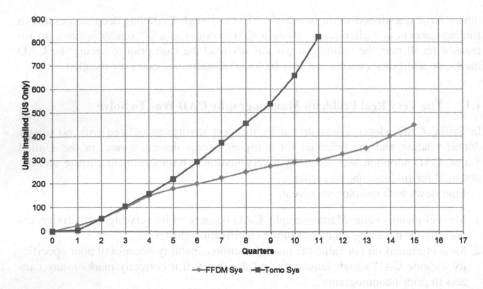

Fig. 1. Adoption of FFDM systems and Tomosynthesis systems in the US from date of first FDA approval[10,11]

within a narrow sweep, Niklason showed that reconstruction of planes within the breast had the potential to mitigate the issues of overlapping tissue.

In the years since that first paper, tomosynthesis has taken root. Now FDA approved, and validated through a series of large, peer-review clinical studies[12,13,14], tomosynthesis is gaining clinical adoption in the United States at a rate almost twice that of digital mammography (**Fig. 1**).

The recent and large studies referenced above confirm clinical evidence from earlier, smaller studies. All told, tomosynthesis has demonstrated the potential to increase the detection of invasive cancers by as much as 40%[12], and decrease the recall rate by as much as 37%[14].

9   Niklason L et al. Digital tomosynthesis in breast imaging. Radiology. 1997 Nov;205(2):399-406.

10 http://www.auntminnie.com/default.asp?Sec=sup&Sub=wom&Pag=dis&ItemId=51831

11 http://www.bizjournals.com/milwaukee/stories/2002/04/15/daily40.html

12 Skaane P et al. Comparison of Digital Mammography Alone and Digital Mammography Plus Tomosynthesis in a Population-based Screening Program. Radiology. 2013 Apr; 267(1):47-56.

13 Ciatto S et al. Integration of 3D digital mammography with tomosynthesis for population breast-cancer screening (STORM): a prospective comparison study. The Lancet Oncology, Volume 14, Issue 7, Pages 583 - 589, June 2013.

14 Rose SL et al. Implementation of breast tomosynthesis in a routine screening practice: an observational study. AJR Am J Roentgenol. American Journal of Roentgenology. 2013;200: 1401-1408.

Most of the work in these studies was done using "Combo" mode (3D+2D). The breast is compressed while both a tomosynthesis scan and a conventional 2D image are acquired. Combo mode was a means to study tomosynthesis while ensuring that the "standard of care" 2D mammogram was also available. Clinical studies showed significantly better reader performance with 3D+2D compared to 2D alone.

What, if any, is the clinical problem that tomosynthesis cannot solve, and which could be helped with a new CAD methodology? Masses and architectural distortions are better appreciated in tomosynthesis due to the removal of overlapping tissue; individual calcifications actually have higher local contrast in many cases than in 2D, yet may be distributed over many slices so the clusters may not be as well appreciated.

Determining that a microcalcification is in fact part of a three-dimensional cluster spread across several (potentially non-adjacent) slices is a very real challenge. For a human observer it may mean jogging up and down through the stack of slices to build a model of the cluster in the clinician's mind, slowing down reading and contributing to fatigue, which is proven to lead to reduced accuracy of reading mammograms[15].

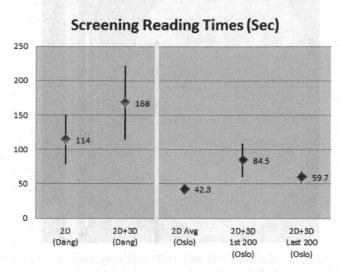

Fig. 2. A Comparison of Reading Times in Screening[16,17]

2.1   Tomosynthesis Reading Time

Reading time is important in screening. Two recent papers provide differing pictures of reading time ranges (one is single-reading, one is double-reading with consensus).

[15] Krupinski EA. Reader Fatigue Interpreting Mammograms, Digital Mammography Lecture Notes in Computer. Science. Vol 6136, 2010, pp 312-318.

[16] Dang PA et al. Addition of tomosynthesis to conventional digital mammography: effect on image interpretation time of screening examinations. Radiology. 2014 Jan;270(1):49-56.

[17] Skaane P et al. Trends in Time to Interpretation of Tomosynthesis Based Screening Examinations with Increasing Experience. RSNA 2013 Presentation SSK01-04, Weds, 2013-12-04 10:30 – 12:00, Arie Crown Theater.

Both studies (**Fig. 2**) demonstrated an increase in reading time when tomosynthesis was added, but the Oslo study goes further by showing that reading time dropped 30% over the course of the study, as the radiologists gained experience.

These studies, though, do not break down the tasks involved in reading. What fraction of their time is spent trying to perceive microcalcification clusters?

2.2   Introduction of Tomosynthesis Calcification CAD

The first commercially-available Tomosynthesis CAD product was a calcification cluster detection tool[18]; it provided marking of clusters and individual calcifications detected (**Fig. 3**) in tomosynthesis slices.

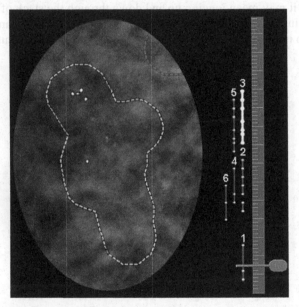

Fig. 3. Tomosynthesis Calcification CAD mark (left) indicating a detected cluster of calcifications; the outline indicates the X/Y extent of the cluster

Because of the additional reading time associated tomosynthesis slices, the success of tomosynthesis CAD will be closely tied to the efficiency of tools offered by workstation vendors. Adding CAD marks on individual slices may help with perception of clusters of calcium, but will it provide the efficiency needed to use tomosynthesis and Tomosyntheses CAD in screening?

2.3   Introduction of C-View 2D Generated Images

During the FDA's presentation to the Radiological Devices Panel reviewing Tomosynthesis, FDA stated that the benefit from tomosynthesis in screening "outweighed

---

18 Hologic® ImageChecker® 3D Calc CAD.

any risk from the additional X-ray dose". But, despite the relatively low dose of Combo mode, at least compared to screen film, clinicians remain concerned about the dose of tomosynthesis Combo mode.

A new technology for generating a 2D image from tomosynthesis slices (known as "C-View") was developed to preserve the primary benefit of tomosynthesis -- reduced impact of super-imposed tissue – and still provide a 2D image for use in temporal comparison in future years. Ideally, reading tomosynthesis slices plus generated 2D images would give clinical benefit equivalent to reading a Combo mode study, but at half the dose.

Most tomosynthesis-ready workstations provide the ability to "slab" together adjacent slices using the Maximum Intensity Projection (MIP) method. When applied to tomosynthesis images, MIP has the unfortunate side-effect of re-introducing tissue super-imposition from other slices, which makes the 2D MIP image blurry. For that reason, MIP should probably not be used in the context of digital breast tomosynthesis, although it can help make appreciation clustered calcifications easier.

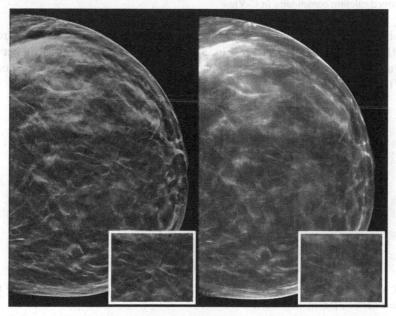

Fig. 4. C-View 2D image (left) and Tomo MIP image (right) taken from of all slices of the breast

C-View is different – it uses a series of complex filters to preserve the local contrast of "interesting" structures in tomosynthesis slices, such as bright spots, linear structures, and the edges of lobulated and microlobulated forms. A weighted sum then integrates the filtered slices. **Fig. 4** clearly shows the difference between MIP and C-View representations of the same set of tomosynthesis slices.

Clinically, the C-View algorithm results in some types of lesions becoming more conspicuous (such as the stellate lesion central in the breast in **Fig. 4 Insets**) because of the removal of super-imposed tissue due to the weighted sum favoring "interesting" characteristics of the image, such as radiating lines, lobulated density or clusters of bright spots.

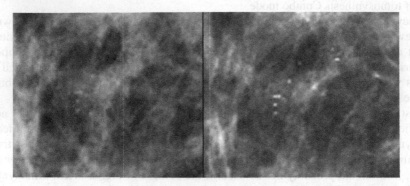

Fig. 5. Close-ups of conventional 2D (left) and C-View (right) images of a breast demonstrating improved calcium conspicuity in C-View

Consider the selected regions from a pair of 2D and C-View images acquired in ComboHD mode (3D+2D+C-View) (**Fig. 5**). There is reasonable similarity between the 2D and C-View images. The calcification cluster is much more conspicuous in the C-View 2D image region.

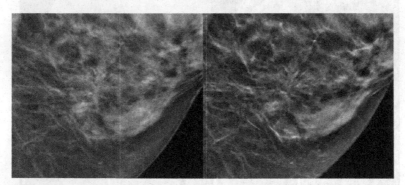

Fig. 6. Close-ups of conventional 2D (left) and C-View (right) images demonstrating better linear structure conspicuity in C-View

Fig. 6 shows a large stellate lesion that might be unappreciated in the conventional 2D image –a notable area of high density slightly inferior may distract the reader. But the C-View image clearly demonstrates a large area of architectural distortion, with linear structures radiating from a central area.

The first large study performed with C-View was the Oslo study[19]. Dr. Skaane reported that reading tomosynthesis images with C-View 2D images "performed comparably" to

---

[19] Skaane et al. Two-View Digital Breast Tomosynthesis Screening with Synthetically Reconstructed Projection Images: Comparison with Digital Breast Tomosynthesis with Full-Field Digital Mammographic Images. Radiology. January 2014, ePub ahead of print.

Combo imaging "in terms of cancer detection and false-positive scores" and should be considered "acceptable for routine use in mammography screening".

3 A New and Different CAD for Tomosynthesis

The development of C-View images led to an alternative solution for CAD in tomosynthesis imaging ... simply apply Mammography CAD algorithms to C-View images. The approach had some attractive advantages: first, it might be possible to adapt existing 2D CAD algorithms to C-View, rather than developing a new algorithm from the ground up; second, the concept would preserve the well-accepted CAD reading paradigm (marks on 2D images).

Our solution was to create a CAD system architecture that would transform C-View image pixels into a "For Processing" equivalent use solely for 2D CAD processing. The C-View CAD algorithm received US FDA approval in early 2014.

This method, while expedient, can certainly be improved further. The existing Mammography CAD algorithms have been trained on images where lesions include the effects of super-imposed tissue; our next step will be to re-train the CAD algorithm on C-View cases alone.

4 Conclusion

The demonstrated clinical benefits of tomosynthesis are putting very strong pressure on breast imagers to shift away from conventional digital mammography; Mammography CAD developers must adapt in the same way. We suspect that human readers are still prone to the same sorts of perceptual errors when reading tomosynthesis (E.g., satisfaction of search) that caused the development of Mammography CAD in the first place, so there presumably is room for a new CAD of some form.

It is now up to us, the CAD developers of the world, to put our heads together and invent the next perception aid tool that will help radiologists efficiently read tomosynthesis and C-View images with fewer perceptual errors. Whether it be CAD as in the past, or a new generation of C-View image in the future, radiologists still need our help.

Advanced Telecommunications in Breast Imaging – Streamlining Telemammography, Telepathology and Teleoncology Services to Improve Patient Care

Elizabeth A. Krupinski

Department of Medical Imaging, University of Arizona, Tucson, AZ USA
krupinski@radiology.arizona.edu

Abstract. Teleradiology services are very common worldwide, and Full Field Digital Mammography (FFDM) systems have made it possible to include mammography. This is important because breast cancer is the most common cancer in women in many parts of the world and it is the second leading cause of cancer deaths. In rural and medically underserved areas, mammography rates are lower than in urban areas for a variety of reasons, including lack of dedicated screening facilities and/or personnel, poor compliance, and large distances between patients and clinics (making it difficult to return for follow-up care). Once possible cancers are detected, biopsies are performed but in many cases reports are very slow to get back to the patient and/or local clinician impacting treatment and follow-up. Telepathology can address this situation. Patients may also require oncology services and in rural areas they are often limited or non-existent. Real-time teleoncology services can facilitate treatment and counseling. Finally, breast care support and education can be facilitated by virtual support groups and broadcasting education lectures.

Keywords: telemammography, telepathology, teleoncology, virtual support groups, distance education.

1 Introduction

Breast cancer is the most common cancer in women in many parts of the world and it is the second leading cause of cancer deaths. [1] Cancer prevention services are generally provided by primary care health professionals, but specialized genetic and high-risk follow-up and prevention is generally provided in cancer centers by cancer specialists. For many patients, however, getting access to specialized cancer services is a significant challenge. For example, Onega et al. studied access to oncology care in the US and found that travel to a National

Cancer Institute (NCI)-designated cancer center was an hour or more for the majority of patients. [2] Travel times are even greater for Native American, suburban and rural populations, to both NCI-designated cancer centers and any other cancer treatment center. Since about 25% of the US population lives in remote or rural areas, there are significant

H. Fujita, T. Hara, and C. Muramatsu (Eds.): IWDM 2014, LNCS 8539, pp. 38–43, 2014.
© Springer International Publishing Switzerland 2014

Limitations to access to medical care exist around the world so ways to extend and improve access to care using telemedicine is a valuable opportunity to improve health outcomes.

2   Telemammography

The Department of Radiology at the University of Arizona has been providing tele-mammography services since 2001 to seven communities around the state as part of its teleradiology outreach program. The outreach service was initiated in 1997, and operates using the telemedicine network infrastructure that was designed, built and is now maintained by the Arizona Telemedicine Program (ATP). The Arizona Teleme-dicine Program is a private Asynchronous Transfer Mode (ATM) network from commercial carriers. [3-5]

The ATP was created in 1996 by the Arizona State Legislature as a multidiscipli-nary, university-based program to provide telemedicine services, distance learning, informatics training, and telemedicine technology assessment throughout the state. It was mandated by the Legislature that the program provide services to a range of healthcare service users including geographically isolated communities, Native Amer-ican communities, and the Department of Corrections' rural prisons. After initial implementation in 1997 with eight pilot sites, the ATP now operates a broadband telecommunications network that links over 150 not-for-profit and profit healthcare organizations, functioning as a "virtual corporation". The ATP's core mission is to provide access to specialty health care services for medically underserved communi-ties in the rural areas of the state, and to date nearly 250,000 Arizonians have received healthcare services via telemedicine. These services are provided over a private ATM network, operating over an infrastructure of T-1 and T-3 circuits leased from com-mercial vendors. Both store-and-forward and real-time interactive applications are used, providing clinical consultations in over 55 sub-specialties.

The telemammography service provides image interpretations to very rural areas that generally have no sub-specialty radiologists such as mammographers or even have no on-site radiologists at all. Prior to telemammography being available, mam-mography services were sporadic and many women did not receive necessary screen-ing and/or follow-up imaging and care. If they did get a screening exam at their local clinic or via a mobile van service, neither provided rapid turn-around interpretations. Women often went home after being imaged and it was very difficult to contact them if additional images or tests were required because they often have no phones or reliable mail service.

To address this issue, the telemammography service requires that once a case is transmitted from the acquisition site, screening exams must be interpreted within 45 minutes and diagnostic exams must be interpreted within 30 minutes. Most women are willing to wait for this amount of time and follow-up services (e.g., additional imaging or biopsies) are provided in a much more efficient and timely manner.

To date we have done nearly 30,000 cases and the telemammographers have been able to meet the turn-around time requirements in over 95% of cases transmitted. Longer times have occurred mostly due to transmission difficulties, not because of prolonged times once the images arrived at the interpretation workstation.

Mammographic interpretation is only one link in the breast care chain. If something is found on mammography follow-up imaging is generally required. Most of these rural sites do not have MRI, but ultrasound is available and very useful in many situations. Thus, the telemammography program also provides interpretations of breast ultrasound images, and to date we have done nearly 3,000 breast ultrasound interpretations via teleradiology.

3   Telepathology

When biopsies are required the same challenges regarding getting results to the local clinician and the patient in these rural areas exist with pathology services as with radiology. When a finding suspicious of breast cancer is found, the process from mammography to clinical consultation with the oncologist generally takes about 28 days before treatment begins. It is even longer for women in rural areas because they typically need to travel to an urban hospital for care, but in both scenarios (urban or rural), there are long waiting time between initial diagnosis, getting the pathology results, and receiving an oncology consultation. All of this waiting and uncertainly can be extremely stressful for the patient. To help reduce these waiting times, we have evaluated rapid-processing and digitization of breast biopsy samples for telepathology interpretation.

Prior to investing in starting up a telepathology service for this application area, we had to consider the business model. Therefore as an initial step we surveyed patients at the university breast clinic to determine if and how much they would be willing to pay for faster biopsy results, since it was not clear if insurance companies and other payers would be willing to pay. The study had 312 breast center clients responding. If diagnosed with cancer, 92% of the respondents said they would seek an expert second opinion. Asked if they would pay a co-payment for a second opinion if their insurance covered the benefit, 97% responded yes. Thirty-five percent reported they would pay more than $50, although significantly more would be willing to pay only $25 or less. When asked how far they would be willing to travel for such a service, 33% reported a willingness to travel over 50 miles and 47% were willing to travel between 11 and 50 miles.

For the telepathology component, biopsy tissue specimens are acquired and processed by a Vacuum Histoprocess and ultra-rapid fixation system. They are converted to a digital image by a DMetrix scanner, and sent via the telemedicine network to the pathology department. In the program, patients receiving a biopsy before noon can utilize this Ultra-Clinic® process and the telepathology reports are relayed back to the breast center later that day in the majority of cases. [6]

4   Teleoncology

If the pathology report comes back positive, the patient then needs to receive treatment. In many cases the patient still needs to travel to a dedicated oncology and/or radiation oncology site, but some of the preliminary and post-treatment meeting travel can be avoided using teleoncology. In rural areas many women do not have the time or transportation to make these trips and often end up going untreated. Teleoncology uses the real-time videoconferencing capabilities of the network to connect the rural patient with the teleoncologist. A healthcare provider (often a nurse or promotora) is generally located in the room with the patient to provide additional support and advice while the teleoncologist explains the diagnosis, prognosis, and treatment options to the patient. Ideally this occurs during the same day as the telemammography and telepathology services but is often the hardest to schedule as it is real-time and requires the oncologist to arrange her schedule to make the meeting which can be difficult. [7]

5   Counseling and Patient Education

There is a known sub-set of women who are at increased risk for breast cancer (BRCA1/BRCA2), but in order to verify whether or not someone has this particular genetic risk testing is required. Once the risk is known, counseling is often required as well. Again however, genetic counseling services are not often available outside of a university or tertiary care center. Genetic health-care delivery often relies on a specialists traveling to communities in need. Unfortunately, this results in sporadic care that can leave patients and families unsupported for long periods of time.

The Arizona Telemedicine Program established a telegenetics program to provide genetic counseling. These are real-time telecounseling sessions in which a certified genetic counselor meets virtually with the patient (and family on many occasions), providing advice and options with respect to living with a significant genetic risk for cancer. The service was evaluated and patients strongly agreed that they found telegenetics consultation to be beneficial; that having the telemedicine visit was preferable to waiting for a face-to-face appointment with the same doctor; and patients did not see a need to seek in-person genetic counseling services in the future as they were so satisfied with the telegenetics service. [8,9]

We have also investigated the use of virtual support groups for breast cancer patients. [9] In many cases a breast cancer patient may be the only one of one of very few in their community if they live in a rural area. This makes it very difficult for them to form or attend a support group. Virtual support groups help alleviate this problem to some extent by bringing patients together virtually in real-time. Success of these virtual groups depends a bit more on the group members and the level of interaction than in-person groups – sometimes members in the virtual group take more time to "warm up" to each other and get used to sharing without being in the same physical location.

Finally we have developed a breast cancer health education series as part of our overall distance learning program [4] that is offered to patients, families, and primary care providers using statewide simultaneous teleconferencing in English and Spanish. The program is called Vida! and was started in 2008. Since then there have been 28 broadcast lectures with 456 attendees from 11 sites. As this is a CME accredited activity for healthcare providers we collect evaluation data and overall the attendees find the lectures to be very useful, provide new information, and will likely provide them with the knowledge and skills to better care for breast cancer patients. Topics have included body image concerns, diet and nutrition, links between breast and ovarian cancers, exercise, heredity issues, depression, and many more issues of relevance to breast cancer patients and providers.

6   Challenges

There are some components of this "bundled" telebreast care service that have been easier to implement and sustain than others. The easiest has been telemammography as many rural sites have invested in FFDM technologies, are connected to the ATP and thus our Department of Medical Imaging for efficient and effective interpretation of mammograms and ultrasound exams. Telepathology has had some challenges for two reasons. The first is that there is not always someone at the rural site qualified to do the biopsy. If there is, the second challenge has been the cost to the sites for purchasing the units required to prepare the biopsies (Vacuum Histoprocess and ultra-rapid fixation system) and scan and transmit the images to the pathology department. This equipment is rather costly and use is limited to a few cases per month making it difficult to convince financially strapped clinics and hospitals to purchase.

The virtual support groups have waxed and waned over the years, as noted above depending on the make-up of the individual group members, how well they interact with each other, and how well they maintain meeting attendance. What has been interesting is the mix of cultures – Native American, Hispanic, Caucasian, Asian and African American women have participated and found numerous common topics, feelings and challenges to discuss. The Vida! education series has also been very successful with an average of 6 healthcare providers (range 1-18) attending each broadcast for CME credit and about 12 patients attending each one.

In order to further expand the program and truly provide one-day breast care tele-services we would require a rather significant investment in the accessory technologies required to do the telepathology component. Getting clinicians motivated to participate is a minor challenge but could be overcome by volume. If the patient volume was high enough to establish a set teleoncology clinic (like our other real-time clinics), the tele-oncologist would be better able to fit the sessions into her schedule on a regular basis. Overall however this innovative approach to providing care across the spectrum of clinical areas associated with breast care has been successful in terms of providing patients with timely and expert breast care that they otherwise would not have likely received.

References

1. National Cancer Institute.: Breast Cancer Facts and Figures (2005), https://www.cancer.gov/cancertopics/breast
2. Onega, T., Duell, E.J., Shi, X., Wang, D., Demidenko, E., Goodman, D.: Geographic access to cancer care in the U.S. Cancer 112, 909–918 (2008)
3. McNeill, K.M., Weinstein, R.S., Holcomb, M.J.: Arizona Telemedicine Program: implementing a statewide health care network. J. Am. Med. Informatics. Assn. 5, 441–447 (1998)
4. Krupinski, E.A., Weinstein, R.S.: Telemedicine in an academic center – the Arizona Telemedicine Program. Telemed. e-Health. 19, 349–356 (2013)
5. Krupinski, E., McNeill, K., Ovitt, T.: High-volume teleradiology service: focus on radiologist satisfaction. J. Digit. Imag. 16, 203–209 (2003)
6. Weinstein, R.S., Lopez, A.M., Barker, G.P., Krupinski, E.A., Descour, M.R., Scott, K.M., Richter, L.C., Beinar, S., Holcomb, M.J., Bartels, P.H., et al.: The innovative bundling of teleradiology, telepathology and teleoncology services. IBM Syst. J. 46, 69–84 (2007)
7. Lopez, A., Venker, C.C., Howerter, A., Barker, G.P., Bhattacharyya, A., Scott, K.M., Descour, M.R., Richter, L.C., Krupinski, E.A., Weinstein, R.S.: Demonstration of an expedited breast care (EBC) clinic. J. Clin. Onc. 24,18S (2006)
8. Cunniff, C., Lopez, A.M., Webster, P.D., Weinstein, R.S.: Tele-genetics: Novel Application to Address Health Care Disparities in Pediatrics. Paper presented at the 12th Annual Meeting American Telemedicine Association Meeting, Nashville, TN (2007)
9. Lopez, A.M.: Telemedicine, telehealth, and e-health technologies in cancer prevention. In: Alberts, D., Hess, L.M. (eds.) Fundamentals of Cancer Prevention, pp. 259–277. Springer, Berlin (2014)

Predicting the Benefit of Using CADe in Screening Mammography

Robert M. Nishikawa[1] and Andriy Bandos[2]

[1] Department of Radiology, University of Pittsburgh, Pittsburgh, USA
nishikawarm@upmc.edu
[2] Department of Biostatistics, University of Pittsburgh, USA
anb61@pitt.edu

Abstract. The goal of computer-aided detection (CADe) in screening mammography is to help radiologist avoid missing breast cancer. Thus when designing a CADe system it is important to know how different methods and parameters would affect radiologists' ability to use the system effectively. Short of conducting an observer study or a clinical trial, this is not possible. In this paper, we present preliminary results on a model that can predict how many additional cancers a radiologist would detect, if they used a CADe system. The model uses the results of radiologists' reading of a set of screening mammograms without using CADe to predict the probability that a radiologist would miss a cancer when reading without CADe and the probability that the radiologist would recall the woman if CADe flagged the missed cancer. In our initial study, 8 radiologists read 300 screening mammograms containing 69 cancers with and without CADe. Our model predicted that on average a radiologist would detect 4.7 extra cancers while the actual number of extra cancers detected per radiologist was 3.6. Bootstrapping across readers, the 95% CI for the difference between the predicted and actual number of extra cancers was [-1.52, 3.30]. The overall ability of the model to discriminate between lesions detected as a result of CAD flag and other lesion examinations was moderately high, with c-index of 0.77 (95% CI of [0.6, 0.91]). We are currently conducting a study with larger number of radiologists and cases to obtain better estimates of the accuracy of our model.

Keywords: computer-aided detection, screening, mammography, modeling.

1 Introduction

Computer-aided detection (CADe) is being used to assist radiologists in detecting breast cancer in mammographic screening. It is important, then, that CADe algorithms be developed with the specific goal of assisting radiologists. This is not practical currently. CADe systems are developed to have high sensitivity for detecting breast cancer while maintaining a reasonably low false-detection rate. It is not known whether this approach actually produces a CADe system that is optimally beneficial to radiologists. We are developing a method that can be used to optimize a

H. Fujita, T. Hara, and C. Muramatsu (Eds.): IWDM 2014, LNCS 8539, pp. 44–49, 2014.

CADe algorithm so that it provides maximum benefit to the radiologist (i.e., increases their sensitivity without a large increase in their callback rate). In our initial method, we estimate the probability that a radiologist will miss a cancer and the probability that if the radiologist missed a cancer and CADe marked the cancer, the radiologist would recall the woman. We propose to estimate both of these probabilities from a single reading of a mammogram by a group of radiologists reading without CADe.

2   Method

2.1   Observer Study

We conducted an observer study to measure the benefits of using CADe in screening mammography [1]. Eight MQSA radiologists read 300 cases that contained 69 biopsy-proven cancers. Each case consisted of the standard 4-view screen-film mammograms of the index exam and, when available, a previous exam. The index cancer cases were selected based on the presence of a cancer that was missed clinical, but was visible retrospectively.

For each case, the radiologist first read the mammograms without CADe and recorded the location of any suspicious lesions and whether they would recall the woman for a diagnostic workup of the lesion. The radiologist were then shown the results of the CADe system and rescored the case.

We used a commercial CADe system in our study. For the 300 cases, the CADe system had a sensitivity of 55% with an average of 2.4 false detections per case.

2.2   Model

The objective is to measure the change in the number of cancers detected (ΔN_{Ca}) when CADe is used. In its simplest form, which assumes only 1 lesion per case (these equations can be generalized to an arbitrary number of cancers per case):

$$\Delta N_{Ca} = \sum_{i=1}^{N_c} \Pr_i(miss)\Pr_i(\det | CADe+,miss)\Pr_i(CADe+ | miss) \tag{1}$$

where N_c is the number of cases with cancer. $\Pr_i(miss)$ is the probability that the radiologists will miss the lesion in the ith case when reading unaided. $\Pr_i(\det|CADe+,miss)$ is the probability that the radiologist will detect the originally missed lesion in the ith case, if it is marked by CADe. $\Pr_i(CADe+|miss)$ is the probability that CADe detects the lesion in the ith case, if the radiologist missed the cancer. Each product is the probability that a given lesion is detected due to the CADe output (i.e., missed before CAD, detected by CAD, and reported by a radiologist after CAD). However, the probability of the CADe system detecting the given cancer is independent of whether the radiologist detected or missed that cancer. Therefore, $\Pr_i(CADe+|miss) = \Pr_i(CADe+)$ and Eq. (1) becomes:

$$\Delta N_{Ca} = \sum_{i=1}^{N_C} \mathrm{Pr}_i(miss)\,\mathrm{Pr}_i(\det \mid CADe+, miss)\,\mathrm{Pr}_i(CADe+) \ , \qquad (2)$$

where $\mathrm{Pr}_i(CADe+)$ is the probability that CADe detects the lesion in the ith case. It is either 0 or 1. This is easily measured by running the case through the CADe system.

In their landmark paper, Berhenne *et al.* estimated $\mathrm{Pr}_i(\det|CADe+,miss)$ as the probability that a radiologist would detect the lesion unaided [2]. Their rationale was that a radiologist is more likely to react to a CADe prompt if the CADe-marked lesion looks more like a cancer. However, their analysis does not account for the probability that a radiologist would miss the cancer, $\mathrm{Pr}_i(miss)$. We estimate that as 1.0 minus the probability the lesion is detected (without CADe), which is the number of radiologists detecting the lesion divided by the total number of radiologists.

We will show that Eq. 2 can estimate the actual increase in the number of cancers detected when a radiologist uses CADe using data from the observer study.

2.3   Statistical Analysis

We performed two analyses to evaluate the model. The first was to compare the predicted and actual number of extra cancers found by a radiologist using CADe. We used bootstrapping across both readers and cases to measure the 95% CI in the difference between predict and actual values.

For second analysis, we evaluated the ability of discriminative ability of the model using c-index as a figure of merit. We examined each decision made the eight radiologists on the 69 cancers, a total of 552 decisions. The 552 decisions were grouped into cancers that the radiologist found only by using CADe (designated as positive cases) of which there were 29 cases; and all other cases (designated as negative cases). We then rank-ordered the cases based on the predicted probability that a radiologist would detect the cancer by using CADe (Eq. 2). We computed the corresponding c-statistic and the corresponding 95% confidence interval using bootstrap over readers and cases. Values of the c-statistic above 0.5 indicate a nontrivial (better-than-chance) performance of the model (or that lesions detected with CAD tend to have higher probability predicted by the model

3   Results

Table 1 summarizes the results of the observer study with regards to the model. The model predicted that on average each radiologist would detect 4.6 additional cancers when using CADe, whereas the actual number from the observer study was 3.6 cancers. The difference was 0.98 with 95% CI of [-1.52, 3.30].

Computing the c-statistic, which is a measure of the accuracy of the model, a value of 0.77 was found with 95% CI of [0.60, 0.91].

Table 1. The predicted benefit and actual benefit of using CADe

# of Rad. detecting a given Ca unaided	Total # of Ca detected by Rad. unaided	Prob Rad. misses Ca unaided	Prob Rad. detects missed Ca with CADe	Total # of Ca detected by CADe	Prob CADe detects Ca	Model prediction*	Total # of Ca detected by Rad. using CADe	Actual Benefit*
0	12	1	0	5	0.42	0.00	6·	0.75
1	5	0.875	0.125	1	0.2	0.11	0	0.00
2	5	0.75	0.25	1	0.20	0.19	0	0.00
3	4	0.625	0.375	1	0.25	0.23	1	0.13
4	3	0.5	0.5	2	0.67	0.50	6	0.75
5	6	0.375	0.625	5	0.83	1.17	7	0.88
6	12	0.25	0.725	7	0.58	1.31	5	0.63
7	14	0.125	0.875	10	0.71	1.09	4	0.50
8	8	0	1	5	0.625	0	0	0
Total	69			37		4.61	29	3.63
95% CI				[28,46]		[3.1,6.2]	[11,51]	[1.4,6.4]
A	B	C=1-A/8	D=A/8	E	F=E/B	‡G=C*D *F*B	H	I=H/8
		P(miss)	P(det|CADe+,miss)		P(CADe+)	ΔN_{cancer}		

* cancers (Ca) per radiologist (Rad.); prob=probability

Column B is the number of cancers of the category given in Col A that radiologists detected (e.g., there were 12 cancers that were detected by exactly 6 radiologists).

Column E and H need to be interpreted together (e.g., in the second row, CADe marked 5 cancers and the 8 readers reading those 5 cases found 6 cancers out of the total of 40 opportunities [8 radiologists times 5 CADe-marked cancers]).

‡ By multiplying by B, each row is a sum over a subset of cases that depends on the number of Rad. detecting the cancer unaided. Then summing column G produces a sum over all the cancers, Eq. 2.

4   Discussion

The model was fairly accurate at discriminating lesions-examinations that would benefit from CAD from the rest (c-index of 0.77). The predicted number of cancer-detection added due to CAD was predicted up to within 1 cancer per radiologists; however the current study does not exclude the possibility for the difference to be anywhere in (-1.55, 3.30) range. We are in the process of conducting a larger experiment with 30 radiologists and 100 cancers.

In addition to the low statistical power, the relatively small number of radiologists in our study limits the accuracy of the probability estimates needed in Eq. (2). That is, the probability estimates are quantized into 8 values. With more radiologists discrepancies between the predicted and actual number of additional cancers detected by using CADe can be reduced. For example, for the data line in Table 1, cancers that were missed by all 8 radiologists contribute 0 to the predicted benefit because the probability that a radiologist detects a missed cancer flagged by CADe is 0. However, the actual benefit of CADe for those cancers was 0.75. With more readers, we anticipated that the number of cases with all radiologists missing the cancer will be reduced. In the study that is currently underway, 30 radiologists will quantize the probabilities in increments of 0.033 compared to 0.125 with 8 radiologists used in the study reported here.

Currently the model is relatively simple. The model could potentially be improved by adding factors related to the whether the cancer is marked by CADe in both views (assuming the cancer is visible in both views) and the number of false detections per case. Both these factors have been report in the literature to influence radiologists' ability to use CADe effectively [3-5]

In the initial that we present here, we have only modeled detection of cancers. It is also necessary and important to model radiologists' detection of false positives and the effect that CADe has on increasing radiologists' false detection rate. We anticipate that this will require a different model or at least an additional term to the model for cancer detection presented in this paper. Whereas, cancers detected by a radiologist correspond to an actual lesion, some false detections correspond to a superposition of normal breast tissue that looks like a cancer. Since there is no actual lesion, these types of detection tend to be more random when comparing false detections from different radiologists. There may be a based line of "random" detections that needs to be added to the model proposed here. That is a number of detections that only 1 radiologist would detect. We will be able to estimate this baseline from the larger experiment that we are currently collecting.

Obuchowski has published a multiple-variable logistic regression model to predict the performance of an improved CADe scheme for detection of lung nodules in chest radiographs based on results of observer study of the original CADe scheme [6]. Her method is analogous to our method described here. The main difference with her approach is that she infers the factors that influence radiologists' ability to use CADe.

A model of CADe, such as the one proposed here, has several potential applications. It could be used to optimize a CADe algorithm to maximize the benefit to the radiologist as oppose to optimizing stand-alone performance (sensitivity and false detection rate) as is done now. Further, the model could be used to assist in deciding the operating point on the CADe algorithms FROC curve. Currently this is done in a very subjective manner.

In summary, we present preliminary results of a model that helps assess the benefit of use CADe in screening mammography. Although this initial study was relatively small, the model demonstrated good discriminative ability. The larger study we are currently conducting will help better evaluate the model, in particular in terms of the accuracy of the predicted total number of extra lesions.

Acknowledgments and Disclosures. RM Nishikawa receives royalties from Hologic, Inc. This work was funded in part from a grant from the NIH/NIBIB R01 EB013680.

References

1. Nishikawa, R.M., Schmidt, R.A., Linver, M.N., Edwards, A.V., Papaioannou, J., Stull, M.A.: Clinically Missed Cancer: How Effectively Can Radiologists Use Computer-Aided Detection? American Journal of Roentgenology 198, 708–716 (2012)
2. Warren-Burhenne, L.J., Wood, S.A., D'Orsi, C.J., Feig, S.A., Kopans, D.B., O'Shaughnessy, K., Sickles, E.A., Tábar, L., Vyborny, C.J., Castellino, R.A.: Potential contribution of computer-aided detection to the sensitivity of screening mammography. Radiology 215, 554–562 (2000)
3. Chan, H.-P., Doi, K., Vyborny, C.J., Schmidt, R.A., Metz, C.E., Lam, K.L., Ogura, T., Wu, Y., MacMahon, H.: Improvement in radiologists' detection of clustered microcalcifications on mammograms: The potential of computer-aided diagnosis. Investigative Radiology 25, 1102–1110 (1990)
4. Zheng, B., Swensson, R.G., Golla, S., Hakim, C.M., Shah, R., Wallace, L., Gur, D.: Detection and classification performance levels of mammographic masses under different computer-aided detection cueing environments. Acad. Radiol. 11, 398–406 (2004)
5. Nishikawa, R., Edwards, A., Schmidt, R., Papaioannou, J., Linver, M.: Can radiologists recognize that a computer has identified cancers that they have overlooked? In: Proc. SPIE, vol. 6146, pp. 1–8 (2006)
6. Obuchowski, N.A.: Predicting Readers' Diagnostic Accuracy with a New CAD Algorithm. Academic Radiology 18, 1412–1419 (2011)

Modeling Breast Cancer Screening Outcomes

Martin J. Yaffe[1,2], Nicole Mittman[3], Natasha Stout[4], Pablo Lee[5], and Anna Tosteson[6]

[1] Physical Sciences, Sunnybrook Research Institute, Toronto, Canada
[2] Department of Medical Biophysics, University of Toronto, Toronto, Canada
[3] Health Outcomes and PharmacoEconomic (HOPE) Research Centre, Sunnybrook Research Institute, Toronto, Canada
[4] Department of Population Medicine, Harvard Medical School, Boston, USA
[5] Institute for Technology Assessment, Massachusetts General Hospital, Boston, USA
[6] The Dartmouth Institute for Health Policy and Clinical Practice, Geisel School of Medicine at Dartmouth, Hanover, USA
martin.yaffe@sri.utoronto.ca

Abstract. There is currently rapid development of imaging technologies for breast cancer screening. In addition there is considerable controversy regarding the optimal screening strategy, including the ages at which screening should begin and end, the interval between screens and the imaging modality or modalities which should be used. Furthermore, there are major economic considerations related to whether screening should be done and how it should be done. Here, we describe the use of the Wisconsin CISNET computer model of breast cancer development to predict key outcomes associated with breast cancer, including incidence, mortality and life-years lost due to breast cancer. The sensitivity and specificity of the detection method and their dependence on factors such as age and breast density are implemented in the model through use of empirical data. Distributions of cancer characteristics are used to determine the type of modern therapy utilized and its effectiveness. Using this framework, the effectiveness of a particular screening strategy can be compared with other scenarios such as not screening at all or following published recommendations. The model can directly inform a cost-effectiveness or cost-utility analysis.

Keywords: breast cancer screening, modeling, mammography, outcomes, cost-effectiveness.

1   Introduction

The efficacy and effectiveness of mammography screening have been topics of heated debate for many years. Part of the underlying motivation of such debate is that screening programs utilize very substantial resources, resources that might be applied to other challenges in health. Decisions regarding whether to screen, who to screen, what modalities should be used and how frequently screening should occur are best made when there is an understanding of the trade-offs between improved health outcomes, potential harms, limitations and monetary costs of the intervention. There have been several previous cost-effectiveness analyses of mammography screening.[1–3] Most of these were conducted some time ago and do not reflect the performance of the

H. Fujita, T. Hara, and C. Muramatsu (Eds.): IWDM 2014, LNCS 8539, pp. 50–55, 2014.
© Springer International Publishing Switzerland 2014

methods currently used for detection or for treatment of breast cancer. Here we describe work using a validated model of breast cancer development to predict cancer outcomes associated with various screening strategies. We consider benefits in terms of lives saved and women-years saved through screening and limitations in terms of missed cancers and women recalled for further examination when they don't have breast cancer. The model is being employed to drive cost-effectiveness and cost-utility analyses for mammography screening, which will be reported elsewhere.

2   Methods

2.1   Breast Cancer Model

To model the development of cancer in a cohort of women, we used the University of Wisconsin Breast Cancer Epidemiology Simulation Model[4], developed under the US National Cancer Institute-funded Cancer Intervention and Surveillance Modeling Network (CISNET) program[5]. The model was originally developed and calibrated such that it reflected US breast cancer incidence and mortality trends from 1975-2000[4]. Details of the model have been described elsewhere and are available at www.cisnet.cancer.gov. We recalibrated the model to describe cancer incidence in Canada[6].

We began with a cohort of 2,000,000 women, born in 1960. The model "follows" them through their lives, randomly "seeding" breast cancers with a distribution of frequencies and growth characteristics derived from population statistics. Cancers are modeled as spheres that grow according to a Gompertz type growth function. Four "stages" of cancer – *in situ*, local, regional and distant – are defined according to the size of the sphere at detection. Treatment options are based on these stages, which also influence survival. Women are followed through the model until they die of breast cancer, some other cause or reach age 99.

2.2   Cancer Detection and Treatment

Although the model could be applied to any mode of cancer detection, here we only considered screening mammography. Empirical data on the sensitivity and specificity of mammography from The Breast Cancer Surveillance Consortium[7] and from The Screening Mammography Program of British Columbia[8] were used to inform the model. Sensitivity and specificity data of modern digital mammography were used and these were available for age bands over the range 40 to 80 years, for the four BIRADS breast density categories and for initial and recurring screening examinations.

The model also randomly assigned prognostic characteristics to each cancer that developed according to population frequencies for these characteristics. The original CISNET model included hormone receptors ER and PR; as part of our modifications we have added HER2/neu[9]. In the treatment section of the model, therapies including surgery, radiation therapy and adjuvant chemotherapy are assigned according to modern clinical practice guidelines, with the use of tamoxifen, aromatase inhibitors and trastuzumab where there was receptor positivity for these drugs[10].

2.3   Screening Outcomes

From the model, age-specific incidence and mortality can be estimated. In addition, we can calculate age-specific incidence-based mortality, i.e., the number of breast cancer deaths that would eventually occur, associated with the detection of breast cancer at a particular age, and this was done for a number of screening strategies (Table 1) that are either used in some jurisdictions or that have been suggested. We also included "no screening", i.e. women receive no routine mammography screening at all during their lifetimes, as a reference. In addition to mortality (lives lost), we calculated the number of women-years of life lost for cancer detected at each age.

Table 1. Screening scenarios modeled

No Screening	
Digital Mammography	**Film Mammography**
Annual 40-49	Annual 40-49
Annual 40-69	Annual 40-69
Annual 40-74	Annual 40-74
Annual 50-69	Annual 50-69
Annual 50-74	Annual 50-74
Biennial 50-69	Biennial 50-69
Biennial 50-74	Biennial 50-74
Triennial 50-69	Triennial 50-69
Triennial 50-74	Triennial 50-74
Annual 40-49, Biennial 50-69	Annual 40-49, Biennial 50-69
Annual 40-49, Biennial 50-74	Annual 40-49, Biennial 50-74

3   Results

Fig. 1 shows the modeled age and stage specific incidence of breast cancer for the cohort. At left, in the absence of screening, there is a relatively high incidence of "Regional" disease. This would correspond to lymph node positive cancer. At right, for biennial screening with digital mammography from ages 50-74 the Regional and Distant components drop sharply due to earlier detection of localized cancers, while at the same time there is a marked increase in *in situ* cancer, because it can now be detected through microcalcifications seen on mammography. The "spikes" in incidence seen at the initiation of screening represent cancers that had been present in previous years, but undetectable in the absence of screening. To avoid a large oscillation in the incidence between alternate years in which screening is or is not performed, for this graph the cohort was split into two, with each group screened in odd or even years only. In Fig. 2 at left, age-specific mortality is compared between two screening regimens and no screening. At right, the number of breast cancer deaths (at any age) in the cohort is plotted versus the age at which the cancer is diagnosed. This graph describes the burden of breast cancer in terms of when it arises, while both graphs illustrate the impact of screening.

4   Discussion

Screening is seen to shift the detection of breast cancer to an earlier time and to reduce the stage at which it is detected. Note that shortly after screening is discontinued, there is a shift back to the incidence of more advanced cancers. The spike in incidence-based mortality at the onset of screening on the graph right side of Fig.2 indicates that these cancers indeed have the potential to kill and are not just indolent cancers that don't require detection. When a number of screening scenarios are modeled, it is seen from Fig. 3, that in general, the benefit, in terms of number of women-years saved through screening, continues to increase with the total number of screens that a woman receives, over the age range 40-74 years. Clearly, some approaches provide greater benefit for the same number of screens and would therefore be more efficient. Of course, this benefit must be considered in light of the number of times women would be recalled for additional imaging due to suspicious additional findings on screening, the number of additional negative biopsies required and the cost of screening. These are being assessed in ongoing cost-effectiveness and cost-utility studies driven by results from this model. The model can also be used to estimate the amount of overdetection (frequently mistakenly referred to as "overdiagnosis"), *i.e.* the number of cancers that would be detected by screening which would never otherwise appear in a woman's lifetime. Costs can be considered both as those incurred by a health care system or those to society, the latter including the lost productivity of an individual who dies prematurely due to breast cancer.

The current breast cancer growth model is relatively simple; for example there is no growth rate dependence of cancers based on the woman's age. In future work we will consider more sophisticated algorithms and possibly more targeted approaches to screening based on factors such as breast density and risk.

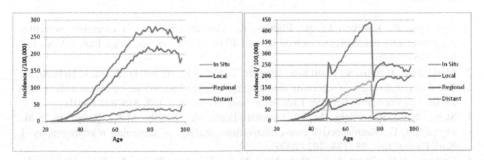

Fig. 1. Incidence for each modeled stage. (L) No Screening, (R) Biennial from 50-74 y.

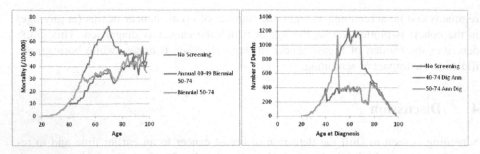

Fig. 2. (L) Mortality rates (per 100,000) for No Screening (blue), annual screening from 40-49 followed by biennial screening from 50-74 (red) and biennial screening from 50 to 74 years of age (green) with digital mammography. (R) Number of deaths (from initial birth cohort of 2,000,000) versus age at which cancer was detected for no screening, for annual screening from 40-74 and for annual screening from 50-74.

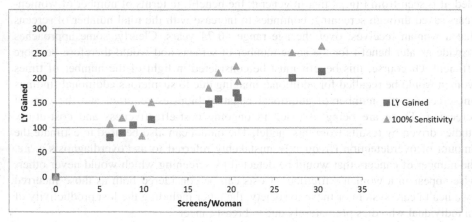

Fig. 3. Number of life-years gained through screening versus the total number of lifetime screens received by each participant. Squares represent current screening methods while triangles indicate the potential performance if the screening sensitivity were 100%.

References

1. Salzmann, P., Kerlikowske, K., Phillips, K.: Cost-effectiveness of extending screening mammography guidelines to include women 40 to 49 years of age. Ann. Intern. Med. 127, 955–965 (1997)
2. Mandelblatt, J., Saha, S., Teutsch, S., Hoerger, T., Siu, A.L., Atkins, D., Klein, J., Helfand, M.: The cost-effectiveness of screening mammography beyond age 65 years: a systematic review for the U.S. Preventive Services Task Force. Ann. Intern. Med. 139, 835–842 (2003)
3. Stout, N.K., Rosenberg, M.A., Trentham-Dietz, A., Smith, M.A., Robinson, S.M., Fryback, D.G.: Retrospective cost-effectiveness analysis of screening mammography. J. Natl. Cancer Inst. 98, 774–782 (2006)
4. Fryback, D.G., Stout, N.K., Rosenberg, M.A., Trentham-Dietz, A., Kuruchittham, V., Remington, P.L.: The Wisconsin Breast Cancer Epidemiology Simulation Model. J. Natl. Cancer Inst. Monogr., 37–47 (2006)

5. Feuer, E.J., Etzioni, R., Cronin, K.A., Mariotto, A.: The use of modeling to understand the impact of screening on U.S. mortality: examples from mammography and PSA testing. Stat. Methods Med. Res. 13, 421–442 (2004)
6. Statistics Canada: Life Tables, Canada, Provinces and Territories, http://www5.statcan.gc.ca/bsolc/olc-cel/olc-cel?catno=84-537-XIE&lang=eng (accessed December 1, 2013)
7. National Cancer Institute: The Breast Cancer Surveillance Consortium, http://breastscreening.cancer.gov/data/ (accessed January 14, 2014)
8. Screening Mammography Program of British Columbia: Screening Mammography Program 2012 Annual Report, http://www.smpbc.ca/NR/rdonlyres/3AF15A7A-B9D4-43C2-A93A-230A634E94AC/60300/SMP_2012AR_WEB.pdf   (accessed February 26, 2013)
9. Marla, S., Cardale, J., Dodwell, D.J., Skene, A., Gojis, O., Palmieri, C., Abram, P., Cleator, S., Bowman, A., Doughty, J.C.: HER2-positive early breast cancers: What proportion are receiving adjuvant trastuzumab therapy- A multicenter audit. J. Clin. Oncol. 28, 668 (2010)
10. Early Breast Cancer Trialists' Collaborative Group: Effects of chemotherapy and hormonal therapy for early breast cancer on recurrence and 15-year survival: an overview of the randomised trials. Lancet. 365, 1687–717 (2005)

The Impact of Introducing Full Field Digital Mammography into a Screening Programme

Thomas Fyall[1], Caroline Boggis[2], Jamie Sergeant[3,4], Elaine Harkness[2,5],
Sigrid Whiteside[6], Julie Morris[6], Mary Wilson[2], and Susan M. Astley[2,5]

[1] Manchester Medical School, University of Manchester, Oxford Road, Manchester,
M13 9PT, UK
[2] Nightingale Centre and Genesis Prevention Centre, University Hospital of South Manchester,
Manchester M23 9LT, UK
[3] Arthritis Research UK Centre for Epidemiology, Institute of Inflammation and Repair, Faculty
of Medical and Human Sciences, Manchester Academic Health Science Centre, University of
Manchester, Oxford Road, Manchester M13 9PT, UK
[4] NIHR Manchester Musculoskeletal Biomedical Research Unit, Central Manchester NHS
Foundation Trust, Manchester Academic Health Science Centre, Manchester, UK
[5] Centre for Imaging Sciences, Institute of Population Health, Faculty of Medical and Human
Sciences, Manchester Academic Health Science Centre, University of Manchester, Oxford
Road, Manchester M13 9PT, UK
[6] Department of Medical Statistics, University Hospital of South Manchester,
Manchester M23 9LT, UK
sue.astley@manchester.ac.uk

Abstract. As digital mammography has largely replaced analogue mammography for screening, we examine the impact of the change on clinical outcomes. Data were obtained for 62,599 women undergoing routine screening mammography between January 2010 and March 2012 during the transition from analogue to digital screening, and on a monthly basis for the two years following complete conversion to digital mammography. With digital mammography, the recall rate increased from 3.58% to 4.69% (p<0.001) and the biopsy/cytology referral rate increased from 1.49% to 1.88% (p=0.01) whilst the cancer detection rate did not change significantly. The recall rate showed a strong positive correlation with time (r=0.71, p<0.001) and biopsy rate showed a moderate positive correlation (r=0.52 p=0.011). The cancer detection rate showed a moderate negative correlation with time (r=-0.567 p=0.05). Whilst all the outcome measures reported meet the standards set by the national screening programme, these results indicate a need for regular monitoring following changes to screening technology.

Keywords: Screening, recall, biopsy, cancer detection, film, digital, mammogram.

H. Fujita, T. Hara, and C. Muramatsu (Eds.): IWDM 2014, LNCS 8539, pp. 56–63, 2014.
© Springer International Publishing Switzerland 2014

1 Introduction

1.1 Breast Screening

Despite recent controversies, the UK national breast screening programme has been shown to significantly decrease mortality, offering an estimated 20% relative risk reduction to women who are screened every three years over a 20 year period and thus saving one breast cancer death for every 250 women invited for screening [1]. This equates to an estimated 1300 deaths from breast cancer saved per year. Nearly 2.2 million women aged between 45 and 74 were screened in 2010-11, with on average, 4.1% of women recalled for assessment [2]. For those women undergoing their first screening examination (the prevalent screen), the recall rate was 7.9% with 1.8 benign biopsies per 1000 women and 5.0 invasive cancers per 1000 women. The published standards are <10%, <=3.6 and >=2.7 respectively. For women undergoing a subsequent (incident) screen, the recall rate was 3.1% and the benign biopsy and invasive cancer rates were 0.5 and 6.1 respectively. Published standards are <7%, <2.0 and >=1.6 respectively.

Nationally, between 2008-9 and 2010-11 recall rates for age 45-74 (prevalent screen) fell from 8.7% to 7.9%, whilst the benign biopsy rate dropped from 2.0 to 1.8 per 1000 and invasive cancer rate from 5.3 to 5.0 [2,3]. For incident screens, the recall rate fell from 3.4% to 3.1% with the benign biopsy rate dropping from 1.0 to 0.5 and the invasive cancer rate from 6.2 to 6.1. During the earlier period almost all screening was undertaken using film-screen systems, although by July 2011 85% of screening units had at least one Full Field Digital Mammography (FFDM) system [2].

Rates vary across the country, and in the region studied in this paper, in the 50-70 age group at the 2010-11 prevalent screen the recall rate was 8.5%, benign biopsies were carried out in 1.9 per 1000 women screened and 5.2 cancers were detected for every 1000 women screened. For incident round screening these figures were 3.3%, 0.05 and 6.4 respectively [2].

1.2 The Introduction of Full Field Digital Mammography

FFDM has several inherent practical advantages over screen film (analogue) mammography including the possibility of electronic archiving and image transfer between sites, on-screen image manipulation, reduction in storage requirements and reduction in dose [4,5]. In terms of diagnostic performance, initial studies in the U.S.A. found that FFDM was at least as good at detecting cancer in women with an abnormal analogue screening mammogram [6]. The American College of Radiology Imaging Network subsequently set up the Digital Mammographic Imaging Screening Trial (DMIST) in which each woman received both forms of mammogram [7]. The results showed for the screening population as a whole, screen film mammography (SFM) and FFDM had very similar screening accuracy and no significant difference in recall rate (8.4% for both). FDDM was however shown to be more accurate for three population subgroups: those under 50, those with very dense breasts and those who are pre or peri-menopausal. Several further studies have since been conducted, and the consensus is that FFDM is at least as good as, if not better than analogue mammography for cancer detection [8].

Recalls due to poor quality images or technical problems are widely reported as being lower in FFDM since the mammograms are available for review by the radiographer at the time of imaging [9, 10]. Despite this, out of ten studies reviewed by Skaane in 2009, in two the overall recall rate was found to be lower with FFDM, in five higher and in three there was no significant difference [8]. More recent studies suggest that the introduction of FFDM does lead to increased recall rates. In Europe, a retrospective analysis of the effects of introducing FFDM showed a significant increase in both cancer detection and recall rates the year after FFDM was introduced. Subsequently recall rates decreased, but remained higher than the original pre-FFDM levels [11]. The authors postulated that the use of analogue mammograms for reference may have contributed to the increase in recall rates. In 2011, a U.S. study demonstrated an increase in recall rate with the introduction of FFDM, and the rate continued to increase over the next two years [12]. The cancer detection rate also increased for the first two years of digital screening, but then dropped to a level that was not significantly greater than the previous screen film mammography level. The authors suggested that the increase was due to readers learning how to interpret the digital images.

2   Aims

The aims of this research were to determine whether digital and film-screen mammography yielded significantly different recall rates, biopsy/cytology referral rates and cancer detection rates in a large screening programme making the transition from analogue to digital mammography, and to determine whether any changes persisted over time.

3   Method

We retrospectively compiled breast screening data gathered from January 2010 to March 2012 by the Nightingale Breast Centre, which is responsible for National Health Service breast cancer screening and diagnosis for over 50,000 women per year in Greater Manchester, UK. During this period the screening service made the transition from screen film mammography to FFDM. Data were compiled from standardised statistical reports produced to enable ongoing assessment of performance by the Department of Health. Data were gathered from four Primary Care Trusts (PCTs) covered by the screening programme, all of which converted to digital mammography between March and July 2010.

The clinical outcomes measured were recall rate, biopsy referral rate and cancer detection rate. Recall rate is generally expressed as a percentage of the total number of women screened. The cancer detection rate is the number of cancers detected per 1000 women screened and the biopsy/cytology referral rate is expressed as a percentage.

The data were grouped into monthly intervals, covering the periods prior to, during and after the conversion to FFDM. All women who underwent breast screening during the 26 months from January 2010 to March 2012 were included in the study: incident and prevalent; all ages and all referral pathways. For each PCT, data from the month of transition from SFM to FFDM contains a mixture of both forms of mammogram and was excluded from analyses.

The FFDM images were all taken using GE Senographe Essential digital mammography equipment, from both static sites and mobile screening units. Reader experience varied, but all readers had at least four years experience reading mammograms.

Since we were not able to gather retrospective data regarding the use of prior mammograms, in order to assess whether the interpretation of priors influenced the outcome measures, the analysis was performed separately for prevalent screens where no prior mammograms exist for comparison, and for incident screens.

3.1   Analysis

Overall recall rates and core biopsy/cytology referral rates were recorded. Direct comparisons of aggregate outcome measures between analogue and digital mammography were performed using chi-squared tests. Analogue rates were calculated from data pertaining to the months preceding digital mammography and digital rates were calculated using data after the transition.

Data starting immediately after the transition to digital mammography was aggregated for the 4 PCTs using months post conversion as a measure of time. Least squares regression lines were plotted and Pearson's correlation coefficient calculated for each outcome measure. The final 2 months were excluded from the regression analysis as only 2 of the 4 PCTs had data covering this length of time post conversion to digital mammography.

4   Results

Recall rate results are presented in Table 1. Whilst there was a significant difference (p<0.001) in recall rates overall and for incident screens, with a higher proportion recalled from digital screening, the difference between recall rates for prevalent screens was not significant. For biopsy/cytology referral rates (Table 2), the difference was statistically significant overall (p=0.01), with a higher percentage of biopsies with FFDM. There was a significant increase in incident screening (p<0.001), but not in prevalent screening. Cancer detection rates for the two modalities are shown in Table 3. There were no significant differences between modalities.

Table 1. Recall rates for digital and analogue mammography. * denotes a statistically significant difference between the two modalities.

	Total		Prevalent		Incident	
	Analogue	Digital	Analogue	Digital	Analogue	Digital
Number Recalled	328	2505	162	976	166	1529
Number Screened	9155	53444	1898	10462	7257	42982
% Recall Rate	3.58%*	4.69%*	8.54%	9.33%	2.29%*	3.56%*

Table 2. Biopsy/cytology referral rates for digital and analogue mammography. * denotes a statistically significant difference between the two modalities.

	Total		Prevalent		Incident	
	Analogue	Digital	Analogue	Digital	Analogue	Digital
Number Biopsy/Cytology	136	1005	68	382	68	623
Number Screened	9155	53444	1898	10462	7257	42982
Biopsy/Cytology Rate (%)	1.49%*	1.88%*	3.58%	3.65%	0.94%*	1.45%*

Table 3. Cancer detection rates for digital and analogue mammography

	Total		Prevalent		Incident	
	Analogue	Digital	Analogue	Digital	Analogue	Digital
Cancers Detected	56	358	15	64	41	294
Number Screened	9155	53444	1898	10462	7257	42982
Cancer Detection Rate/1000	6.15	6.74	7.97	6.16	5.68	6.89

Figure 1 shows the recall rate plotted as a function of time since conversion to digital mammography. The recall rate is positively correlated with months post conversion: for total screens (r=0.71, p<0.001). The biopsy/cytology referral rates were positively but only moderately correlated with months post conversion to digital mammography for total screens (r=0.52, p=0.011); this is illustrated in figure 2. There was a moderate negative correlation between cancer detection and time post digital conversion for total screens (r=-0.567, p=0.05). This was evident in the incident screens (r=-0.643, p=0.001); there was no statistically significant correlation for the prevalent screens.

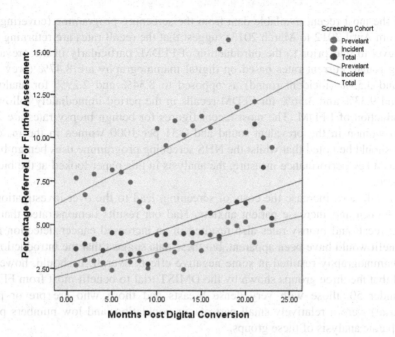

Fig. 1. Recall rates post conversion from analogue to digital mammography

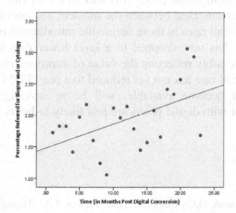

Fig. 2. Biopsy referral rates post conversion from analogue to digital mammography

5   Discussion

Our results indicate that the introduction of FFDM resulted in an increase in recall and biopsy/cytology referral rates (statistically significant in incident round screening) but with no corresponding increase in cancer detection. The biopsy rate and recall rate continued to increase for the two years after conversion to digital mammography, however the most recent available data from the screening programme (covering the period from April 2012 to March 2013) suggest that the recall rates are returning to a similar level to that prior to the introduction of FFDM, particularly in the prevalent screening round: current rates based on digital mammography are 8.47% (prevalent round) and 3.53% (incident round) as opposed to 8.54% and 2.29% for analogue recalls and 9.33% and 3.56% for FFDM recalls in the period immediately following the introduction of FFDM. The most recent figures for benign biopsy rates are 2.06 per 1000 women in the prevalent round and 0.31 per 1000 women in the incident round. It should be noted that whilst the NHS screening programme uses benign biopsy rates as a key performance measure, the analysis in this paper looked at the biopsy referral rate.

High recall rates increase the costs of screening, lead to the over-investigation of healthy women and increase patient anxiety. Had our results demonstrated that the increased recall and biopsy rates also resulted in an increased cancer detection rate, some benefit would have been apparent, but these data suggest that the introduction of digital mammography resulted in some negative effects overall. It should, however, be noted that the three groups shown by the DMIST trial to benefit most from FFDM (those under 50, those with very dense breasts and those who are pre or peri-menopausal) were a relatively small part of our population, and low numbers precluded separate analysis of these groups.

It is of interest that the effects were most apparent in the incident group, where comparison with previous mammograms involved the use of film priors. The current recall rate for the incident round (3.53%) is still based on film priors, so this could explain the differences observed between the incident and prevalent rounds in terms of achieving similar recall rates to those before the introduction of FFDM. The prevalent round recall rate has now dropped to a level lower than that observed during analogue screening, possibly reflecting the value of improved image quality, whereas the incident round recall rate has not yet reduced to a pre-FFDM level. Our next step, when sufficient data become available, will be to investigate whether women screened using FFDM with digital priors are less likely to be recalled than those with film priors.

References

1. Marmot, M.G., Altman, D.G., Cameron, D.A., Dewar, J.A., Thompson, S.G., Wilcox, M.: The Independent UK Panel on Breast Cancer Screening. The benefits and harms of breast cancer screening: an independent review. A report jointly commissioned by Cancer Research UK and the Department of Health (England), October 2012. British Journal of Cancer 108, 2205–2240 (2013), doi:10.1038/bjc.2013.177
2. The National Health Service Breast Screening Programme Annual Review 2012 (2012), http://www.cancerscreening.nhs.uk/breastscreen/publications/nhsbsp-annualreview2012.pdf, ISBN: 978-1-84463-093-6
3. The National Health Service Breast Screening Programme Annual Review 2010 (2010), http://www.cancerscreening.nhs.uk/breastscreen/publications/nhsbsp-annualreview2010.pdf, ISBN: 978-1-84463-075-2

4. Hauge, I.H.R., Pedersen, K., Sanderud, A., et al.: Patient Doses From Screen Film and Full Field Digital Mammography in a Population Based Screening Programme. Radiation Protection Dosimetry 148(1), 65–73 (2012)
5. Hendrick, R.E.: Comparison of Acquisition Parameters and Breast Dose in Digital Mammography and Screen Film Mammography in the American College of Radiology Imaging Network Digital Mammographic Imaging Screening Trial. Am. J. Roentgenol. 194(2), 362–369 (2010)
6. Pisano, E.D., Yaffe, M.J., Hemminger, B.M., Edward Hendrick, R., Niklason, L.T., Maidment, A.D.A., Kimme-Smith, C.M., Feig, S.A., Sickles, E.A., Patricia Braeuning, M.: Current status of full-field digital mammography. Academic Radiology 7(4), 266–280 (2000)
7. Pisano, E.D., Gatsonis, C., Hendrick, E., Yaffe, M., Baum, J.K., Acharyya, S., Conant, E.F., Fajardo, L.L., Bassett, L., D'Orsi, C., Jong, R., Rebner, M.: Digital Mammographic Imaging Screening Trial (DMIST) Investigators Group 2005 Diagnostic Performance of Digital versus Film Mammography for Breast-Cancer Screening. N. Engl. J. Med. 353, 1773–1783 (2005), doi: 10.1056/NEJMoa052911
8. Skaane, P.: Studies comparing screen film mammography and full field digital mammography in breast cancer screening: updated review. Acta Radiol. 50(1), 3–14 (2009)
9. Del Turco, M.R., Mantellini, P., Ciatto, S., Bonardi, R., Martinelli, F., Lazzari, B., et al.: Full-field digital versus screen-film mammography: comparative accuracy in concurrent screening cohorts. Am. J. Roentgenol. 189, 860–866 (2007)
10. Vigeland, E., Klaasen, H., Klingen, T.A., Hofvind, S., Skaane, P.: Full field digital mammography compared with screen film mammography in the prevalent round of a population based screening program: the Vestfold County study. Eur. Radiol. 18, 183–191 (2008)
11. Vernacchia, F.S., Pena, Z.G.: Digital mammography: its impact on recall rates and cancer detection rates in a small community based radiology practice. AJR Am. J. Roentgenol. 193(2), 582–585 (2009)
12. Glynn, C., Farria, D., Monsees, B., et al.: Effect of transition to digital mammography on clinical outcomes. Radiology 260, 664–670 (2011)

Fully Automated Nipple Detection in 3D Breast Ultrasound Images

Lei Wang[1], Tobias Böhler[1], Fabian Zöhrer[1], Joachim Georgii[1], Claudia Rauh[2],
Peter A. Fasching[2], Barbara Brehm[3], Rüdiger Schulz-Wendtland[3],
Matthias W. Beckmann[2], Michael Uder[3], and Horst K. Hahn[1]

[1] Fraunhofer MEVIS - Institute for Medical Image Computing, Bremen, Germany
[2] Frauenklinik des Universitätsklinikums Erlangen, Germany
[3] Institut für Diagnostische Radiologie des Universitätsklinikums Erlangen, Germany

Abstract. Nipple position provides useful diagnostic informations in
reading automated 3D breast ultrasound (ABUS) images. The identification of nipples is required to localize and determine the quadrants
of breast lesions. Additionally, the nipple position serves as an effective landmark to register an ABUS image to other imaging modalities,
such as digital mammography, breast magnet resonance imaging (MRI),
or tomosynthesis. Nevertheless, the presence of speckle noise induced
by interference waves and variant imaging directions in ultrasonography poses challenges to the task. In this work, we propose a fast and
automated algorithm to detect nipples in 3D breast ultrasound images.
The method fully takes advantages of the consistent characteristics of
ultrasonographic signals observed at nipples and employs a multi-scale
Laplacian-based blob detector to eventually identify nipple positions.
The accuracy of the proposed method was tested on 113 ABUS images,
resulting in a distance error of 6.6 ± 8.9 mm (*mean ± std*).

1 Introduction

In complement to mammography, automated 3D breast ultrasound (ABUS)
emerges as an important imaging modality applied in breast cancer, especially
on patients with dense breasts where the sensitivity of mammography is poor.
Recent studies reported that supplemental ABUS increases detection rate of
small and mammography occult breast cancers [1,2]. Hence, the interpretation of
ABUS data has gained significant interests in computer-aided diagnosis (CAD) of
breast cancer [3,4,7]. In a CAD system, nipple position is an important reference
marker which allows for localizing the quadrants of breast lesions. Furthermore,
given data acquired in other imaging modalities, such as mammography, MRI
or tomosynthesis, registering images across multiple modalities requires nipple
positions as effective reference landmarks to improve registration accuracy. In
this work, a fast and automated method that focuses on precise detection of
nipple positions in ABUS is implemented and tested.

H. Fujita, T. Hara, and C. Muramatsu (Eds.): IWDM 2014, LNCS 8539, pp. 64–71, 2014.

2   Materials and Methods

2.1   Dataset

We collected 113 ABUS image sequences acquired by Siemens S2000 ABVS systems as part of the iMODE-B (imaging and molecular detection for breast cancers) study at the University Breast Center Franconia, University Hospital Erlangen, Germany. The study was approved by the Ethics Committee of the Medical Faculty, Friedrich-Alexander University Erlangen Nuremberg and all patients gave written informed consent. Breasts were scanned in five possible imaging views: anterior-posterior (AP), medial (MED), lateral (LAT), superior (SUP) and inferior (INF) (as shown in Fig. 1). Acquisitions in different views involve different compressions of breasts, which leads to variant imaging characteristics of nipples. The presence of nipples varies according to different acquisition views. The locations of nipples were clearly identified in AP views and distributed in peripheral regions in other views. For several extreme cases where the nipples were pushed to the image borders, a portion of the nipples were still visible. The image resolution of the collected ABUS volumes is $719 \times 516 \times 318$, associated with in-plane voxel spacing of 0.2×0.07 mm and slice thickness of 0.525 mm. To validate the performance of our method, an experienced radiologist annotated all images by pinpointing the tip points of nipples (a tip point is the most anterior point of a nipple in coronal planes), serving as the ground truth.

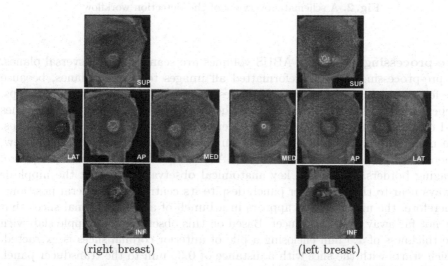

(right breast)   (left breast)

Fig. 1. ABUS scans for the right and left breasts of a patient, illustrating nipple positions in different imaging views: AP, MED, LAT, SUP and INF

2.2 Methods

The method is comprised of several pre-processing steps to find the region of interest (ROI) of the nipple and build a binary mask that excludes background. Then, a multi-scale blob detector is employed to detect the nipple tip point. A schematic overview of the entire detection workflow is illustrated in Fig. 2.

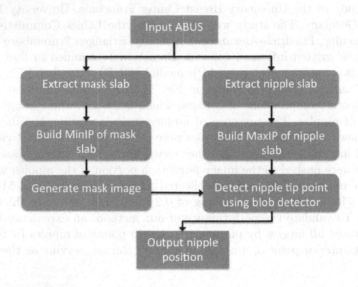

Fig. 2. A schematic overview of the detection workflow

Pre-processing. Normally, ABUS volumes are scanned in transversal planes. In pre-processing step, we reformatted all images to coronal planes, because the features extracted from coronal planes will be analyzed in subsequent steps. Depending on different scanning views, the ultrasound transducer panel touches and compresses the target breast in different ways. Usually, in coronal planes, the nipple is imaged in the center of an ABUS volume scanned in AP view, whereas other views, such as MED or LAT, can push the nipple to peripheral imaging borders. One of the key anatomical observations is that the nipple is always near to the transducer panel, despite its centric or peripheral positions. Therefore, the nipple always appears in a bunch of anterior coronal slices that are not far away from transducer. Based on this observation, a nipple slab with the thickness of 1.5 mm enclosing a pile of anterior coronal slices is extracted, which starts with the slice with a distance of 0.35 mm to the transducer panel. The nipple slab defines a ROI, where subsequent nipple detection algorithms are applied to localize nipple tip points. In addition, to get rid of background, another mask slab with the same thickness of 1.5 mm following the nipple slab is extracted (see Fig. 3).

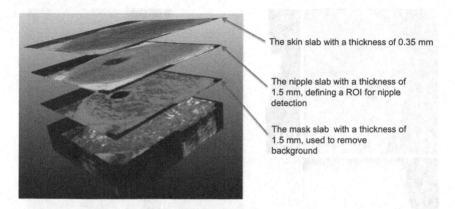

The skin slab with a thickness of 0.35 mm

The nipple slab with a thickness of 1.5 mm, defining a ROI for nipple detection

The mask slab with a thickness of 1.5 mm, used to remove background

Fig. 3. 3D visualization of the extracted nipple slab (yellow) and mask slab (green)

Then, the minimum intensity projection (MinIP) image over all slices of the mask slab is calculated, resulting in a 2D projected image where the intensities of background areas are almost zero (Fig. 4(1)). By a simple thresholding process, a binary mask containing the pixels with intensities larger than 1 is obtained. Followed by a morphological closing operation with a kernel size 5×5, possible holes and gaps of the binary mask are filled (Fig. 4(2)). Similarly, the maximum intensity projection (MaxIP) image of the nipple slab is computed, resulting in a 2D map, in which the nipple tip point will be searched for (Fig. 4(3)). To reduce computational expense, the MaxIP image of the nipple slab and the mask image are down-sampled to a lower in-plane resolution defined by a fixed scale factor: 0.125×0.125. To eliminate disturbing structures, the MaxIP image is further smoothed by a Gaussian kernel with $\sigma = 3$ (Fig. 4(4)).

Blob Detection. A key observation is that the nipple appears as a 2D dark blob structure in the MaxIP image of the nipple slab, which can be enhanced by a commonly used blob descriptor: Laplacian of Gaussian filter (LoG) [5]. Given a MaxIP image $I(x,y)$ and a Gaussian kernel at scale σ: $g(x,y,\sigma)$, the MaxIP image convolved with multiple Gaussian kernels with variant sizes leads to a scale-space representation: $L(x,y,\sigma) = I(x,y) \star g(x,y,\sigma)$ [6]. The Laplacian operator $\nabla^2 L = L_{xx} + L_{yy}$ is then calculated at each scale σ, which produces strong negative response in dark blob regions (Fig. 4(5)). We adopted a multi-scale LoG filter with variant σ ranging from 1.5 to 15 mm with a step size of 1.5 mm. The optimal scale that delivers the global minimal response is selected, and the corresponding 2D coordinate in the MaxIP image is recorded as the nipple position in X and Y dimensions. To fetch the Z dimension, we projected the 2D point back to the middle slice of the nipple slab, which reconstructs the 3D position of the nipple (Fig. 4(6)).

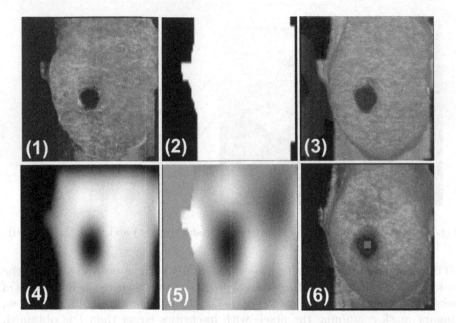

Fig. 4. workflow of blob structure detection: (1) MinIP image of the mask slab; (2) generated binary mask; (3) MaxIP image of the nipple slab; (4) down-sampled and smoothed MaxIP image; (5) response of LoG filter at scale $\sigma = 6$; (6) extracted global minima and detected nipple position (red).

3   Evaluations and Results

We ran the algorithm on 113 ABUS volumes in the testing data set. The average computation time per ABUS volume was 0.6 seconds on a machine with a 3.7GHz CPU. The detection accuracy was quantitatively measured by calculating the root-mean-square distance in mm (RMSD) between detected nipple positions and annotated ground truth in 3D. Statistical analysis of the distance error were conducted, obtaining a result of 6.6 ± 8.9 mm ($mean\pm std$). Figure 5 demonstrates the histogram analysis of RMSD, showing the majority of distance deviation falls in the interval of $(0, 15)$ mm. Moreover, the distribution of detection rates against variant tolerant thresholds of distance errors is depicted in Fig. 5. It is noticed that nearly half of the test images achieved a distance error less than 4 mm, and more specifically when setting tolerance as 8 mm, where is the average size of the nipples in our database, nearly 78% of test images were correctly detected. Several successfully detected cases with various nipple positions are demonstrated in Fig. 6.

Nevertheless, one can easily notice that there were two outliers with extreme large errors observed in the diagram of distance histogram (see again Fig. 5).

By investigating these two cases, we find that the method might fail when nipples were pushed to image borders during acquisition and imaged partially in extracted nipple slabs (see Fig. 7 (a)). Besides, the LoG filter was proved to perform stably in detecting global minimal response that is supposed to associate with the target nipple position. However, when the breast mask extracted from mask slab is not sufficiently accurate, or a lesion that mimics the features of the nipple appears in the nipple slab, the LoG filter might be attracted by the spurious structure and recognizes it as the nipple position (see Fig. 7(b)).

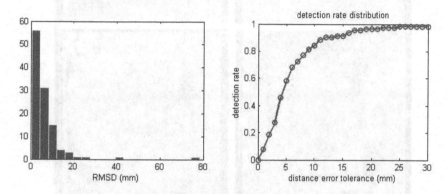

Fig. 5. Histogram analysis of RMSD (left). Detection rates against variant tolerant distance errors (right).

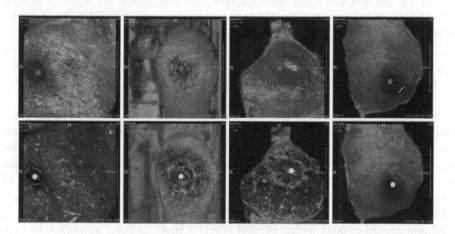

Fig. 6. Four successful cases overlaid with the detected nipples (red) and the annotated markers (yellow); each column represents one case

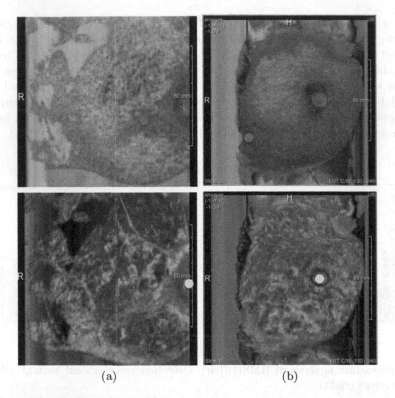

(a)   (b)

Fig. 7. Two failed cases overlaid with the detected nipples (red) and reference markers (yellow): (a) the first failed case with RMSD= 43.1 mm, where the nipple is imaged partially and very close to borders; (b) the second failed cases with RMSD= 78.4 mm, where the minimal detected by LoG filter does not correspond to the nipple

4   Conclusion and Discussions

In this work, we presented a fast and automated method to detect nipple positions in ABUS scans. The method fully takes advantages of anatomical and ultrasonographic properties of nipples in coronal planes. A multi-scale blob detector based on Laplacian filters permits the detection of nipples with variant sizes and signal strengths. A test on 113 ABUS volumes shows its capability of precisely detecting nipples.

The proposed method assumes that nipple is imaged near to the transducer panel and should appear within several anterior slices in coronal planes. In case the nipple is not sufficiently scanned in the field of view, or the structures, such as lesions, which mimic the properties of nipples, exist in the nipple detection slab, the LoG filter might be attracted to these spurious regions and deliver false results. Normally, for these cases, the second minimal points are associated with the nipples. Therefore, a natural improvement is to take more candidate minimal points into account instead of always choosing the first one. By analyzing features of these candidates and selecting the one with the best fitting with the target nipple, the detection rate could be further improved.

Acknowledgments. This work was supported by the German Federal Ministry of Education and Research (BMBF), project grant No. 13EX1012D. The research leading to these results has received co-funding from the European Unions Seventh Framework Programme FP7 under grant agreement No. 306088.

References

1. Giuliano, V., Giuliano, C.: Improved breast cancer detection in asymptomatic women using 3D-automated breast ultrasound in mammographically dense breasts. Clinical Imaging, 480–486 (2013)
2. Nothacker, M., Duda, V., Hahn, M., Warm, M., Degenhardt, F., Madjar, H., Albert, U.-S.: Early detection of breast cancer: benefits and risks of supplemental breast ultrasound in asymptomatic women with mammographically dense breast tissue. A systematic review. BMC Cancer 9, 335 (2013)
3. Tan, T., Platel, B., Mus, R., Tabar, L., Mann, R.M., Karssemeijer, N.: Computer-aided detection of cancer in automated 3-D breast ultrasound. IEEE Transactions on Medical Imaging 32(9), 1698–1706 (2013)
4. Tan, T., Platel, B., Twellmann, T., van Schie, G., Mus, R., Grivegnee, A., Mann, R.M., Karssemeijer, N.: Evaluation of the Effect of Computer-Aided Classification of Benign and Malignant Lesions on Reader Performance in Automated Three-dimensional Breast Ultrasound. Academic Radiology 20, 1381–1388 (2013)
5. Huertas, A., Medioni, G.: Detection of intensity changes with sub pixel accuracy using Laplacian-Gaussian masks. IEEE Trans. on Pattern Analysis and Machine Intelligence 8, 651–664 (1986)
6. Lindeberg, T.: Feature detection with automatic scale selection. International Journal of Computer Vision 30(2), 77–116 (1998)
7. Wang, L., Zoehrer, F., Friman, O., Hahn, H.K.: A fully automatic method for nipple detection in 3D breast ultrasound images. Computer Assisted Radiology and Surgery 6(suppl. 1), 191–192 (2011)

Breast Imaging with 3D Ultrasound Computer Tomography: Results of a First In-vivo Study in Comparison to MRI Images

Torsten Hopp[1], Lukas Šroba[2], Michael Zapf[1], Robin Dapp[1], Ernst Kretzek[1], Hartmut Gemmeke[1], and Nicole V. Ruiter[1]

[1] Karlsruhe Institute of Technology
Institute for Data Processing and Electronics
torsten.hopp@kit.edu
http://www.ipe.kit.edu
[2] Slovak University of Technology
Institute of Electrical Engineering

Abstract. Ultrasound Computer Tomography (USCT) is a promising modality for breast imaging. We developed and tested the first full 3D USCT system aimed at in-vivo imaging. It is based on approx. 2000 ultrasound transducers surrounding the breast within a water bath. From the acquired signal data, reflectivity, attenuation and sound speed images are reconstructed. In a first in-vivo study we imaged ten patients and compared them to MRI images. To overcome the considerably different breast positioning in both imaging methods, an image registration and image fusion based on biomechanical modeling of the buoyancy effect and surface-based refinement was applied. The resulting images are promising: compared with the MRI ground truth, similar tissue structures can be identified. While reflection images seem to image even small structures, sound speed imaging seems to be the best modality for detecting cancer. The registration of both imaging methods allows browsing the volume images side by side and enables recognition of correlating tissue structures. The first in-vivo study was successfully completed and encourages for a second in-vivo study with a considerably larger number of patients, which is currently ongoing.

Keywords: Ultrasound Computer Tomography, 3D Breast Imaging, Multimodal Image Registration.

1 Introduction

Ultrasound Computer Tomography (USCT) is a promising modality for breast imaging. Although the principle is known since the 1970s [1], increasing computational power just recently made it possible to develop systems capable of in-vivo imaging. First USCT systems are currently evaluated in first clinical trials [2,3]. In contrast to slice-acquiring 2D systems [3,4], we have developed the first full 3D USCT system aimed at in-vivo imaging (Fig. 1) [5,6]. USCT allows simultaneous acquisition of reflection, attenuation and sound speed images,

H. Fujita, T. Hara, and C. Muramatsu (Eds.): IWDM 2014, LNCS 8539, pp. 72–79, 2014.

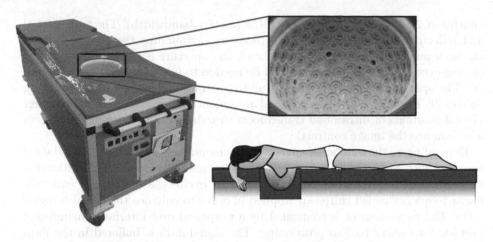

Fig. 1. Left: 3D USCT device. Top right: Detailed view of the transducer aperture. Bottom right: Illustration of the patient positioning during image acquisition.

and offers high image quality compared to conventional ultrasound. Due to the defined patient positioning, images are reproducible. Our 3D USCT overcomes the large slice thickness respectively anisotropic resolution of 2D systems and promises a considerably faster data acquisition since the raw data for a 3D image volume is acquired in parallel.

Recently we conducted a first in-vivo study with ten patients at the University Hospital of Jena, Germany [7]. For comparison MRI images of the same patients were acquired. In this paper we briefly describe the system setup, imaging principle and image reconstruction methods before presenting clinical results of our first pilot in-vivo study. For evaluation of the diagnostic value, a visual comparison with MRI images was carried out. Due to the different imaging conditions (e.g. buoyancy in USCT) this turned out to be challenging. To support the comparison, an image registration respectively image fusion was developed and applied to overcome the considerably different breast positioning. The focus of this work is to carry out a first visual comparison of USCT images and MRI images using the proposed image registration method.

2 Methods

2.1 Data Acquisition and Image Reconstruction

The KIT 3D USCT has a semi-ellipsoidal aperture filled with water, which acts as coupling medium. The aperture has an inner diameter of 26 cm and a height of 18 cm. It is equipped with 628 ultrasound emitters and 1413 receivers (Fig. 1). The aperture and data acquisition hardware as well as the electric and water supplies are integrated into a patient bed, on which the patient lies prone with one breast freely immersed into the aperture. The data acquisition is carried out by sequentially sending out an approx. spherical wave front from a single emitter at 2.5 MHz center frequency (50% relative bandwidth). The transmitted and reflected wave is recorded by all receivers surrounding the breast. Despite the high number of emitters and receivers, the aperture is sparse as two orders of magnitude more transmitters would be needed to fulfill the sampling theorem [8]. The sparsity results in artifacts due to grating lobe effects in the resulting images [9]. Rotational and translational movement of the aperture creates further virtual positions of ultrasound transducers to reduce the sparsity of the system and enhance the image contrast.

Depending on the number of aperture movements, up to 80 GB of signal data is acquired with an FPGA-based system using 480 parallel channels for digitization at 12 Bit and 20 MHz sampling frequency. To excite the ultrasound emitters, linear frequency coded chirps are applied in order to enhance the signal-to-noise ratio. The measurement is controlled by a graphical user interface, including a preview for correct patient positioning. The signal data is buffered in the data acquisition system and afterwards transferred to a image reconstruction server.

From the acquired signal data, three types of images can be reconstructed: reflection images displaying the morphology of the breast as well as attenuation and sound speed images, which are expected to quantitatively characterize different types of tissue [10]. The applied reconstruction algorithm for reflectivity imaging is a 3D synthetic aperture focusing technique (SAFT) [11]. It calculates at each image voxel the mean of all reflections which might originate from its spatial position. Before the SAFT reconstruction is applied, the acquired signal data is pre-processed using a matched filter, an envelope transformation followed by a maximum detection and a convolution with an optimal pulse [12]. The reflection imaging reconstruction runs on a GPU cluster to reduce the computation time considerably [13].

Attenuation and sound speed imaging uses a ray-based approach for reconstruction. The transmission signals are detected and the relative signal energy resp. time-of-flight are applied in an algebraic reconstruction technique. Compressive sampling, i.e. a 3D adaption of TVAL3 using total variation minimization is employed for optimization [14].

After performing the reconstruction of reflection, sound speed and attenuation images, the water background is removed for improved visualization and further processing using a segmentation method applied to the reflection image. The method is based on detecting the breast boundary in a subset of coronal slices using a Canny edge detection algorithm followed by a surface fitting to inter- resp. extrapolate the 3D breast surface [15].

2.2 Image Registration and Image Fusion

For comparison of the reconstructed USCT images to an established modality, MRI images of all patients included in the first in-vivo study were acquired at the same day. In MRI the breast is positioned pendulous in prone position within a dedicated breast coil. However due to buoyancy in USCT and deformations of breast when contacting the MRI coil, direct voxel comparison is not possible. Due to immersing the breast into the water bath, it buoys up resulting in e.g.

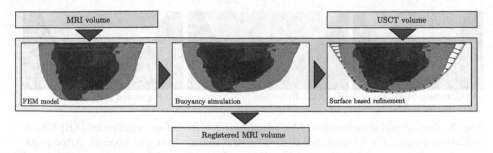

Fig. 2. Illustration of the registration processing steps. The images show semi-transparent renderings of the FEM model, which is built based on the segmented MRI volume representing fat (blue) and glandular tissue (red/purple). After the buoyancy simulation is applied, the surface of the deformed FEM model is compared to the surface of the USCT volume (green) and displacement vectors are defined. For better visualization this process is illustrated in 2D.

a shortening of approx. 15% in anteroposterior direction while it is broadened at the chest wall. Complex interactions within the breast result in nonlinear deformations of tissue structures.

We developed and applied an image registration to minimize the differences of the deformation state. The registration is based on biomechanical modeling of the breast using the MRI volume. The biomechanical model originates from our earlier work; for more details refer to [16]. To build up the model, the MRI is segmented into background, fat and glandular tissue using a combination of a Level-Set-Evolution algorithm based on [17] and Fuzzy-C-Means clustering. To simulate the effect of buoyancy, a gravity load is applied in anteroposterior direction using a Finite Element simulation (Fig. 2). Nodes at the back of the breast model are fixated to model the connection of the breast at the chest wall. The mechanical parameters are optimized based on surface agreement of deformed MRI volume and USCT volume with an exhaustive search. Due to the complexity of the deformation, not all effects of the different breast deformation states can be modeled with the buoyancy simulation since e.g. manual adjustments of the breast positioning as well as the contact interaction of the breast with the MRI coil are unknown. A surface-based refinement simulation is carried out afterwards to compensate for these effects and obtain overlapping breast boundaries. In this simulation displacement vectors between the outcome of the buoyancy simulation and the USCT volume are defined based on the surface normals of the breast shape and a closest point assumption (Fig. 2, right). The finally registered MRI image is reconstructed by applying the computed deformation fields to the voxel images using a three-dimensional linear interpolation.

Diagnostic information of USCT may thereafter be superimposed on MRI images for evaluation of corresponding structures, i.e. an image fusion can be carried out. In this work we combine the quantitative sound speed values measured in USCT with the MRI images. The sound speed is color-coded and then semi-transparently rendered on top of the gray scale MRI images. Thresholds

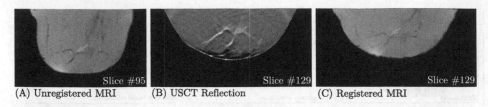

(A) Unregistered MRI   (B) USCT Reflection   (C) Registered MRI

Fig. 3. Transversal slice image of (A) T1 weighted MRI before registration, (B) USCT reflection image, (C) T1 weighted MRI after the registration was applied. After registration, the corresponding tissue structures are depicted at the same slice position and the breast shape in the MRI image equals the breast shape in the USCT image. Note the different slice position in the unregistered MRI image, which necessitates individual browsing of the image stack.

on the sound speed overlay can be applied to highlight only tissue with a suspiciously high sound speed.

3 Results

The first in-vivo study was carried out successfully with ten patients (mean age: 55.6 years $\pm$ 13.5 years, breast sizes: B-, C-, D-cup). The study was aimed on testing the image acquisition and reconstruction methods in a clinical setup. For most patients, the breast diagnosed with lesions was imaged with ten aperture positions. The contra-lateral breast was imaged with four aperture positions. In average, the image acquisition took 7 min. 30 sec. using ten aperture positions resp. 3 min. using four aperture positions, which is already in a clinically applicable range.

Reflection volumes were reconstructed with a main lobe width of the optimal pulse of $2\,\mu s$ which corresponds to a Full Width Half Maximum (FWHM) of the point spread function of approx. $1.5\,mm$. The voxel size was set to isotropic $0.7\,mm$ to fulfill the sampling theorem and approximately match the in-plane resolution of the MRI images (voxel size $(0.9\,mm)^2$, spacing between slices: $3.0\,mm$). Transmission volumes, i.e. sound speed and attenuation volumes were reconstructed with an isotropic voxel size of $2.7\,mm$.

We found out that patient movement seems to be a minor problem. No definite movements between reconstructions of the single aperture positions could be detected. Furthermore breathing motion seems to have no effect on the breast. This might be due to the patient position on the USCT device (Fig. 1) and the water bath, which damps breast movements.

After reconstructing all USCT modalities, the registration and image fusion were applied to achieve comparable images and visually evaluate the USCT images against the ground truth MRI (Fig. 3).

For two patients diagnosed with a large carcinoma, USCT was able to depict a region of high sound speed at the corresponding position. Fig. 4 shows a transversal slice image of a 64 year old patient with a large inflammatory carcinoma. The fused image (right) combines the gray scale MRI image with the

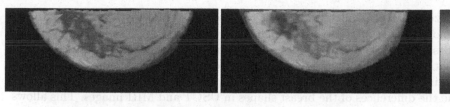

Sound speed in m/s 1600 — 1300

Fig. 4. Transversal slice image of a patient with an inflammatory carcinoma (green marker) in the registered T1 weighted MRI image (left) and fused image of the MRI with the USCT sound speed image (right). The sound speed information is color-coded and rendered semi-transparently on the MRI slice.

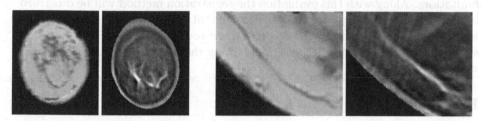

Fig. 5. Coronal slice image of a non-cancerous patient (left) and enlargement of a tiny tissue structure in a transversal slice (right). Each case depicts the registered T1 weighted MRI image and the corresponding USCT reflection image.

color coded USCT sound speed image. A high sound speed value (red) indicates the cancer at approx. the same position it is positioned in the registered MRI image.

The image registration allowed us to identify corresponding tissue structures in USCT and MRI images at the same slice position. Fig. 5. (left) depicts coronal slice images of a 39 year old patient. The predominant structures visible in the MRI image can as well be identified in the reflection USCT image. Fig. 5 (right) shows an enlarged detail of a transversal slice of the same patient, in which a tiny tissue structure can be identified in both images.

4 Discussion and Conclusion

We successfully developed and tested a 3D Ultrasound Computer Tomography system for dedicated breast imaging and achieved our initial design goals. The imaging process, i.e. data acquisition, data pre-processing and image reconstruction, could be successfully evaluated in a first in-vivo pilot study with ten patients. The feedback of patients indicates a convenient patient comfort. The resulting images are promising: compared to the MRI ground truth, similar tissue structures can be identified. While reflection images seem to image even small structures, sound speed imaging seems to be the best indicating modality for detecting carcinomas at the current status. A second in-vivo study with a considerably larger number of patients is currently launched to systematically analyze the applicability to different tumor entities and further investigate the diagnostic value of the three modalities provided by USCT. Furthermore the results of this first in-vivo study will lead to future optimization of the system.

Without registration it was difficult to recognize corresponding inner structures in both imaging methods. Hence we applied an image registration to overcome the differences of the breast shapes in USCT and MRI images. This allows browsing the volume images side by side and makes it easier to identify correlating structures. It is currently used for further investigation of the diagnostic value of USCT images. In our ongoing work we are focusing on an evaluation of the proposed image registration method in terms of registration accuracy and limitations. Along with this evaluation the registration method will be described in more detail. Challenges for the registration still remain in cases with large deformations of the breast in MRI due to narrow breast coils resulting e.g. in skin strains. Our future work will focus on adapting the registration to such cases as well.

References

1. Schomberg, H.: An improved approach to reconstructive ultrasound tomography. Journal of Physics D: Applied Physics 11, L181 (1978)
2. Duric, N., Littrup, P., Chandiwala-Mody, P., Li, C., Schmidt, S., Myc, L., Rama, O., Bey-Knight, L., Lupinacci, J., Ranger, B., Szczepanski, A., West, E.: In-vivo imaging results with ultrasound tomography: report on an ongoing study at the Karmanos Cancer Institute. In: Proceedings SPIE Medical Imaging (2010)
3. Wiskin, J., Borup, D., Johnson, S., Berggren, M., Robinson, D., Smith, J., Chen, J., Parisky, Y., Klock, J.: Inverse Scattering and Refraction Corrected Reflection for Breast Cancer Imaging. In: Proceedings SPIE Medical Imaging 2010 (2010)
4. Duric, N., Littrup, P., Poulo, L., Babkin, A., Pevzner, R., Holsapple, E., Rama, O., Glide, C.: Detection of Breast Cancer with Ultrasound Tomography: First Results with the Computerized Ultrasound Risk Evaluation C.U.R.E. Medical Physics 34(2), 773–785 (2007)
5. Gemmeke, H., Ruiter, N.: 3D ultrasound computer tomography for medical imaging. Nuclear Instruments and Methods in Physics Research Section A: Accelerators, Spectrometers, Detectors and Associated Equipment 580(2), 1057–1065 (2007)
6. Ruiter, N., Zapf, M., Dapp, R., Hopp, T., Gemmeke, H.: First in vivo results with 3D Ultrasound Computer Tomography. In: Proceedings IEEE Ultrasonics Symposium (2012)
7. Ruiter, N.V., Zapf, M., Dapp, R., Hopp, T., Kaiser, W., Gemmeke, H.: First Results of a Clinical Study with 3D Ultrasound Computer Tomography. In: Proceedings IEEE Ultrasonics Symposium (2013)
8. Ruiter, N., Zapf, M., Hopp, T., Gemmeke, H.: Experimental evaluation of noise generated by grating lobes for a sparse 3D ultrasound computer tomography system. In: Proceedings SPIE Medical Imaging (2013)
9. Ruiter, N., Dapp, R., Zapf, M., Gemmeke, H.: A new method for grating lobe reduction for 3D synthetic aperture imaging with ultrasound computer tomography. In: Proceedings IEEE Ultrasonics Symposiums (2010)
10. Greenleaf, J.F., Bahn, R.C.: Cinical Imaging with Transmissive Ultrasonic Computerized Tomography. IEEE Transactions on Biomedical Engineering 28(2), 177–185 (1981)

11. Norton, S., Linzer, M.: Ultrasonic reflectivity imaging in three dimensions: Reconstruction with a spherical array. Ultrasonic Imaging 1(3), 210–231 (1979)
12. Ruiter, N., Schwarzenberg, G., Zapf, M., Gemmeke, H.: Improvement of 3D ultrasound computer tomography images by signal pre-processing. In: Proceedings IEEE Ultrasonics Symposium (2008)
13. Kretzek, E., Zapf, M., Birk, M., Gemmeke, H., Ruiter, N.: GPU based acceleration of 3D USCT image reconstruction with efficient integration into MATLAB. In: Proceedings SPIE Medical Imaging (2013)
14. Birk, M., Dapp, R., Ruiter, N., Becker, J.: GPU-based iterative transmission reconstruction in 3D ultrasound computer tomography. Journal of Parallel and Distributed Computing 74(1), 1730–1743 (2014)
15. Hopp, T., Zapf, M., Ruiter, N.: Segmentation of 3D Ultrasound Computer Tomography Reflection Images using Edge Detection and Surface Fitting. In: Proceedings SPIE Medical Imaging (2014)
16. Hopp, T., Dietzel, M., Baltzer, P., Kreisel, P., Kaiser, W., Gemmeke, H., Ruiter, N.: Automatic multimodal 2D/3D breast image registration using biomechanical FEM models and intensity-based optimization. Medical Image Analysis 17(2), 209–218 (2013)
17. Li, C., Huang, R., Ding, Z., Gatenby, J., Metaxas, D., Gore, J.: A Level Set Method for Image Segmentation in the Presence of Intensity Inhomogeneities With Application to MRI. IEEE Transactions on Image Processing 20(7), 2007–2016 (2011)

Factors Affecting Agreement between Breast Density Assessment Using Volumetric Methods and Visual Analogue Scales

Lucy Beattie[1], Elaine Harkness[2,3,4,*], Megan Bydder[3], Jamie Sergeant[2,5,6], Anthony Maxwell[2,3,4,8], Nicky Barr[3], Ursula Beetles[3], Caroline Boggis[3], Sara Bundred[3], Soujanya Gadde[3], Emma Hurley[3], Anil Jain[3], Elizabeth Lord[3], Valerie Reece[3], Mary Wilson[3], Paula Stavrinos[3,4], D. Gareth Evans[3,4,7,8], Tony Howell[3,4,8], and Susan M. Astley[2,3,4,8]

[1] Manchester Medical School, University of Manchester, Stopford Building, Oxford Road, Manchester, M13 9PT
[2] Centre for Imaging Sciences, Institute of Population Health, University of Manchester, Stopford Building, Oxford Road, Manchester, M13 9PT
[3] Genesis Breast Cancer Prevention Centre, University Hospital of South Manchester NHS Trust, Wythenshawe, Manchester M23 9LT, UK
[4] The University of Manchester, Manchester Academic Health Science Centre, University Hospital of South Manchester NHS Foundation Trust, Wythenshawe, Manchester M23 9LT, UK
[5] Arthritis Research UK Centre for Epidemiology, Institute of Inflammation and Repair, Faculty of Medical and Human Sciences, Manchester Academic Health Science Centre, University of Manchester, Oxford Road, Manchester M13 9PT, UK
[6] NIHR Manchester Musculoskeletal Biomedical Research Unit, Central Manchester NHS Foundation Trust, Manchester Academic Health Science Centre
[7] Manchester Centre for Genomic Medicine, Central Manchester Foundation Trust, St. Mary's Hospital, Oxford Road, Manchester M13 9WL, UK
[8] Manchester Breast Centre, Manchester Cancer Research Centre, University of Manchester, Christie Hospital, Withington, Manchester, M20 4BX, UK
Elaine.F.Harkness@manchester.ac.uk

Abstract. Mammographic density in digital mammograms can be assessed visually or using automated volumetric methods; the aim in both cases is to identify women at greater risk of developing breast cancer, and those for whom mammography is less sensitive. Ideally all methods should identify the same women as having high density, but this is not the case in practice. 6422 women were ranked from the highest to lowest density by three methods: Quantra[TM], Volpara[TM] and visual assessment recorded on Visual Analogue Scales. For each pair of methods the 20 cases with the greatest agreement in rank were compared with the 20 with the least agreement. The presence of microcalcifications, skin folds, suboptimally positioned inframammary folds, and whether or not the nipple was in profile were found to affect agreement between methods ($p<0.05$). Careful positioning during mammographic imaging should reduce discrepancy, but a greater understanding of the relationship between methods is also required.

---

* Corresponding author.

H. Fujita, T. Hara, and C. Muramatsu (Eds.): IWDM 2014, LNCS 8539, pp. 80–87, 2014.
© Springer International Publishing Switzerland 2014

Keywords: Digital, mammogram, breast density, agreement, radiographic features.

1   Introduction

Breast density is usually assessed in X-ray mammograms. It varies greatly between women and is influenced by a number of factors including genetics, menopausal status, age and body mass index (BMI) [1]. There are several methods for measuring breast density including subjective area-based methods such as Visual Analogue Scales (VAS), and Breast Imaging and Reporting Data System (BI-RADS) categories for breast density [1,2]. More recently objective volumetric methods have been developed including Quantra™ [3] and Volpara™ [4]. The exact methods for quantifying density used by the manufacturers of Quantra™ and Volpara™ are commercially sensitive, but it is known that different calibration methods are employed, and that the contribution of the skin is disregarded when calculating density measures for Volpara™ therefore we expect the results for Volpara™ to be lower than those for Quantra™. The aim of this study was to identify differences in breast density assessments by Quantra™, Volpara™ and VAS, and to seek to identify patient characteristics, mammographic features and imaging parameters associated with these differences.

2   Methods

Women were recruited from the Predicting Risk of Cancer At Screening (PROCAS) study [3]. PROCAS includes approximately 50,000 women invited for routine breast screening who consented to participate and provided additional information on risk factors for breast cancer by completing a 2-page questionnaire at the time of screening. Women were included if they had density measurements from Quantra™ version 1.3 and Volpara™ version 1.4.0, and from VAS as assessed by two independent readers (VAS1 and VAS2) from a pool of consultant radiologists and advanced radiographic practitioners. VAS forms consisted of four 10cm lines (one for each mammographic view) marked 0% and 100% at each end. Readers place a vertical mark on the line to indicate their assessment of percentage density for each view. Women with missing data for BMI, or with BMI values out with the range 16 to 60 were excluded.

For each measurement method (Quantra™, Volpara™, VAS1, VAS2, VAS average (the average of VAS1 and VAS2)) densities were ranked in ascending order. The range of density measures is different for each method, therefore calculating the difference in breast density between methods would not necessarily identify the most discrepant cases. On the other hand, discrepancies in ranking enable the identification of subjects where one method assigned a high density score and another method a low density score for the same case. A similar method was used to find the least discrepant cases for each of the pairs of methods. Differences in rank between each pair of methods were sorted in descending order and the cases with the 20 largest and smallest differences for each pair of methods (Quantra™ vs Volpara™; Quantra™ vs VAS average; Volpara™ vs VAS average; and VAS1 vs VAS2) were selected. Where there were ties in the differences in rank between methods these were included, so some groups contain more than 20. Mammograms for each of these women were retrieved and information was extracted by one film reader using a pro-forma.

The pro-forma gathered information on: patient details (age, body mass index); mammographic abnormalities (masses, calcification, distortion, asymmetry, previous breast surgery, previous biopsy (including markers from biopsy)); density results (VAS1, VAS2, Quantra™, Volpara™); positioning (pectoralis muscle – optimal/suboptimal, inframammary folds (IMFs) – optimal/suboptimal, nipple in profile, skin folds, image blurred); radiographic parameters (tube voltage(kV), tube current (mA), breast compression thickness (mm), compression force (N)); and other parameters (visible skin texture, objects in film, non-uniform glandular tissue distribution, prominent vascular markings, prominent lymph nodes). T-tests were carried out for continuous data and Chi-square tests were carried out for categorical data for each of the pairs of methods. Results were considered significant if the p-value was ≤ 0.05.

3   Results

In total, 6422 women met the entry criteria and had density readings for all three methods. The mean age was 59.3 years (SD 6.7) and mean BMI was 27.9 kg/m^2 (SD 5.5). Mean densities were 6.8 (SD 3.7), 15.5 (SD 5.7), 29.6 (SD 17.3) and 26.9 (SD 20.0) for Volpara™, Quantra™, VAS1 and VAS2 respectively. Figure 1 shows the level of agreement between the ranks for each pair of methods as well as the least and most discrepant cases selected for the study.

Comparison between Quantra™ and Volpara™
When comparing Quantra™ and Volpara™, presence of calcification was significantly different between the two measurement methods with those in the most discrepant group having more calcifications than those in the least discrepant group. There were also significantly more suboptimally imaged IMFs in the most discrepant group (Table 1). In addition, there was a significant difference in age between the most and least discrepant groups (p=0.036) with those in the most discrepant group being older (mean 61.5) than those in the least discrepant group (mean 56.6).

Comparison between Quantra™ and VAS Average
For the comparisons between Quantra™ and average VAS scores, the nipple was not in profile for the LCC view significantly more in the most discrepant group compared to the least discrepant group (Table 2). Similarly, skin folds for the LMLO view were present significantly more in the most discrepant group. Breast thickness (mm) after

compression was significantly higher in the most discrepant group for three out of the four mammographic views (RMLO, RCC and LCC) when comparing the difference between Quantra™ and average VAS scores (Table 3). There were no other significant results between Quantra™ and VAS .

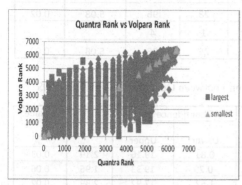
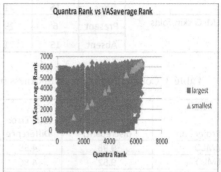
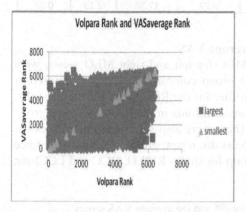
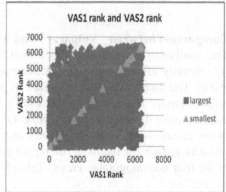

Fig. 1. Ranks for each pair of methods (eg. Quantra™ with Volpara™). Those selected for the current study are highlighted-least discrepant cases shown in green and most discrepant cases in red.

Table 1. Comparisons between Quantra™ and Volpara™

Image feature		Most discrepant		Least discrepant		Chi-Square	p-value
		n	%	n	%		
Calcification	No	16	80	21	100		
	Yes	4	20	0	0	4.65	0.031
RMLO Inframammary Fold	Optimal	8	40	15	71		
	Suboptimal	12	60	6	29	4.11	0.043
LMLO Inframammary Fold	Optimal	8	40	18	86		
	Suboptimal	12	60	3	14	9.23	0.002

Table 2. Comparisons between Quantra™ and VAS average

Image feature		Most discrepant		Least discrepant		Chi-Square	p-value
		n	%	n	%		
LCC nipple in profile	No	6	29	1	4		
	Yes	15	71	23	96	5.08	0.02
LMLO skin folds	Present	6	29	1	4		
	Absent	15	71	23	96	5.08	0.02

Table 3. Comparison of breast thickness (mm) between Quantra™ and average VAS

Projection	Mean Difference (most – least discrepant)	Std. Error Difference	95% Confidence Interval		t	p-value
			Lower	Upper		
RMLO	9.98	4.55	0.81	19.16	2.19	0.03
LMLO	9.52	4.86	-0.29	19.33	1.96	0.06
RCC	9.72	4.07	1.52	17.92	2.39	0.02
LCC	9.05	4.13	0.72	17.38	2.19	0.03

Comparison between Volpara™ and Average VAS

The number of women with suboptimal IMFs, for left and right MLO views, were significantly higher in the most discrepant group compared to the least discrepant group. The nipple was also less often in profile, for the RCC view, for the most discrepant group. There were significantly more skin folds in the least discrepant group than the most discrepant group (Table 4). There were also significant differences between compression force for the most and least discrepant groups. Compression force (N) was greater for the most discrepant group for three (RMLO, RCC and LCC) out of the four mammographic views (Table 5).

Table 4. Comparison between Volpara™ and the average VAS scores

Image feature		Most discrepant		Least discrepant		Chi Square	p-value
		n	%	n	%		
RMLO Inframammary Fold	Optimal	8	40	16	73		
	Suboptimal	12	60	6	27	4.58	0.03
LMLO Inframammary Fold	Optimal	8	40	16	73		
	Suboptimal	12	60	6	27	4.58	0.03
RCC nipple in profile	no	5	25	0	0		
	yes	15	75	22	100	6.24	0.01
RMLO skin folds	Present	2	10	10	45		
	Absent	18	90	12	55	6.45	0.01

Table 5. Comparison of compression force (N) between Volpara™ and average VAS

Projection	Mean Difference (most – least discrepant)	Std. Error Difference	95% Confidence Interval		t	p-value
			Lower	Upper		
RMLO	20.77	7.88	4.84	36.71	2.64	0.01
LMLO	12.18	7.98	-3.94	28.30	1.53	0.13
RCC	15.59	7.38	0.67	30.51	2.11	0.04
LCC	26.00	7.09	11.67	40.33	3.67	0.001

Table 6. Difference in tube current (mAs) between VAS1 and VAS2

Projection	Mean Difference (most – least discrepant)	Std. Error Difference	95% Confidence Interval		T	p-value
			Lower	Upper		
RMLO	-14.76	7.25	29.41	-0.11	2.04	0.05
LMLO	-16.29	10.60	37.72	5.14	0.54	0.13
RCC	22.09	26.03	0.51	74.69	0.85	0.40
LCC	-7.72	3.36	14.51	-0.93	2.30	0.03

Comparison between VAS1 and VAS2

There was a statistically significant difference between the tube current recorded for the RMLO and LCC views, with the mean being significantly higher in the least discrepant group. There were no other significant results between VAS1 and VAS2.

4   Discussion

When comparing the different methods for density measurement in the most and least discrepant cases there were a number of interesting findings. Calcification and IMFs were found to be present more often in the most discrepant group when comparing Quantra™ and Volpara™, implying that the two technologies do not agree. How these are dealt with by the computer software designed to measure volumetric density is not publicly known. Those in the most discrepant group also tended to be older than those in the least discrepant group suggesting that volumetric methods may find it more difficult to agree on density of older women's mammograms. Generally, the volume of fibroglandular tissue decreases with age, therefore it is possible that volumetric technologies find smaller volumes of fibroglandular tissue more difficult to interpret, although interestingly, there were no such differences between volumetric methods and VAS density results.

When comparing densities between Quantra™ and VAS average considerably fewer nipples were in profile in the most discrepant group than the least discrepant group for the LCC view. In some images the automated method may have interpreted the nipple as fibroglandular tissue whereas VAS readers would recognise this as a positioning issue. However, this was not found in the three other mammographic views. There was a similar finding for the presence of skin folds. Compression thickness was also significantly different for three mammographic views when Quantra™ and VAS were compared. Compressing the breast minimises movement and spreads the fibroglandular tissue, and dense tissue may be more difficult to assess accurately in a projection image when less compression is used. Interestingly, differences in compression force were not significant in any of the views when comparing these two methods.

Like the comparisons between Quantra™ and VAS, there were a number of significant differences between Volpara™ and VAS for IMFs, nipple not in profile and skin folds. Compression force was found to be higher in the most discrepant group for all four views suggesting less agreement when a larger force is applied.

A limitation of the current study was that density methods were measured across all four views, however the assessment of positioning and information extracted on radiographic parameters from the DICOM headers was for individual mammographic views. It would be interesting to see whether the discrepancies in density are specific to individual mammographic views. Furthermore, assessment of image positioning relied on the interpretation of a single film reader. However images were anonymised and assessed in random order so the reader was blind to which group they came from.

5   Conclusions

This study looked at different methods of measuring breast density: Quantra™, Volpara™ and VAS. There was significantly more calcification and suboptimal IMFs in the most discrepant group when comparing Quantra™ and Volpara™. We also found significant results when comparing the computerised methods with VAS. There were more skin folds in the most discrepant group when comparing Quantra™ and VAS, and the compressed breast thickness was also significantly larger in the most discrepant group. Comparing Volpara™ and VAS found that suboptimal IMFs contributed to disagreement in breast density. Compression force was also significantly higher in the most discrepant group.

At present, there are important differences between different methods of breast density assessment. A greater understanding of the reasons behind such differences coupled with careful radiographic technique should lead to a reduction in these discrepancies.

Acknowledgements. We acknowledge the support of the National Institute for Health Research (NIHR) and the Genesis Prevention Appeal for their funding of the PROCAS study. We would like to thank the women who agreed to take part in the study, the study radiologists and advanced radiographer practitioners for VAS reading, the radiographers involved in the Greater Manchester Breast Screening Programme and the study staff for recruitment and data collection,. We also thank Hologic Inc. for providing Quantra™ and Matakina Technology Limited for providing Volpara™. This paper presents independent research funded by the National Institute for Health Research (NIHR) under its Programme Grants for Applied Research programme (reference number RP-PG-0707-10031: "Improvement in risk prediction, early detection and prevention of breast cancer"). The views expressed are those of the author(s) and not necessarily those of the NHS, the NIHR, or the Department of Health.

References

1. Boyd, N.F., Dite, G.S., Stone, J., Gunasekara, A., English, D.R., McCredie, M.R., et al.: Heritability of mammographic density, a risk factor for breast cancer. N. Engl. J. Med. 347(12), 886–894 (2002)
2. Boyd, N.F., Guo, H., Martin, L.J., Sun, L., Stone, J., Fishell, E., et al.: Mammographic Density and the Risk and Detection of Breast Cancer. N. Engl. J. Med. 356(3), 227–236 (2007)
3. Hologic- Quantra Volumetric Assessment (2012),
   http://www.hologic.com/en/breast-screening/
   volumetric-assessment/
4. Volpara Density (2013), http://www.volparadensity.com/
5. Evans G. PROCAS study (2011),
   http://www.uhsm.nhs.uk/research/Pages/PROCASstudy.aspx
   (June 16, 2013)
6. Sergeant, J.C., Warwick, J., Evans, D.G., Howell, A., Berks, M., Stavrinos, P., Sahin, S., Wilson, M., Hufton, A., Buchan, I., Astley, S.M.: Volumetric and Area-Based Breast Density Measurement in the Predicting Risk of Cancer at Screening (PROCAS) Study. In: Maidment, A.D.A., Bakic, P.R., Gavenonis, S. (eds.) IWDM 2012. LNCS, vol. 7361, pp. 228–235. Springer, Heidelberg (2012)

Breast Tissue Segmentation and Mammographic Risk Scoring Using Deep Learning

Kersten Petersen[1], Mads Nielsen[1,2], Pengfei Diao[1],
Nico Karssemeijer[3], and Martin Lillholm[2]

[1] Department of Computer Science, University of Copenhagen, Denmark
[2] Biomediq A/S, Copenhagen, Denmark
[3] Department of Radiology, Radboud University Nijmegen, Netherlands

Abstract. Mammographic scoring of density and texture are established methods to relate to the risk of breast cancer. We present a method that learns descriptive features from unlabeled mammograms and, using these learned features as the input to a simple classifier, address the following tasks: i) breast tissue segmentation ii) scoring of percentage mammographic density (PMD), and iii) scoring of mammographic texture (MT). Our results suggest that the learned PMD scores correlate well to manual ones, and that the learned MT scores are more related to future cancer risk than both manual and automatic PMD scores.

Keywords: Unsupervised feature learning, deep learning, breast cancer, mammograms, prognosis, risk factor, segmentation.

1 Introduction

Breast cancer is the most common cancer (non-melanoma skin cancer excluded) worldwide, with more than 430,000 deaths in 2010 alone [1]. In order to reduce breast cancer mortality, it is important to identify, monitor, and possibly treat high risk patients early. One of the strongest known risk factors for breast cancer is the relative amount of radiodense tissue in the breast, expressed as mammographic density (MD) [2][3]. Widespread MD scores range from manual categorical (e.g., BI-RADS, Wolfe [4], Tabár [5]) to continuous scores (e.g., Cumulus-like thresholding). A major problem is that fully manual or user-assisted scoring is subjective and time-consuming. There has been a trend towards fully automating MD scoring, but most of these approaches rely on handcrafted features with several adjustable hyperparameters. Similarly, mammographic texture (MT) scoring methods, describing mammographic heterogeneity, have used manually encoded and selected features.

In this paper, we investigate a method to automatically learns features that best describe mammogram appearance patterns. These data-driven features can be used to address three breast cancer risk related tasks that have previously been modeled in very different ways: breast tissue segmentation, percentual mammographic density (PMD) scoring, and mammographic texture (MT) scoring.

H. Fujita, T. Hara, and C. Muramatsu (Eds.): IWDM 2014, LNCS 8539, pp. 88–94, 2014.
© Springer International Publishing Switzerland 2014

2   Materials and Method

2.1   Materials

We have evaluated our method on 495 right and corresponding left mediolateral (RMLO and LMLO) mammograms from a previously published case-control study from the Dutch screening program. This study was originally designed for investigating the effect of recall rate within the Dutch biennial breast screening program [7]. Selected mammograms from this study contained 250 controls and 245 cases of which 123 were diagnosed with an interval cancer and 122 with a screen-detected cancer. The case mammograms were selected 4 years prior to a screen detected and 2-4 years prior to an interval cancer. The mammograms of the controls remained cancer free in the subsequent 4 years. The participants of the study were between 49 and 81 years old and the study groups were matched for age. The mammograms were digitized with a Vidar scanner that provided an image resolution of roughly 1500×2500 pixels on 12-bit gray scale and 50×50 microns. On the RMLO mammograms, a trained radiologist annotated the skin-air boundary and the pectoral muscle by a polygon tool, and estimated BI-RADS and PMD using a Cumulus-like approach.

2.2   Methods

The employed texture scoring method learns a deep hierarchy of increasingly more abstract features from unlabeled data and maps the final feature representation to the label of interest. Depending on the task, these per pixel labels are i) segmentation: background (BG), pectoral muscle (PM), and breast tissue (BT) ii) PMD scoring: fatty tissue, and dense tissue iii) MT scoring: healthy, and diseased (each pixel is associated with the cancer outcome label). The employed model is called a convolutional sparse autoencoder (CSAE [6]) and processes small patches at multiple image scales from the mammogram.

The training data is collected by randomly drawing 50,000 patches across a set of training mammograms and by associating them with the label of interest. An unseen mammogram is segmented or scored by applying the trained model in a sliding window approach. At the image boundary, the image is padded with a constant value. A label posterior of the disease class is gained for each location, and afterwards averaged to produce a single score per mammogram. In the following, we summarize the ingredients of the CSAE model: a convolutional architecture as the model representation, and a sparse autoencoder for learning the model parameters.

Convolutional architecture A *convolutional Architecture.* is suited for learning a deep feature hierarchy from structured data [8]. It is similar to neural networks, but has two advantages: First, convolutional architectures model the topology of the input in each layer, e.g., images as a 2D grid. Second, they are able to scale to much larger inputs by constraining the number of trainable parameters.

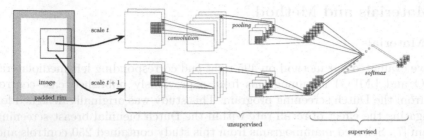

Fig. 1. Deep convolutional architecture. Patches are extracted from multiple scales of the image and fed to the convolutional architecture. The patch (or *feature map*) at scale $t + 1$ only considers every second pixel, such it has the same size as the patch from scale t. The small subregions within the extracted patches are referred to as *local receptive fields*. We refer to the text for more details.

The hidden layers of a convolutional architectures consist of *convolutional* and *pooling* layers, usually in alternating order. In our convolutional architecture, we have replaced one pooling layer by a convolutional layer to have invariance to noise, but still pick up details that could benefit the segmentation or scoring task. This design choice was confirmed by slightly better results.

Convolutional layers are similar to hidden layers in a traditional neural network. They are parameterized by trainable weight parameters that can be interpreted as *features*. However, rather than connecting each unit to all input units, convolutional units are only connected to spatially close units. Each set of input units usually corresponds to a small squared subregion of the input grid and is collectively referred to as a *local receptive field*. In Figure 1, the local receptive fields are connected with red, blue, or green lines to a unit of an output feature map. Weighting the units within a local receptive field is equivalent to a convolution of the input feature map.

In a convolutional architecture, the layer units are not stored as a vector, but in a multi-channel grid structure. The convolutional layer convolves the input of each channel, sums the responses, adds a bias term, and sends the result through a scalar-wise nonlinear activation function to create one output feature map. This nonlinear multi-channel processing is repeated with different filter weights to create multiple output feature maps. Thus, each convolutional layer is fed with multiple input feature maps and applies different convolutions to create multiple output feature maps. Formally, the jth output feature map of a convolutional layer is given by

$$z_j^{\text{out}} = \sigma(w_j * z + b_j \mathbf{1}_{m'}), \tag{1}$$

where w_j denotes the filter for the jth output map, z all input feature maps as a tensor, b_j the bias for the jth map, and $\mathbf{1}_{m'}$ denotes an $m' \times m'$ matrix of ones. The activation function is denoted by $\sigma(x) = \max(x, 0)$.

Table 1. Comparison of expert's PMD scores with expert's BI-RADS and automated CSAE PMD scores

Method	Case	Control	R_{PMD}	AUC (95% CI)
PMD	0.20 ± 0.13	0.18 ± 0.13	-	0.56 (0.51, 0.61)
BI-RADS	2.23 ± 0.72	2.10 ± 0.76	0.87	0.55 (0.50, 0.60)
PMD$_{CSAE}$	0.21 ± 0.11	0.18 ± 0.13	0.87	0.56 (0.51, 0.61)

The output of the convolutional layer is often fed to a pooling layer which summarize the distributions within small (non-overlapping) spatial regions. The final architecture layer maps the output of the last hidden layer to the labeled data, in the same way as it is modeled in a neural network.

Figure 1 illustrates our convolutional architecture for processing multiscale input patches. The large rectangles denote feature maps, whereas the small rectangles represent local receptive fields. We employ one pooling layer (blue) and three convolutional layers (red), which are trained in an unsupervised way by sparse autoencoders (see next Section). The last two layers are finally trained by a classifier to map the output to the labels of interest.

Sparse Autoencoder. Here, we describe how the w_j weights from the convolutional layer described above are trained by reconstructing the inputs of a convolution operation, i.e., patches of the size of local receptive fields, using an encoder-decoder architecture [9]. The *encoder* maps the input to a hidden layer and uses the same activation function that was defined in the convolutional layer. The *decoder* maps the hidden layer to the output layer, which is set to be the same as the input. This autoencoder structure enables to learn features without using the label information. As a refinement to this architecture, we have incorporated a sparsity regularizer to control the capacity of this model.

3 Results

3.1 Breast Tissue Segmentation

The mean and standard deviation of the Dice coefficient for automated vs. expert's breast tissue segmentation (BG: 0.99 ± 0.01, PM: 0.95 ± 0.08, and BT: 0.98 ± 0.01).

In the following, the automated breast tissue mask is used as a region of interest in both scoring tasks.

3.2 Mammographic Density Scoring

The CSAE model was trained to automatically compute PMD. Table 1 presents i) mean and standard error for cancers and controls, ii) Pearson's R correlation

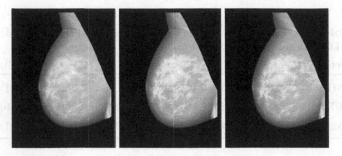

Fig. 2. Automated PMD. From let to right: original image; dense tissue (in red) based on expert Cumulus-like score; PMD$_{CSAE}$ posterior of dense tissue class.

Table 2. Comparison of automated texture scores

Method	AUC (95% CI)
MT$_{kNN}$ (R)	0.62 (0.57, 0.67)
MT$_{CSAE}$ (R)	0.65 (0.60, 0.70)
MT$_{CSAE}$ (L)	0.65 (0.60, 0.70)

coefficient between automated and manual PMD scores, and iii) the area under the ROC curve (*AUC*). We see that our automated PMD scores are well correlated to manual PMD and equally discriminative. A typical density segmentation result is shown in Fig. 2.

3.3   Mammographic Texture Scoring

The CSAE model has been evaluated on the LMLO and RMLO mammograms of the Nijmegen dataset. Since manual breast segmentations were only available for the RMLO view, we applied the segmentation model trained on the RMLO view to the LMLO mammograms. The obtained automated segmentations were scored with the texture model that was trained on the RMLO mammograms as well. In both experiments, the RMLO mammograms in the cross validations folds were replaced with their LMLO counterparts.

Table 2 summarizes the obtained AUCs for our model applied to RMLO, MT$_{CSAE}$ (R), and LMLO, MT$_{CSAE}$ (L). We also compared these models to the previously best performing MT scoring method by Nielsen et al., MT$_{kNN}$ (R)[10]. Pearson's R correlation of the two automated MT scores to manual PMD is low (both $R_{PMD} = 0.10$), suggesting that our MT scores add to manual PMD in terms of risk segregation.

Figure 3 illustrates the correlation of the automated MT scores on LMLO and RMLO view (Pearson's $R = 0.85$), which compares to widespread volumetric density scores like Volpara^{TM} ($R = 0.92$ on 2217 mammograms) [11].

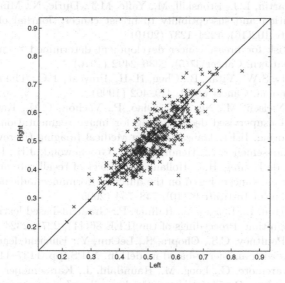

Fig. 3. Correlation of texture scores between left and right breast. The black line is the identity line. The corresponding Pearson's R correlation coefficient is 0.85.

4   Conclusion

We have presented an unsupervised feature learning method for breast region segmentation, automatic PMD scoring, and automatic MT scoring. The model learns features across multiple scales and harnesses correlations in the target values. Once the features are learned, they are fed to a simple classifier that is specific to the task of interest. The CSAE model achieved state-of-the-art results on each of the three different breast cancer related tasks.

Acknowledgements. This work was supported by the Danish National Advanced Technology Foundation under the grant Personalized Breast cancer Screening, the Danish Cancer Society, and the European Unions Seventh Framework Programme FP7 under grant agreement no 306088.

References

1. Lozano, R., Naghavi, M., Foreman, K., Lim, S., Shibuya, K., Aboyans, V., Abraham, J., Adair, T., Aggarwal, R., Ahn, S.Y., et al.: Global and regional mortality from 235 causes of death for 20 age groups in 1990 and 2010: a systematic analysis for the global burden of disease study 2010. The Lancet 380(9859), 2095–2128 (2013)
2. McCormack, V.A., dos Santos Silva, I.: Breast density and parenchymal patterns as markers of breast cancer risk: A meta-analysis. Cancer Epidemiology Biomarkers & Prevention 15(6), 1159–1169 (2006)

3. Boyd, N.F., Martin, L.J., Bronskill, M., Yaffe, M.J., Duric, N., Minkin, S.: Breast tissue composition and susceptibility to breast cancer. Journal of the National Cancer Institute 102(16), 1224–1237 (2010)
4. Wolfe, J.N.: Risk for breast cancer development determined by mammographic parenchymal pattern. Cancer 37(5), 2486–2492 (1976)
5. Tabár, L., Duffy, S.W., Vitak, B., Chen, H.-H., Prevost, T.C.: The natural history of breast carcinoma. Cancer 86(3), 449–462 (1999)
6. Petersen, K., Nielsen, M., Ng, A.Y., Diao, P., Vachon, C.M., Karssemeijer, N., Lillholm, M.: Unsupervised deep learning for image segmentation and mammographic risk scoring. IEEE Transactions on Medical Imaging (in review)
7. Otten, J.D., Karssemeijer, N., Hendriks, J.H., Groenewoud, J.H., Fracheboud, J., Verbeek, A.L., de Koning, H.J., Holland, R.: Effect of recall rate on earlier screen detection of breast cancers based on the dutch performance indicators. Journal of the National Cancer Institute 97(10), 748–754 (2005)
8. LeCun, Y., Bottou, L., Bengio, Y., Haffner, P.: Gradient-based learning applied to document recognition. Proceedings of the IEEE 86(11), 2278–2324 (1998)
9. Ranzato, M., Poultney, C.S., Chopra, S., LeCun, Y.: Efficient learning of sparse representations with an energy-based model. In: NIPS, pp. 1137–1144 (2006)
10. Nielsen, M., Karemore, G., Loog, M., Raundahl, J., Karssemeijer, N., Otten, J., Karsdal, M., Vachon, C., Christiansen, C.: A novel and automatic mammographic texture resemblance marker is an independent risk factor for breast cancer. Cancer Epidemiology 35(4), 381–387 (2011)
11. Highnam, R., Brady, S.M., Yaffe, M.J., Karssemeijer, N., Harvey, J.: Robust breast composition measurement - volpara™. In: Martí, J., Oliver, A., Freixenet, J., Martí, R. (eds.) IWDM 2010. LNCS, vol. 6136, pp. 342–349. Springer, Heidelberg (2010)

Optimization of X-Ray Spectra for Dual-Energy Contrast-Enhanced Breast Imaging: Dependency on CsI Detector Scintillator Thickness

Pablo Milioni de Carvalho[1,2], Ann-Katherine Carton[2], Sylvie Saab-Puong[2], Răzvan Iordache[2], and Serge Muller[2]

[1] IR4M (UMR8081), Université Paris-Sud, CNRS; Orsay, France
[2] GE Healthcare, 283 rue de la Minière, 78533 Buc, France
pablo.milionidecarvalho@ge.com

Abstract. Columnar structured cesium iodide (CsI) scintillators doped with Thallium (Tl) have been used extensively for indirect X-ray imaging detectors. Here, theoretical modeling was performed to assess the impact of CsI thickness on optimal acquisition spectra for dual-energy iodine-enhanced breast computed tomography (bCT). Contrast-to-noise ratio (CNR) between iodine-enhanced and non-enhanced breast tissue normalized to the square root of the total average glandular dose (AGD) was computed as a function of the fraction of the AGD allocated to the low-energy images. Peak CNR/√AGD and optimal low-energy AGD allocations were identified for small, average and large uncompressed breasts. Optimal high-energy spectra were found to be almost independent of CsI thickness and occurred just above the Cs and I K-edges (range 34 to 36 keV), while optimal low-energy spectra varied largely with CsI thickness, ranging from 25 keV to 33 keV for 100 μm to infinite CsI scintillator thicknesses.

Keywords: breast, computed tomography, dual energy, scintillator.

1 Introduction

Indirect flat-panel imagers with CsI:Tl scintillators have been widely used for digital breast X-ray imaging since last decade. Several publications have investigated their imaging performance at typical X-ray spectra for conventional digital mammography, digital breast tomosynthesis and dedicated breast computed tomography [1–4]. So far, no study has been dedicated to the energy-dependent imaging performance of CsI as a function its thickness for dual-energy applications. Here, we investigate the impact of CsI scintillator thickness on the optimal spectra for dual-energy breast imaging combined with a vascular iodine-based contrast agent. Theoretical modeling was performed to assess optimally enhanced iodine-equivalent images, with contrast-to-noise ratio (CNR) between iodine-enhanced and unenhanced tissue normalized to the square root of the average glandular dose (AGD) as Figure-of-Merit. Our investigation is demonstrated for dual-energy contrast-enhanced breast CT (CE-bCT).

H. Fujita, T. Hara, and C. Muramatsu (Eds.): IWDM 2014, LNCS 8539, pp. 95–102, 2014.

2   Theory

2.1   X-ray Photon Detection

Assuming a mono-energetic X-ray beam, a breast image formed only by primary X-rays photons and an energy-integrating quantum-noise limited detector which does not introduce any blurring can be calculated as:

$$I(i) = k \cdot E \cdot \mathcal{P}\left\{\eta(E)I_0(E,i)e^{-\int \mu(r,E)dl}\right\} \tag{1}$$

where $I(i)$ is the per-pixel signal intensity, k is a constant representing optical quanta generation and other scaling factors, E is the X-ray energy, $\mathcal{P}\{\cdot\}$ denotes a Poisson distribution, $I_0(E,i)$ is the photon fluence at energy E generated by a monochromatic point source s towards a detection element i, $\mu(r,E)$ is the linear attenuation of the imaged breast at energy E and position r in its volume, dl is the incremental thickness of the traversed breast in the path s to i and $\eta(E)$ is the quantum efficiency of the detector at energy E.

The function $\eta(E)$ can be extremely complex accounting for different energy-dependent inefficiencies during the detection process. In this work we assumed $\eta(E)$ to depend only on CsI scintillator thickness:

$$\eta(E) = 1 - e^{-\mu_{CsI}(E)t_{CsI}(i)} \tag{2}$$

where $\mu_{CsI}(E)$ is the linear attenuation coefficient at energy E of a continuous and homogenous CsI layer and $t_{CsI}(i)$ is the oblique thickness of the scintillator at detector element i. For simplicity, X-ray beam obliquity was disregarded in $\eta(E)$ calculation since it would entail only small differences in signal intensities for small incident angles [5]. Therefore, t_{CsI} values are same at all detector positions.

2.2   Image-Based Dual-Energy Recombination

In an iodine-enhanced dual-energy breast imaging setup, the breast can be approximated as being composed of three basis materials: adipose, fibroglandular tissue and the injected iodine. Moreover, the composition of every unit of volume in the breast can be assumed to be an ideal solution of these three materials, *i.e.* with final volume equal to the volume of its constituent parts (volume conservation):

$$f_{adipose}(r) + f_{gland}(r) + f_{iodine}(r) = 1 \tag{3}$$

where $f_{adipose}(r)$, $f_{gland}(r)$ and $f_{iodine}(r)$ are the volume fractions of adipose, fibroglandular tissue and iodine, respectively, at position r in the breast volume.

After tomographic reconstruction, low-energy (LE) and high-energy (HE) cross-sectional images can be described by the expressions:

$$\begin{cases} \tilde{\mu}^{LE}(r) = \mu_{adipose}^{LE} \cdot f_{adipose}(r) + \mu_{gland}^{LE} \cdot f_{gland}(r) + \mu_{iodine}^{LE} \cdot f_{iodine}(r) \\ \tilde{\mu}^{HE}(r) = \mu_{adipose}^{HE} \cdot f_{adipose}(r) + \mu_{gland}^{HE} \cdot f_{gland}(r) + \mu_{iodine}^{HE} \cdot f_{iodine}(r) \end{cases} \tag{4}$$

where $\tilde{\mu}^{LE}(r)$ and $\tilde{\mu}^{HE}(r)$ are the measured linear attenuation coefficients of the breast at LE and HE at position r in their respective volume, and $\mu_{adipose}^{LE,HE}$, $\mu_{gland}^{LE,HE}$ and $\mu_{iodine}^{LE,HE}$ are the linear attenuation coefficients of adipose, fibroglandular tissue and of iodine uptake at LE and HE.

The slice images obtained by solving the system of the three above equations for f_{iodine} are hereafter referred to as *iodine-equivalent images*, as their intensity values are proportional to the quantity of iodine inside each voxel.

3   Materials and Methods

3.1   Breast Phantom and X-ray Image Simulation

To mimic small, average and large uncompressed breasts of a woman in prone position, three 50% fibroglandular equivalent analytic cylindrical phantoms with a 10, 14 and 18-cm diameter and a height equal to three-quarters of their respective diameter were simulated [6]. The phantom includes 10-mm diameter spherical inserts, distributed in a coronal plane at mid-depth of the cylinder (Fig. 1a). The inserts are composed of homogeneous mixtures of fibroglandular and adipose-equivalent tissues, as well as homogeneous mixtures of 50% fibroglandular equivalent tissue and 0.5, 1.0, 2.5 and 5.0 mg/cm^3 iodine concentrations. All homogeneous mixtures in the phantom were obtained respecting volume conservation (Equation 2).

A cone-beam breast CT topology similar to that published by Boone *et al.* [7] was considered (cf. Fig. 1b) assuming a quantum-limited, energy-integrating (Equation 1) detector with 0.776 mm detector element pitch. CsI scintillators with 100, 250, 400, 600 and 780 μm thicknesses, as well as a perfect energy-integrating detector with $\eta(E) = 1$ regardless of the energy value, were investigated. Per scan, three-hundred projection images were acquired using an analytic ray-tracing projector and monoenergetic, primary X-rays only. The projections were reconstructed by filtered

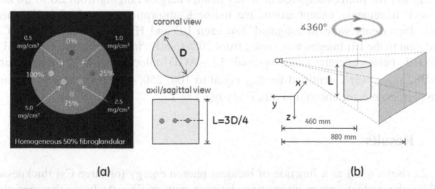

(a)   (b)

Fig. 1. Illustration of (a) a cylindrical phantom with spherical iodine inserts and (b) the cone-beam CT geometry used to assess the effect of CsI scintillator thickness on optimal acquisition spectra for dual-energy iodine-enhanced bCT

back-projection with ideal ramp filter, to obtain 512×512 coronal images with $0.41 \times 0.41 \ mm^2$ pixel size, and $1 \ mm$ slice thickness.

Average Glandular Dose (AGD) was estimated using a Monte Carlo simulator; two million photons undergoing Rayleigh, Compton and photoelectric interactions were tracked in voxelized versions of the analytical phantoms, sampled at $2 \times 2 \times 2 \ mm^3$ voxel sizes. X-ray beam fluence was adjusted to provide a total AGD of 100 mGy and achieve adequate detector incident X-ray photon fluence and the desired quantum statistics for all experimental conditions.

Analytical projections, tomographic reconstructions and radiation dose were simulated using CatSim, an X-ray imaging system simulation platform previously developed and validated at General Electric [8].

3.2   Optimization Criteria

Contrast-to-Noise-Ratio per pixel between iodine-enhanced breast tissue and background breast tissue normalized to the square root of the total AGD (CNRD) was used as the Figure-of-Merit for the detectability of iodine in iodine-equivalent images:

$$CNRD_{iodine-bg} = \left(SI_{iodine} - SI_{bg}\right) \Big/ \sigma_{bg} \sqrt{AGD_{LE+HE}} \qquad (5)$$

where SI_{iodine} and SI_{bg} are the mean per-pixel signal intensities (SI) in an iodine-enhanced region-of-interest (ROI) and a non-iodine enhanced neighboring ROI, σ_{bg} is the standard deviation of the SI in the non-iodine enhanced ROI and AGD_{LE+HE} is the sum of AGD delivered during LE and HE acquisitions.

Assuming quantum noise only, the standard deviations of the signal intensities in LE and HE images are inversely proportional to $\sqrt{AGD_{LE}}$ and $\sqrt{AGD_{HE}}$, respectively. If $R = AGD_{LE}/AGD_{LE+HE}$ is the LE dose allocation, it can be shown that $CNRD_{iodine-bg}$ is independent of the total AGD and depends only on R [9, 10].

$CNRD_{iodine-bg}$ was calculated in iodine-equivalent images obtained by recombining LE and HE images acquired at X–ray beam energies ranging from 20 to 80 keV in 5 keV increments, except around the iodine K-absorption edge (33.2 keV) where 1 keV increments were investigated. For each LE and HE X-ray beam pair, AGD allocation to the LE images was varied from 20% to 80% in 5-10% steps. Optimal LE and HE beam energies and optimal LE AGD allocation, R_{opt}, maximizing $CNRD_{iodine-bg}$ were identified for t_{CsI} equal to 100, 250, 400, 600 and 780 μm and for a perfect detector absorption efficiency $\eta(E) = 1$.

4   Results

Fig. 2a shows $\eta(E)$ as a function of incident photon energy for three CsI thicknesses and for the perfect energy-integrating detector with $\eta(E) = 1$. It can be seen that $\eta(E)$ increases with scintillator thickness and all curves show discontinuities at the K-edges of Cs (36 keV) and I (33.2 keV), due to the sudden increase in their attenuation coefficients.

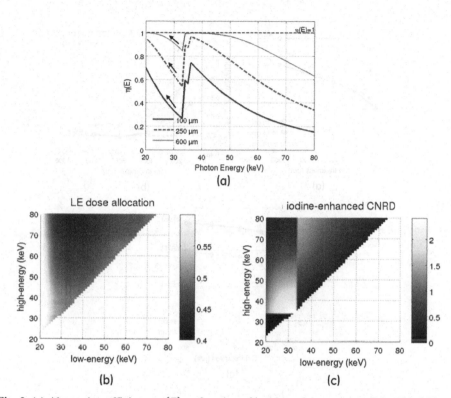

Fig. 2. (a) Absorption efficiency $\eta(E)$ as function of incident photon energy E for 100, 250 and 600 μm CsI thicknesses. (b) Optimal LE dose allocation, R_{opt}, and (c) $CNRD_{iodine-bg}$ at R_{opt} for the 14 cm diameter phantom assuming $\eta(E) = 1$

Fig. 2b and 2c illustrate optimal LE dose allocation, R_{opt}, and the corresponding optimal $CNRD_{iodine-bg}$ values, for all studied LE/HE pairs and for the 14 cm diameter phantom when assuming perfect detector absorption efficiency $\eta(E) = 1$. Optimal LE dose allocation varies around 50% for a large range of LE and HE pairs. However, optimal dose allocation increases rapidly for LE smaller than ~25 keV, such as to compensate the lack of transmitted quanta, and decreases slowly with increasing HE values. $CNRD_{iodine-bg}$ is higher for LE and HE pairs just below and above the iodine K-edge, than for LE and HE pairs with energies farther away from the iodine K-edge discontinuity. Similar trends in LE dose allocation and $CNRD_{iodine-bg}$ as function of the LE and HE X-ray beam pairs were found for all experimental conditions.

Fig. 3a, 3b and 3c show optimal LE, R_{opt}, and the corresponding optimal $CNRD_{iodine-bg}$ values for all studied CsI thicknesses and for the perfect energy-integrating detector. Fig. 3a and 3b show that optimal LE values increase as a function of CsI thickness, while R_{opt}, decreases as a function of CsI thickness. This effect is more pronounced for small CsI thicknesses. For all studied cases, optimal HE beam energy occur just above the K-edges of I or Cs (range 34 to 36 keV). Fig. 3a

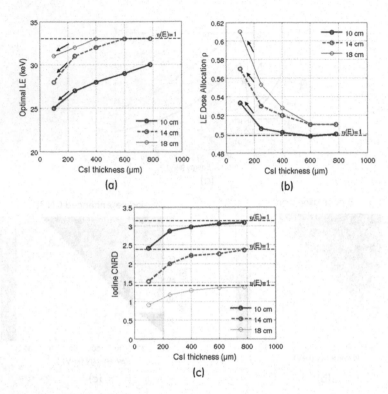

Fig. 3. (a) Optimal LE, (b) optimal LE dose allocation R_{opt} and (c) optimal $CNRD_{iodine-bg}$ as a function of CsI scintillator thickness

shows that optimal $CNRD_{iodine-bg}$ increases monotonically with increasing scintillator thickness and converges to $CNRD_{iodine-bg}$ obtained with the perfect energy-integrating detector. For an average sized breast, $CNRD_{iodine-bg}$ increases from 64% to 95% of the $CNRD_{iodine-bg}$ obtained with the perfect energy-integrating detector, when passing from a 100 to 600 μm thick CsI layer.

5   Discussion

Under the assumptions of primary mono-energetic X-rays and an energy-integrating, quantum-noise limited, blur-free detector with the same absorption efficiency at all incident beam angles, it was shown that optimal LE and optimal dose allocation vary greatly with CsI layer thickness and that optimal iodine detectability monotonically increases with increasing scintillator thickness. It was observed that optimal LE values increase as a function of CsI thickness while optimal LE dose allocation decreases as a function of CsI thickness. This trend can be seen as compensation for the loss in absorption efficiency for energies values just below the iodine K-edge (cf. black arrows in Fig. 2a, 3a and 3b).

In this study, simplified assumptions on X-ray image generation were made. A point source, emitting mono-energetic X-ray beams was assumed. Although the adoption of polychromatic spectra would degrade iodine uptake detectability, our results can be used as a preliminary detectability evaluation for polychromatic X-ray beams with average energy coincident with the studied monochromatic energies. X-ray scatter was not modeled. As shown by Glick et al. [11], X-ray scattering has a moderate degradation effect on lesion detectability. Nonetheless, this effect showed little energy-dependency and has thus little impact on optimal dual-energy spectra.

Idealistic hypothesis for the detector model were also made. Optical glare, the scatter of optical photons within the phosphor layer of the detector, and its degrading effect on the detector pre-sampling MTF was disregarded. Our results showed that CNRD increases with increasing scintillator thickness. However, it is known that the detector pre-sampling MTF degrades with increasing scintillator thickness, especially at high-frequency components. A blur-free assumption would in this case be interesting to evaluate iodine uptake detectability through low-frequency metrics such as CNRD, but would possibly be insufficient for the assessment of iodine uptake morphology and other Figures-of-Merit sensible to high-frequency variations in signal intensity.

X-ray beam obliquity was not taken into account when computing in $\eta(E)$. By geometric calculation, it can be demonstrated that oblique X-ray beam incidence entails up to ~5% increase in t_{CsI} values (at the largest obliquity, for the largest phantom) and, as consequence, ~3% average increase in $\eta(E)$. In cross-sectional images reconstructed at the phantom's mid-depth, differences in lesion CNRD values would be below 1% and, therefore, with imperceptible impact on the results presented above. Further studies including more realistic detector models will provide better understanding on the impact of different CsI scintillators on iodine uptake detectability and characterization.

In this work, results were shown for a cone-beam breast CT geometry, for which the breast is not compressed during imaging (10 to 18 cm in diameter). These findings can explain the behavior of optimal spectra previously found for dual-energy contrast-enhanced mammography with compressed breasts (2 to 8 cm thick) [9, 12].

6   Conclusions

Several research papers on optimizing LE and HE X-ray spectra for dual-energy contrast-enhanced iodine breast imaging found counter-intuitive results; optimal spectra do not bracket the K-edge of iodine as closely as expected. Our work presents preliminary evidence that optimal X-ray spectra strongly depend on detector scintillator thickness. Detector energy-dependent absorption inefficiencies should therefore be taken into account when designing X-ray imaging systems for spectral applications.

Acknowledgements. This study was funded by the ANRT, under the PhD CIFRE convention 2010/756.

References

1. Ghetti, C., Borrini, A., Ortenzia, O., Rossi, R., Ordóñez, P.L.: Physical characteristics of GE Senographe Essential and DS digital mammography detectors. Med. Phys. 35, 456 (2008)
2. Liaparinos, P., Bliznakova, K.: Monte Carlo performance on the x-ray converter thickness in digital mammography using software breast models. Med. Phys. 6, 6638–6651 (2012)
3. Carton, A.-K., Acciavatti, R., Kuo, J., Maidment, A.D.A.: The effect of scatter and glare on image quality in contrast-enhanced breast imaging using an a-Si/CsI(Tl) full-field flat panel detector. Med. Phys. 36, 920–928 (2009)
4. Shen, Y., Zhong, Y., Lai, C.-J., Wang, T., Shaw, C.C.: Cone beam breast CT with a high pitch (75 μm), thick (500 μm) scintillator CMOS flat panel detector: visibility of simulated microcalcifications. Med. Phys. 40, 101915 (2013)
5. Mainprize, J.G., Bloomquist, A.K., Kempston, M.P., Yaffe, M.J.: Resolution at oblique incidence angles of a flat panel imager for breast tomosynthesis. Med. Phys. 33, 3159 (2006)
6. Boone, J.M., Kwan, A.L.C., Seibert, J.A., Shah, N., Lindfors, K.K., Nelson, T.R.: Technique factors and their relationship to radiation dose in pendant geometry breast CT. Radiology, 3767–3776 (2005)
7. Boone, J.M., Nelson, T.R., Lindfors, K.K., Seibert, J.A.: Dedicated Breast CT: Radiation Dose and Image Quality Evaluation. Radiology 221, 657 (2001)
8. De Man, B., Basu, S., Chandra, N., Dunham, B., Edic, P., Iatrou, M.: CatSim: a new computer assisted tomography simulation environment. In: Proc. SPIE, vol. 6510, pp. 1–8 (2007)
9. Puong, S., Bouchevreau, X., Patoureaux, F., Iordache, R., Muller, S.: Dual-energy contrast enhanced digital mammography using a new approach for breast tissue canceling. In: Proc. SPIE, vol. 33, pp. 65102H–65102H–12 (2007)
10. de Carvalho, P., Carton, A.-K., Saab-Puong, S., Iordache, R., Muller, S.: Spectra optimization for dual-energy contrast-enhanced breast CT. SPIE Med. Imaging (2013)
11. Liu, B., Glick, S., Groiselle, C.: Characterization of scatter radiation in cone beam CT mammography. In: Proc. SPIE Med. Imaging, vol. 5745, pp. 818–827 (2005)
12. Karunamuni, R., Maidment, A.: Quantification of a silver contrast agent in dual-energy breast x-ray imaging. In: Proc. SPIE Med. Imaging, pp. 1–4 (2013)

Dose-Saving Potential of Linear- and Non-Linear Energy Weighting in Photon-Counting Spectral Mammography

Udo van Stevendaal[1], Hanno Homann[1], Ewald Roessl[1],
Klaus Erhard[1], and Björn Cederström[2]

[1] Philips Technologie GmbH, Innovative Technologies,
Philips Research Laboratories,
Roentgenstrasse 24, 22335 Hamburg, Germany
udo.van.stevendaal@philips.com
[2] Philips Healthcare,
Mammography Solutions, SE-171 41 Solna, Sweden

Abstract. Energy weighting techniques are known to improve the contrast-to-noise (CNR) ratio in energy-sensitive, x-ray photon detection, in particular in the absence of scattered radiation. In spite of the rather moderate reported improvements in CNR, typically ranging between 5-10%, it is of high relevance to quantify the potential for saving radiation dose in a mammography screening environment. In this paper we experimentally investigate the possible improvements to be obtained by energy-weighting of data acquired with a Philips MicroDose SI mammography system. We compare three schemes to combine the raw data consisting of counts registered in the low- and high-energy bins, respectively: conventional summation, linear weighting and non-linear weighting of the two energy bins. Measurements on a dedicated phantom were analyzed to quantify the potential for reduction of patient dose of linear and non-linear energy weighting. By averaging improvements of CNR achieved over several pairs of regions-of-interest (ROI) we report a potential to reduce the patient dose by 7% for linear- and 9% for non-linear energy weighting, in good agreement with expectation.

Keywords: Energy weighting, digital mammography.

1 Introduction

Contrast in radiographic x-ray imaging is a strongly decreasing function of energy [1]. The acquisition of two, spectrally different attenuation measurements in the Philips MicroDose SI mammography system (see Refs. [2,3,4]) offers the possibility to give higher weight to the low energy measurement and, thus, increase the contrast in the resulting image compared to an equally (energy-)weighted summation image [5,6]. The latter is derived from the sum of the counts registered in the low- and high-energy bins. Noise limits the gains expected by this procedure, called energy-weighting. Image noise affects the low-energy bin more

H. Fujita, T. Hara, and C. Muramatsu (Eds.): IWDM 2014, LNCS 8539, pp. 103–108, 2014.

strongly than the high-energy bin. This is due to the beam-hardening effect that deprives the transmitted spectrum predominantly of low-energy photons. This effect will be most dominant for thick and/or dense breasts, when the low-energy bin will receive much fewer counts than the high-energy bin. Therefore, the gain in contrast has to be put in proportion to the increase of image noise [7]. It should be mentioned that in the MicroDose SI mammography system the thresholds are optimized depending on breast thickness and corresponding kVp setting of the scan. This compensates for the loss of low-energy counts for thicker or dense breasts.

This paper is structured in the following way: in Section 2 we outline the linear- and non-linear image weighting schemes we employed in this work. We furthermore describe the dedicated phantom scanned to investigate the contrasts and noise in various regions of different tissue composition and define the figure-of-merit (FOM) used to optimize the energy-weighting image. Note that the phantom is designed such that it almost completely covers the range of breast tissue thickness compositions which are expected in clinical practice. In Section 3 we put together the gains measured in the FOM by linear- and non-linear energy weighting. As a reference, we used the conventional "sum-image" obtained by a simple addition of counts from low- and high-energy bins. We summarize our results in Section 4 and also discuss possible shortcomings and future extensions of this approach.

2   Methods

2.1   Image Weighting Schemes

Let us denote the number of counts registered for a given detector pixel in the low- and high-energy bins by l_1 and l_2, respectively. We then choose to parameterize a non-linear combination of low-energy counts l_1 and high-energy counts l_2 in the following way [8,9]:

$$L^{NL} = Al_1 + (1 - A)l_2 + B_{11}l_1^2 + B_{12}l_1l_2 + B_{22}l_2^2, \tag{1}$$

where the double appearance of the constant A is reminiscent of the reduction of the degree of freedom related to the scaling of the image L^{NL} by a global factor. In this work we will be concerned exclusively with image combinations of the form (1). Note that in the case $B_{11} = B_{12} = B_{22} = 0$, the above equation reduces to

$$L^L = Al_1 + (1 - A)l_2, \tag{2}$$

which is the case of linear energy-weighting. When choosing $A = 1/2$, we obtain, up to scaling by a factor of 2, the case of the "sum-image" conventionally used for image presentation:

$$L^S = \frac{1}{2}(l_1 + l_2). \tag{3}$$

In order to quantify the potential improvements in image quality by energy weighting, we define the following figure-of-merit (FOM) function

$$\text{FOM}^{M}_{\mathcal{R}_1\mathcal{R}_2}(A, B_{11}, B_{12}, B_{22}) = 2\frac{(L^M_{\mathcal{R}_1} - L^M_{\mathcal{R}_2})^2}{\sigma^2_{L^M_{\mathcal{R}_1}} + \sigma^2_{L^M_{\mathcal{R}_2}}} \tag{4}$$

for each pair of regions-of-interest (ROI) $\mathcal{R}_1$ and $\mathcal{R}_2$. This FOM takes the two dominant effects of energy weighting into account, namely contrast enhancement and noise increase.

In Eq. (4) $M = S, L, NL$ stands for the weighting method used, denoting the sum-image, linear weighting and non-linear weighting, respectively. The dependence on the parameters $A, B_{11}, B_{12}, B_{22}$ is via all four terms with $\sigma^2_{L^M_{\mathcal{R}_1}}$ and $\sigma^2_{L^M_{\mathcal{R}_2}}$ denoting the noise in the weighted images in the two ROIs. The FOM defined above is given by the square of the contrast between the image values in the weighted images in the two ROIs $\mathcal{R}_1$ and $\mathcal{R}_2$ divided by the average noise variance in the two ROIs. The optimization of the parameters is based on a Nelder-Mead Simplex Algorithm.

2.2 Phantom Description

The phantom we used to evaluate the improvements in contrast-to-noise ratio (CNR) by energy-weighting consists of three main blocks each containing nine steps of aluminum (Al) heights and eight steps of polyethylene (PE) heights. The Al heights range from 0.0 to 4.0 mm in steps of 0.5 mm while the PE heights are 5.0, 10.0, 16.3, 26.3, 41.3, 56.3, 71.3 and 86.3 mm, respectively. This results in various segments with different combinations of Al and PE heights (see Figs. 1 and 2).

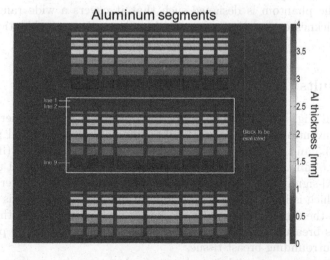

Fig. 1. Aluminum segments of the used phantom. For testing the algorithm only the central block is evaluated.

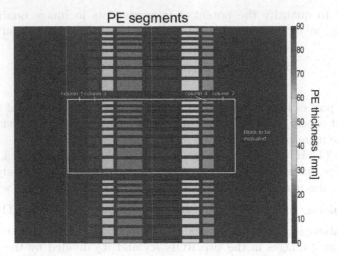

Fig. 2. Polyethylene segments of the used phantom. For testing the algorithm only the central block is evaluated.

For example, the aluminum height is the same for all segments in one row while it increases with the line number. The PE height is the same for all segments in one column. The segments of the leftmost column have the minimum height of 5 mm while the segments of the following PE height of 10 mm are in the rightmost column. The height of the PE segments increases alternatingly regarding the position of the columns.

The phantom consists of three identical blocks of Al- and PE-height combinations while only the central block is evaluated for testing the algorithm. Contrasts were optimized for regions $\mathcal{R}_1$ in one row and $\mathcal{R}_2$ located in the row below. The phantom is designed such that it covers a wide range of realistic breast thicknesses and tissue compositions by various combinations of Al and PE steps.

3 Results

Fig. 3 and Fig. 4 show the values of the optimized figure-of-merit normalized to the conventional FOM from the sum image for four selected pairs of ROIs between 3.5 and 4.0 mm Al (lines 8 and 9), 2.0 and 2.5 mm Al (lines 5 and 6), 1.0 and 1.5 mm Al (lines 3 and 4), and 0 and 0.5 mm Al (lines 1 and 2).

Each Al-signal difference is measured with additional PE material, the thickness of which is increasing with the column index. Therefore, this measurement simulates the signal difference of a lesion in a variety of breast thicknesses and in various breast compositions representing extremely dense to predominantly adipose surrounding breast tissue.

Non-linear energy weighting always produces results superior to the linear energy weighting, as an obvious consequence of Eq. (2) being contained within

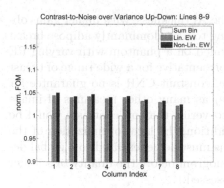
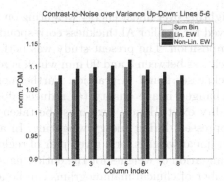

Fig. 3. Figure of merit (FOM) normalized to the sum image for comparison between Al thicknesses of 3.5 and 4.0 mm (left) and 2.0 and 2.5 mm (right)

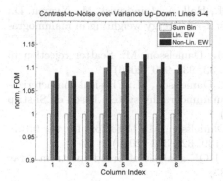
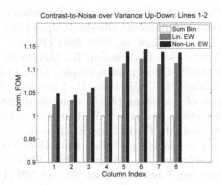

Fig. 4. Figure of merit (FOM) normalized to the sum image for comparison between Al thicknesses of 1.0 and 1.5 mm (left) and 0 and 0.5 mm (right)

the range of parameterizations of Eq. (1). As a reference, the conventional FOM from the sum image is given which is unity by definition. In quantitative terms, this means that the typical gain in FOM is 7% for linear energy weighting and 9% for non-linear energy weighting.

4 Conclusions

We verified the potential to improve CNR by means of linear, and non-linear energy weighting of energy-selective photon-counting raw data acquired in two energy bins on a MicroDose SI spectral mammography imaging unit. The improvements demonstrate well the potential of the technique to further reduce the dose delivered to the breast during digital breast x-ray examinations. Compared to an equally-weighted summation image, a dose reduction of 7% and 9% could be achieved without loss in CNR by linear and non-linear energy weighting, respectively. We noticed a dependence of the improvement from non-linear energy weighting over linear energy weighting on the Al thickness, with higher gains observed for smaller Al thickness corresponding to a predominantly adipose breast composition. The present study was performed on a phantom with varying PE thickness between 5 and 90 mm which is representative for a wide range of breast thicknesses found in practice. Furthermore, constant CNR is no guarantee for unchanged image quality (at reduced dose) as many other measures of image quality exist. Hence, care must be taken to verify, that no contrasts would be suppressed during energy weighting. In addition, the local optimization of the non-linear weights for a given pair of regions must be generalized to a global determination of weights for the entire mammogram before the quality of a larger number of clinical mammograms can be assessed.

References

1. Cahn, R.N., Cederström, B., Danielsson, M., Hall, A., Lundqvist, M., Nygren, D.: Detective quantum efficiency dependence on x-ray energy weighting in mammography. Med. Phys. 26, 2680–2683 (1999)
2. Aslund, M., Cederström, B., Lundqvist, M., Danielsson, M.: Scatter rejection in multislit digital mammography. Med. Phys. 33, 933–940 (2006)
3. Aslund, M., Cederström, B., Lundqvist, M., Danielsson, M.: Physical characterization of a scanning photon counting digital mammography system based on Si-strip detectors. Med. Phys. 34, 1918–1925 (2007)
4. Aslund, M., Fredenberg, E., Telman, M., Danielsson, M.: Detectors for the future of X-ray imaging. Radiat. Prot. Dosimetry 139, 327–333 (2010)
5. Tapiovaara, M.J., Wagner, R.F.: SNR and DQE analysis of broad spectrum x-ray imaging, Phys. Med. Biol. 30, 519–529 (1985)
6. Giersch, J., Niederlöehner, D., Anton, G.: The influence of energy weighting on X-ray imaging quality. Nucl. Instrum. Meth. Phys. Res. A 531, 68–74 (2004); Proceedings of the 5th International Workshop on Radiation Imaging Detectors
7. Wagner, R.F., Brown, D.G.: Unified SNR analysis of medical imaging systems. Phys. Med. Biol. 30, 489 (1985)
8. Niederlöhner, D., Karg, J., Giersch, J., Anton, G.: The energy weighting technique: measurements and simulations. Nucl. Instrum. Meth. Phys. Res. A 546, 37–41 (2005); Proceedings of the 6th International Workshop on Radiation Imaging Detectors
9. Shikhaliev, P.: Energy-resolved computed tomography: first experimental results. Phys. Med. Biol. 53, 5595–5613 (2008)

Compositional Three-Component Breast Imaging of Fibroadenoma and Invasive Cancer Lesions: Pilot Study

Serghei Malkov[1], Fred Duewer[1], Karla Kerlikowske[2], Karen Drukker[3], Maryellen Giger[3], and John Shepherd[1]

[1] Dept. of Radiology & Biomedical Imaging, Univ. of California at San Francisco
{Serghei.Malkov,John.Shepherd}@ucsf.edu
[2] Depts. of Medicine and Epidemiology and Biostatistics, Univ. of California at San Francisco
Karla.Kerlikowske@ucsf.edu
[3] University of Chicago, Chicago IL
{kdrukker,m-giger}@uchicago.edu

Abstract. Purpose: To investigate the lesion discrimination ability of compositional 3-component breast imaging technique (3CB) of patients with suspicious breast lesions (BIRADS 4 or greater).

Materials and Methods: A novel dual-energy 3CB imaging technique concludes in quantifying of the lipid, protein, and water thicknesses. The protocol was designed to be performed on a standard full-field digital mammography system by imaging additional high-energy image using a 3-mm Al filter. A pilot study of 43 abnormal breast findings on diagnostic mammography was performed using the 3CB protocol. The lesion groups include fibroadenoma (FA), invasive (IDC), DCIS and benign tissues. The lesions were delineated by the radiologist on CC and MLO views, and the compositional measures of the whole breasts, local areas within lesions and their peripheries were derived. Univariate logistic regression statistics was applied to analyze lesion different group separation. The variable statistical significance of MLO, CC views and their average was also compared.

Results: We found for FA/rest group discrimination that water and lipid difference between lesion and periphery are significant for CC and MLO views. In addition, the breast fibroglandular dense volume are also significant for both views. Lesion to background water difference predicted FA with an odds ratio = 4.4 , ROC area of 0.8. For cancer/non cancer groups there were no variables showing the significance for both views. However, for IDC/rest groups lipid thicknesses within breast and at the periphery normalized by total thicknesses become significant for both views.

Conclusion: Our pilot set data demonstrates that the technique provides biologically meaningful compositional components of lesion, its periphery and breast which are statistically significant for FA/rest and invasive cancers/rest group separation.

Keywords: Breast composition, dual energy digital mammography, cancer lesion, logistic regression.

H. Fujita, T. Hara, and C. Muramatsu (Eds.): IWDM 2014, LNCS 8539, pp. 109–114, 2014.
© Springer International Publishing Switzerland 2014

1   Introduction

X-ray mammography is the primary technique for breast cancer screening, its early detection and diagnostics. However, mammography has some limitations especially for breasts with dense tissue. As only 20% of biopsies are breast cancer, finding a way to avoid biopsies would make an important impact in terms of reducing unnecessary biopsies. We propose to improve the utility of quantitative imaging analysis (QIA) programs for mammography by increasing the number of invasive cancers diagnosed without increasing the harms to women through unnecessary additional imaging and biopsies. To advance CAD/QIA methods, biologically-relevant information is needed from the breast image. We are developing novel mammographic biomarkers, lipid-protein-water signatures [1], to determine if composition alone or combined with an established and validated CAD/QIA methods can improve the diagnostic accuracy of imaging, and reduce the number of unnecessary biopsies. Invasive cancers are expected to show high degrees of vascularity. Because vasculature structures and other tissue components are expected to differ in elemental composition, compositional information from imaging is expected to provide information that may be used to determine whether a tissue is benign or malignant. Moreover, some compositional measurements of ex-vivo breast tissues demonstrate the existance of unique signature of lesion water, lipid and protein content helpful for lesion type discrimination. The purpose of this paper is to investigate the lesion discrimination ability of a compositional 3-component breast imaging technique (3CB) for patients with suspicious breast lesions. We present in vivo results of compositional properties of women with fibroadenama and invasive lesion types.

2   Methods

2.1   Datasets

All selected participants were women with a BIRADS diagnostic category of 4 or greater who were scheduled to receive a biopsy. They were recruited and imaged with the 3BC technique before their biopsies. We use the following exclusion criteria: failure to receive a biopsy, known prior breast cancer, known prior biopsies, protocol failure, inability of our radiologist to identify the breast lesion by mammography, inability to schedule additional imaging prior to biopsy. Breast biopsies were clinically reviewed by our Pathology Department. The lesions were delineated by the radiologist on CC and MLO views, and the compositional measures of the whole breasts, local areas within lesions and their peripheries were derived. In all, there were 43 lesions that satisfied our quality control procedure. All women were imaged using the 3CB protocol. The lesion were classified into four groups: fibroadenoma (FA, n=11), Invasive (IDC, n=9), ductal carcinoma in situ (DCIS, n=5), benign lesions (n=18).

2.2   Method Description

The dual-energy 3CB imaging protocol was designed to be performed on a standard full-field digital mammography system by imaging additional high-energy image using a 3-mm Al filter [2]. The dual-energy X-ray attenuations along with an accurate measure of breast thickness for each pixel provided the means to solve for three unknown materials in the breast. We chose to represent the breast as its molecular compartments of lipid, water, and protein. In more detail, we measured the x-ray attenuation in a standard screening mammography image, the x-ray attenuation in a high energy/low dose mammography image, and modeled thickness using phantom. Then individual thickness compositional maps were extracted by multiple linear regression analysis. We used a single Hologic Selenia full-field digital mammography system (Hologic, Inc., Bedford, MA). The first exposure was made under the regular clinical screening mammogram conditions. The second mammogram was acquired at a 39 kVp/Rh filter combination. An additional 3-mm thick X-ray filter was placed in the beam. The total dose of this procedure to be approximately 10% more than of average screening mammography. Regions containing calcifications, the chest wall, or the breast edge were excluded. The breast edge was defined as the region within one-quarter of the estimated median breast thickness. Three composition maps as an example of the method output are presented at Fig. 1.

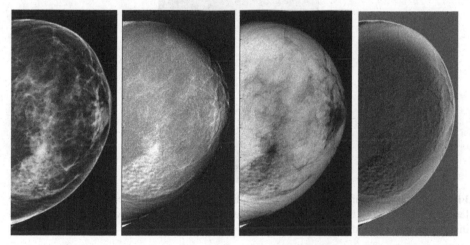

Fig. 1. The method output images from the left to the right: mammogramm, water, lipid, and protein maps

2.3   Variables and Statistics

The lesion compositions were reported as the pixel component thicknesses divided by the total pixel thicknesses averaged within deliniated region (dROIx) where x means

W, L and P for water, thickness and protein respectively. The background compositions were reported as the pixel component thicknesses divided by the total pixel thicknesses averaged in a region of interest 0 to 2.5 mm from the lesion edge (dBCK1x). We use absolute composition thicknesses of lesion (ROIx) and background (BCK1x), and lesion area (ROIA). In addition, the composional differences between lesion and background (tdifROIx = ROIx – BCK1x) were estimated. Fig. 2 demonstrates an example of the mammogram image of the patient diagnosed with IDC. The central part delineation is the lesion boundary drawn by radiologist. Other three delineation lines are located at 2.5 mm equal distance from the boundary. The area between lesion boundary and the further first line characterizes the background. Alongside with local measures, global lesion compositions such as the pixel component thicknesses divide by total pixel thickness averaged for the whole breast (dBreastx) were reported. Other breast measures used in analysis were percent fibroglandular volume (%FGV), fibroglandular tissue volume (FGV) and absolute breast volume (Volume). Univariate logistic regression statistics were applied to analyze the lesion into different groups. The variable statistical significance of MLO, CC views and their averages were also compared. Threshold level of significance was chosen as p-value < 0.05.

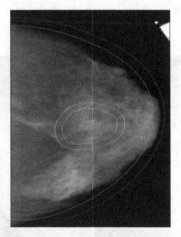

Fig. 2. The mammogram image of the patient diagnosed with IDC. The central part line is the lesion boundary drawn by radiologist. Other three delineation lines are located at 2.5 mm equal distance from the boundary and each other.

3   Results

Table 1 represents odds ratios, ROC areas and p-values of FA/rest group discrimation obtained by univariate logistic regression analysis. Only variables significant (p < 0.05) for one of CC or MLO views are shown. As can be seen, the difference between lesion and background for water and lipid components tdifROIW and tdifROIL were significant for both views. Lesion water tdifROIW parameter predicted FA with an odds ratio = 4.4 , ROC area of 0.8 for average of MLO and CC views. Lesion lipid tdifROIL parameter predicted FA with an odds ratio = 0.31, ROC area of 0.72 for average of MLO and CC views. FGV was also significant for both views with an odds ratio of 2 and ROC area of 0.65. In addtion, lesion area ROIA and protein at the periphery BCK1P are significant for one of veiws and their average. The Table 2 shows odds ratios, ROC areas and p-values of cancer (IDC + DCIS)/rest and IDC/rest group discrimation. As can be seen, no one cancer variable showed significance for both views. At the same time, background water dBCK1W, lipid dBCK1L and %FGV demonstrate significance for one of veiws and their average. But for IDC/ rest separation we can observe two variables: differential lipid lesion dROIL and background dBCK1L which became significant for both views. Other variables which are significant for IDC/rest group are lesion water dBCK1W, breast water dBreastW and lipid dBreastL thicknesses.

Thus, FA/rest group shows the best performance of composition component univariate analysis. The lesion lipid, water and breast dense tissue demonstrated significance. As this is only pilot study with limited number of lesions the more robust study is necessary to exclude random contribution and noise influence. But if we observe the variable for both views it is more likely that we have less probability of random contribution, artifacts or noise. It should be noted that IDC alone demonstrates better results than together with DCIS. The lipid content of lesion and background is found to drive IDC cancer separation from the rest of lesions. In contrary to IDC, the difference between ROI and periphery for lipid and water plays the main role for FA/rest group discrimation.

Table 1. Odds ratios, ROC areas and p-values of FA/rest groups

Effect	CC Views			MLO Views			CC and MLO view averages		
	Odds Ratio	ROC Area	Pr > Chi-Square	Odds Ratio	ROC Area	Pr > Chi-Square	Odds Ratio	ROC Area	Pr > Chi-Square
dBCK1W	0.464	0.699	0.069	0.418	0.692	0.077	0.421	0.703	0.066
tdifROIW	4.610	0.761	**0.009**	2.834	0.749	**0.021**	4.409	0.797	**0.005**
tdifROIL	0.319	0.710	**0.017**	0.355	0.747	**0.015**	0.309	0.719	**0.013**
ROIA	1.871	0.588	0.069	2.440	0.647	**0.024**	2.226	0.636	**0.035**
BCK1P	2.164	0.707	**0.041**	2.009	0.678	0.075	2.083	0.709	**0.047**
FGV	2.008	0.641	**0.049**	2.036	0.649	**0.043**	2.042	0.646	**0.041**
Volume	1.825	0.666	0.089	1.866	0.674	0.077	1.864	0.670	0.075

Table 2. Odds ratios, ROC areas and p-values of cancer/rest and IDC/rest groups

Effect	CC Views			MLO Views			CC and MLO view average		
	Odds Ratio	ROC Area	Pr > Chi-Square	Odds Ratio	ROC Area	Pr > Chi-Square	Odds Ratio	ROC Area	Pr > Chi-Square
dROIW (cancer)	2.508	0.709	**0.026**	1.416	0.548	0.303	1.903	0.622	0.081
dROIW (IDC)	2.910	0.742	**0.022**	1.921	0.597	0.104	2.384	0.671	**0.040**
dROIL (cancer)	0.555	0.611	0.087	0.631	0.619	0.171	0.564	0.622	0.086
dROIL (IDC)	0.456	0.683	**0.043**	0.428	0.727	**0.036**	0.393	0.720	**0.019**
dBCK1W (cancer)	3.112	0.749	**0.012**	1.743	0.614	0.129	2.382	0.693	**0.034**
dBCK1W (IDC)	2.965	0.765	**0.019**	1.975	0.618	0.089	2.403	0.689	**0.036**
dBCK1L (cancer)	0.496	0.675	**0.043**	0.525	0.650	0.062	0.495	0.667	**0.039**
dBCK1L (IDC)	0.473	0.709	**0.042**	0.424	0.724	**0.028**	0.412	0.740	**0.019**
BCK1W (cancer)	3.277	0.746	**0.022**	1.290	0.557	0.452	2.103	0.671	0.057
BCK1W (IDC)	2.081	0.745	0.102	1.348	0.565	0.432	1.702	0.657	0.186
dBreastW (cancer)	1.724	0.650	0.114	1.924	0.626	0.067	1.912	0.633	0.066
dBreastW (IDC)	2.104	0.686	**0.049**	2.033	0.621	0.057	2.267	0.649	**0.033**
dBreastL (cancer)	0.622	0.579	0.144	0.531	0.660	0.061	0.559	0.618	0.073
dBreastL (IDC)	0.565	0.628	0.100	0.471	0.718	**0.036**	0.472	0.709	**0.031**
%FGV (cancer)	1.676	0.621	0.118	2.057	0.676	**0.035**	1.935	0.656	**0.047**
%FGV (IDC)	1.656	0.636	0.156	1.962	0.675	0.056	1.981	0.677	0.051

4   Conclusions

In conclusion, our pilot study demonstrates that multiple compositional compartments are independent associated with fibroadenomas and invasive cancers. The combination of these biologically-relevant compartments may provide additional information to mammograms and lower the risk of unnecessary biopsies.

References

1. Laidevant, A.D., Malkov, S., Flowers, C.I., Kerlikowske, K., Shepherd, J.A.: Compositional breast imaging using a dual-energy mammography protocol. Med. Phys. 37(1), 164–174 (2010)
2. Laidevant, A., Malkov, S., Au, A., Shepherd, J.A.: Dual-Energy X-Ray Absorptiometry Method Using a Full Field Digital Mammography System. In: Krupinski, E.A. (ed.) IWDM 2008. LNCS, vol. 5116, pp. 108–115. Springer, Heidelberg (2008)

Potential Usefulness of Presentation of Histological Classifications with Computer-Aided Diagnosis (CAD) Scheme in Differential Diagnosis of Clustered Microcalcifications on Mammograms

Ryohei Nakayama[1], Kiyoshi Namba[2], Ryoji Watanabe[3], Hiroshi Nakahara[4], and Ralph Smathers[5]

[1] Department of Radiology, Mie University School of Medicine,
2-174 Edobashi, Tsu, 514-8507, Japan
nakayama@clin.medic.mie-u.ac.jp
[2] Center for Breast Diseases and Breast Cancer, Hokuto Hospital and Clinic,
7-5 Inadachokisen, Obihiro, 080-0833, Japan
dreamnamba@me.com
[3] Department of Breast Surgery, Hakuaikai Hospital,
1-28-25 Sasaoka, Fukuoka, 810-0034, Japan
watanabe@hakuaikai.or.jp
[4] Breastopia Namba Hospital, 2-112-1 Maruyama, Miyazaki, 800-0052, Japan
nakahara@breastopia.org
[5] Mammography Specialists Medical Group,
14651 South Bascom Avenue, Suite 210 Los Gatos, CA 95032
rs@mammo.net

Abstract. We compared the usefulness of the presentation of likelihood of histological classifications with that of malignancy evaluated by a CAD scheme in the differential diagnosis of clustered microcalcifications (MCs) on magnified spot mammograms. The likelihood of histological classifications was evaluated by the CAD scheme using 5 objective features that radiologists commonly use for describing MCs. The likelihood of malignancy was evaluated based on the likelihood of histological classifications. Unknown cases for an observer study consisted of 22 benign MCs (15 micro-cysts and 7 mastopathies) and 26 malignant MCs (10 DCISs of comedo type and 16 DCISs of noncomedo type). Thirteen observers independently provided their confidence level regarding the malignancy of the unknown case before viewing the evaluated result by the CAD scheme, after viewing the likelihood of malignancy and after viewing the likelihood of histological classifications. The results were evaluated with multi-reader, multi-case receiver operating characteristic (ROC) analysis. The average area under the curve (AUC) for all observers without CAD, with CAD for malignancy and with CAD for histological calcifications was 0.670, 0.802 and 0.819 ($P < .01$), respectively. The presentation of the likelihood of histological classifications improved radiologists' performance than that of malignancy in the differential diagnosis of MCs.

H. Fujita, T. Hara, and C. Muramatsu (Eds.): IWDM 2014, LNCS 8539, pp. 115–120, 2014.
© Springer International Publishing Switzerland 2014

Keywords: Computer-aided Diagnosis, Clustered Microcalcifications, Magnified spot mammogram.

1   Introduction

Computer-aided diagnosis (CAD) is one of the solutions for improving radiologists' performance [1]. The usefulness of the CAD scheme for distinguishing between benign and malignant lesions at mammography has been shown on many studies. Jiang *et al.* conducted the observer studies for distinguishing between benign and malignant MCs with and without the computer output indicating the likelihood of malignancy. The AUC was thus found to increase from 0.61 to 0.75 by the computer aid ($P < .0001$) [2]. Timps et al. showed the radiologists' performances to improve significantly ($P < .05$) when they used the computer output for the characterization of benign and malignant masses on mammograms using a temporal change analysis [3].

In differential diagnosis on medical images such as X-ray image, CT image and MR image, experienced radiologists usually take into account the histopathological images associated with a lesion. To reduce the number of unnecessary biopsies, clinical decisions for biopsy or follow-up on clustered microcalcifications are also made by taking into account possible histological classifications on magnification mammograms [4,5]. Therefore, the computerized analysis of lesions in determining not only the likelihood of malignancy but also the likelihood of histological classifications may be helpful to radiologists for their decisions on patient management. We have developed a CAD scheme for determining the histological classification of MCs on mammograms based on the approach employed for clinical diagnosis [6]. Our CAD scheme can evaluate the likelihood of micro-cysts, mastopathies, DCISs of comedo type and DCISs of noncomedo type when analyzing MCs on magnified spot digital mammograms. In this study, we compared the usefulness of the presentation of the likelihood of histological classifications with that of malignancy evaluated by the CAD scheme in the differential diagnosis of MCs.

2   Materials

Our database consisted of 48 regions of interest (ROIs) with MCs which were obtained at Hokuto breast cancer center from May 2011 to March 2013. It included 22 benign MCs (15 micro-cysts and 7 mastopathies) and 26 malignant MCs (10 DCISs of comedo type and 16 DCISs of noncomedo type). These images were obtained from 48 patients using a digital mammography system (Senographe DS, GE Healthcare). All cases had already been pathologically proven.

3   Method

In our CAD scheme, individual microcalcifications were first segmented by use of a novel filter bank and a thresholding technique [7]. Five objective features on MCs were determined by taking into account subjective features that experienced radiologists commonly use to identify possible histological classifications. These objective features were: (1) the variation in the size of microcalcifications within a cluster, (2) the variation in pixel values of microcalcifications within a cluster, (3) the irregularity measure in the shape of microcalcifications within a cluster, (4) the extent of linear and branching distribution of microcalcifications, and (5) the distribution of microcalcifications in the direction toward the nipple. The Bayes decision rule with five objective features was employed for distinguishing between four histological classifications. The classification accuracies of the CAD scheme based on the leave-one-out testing method for the 48 MCs were 86.6% (13/15) for micro-cysts, 71.4% (5/7) for mastopathies, 70.0% (7/10) for DCISs of comedo type, and 81.3% (13/16) for DCISs of noncomedo type, respectively. The sensitivity and the specificity based on the classification results of the histological classification were 86.3% (19/22) and 84.6% (22/26), respectively.

3.1   Observer Study

In the observer study for comparing the usefulness of the presentation of the likelihood of histological classifications with that of malignancy evaluated by the CAD scheme in the differential diagnosis of MCs, an unknown image was first displayed in the center of monitor, as shown in Fig.1. The observer was then asked to mark his or her confidence level regarding the malignancy of the unknown case on a continuous rating scale from 0 to 1 corresponding "definitely benign" and "definitely malignant", respectively. The likelihood of malignancy for the unknown case evaluated by the CAD scheme was then displayed after the observer marked the initial confidence level. The observer was asked again to mark his or her confidence level. The likelihood of histological classifications for the unknown case evaluated by the CAD scheme was displayed after the observer marked the second confidence level. The observer was asked again to mark his or her confidence level. Thirteen radiologists independently participated in the observer study.

The observers were instructed that: 1) The purpose of this study is to compare the usefulness of the presentation of the likelihood of histological classifications with that of malignancy evaluated by a CAD scheme in distinguishing between benign and malignant MCs on magnified spot digital mammograms. 2) You are asked to provide your confidence level regarding the malignancy (or benignity) of MCs on a bar using a mouse first, and then the system shows the evaluated likelihood of malignancy and histological classifications. You are asked to provide your confidence levels again after viewing the estimated likelihood of malignancy and after viewing the estimated likelihood of histological classifications. 3) Forty eight unknown cases are included in this study. 4) There is no time limit.

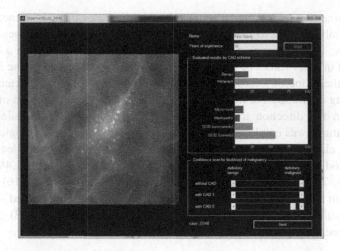

Fig. 1. Observer interface for obtaining observer's confidence level regarding the malignancy of the unknown case before viewing the evaluated result by the CAD scheme, after viewing the likelihood of malignancy, and after viewing the likelihood of histological classifications based on the ROC analysis

3.2   Statistical Analysis

A receiver operating characteristic (ROC) with a sequential-test method [8,9] was employed to compare the usefulness of the presentation of the likelihood of histological classifications with that of malignancy evaluated by the CAD scheme in distinguishing between benign and malignant MCs. The areas under the ROC curve (AUCs) and the 95% confidence intervals were obtained by using the DBM MRMC software package [10,11] that was developed by researchers at the University of Iowa and the University of Chicago. The significances of the differences in the AUCs between observers readings performed without CAD, with CAD for malignancy and with CAD for histological classifications were tested with the Dorfman-Berbaum-Metz method [10,11]. A p-value of less than .05 was considered to indicate a significant difference. The study also assumed that the computer output had either a beneficial or detrimental effect on an observer's diagnosis when the change between the average confidence levels with and without CAD was greater than 0.1.

4   Result

All observers' performances in the differential diagnosis were improved when the CAD scheme was available. Those with CAD for histological classifications were greater than those for malignancy. Figure 2 shows the average ROC curves for all observers in distinguishing between benign and malignant MCs without and with CADs. The average AUCs for all observers without CAD, with CAD for malignancy, and with CAD for histological calcifications was 0.670, 0.802, and 0.819, respectively.

The differences between AUCs without CAD and with CAD for malignancy, between AUCs without CAD and with CAD for histological classifications, and between AUCs with CADs for malignancy and for histological classifications were statistically significant ($P = .0001, .0001$, and $.0062$).

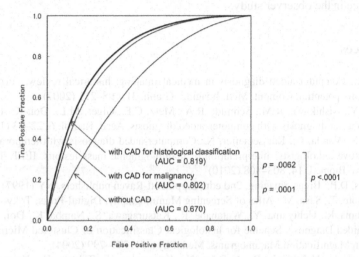

Fig. 2. Comparison of ROC curves for the average performance of 13 radiologists in distinction between benign and malignant clustered microcalcifications without and with CAD schemes

5   Discussion

This study assumed that the computer output had either a beneficial or detrimental effect on an observer's diagnosis when the change between the average confidence levels with and without CAD was greater than 0.1. In the CAD scheme for malignancy, the number of cases with beneficial effects in the average confidence level was 17, whereas the number showing detrimental effects was 3. In the CAD scheme for histological classification, on the other hand, those with beneficial effects in the average confidence level was 21, whereas the number showing detrimental effects was 3. The number of cases with beneficial effects in the CAD scheme for histological classification was greater than those in the CAD scheme for malignancy.

There are some limitations in this study. One limitation is that the CAD scheme used for this study can evaluate the likelihood of only four histological classifications (micro-cysts, mastopathies, DCISs of comedo type and DCISs of noncomedo type) of MCs. It is necessary to make the CAD scheme available for the other histological classifications of MCs in the further study. Another limitation is that we used ROIs instead of whole images as unknown cases in the observer study. However, although the radiologists' performance may be improved by use of the whole image, we believe that the conclusion in this study would not be changed.

6   Conclusion

The presentation of the likelihood of the histological classification evaluated by the CAD scheme showed beneficial effects for most cases, and it improved the clinicians' performance in the observer study.

References

1. Doi, K.: Computer-aided diagnosis in medical imaging: historical review, current status and future potential. Comput. Med. Imaging. Graph. 31, 198–211 (2007)
2. Jiang, Y., Nishikawa, R.M., Schmidt, R.A., Metz, C.E., Giger, M.L., Doi, K.: Improving breast cancer diagnosis with computer-aided diagnosis. Acad. Radiol. 6, 22–33 (1999)
3. Timp, S., Varela, C., Karssemeijer, N.: Computer-aided diagnosis with temporal analysis to improve radiologists' interpretation of mammographic mass lesions. IEEE Trans. Inf. Technol. Biomed. 14, 803–808 (2010)
4. Kopans, D.B.: Breast imaging, 2nd edn. Lippincott-Raven publishers, NY (1997)
5. Morimoto, T., Sasa, M.: Atlas of Screening Mammography. Digital-Press, Tokyo (1996)
6. Nakayama, R., Uchiyama, Y., Watanabe, R., Katsuragawa, S., Namba, K., Doi, K.: Computer-aided Diagnosis Scheme for histological Classification of Clustered Microcalcifications on Magnification Mammograms. Med. Phys. 31, 789–799 (2004)
7. Hizukuri, A., Nakayama, R., Nakako, N., Kawanaka, H., Takase, H., Yamamoto, K., Tsuruoka, S.: Computerized segmentation method for individual calcifications within clustered microcalcifications while maintaining their shapes on magnification mammograms. J. Digit. Imaging. 25, 377–386 (2012)
8. Kobayashi, T., Xu, X.W., MacMahon, H., Metz, C.E., Doi, K.: Effect of a computer-aided diagnosis scheme on radiologists' performance in detection of lung nodules on radiographs. Radiology 199, 843–848 (1996)
9. Uozumi, T., Nakamura, K., Watanabe, H., Nakata, H., Katsuragawa, S., Doi, K.: ROC analysis of detection of metastatic pulmonary nodules on digital chest radiographs with temporal subtraction. Acad. Radiol. 8, 871–878 (2001)
10. Dorfman, D.D., Berbaum, K.S., Metz, C.E.: Receiver operating characteristic rating analysis. Generalization to the population of readers and patients with the jackknife method. Invest. Radiol. 27, 723–731 (1992)
11. Hillis, S.L., Berbaum, K.S., Metz, C.E.: Recent developments in the Dorfman-Berbaum-Metz procedure for multireader ROC study analysis. Acad. Radiol. 15, 647–661 (2008)

Potential Usefulness of Breast Radiographers' Reporting as a Second Opinion for Radiologists' Reading in Digital Mammography

Rie Tanaka[1,*], Miho Takamori[2], Yoshikazu Uchiyama[3], and Junji Shiraishi[3]

[1] School of Health Sciences, College of Medical, Pharmaceutical and Health Sciences, Kanazawa University, Kanazawa, Japan
rie44@mhs.mp.kanazawa-u.ac.jp
[2] Department of Radiology, Ishikawa Prefectural Hospital, Kanazawa, Japan
tanpoppo2006@yahoo.co.jp
[3] Faculty of Life Sciences, Kumamoto University, Kumamoto, Japan
{j2s,y_uchi}@kumamoto-u.ac.jp

Abstract. We investigated a potential usefulness of breast radiographers' reporting, in terms of a second opinion for improving radiologists' diagnostic performance in the detection of microcalcifications in digital mammography. This simulation study was conducted, by use of an existing jackknife free-response receiver operating characteristic (JAFROC) observer study data obtained with 75 cases(25 malignant, 25 benign, and 25 normal cases) of digital mammogram, selected form the digital database for screening mammography (DDSM) provided by University of South Florida. Each of rating scores obtained by 6 breast radiographers was utilized as a second opinion for 4 radiologists' reading with radiographers' reporting. Average figure of merit (FOM) of radiologists' performance was generally improved by use of radiographer's reporting, and significant improvements were found in case of 3 out of 6 radiographers' reporting used.

Keywords: Radiographer reporting, digital mammography, microcalcification, observer study, jackknife free-response receiver operating characteristic (JAFROC).

1 Introduction

The number of mammogram exams has been increasing, and thus, the reading time of radiologist becomes a major concern in screening mammography. The use of computer-aided diagnosis (CAD) system would be expected as one solution for this problem. In fact, many research groups have demonstrated the clinical usefulness of various CADs and they led a common use of CADs in the US [1-3]. On the other hand, as another approach to aid radiologists' reading, utilization of radiographers' reporting (RR) as a second opinion has been recommended in a number of countries [4-7].

---

* Corresponding author.

H. Fujita, T. Hara, and C. Muramatsu (Eds.): IWDM 2014, LNCS 8539, pp. 121–126, 2014.
© Springer International Publishing Switzerland 2014

However, a few studies have been reported for investigating the method to utilize RR in radiologists' interpletations, and for demonstrating the evidence of the clinical utility of RR. The aim of this study is to investigate a practical methodology and potential usefulness of breast radiographers' reporting by use of an existing free-response receiver operating characteristic (FROC) observer study data set.

2   Materials and Methods

This simulation study was conducted by use of an existing free-response receiver operating characteristic (FROC) observer study data set [8], which was obtained with 75 digital mammograms and performed for comparing diagnostic performances between radiologists and breast radiographers. Each of rating scores obtained by 6 breast radiographers was utilized as a second opinion for 4 radiologists' reading with radiographer's report (RR). The radiologists' rating with RR was simulated by combining each of rating scores obtained by a radiologist and a breast radiographer, as described later. Average figure of merit (FOM) of radiologists' performance was statistically analyzed by using jackknife free-response receiver operating characteristic (JAFROC) to verify the effectiveness of RR.

2.1   Dataset

We used 50 digital mammograms with microcalcifications (25 malignant and 25 benign) and 25 normal cases, which were selected from The Digital Database for Screening Mammography (DDSM) provided by University of South Florida (USF) [9, 10].

2.2   Observer Study

Digital mammograms were displayed on a high resolution liquid crystal display (LCD) for mammography (Nio 5M, BARCO) and observed by using a publically available computer interface (ROC Viewer ver 11.4.0.3 developed by Japanese Society of Radiological Technology) [11].

FROC observer study was conducted by 10 observers (4 board-certified radiologists/breast surgeons and 6 board-certified breast radiographers) for detection of malignant microcalcifications. Observers determined the locations and confidence ratings on 75 digital mammograms (4 images /case, R-MLO, L-MLO, R-CC, L-CC). The observers provided written informed consent regarding use of results obtained from the observer study prior to participation.

2.3   Simulation of Radiologists' Rating with Radiographers' Rating

Radiologists' ratings with RR were simulated by combining each rating score of radiologists with those of radiographers, and utilized for JAFROC analysis. Figure 1 shows examples for producing radiologist's rating scores with RR by using the rules employed in this simulation study. In the initial step of combination, a lesion marked by both radiologist and radiographer with a distance less than 20 mm was considered to be the same lesion. If a lesion was marked by both radiologist and radiographer, one mark with higher rating was remained as a rating score with RR (A < A' → A''). If a lesion was marked only by either a radiographer or a radiologist, the mark was remained as a rating score with RR only if the rating was higher than pre-determined threshold value (i.e. 0.20) (B → B'', D→ D''). On the other hand, if a lesion was marked only by either a radiologist or a radiologist with a low rating less than pre-determined threshold value (i.e. 0.20), the mark was rejected in a rating score with RR (C → rejected). In order to investigate the effect of improvement in radiologists' performance, we changed threshold values for the mark selection from 0.1 to 0.5, in increments of 0.1.

| Radiographer's Report (RR) | Radiologist's Rating without RR | Radiologist's Rating with RR |

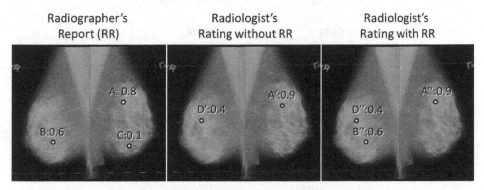

Fig. 1. Example of selections of responses for simulated radiologist's rating with radiographer's reporting (RR)

2.4   Statistical Analysis

Statistical analysis was performed by using JAFROC ver. 4.2, provided by Chakraborty DP et al [8]. Figure of merit (FOM) was calculated as a measure of diagnostic accuracy for the detection of malignant microcalcifications. Average FOM of 4 radiologists' performance with/without RR was statistically analyzed by JAFROC Analysis 3 (Random Readers and Fixed Cases) with one-tailed test (p=0.05).

3   Results and Discussion

Average value of figure of merit (FOM) of radiologists' performance was generally improved by use of radiographer's reporting (Fig. 2), in most of combinations of radiologists and radiographers (Table 1, 2, 3). These results indicated that radiographer's reporting could be used as a second opinion in case of readings of microcalcifications on digital mammography. Significant improvements were found in case of 3 out of 6 radiographers' reporting used (Table 4). In particular, radiologists' performance was significantly improved by using highly skilled radiographers' RR, with high FOM or low FP. When the threshold value of 0.2 was applied, radiologists' performance showed the highest level (Fig. 3). It could be more effective to set criteria for use of rating score provide by radiographers as a second opinion.

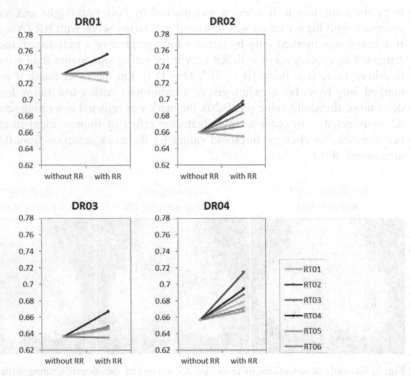

Fig. 2. Change of the figure of merit (FOM) of radiologists' performance with and without each of 6 radiographers' reporting (RR)

Table 1. Diagnostic performances of 4 radiologists without radiographer's reporting (RR) for the detection of microcalcifications

	FOM	TP	Sensitivity	FP	FP [/case]
DR01	0.7316	16	64%	40	0.53
DR02	0.6596	17	68%	79	1.05
DR03	0.6364	12	48%	26	0.35
DR04	0.6568	16	64%	92	1.23
Average	0.6711	15.25	61%	59.25	0.79

Table 2. Diagnostic performances of 6 radiographers for the detection of microcalcifications

	FOM	TP	Sensitivity	FP	FP [/case]
RT01	0.6816	15	60%	41	0.55
RT02	0.7244	19	76%	81	1.08
RT03	0.6364	10	40%	21	0.28
RT04	0.6884	16	64%	44	0.59
RT05	0.6788	14	56%	26	0.35
RT06	0.6680	18	72%	57	0.76
Average	0.6796	15.33	61%	45.00	0.60

Table 3. Average diagnostic performances of 4 radiologists for the detection of microcalcifications by using each of 6 radiographers' reporting (RR)

	FOM	TP	Sensitivity	FP	FP [/case]
RT01	0.6797	15.25	61%	88.25	1.18
RT02	0.6983	16.00	64%	129.00	1.72
RT03	0.6838	15.50	62%	84.50	1.13
RT04	0.7027	16.25	65%	79.75	1.06
RT05	0.6750	15.25	61%	70.00	0.93
RT06	0.6808	15.75	63%	109.25	1.46
Average	0.6867	15.67	63%	93.46	1.25

Table 4. FOM of 4 radiologists with and without each of 6 radiographers' reporting (RR) at the threshold value of 0.2

	without RR	with RR					
		RT01	RT02	RT03	RT04	RT05	RT06
DR01	0.7316	0.7220	0.7328	0.7316	0.7556	0.7312	0.7332
DR02	0.6596	0.6820	0.7032	0.6836	0.7000	0.6700	0.6916
DR03	0.6364	0.6508	0.6536	0.6536	0.6719	0.6516	0.6352
DR04	0.6568	0.7060	0.7104	0.6756	0.6996	0.7088	0.6784
Average	0.6711	0.6902	0.7000	0.6861	0.7068	0.6904	0.6846
P value		0.1066	0.0477	0.0318	0.0017	0.0942	0.0948

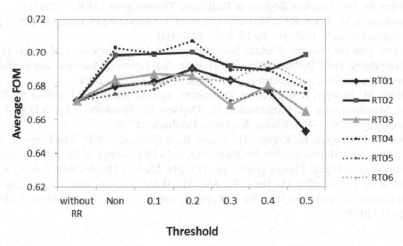

Fig. 3. Relationship between the threshold value for cut-off rating values and average FOM of radiologists with radiographers' reporting

4   Conclusions

We investigated a potential usefulness of breast radiographers' reporting by use of JAFROC analysis employing existing observer study data set. In conclusion, an appropriate use of radiographer's reporting would be useful as a second opinion for improving radiologists' diagnostic performance in the detection of microcalcifications in digital mammography. In order to address clinical effectiveness, further studies for investigating improvements of radiologists' performances with the selected radiographers' reporting determined in this study would be required.

Acknowledgment. This study was partially supported by Foundation for Promotion of Cancer Research.

References

1. Giger, M.L., Karssemeijer, N., Armato III, S.G.: Computer-aided diagnosis in medical imaging. IEEE Trans. Med. Imag. 20, 1205–1208 (2001)
2. Doi, K., MacMahon, H., Katsuragawa, S., Nishikawa, R.M., Jiang, Y.: Computer-aided diagnosis in radiology: potential and pitfalls. Eur. J. Radiol. 31, 97–109 (1999)
3. Vyborny, C.J., Giger, M.L., Nishikawa, R.M.: Computer-aided detection and diagnosis of breast cancer. Radiologic Clinics of North America 38, 725–740 (2000)
4. Radiologist Assistant: Roles and Responsibilities. ACR ASRT Joint Policy Statement (2003)
5. Registered Radiologist Assistant (R.R.A.) In: Certification Handbook and Application Materials, The American Registry of Radiologic Technologists (ARRT) (2003)
6. Paterson, A.M., Price, R.C., Thomas, A., Nuttall, L.: Reporting by radiographers: a policy and practice guide. Radiography 10, 205–212 (2004)
7. Report from the ministry of health, labor and welfare, http://www.mhlw.go.jp
8. Chakraborty, D.P., Berbaum, K.S.: Observer studies involving detection and localization: modeling, analysis, and validation. Med. Phys. 31, 2313–2330 (2004)
9. Heath, M., Bowyer, K.W., Kopans, D.: Current status of the Digital Database for Screening Mammography. In: Karssemeijer, N., Thijssen, M., Hendriks, J. (eds.) Digital Mammography, pp. 457–460. Kluwer Academic, Dordrecht (1998)
10. Heath, M., Bowyer, K., Kopans, D., Moore, R., Kegelmeyer, W.P.: The Digital Database for Screening Mammography. In: Yaffe, M.J. (ed.) Proceedings of the Fifth International Workshop on Digital Mammography, pp. 212–218. Medical Physics Publishing (2001)
11. Shiraishi, J., Fukuoka, D., Hara, T., Abe, H.: Basic concepts and development of an all-purpose computer interface for ROC/FROC observer study. Radiol. Phys. Technol. 6, 35–41 (2013)

Effective Detective Quantum Efficiency (eDQE) Measured for a Digital Breast Tomosynthesis System

Nicholas Marshall, Elena Salvagnini, and Hilde Bosmans

KU Leuven, Department of Imaging and Pathology, Division of Medical Physics and Quality Assessment, Herestraat 49, 3000 Leuven, Belgium
{nicholas.marshall,elena.salvagnini,hilde.bosmans}@uzleuven.be

Abstract. This paper presents effective detective quantum efficiency (eDQE) results for a digital breast tomosynthesis (DBT) system. Poly(methyl methacrylate) (PMMA) blocks of thickness 2, 4, 6 and 7 cm were imaged under automatic exposure control (AEC) in standard 2D digital (planar) mammography (with anti-scatter grid) and DBT mode (without anti-scatter grid). Modulation transfer function (MTF) for the projection images was measured in the front-back and left-right (i.e. tube-travel for DBT) directions using a 0.8 mm thick steel edge at positions 2, 4, 6 and 7 cm above the breast table. NNPS data required for eDQE calculation were calculated from the AEC projection images (the ~0° projection AEC image for DBT). The eDQE at 0.5 mm^{-1} in planar mammography mode was relatively stable at ~0.25 as PMMA thickness changed from 2 to 7 cm. For DBT, blurring from the focus motion and scattered radiation reduced eDQE at 6 and 7 cm PMMA.

1 Background

In the construction of digital breast tomosynthesis (DBT) systems, engineers face a number of design choices including whether to use a moving ("flying focus") or static focus ("step and shoot") during x-ray exposure. It has been shown that the use of a flying focus can severely limit the sharpness of the clinical detail in the DBT projection images [1]. A further choice is whether an anti-scatter grid should be used when acquiring the projection images. Given the direction of x-ray tube motion and the geometry of the standard linear grid used (grid lines running front to back) across the detector, this would require an anti-scatter grid implementation with lamellae running in the direction x-ray tube motion (left-right across the detector). When assessing the image quality performance of x-ray imaging systems, detector performance is normally specified via detective quantum efficiency (DQE) [2], which quantifies the efficiency with which the detector captures the signal-to-noise ratio (SNR) present within the incident x-ray beam. However, DQE is a detector-based metric [2] in which the influence of x-ray source size and scattered radiation on detector efficiency are minimized. In order to assess the impact of focus size and scattered radiation on DBT system efficiency, this paper uses the effective quantum efficiency (eDQE) [3], which gives a measure of system efficiency that includes source size and scattered radiation rejection technique. This was done for standard 2D digital (planar) mammography with anti-scatter grid in place and for the DBT mode, without anti-scatter grid.

H. Fujita, T. Hara, and C. Muramatsu (Eds.): IWDM 2014, LNCS 8539, pp. 127–133, 2014.
© Springer International Publishing Switzerland 2014

2   Methods and Materials

2.1   AEC Settings and Response Function

Data were acquired for a Hologic Selenia Dimensions units (Hologic Inc. Massachussetts, USA) digital breast tomosynthesis mammography system. The Hologic acquires 15 projections over an angular range of 15° in DBT mode. Native pixel pitch of the detector is 0.07mm and this pitch is used for planar 2D mammography; 2x2 pixel binning is applied to the DBT projections. First, the AEC response was assessed using poly(methyl methacrylate) (PMMA) slabs of thickness 2, 4 , 6 and 7 cm, placed on the breast support table. AUTOFILTER mode with AEC sensing region 2 was used. Tube voltage, target/filter (T/F) and tube current-time product (mAs) values are given in table 1. System response was then measured with a 2 mm Al sheet placed at the tube exit port. For the planar mode response, 29 kV W/Rh was set while 29 kV W/Al was used for the DBT mode response. An RTI Barracuda solid state dose detector was placed at the reference position: 6 cm from the chest-wall edge and positioned centrally left-right. The detector air kerma (DAK) per unit mAs was measured using static tube mode (0° DBT). Uniformly exposed (flood) images were acquired over a range of DAK settings for planar and DBT (anti-scatter grid removed for both modes). Pixel value (PV) was measured from DICOM "FOR PROCESSING" images using a 5 x 5 mm ROI placed in the image at the reference position. The PV was plotted against DAK to give a system response curve for each beam quality, for planar and DBT modes.

Table 1. Hologic Dimensions tube voltage, target/filter and mAs set by the AEC for planar and DBT modes. Number of photons q_0 mm^{-2} μGy^{-1} calculated using Boone model [4].

	Planar 2D mammography					DBT				
PMMA (cm)	q photons (mm$^{-2}\mu$Gy^{-1})	kV	TF	target/ filter	mAs	q photons (mm$^{-2}\mu$Gy^{-1})	kV	TF	target/ filter	mAs
2	5320	25	0.155	W/Rh	54	5529	26	0.141	W/Al	48
4	6159	28	0.046	W/Rh	105	7531	30	0.059	W/Al	65
6	6951	30	0.016	W/Rh	259	10421	36	0.036	W/Al	100
7	7441	31	0.013	W/Ag	366	12701	42	0.043	W/Al	95

2.2   Modulation Transfer Function

The system MTF was measured in the projection images using a steel plate MTF tool of dimension 120 mm x 60 mm and thickness 0.8 mm [2]. Images were obtained at 29 kV with a 2 mm thick Al filter placed at the x-ray tube; T/F was W/Rh for planar mode while DBT projection images of the steel plate were acquired using W/Al. The MTF was measured at heights of 0, 2, 4, 6 and 7 cm above the breast table by supporting the edge on small plastic blocks. No PMMA or scattering material was present for these measurements. The steel plate was positioned to give an edge response function in the left-right (i.e. tube-travel direction for the DBT mode) and front-back direction, in separate acquisitions. For DBT mode, edge images were acquired with standard x-ray tube motion and a typical clinical mAs such that the x-ray pulse length per projection was typical for clinical acquisitions; the MTF was calculated from the 0° projection (the 8th projection).

2.3   Noise Power Spectrum, Scatter Fraction and Narrow Beam Transmission

The normalized noise power spectrum (NNPS) was calculated for the different PMMA thicknesses, from regions extracted from the images acquired under AEC control. The regions were positioned 6 cm from the chest wall edge and centrally left-right with respect to the detector. Noise power spectra for planar and DBT mode were linearized and normalized using the respective response function. Scatter fraction data required for the eDQE calculation were taken from literature [5]. Narrow beam transmission of the PMMA blocks was measured using a collimated beam with the RTI Barracuda dosemeter.

2.4   Effective Detective Quantum Efficiency

The eDQE [3] was calculated using the equation:

$$eDQE(u') = \frac{MTF(u')^2}{NNPS(u') \cdot E \cdot TF \cdot q_0}(1-SF)^2 \qquad (1)$$

where u' is spatial frequency scaled to the object plane, $NNPS(u')$ is the normalized noise power spectrum, $MTF(u')$ is the pre-sampled modulation transfer function, SF is the scatter fraction, TF is the narrow beam transmission factor of PMMA, E is the pre-phantom exposure corrected to the detector plane and q_0 is the number of photons μGy^{-1} mm^{-2} (table 1).

3   Results and Discussion

MTF curves measured as a function of height above the breast table are plotted in figure 1. A small reduction in MTF is seen for planar mode in going from 0 cm to 7 cm above the table. This is the increasing influence of focus size (0.3 mm nominal dimension) as the edge is moved towards the source (standard geometric unsharpness). In DBT mode, the MTF curves are notably lower for two reasons. First, the DBT projection images are binned 2x2 to give a 0.14 mm pixel spacing for the projections, a step that reduces the pre-sampled MTF due to the reduced pixel aperture. Second, extended focus size of the tube due to motion of the focus during exposure causes a reduction in MTF [1]. Figure 1 shows this blurring occurs just in the tube-travel direction; this effect is progressively greater as the height of the object above the table increases. This blurring is anisotropic; the effect is absent in the front-back direction where there is no component of focus motion. Exposure pulse length for the DBT exposures was 30 ms, leading to less blurring compared to previously reported data, where a pulse length of 50 ms was measured [1].

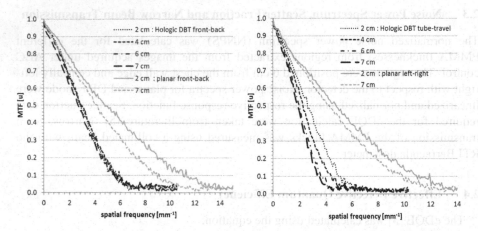

Fig. 1. Hologic pre-sampled MTF measured as a function of height above the table for planar and DBT modes in the left-right (tube travel) direction (left) and front-back direction (right)

Figure 2 plots eDQE for the tube-travel and front-back directions, where a progressive reduction in eDQE is seen in going from 2 cm PMMA to 7 cm PMMA for both directions, from ~0.35 to 0.11. At low spatial frequencies (~0.5 mm^{-1}) there is only a small difference in eDQE and the reduction is largely due to the influence of scattered radiation (SF) on the eDQE. At ~3 mm^{-1}, eDQE in the front-back direction falls

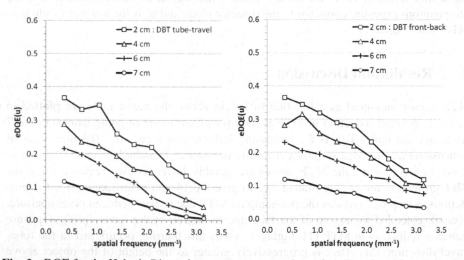

Fig. 2. eDQE for the Hologic Dimensions system measured as a function of position above the table for planar and DBT modes in the left-right (tube travel) direction (left) and front-back direction (right)

from 0.15 to 0.04 while for the tube-travel direction eDQE falls from 0.13 to 0.01, showing the influence of reduced MTF from tube-motion. Overall though, the influence of focus motion blurring is small and eDQE for tube-travel and front-back directions is similar in both shape and magnitude.

Figure 3 compares the eDQE curves at 2 cm and 7 cm PMMA in planar mode (2D with grid) and in DBT mode (without grid). For planar mode, eDQE is reasonably stable in shape and magnitude, showing a small reduction from 0.28 to 0.25 (at 0.5 mm^{-1}). This suggests only a small change in MTF shape and that the grid is controlling scatter well for planar mode. The eDQE at 2 cm PMMA for DBT mode is actually slightly higher than for the planar mode and hence scatter is not a source of image quality loss in DBT image quality when imaging smaller breasts. At 7 cm PMMA, eDQE for the DBT projections is notably lower in both the front-back and left-right directions than planar mode (with grid). This reflects the influence of scattered radiation: the scatter fraction for 7 cm with grid is ~ 0.06 compared to ~0.53 without grid. These data suggest that for binned projections, focus blurring is not

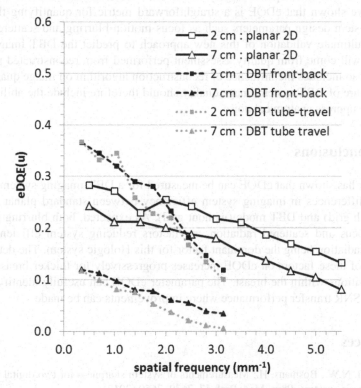

Fig. 3. eDQE for the Hologic system measured as a function of position above the table for planar and DBT modes in the left-right (tube travel) direction (left) and front-back direction (right)

one of the main causes of reduced system SNR efficiency and the main way to improve DBT at thicker breasts for the Hologic would be to reduce the influence of scattered radiation. Note that eDQE is limited to ~3.5 mm^{-1} due to the use of binned projections; projections in planar mode show SNR transfer beyond 5 mm^{-1}.

It should be remembered that eDQE is not an explicit measure of image quality but instead quantifies system SNR transfer efficiency, indicating the potential for the system to produce images of good quality. A system with low eDQE will have to be operated at higher exposures to match the image quality of a system with high eDQE. The term effective noise equivalent quanta (eNEQ) per projection gives the actual number of exposing quanta used to form the projections and determines the quantum noise present in the projections. Future work will compare eNEQ for a planar projection versus the combined eNEQ from the DBT projections. Finally, we note that while eDQE can quantify system SNR transfer efficiency, this parameter is calculated from and applies to the projection image data. One of the fundamental factors affecting object detectability in DBT is the ability of the system to suppress out of plane anatomical noise and this depends largely on the DBT angular range chosen. The above results have shown that eDQE is a straightforward metric for quantifying the influence of system design parameters such as focus motion blurring and scattered radiation. The ultimate validation of this new approach to predict the DBT imaging performance will come from quality assessment performed from reconstructed planes, a step that also includes the influence of reconstruction algorithm on image quality. The final measure of DBT system image quality should therefore include the ability of the system to suppress anatomical noise.

4   Conclusions

This paper has shown that eDQE can be measured for a DBT imaging system and can quantify differences in imaging system efficiency between standard planar imaging mode (with grid) and DBT mode (without grid). As expected, both blurring from the moving focus and scattered radiation, are factors reducing system efficiency, with scattered radiation being the dominant factor for this Hologic system. The detrimental influence of these factors on eDQE increases progressively for thicker breasts and at higher positions within the breast. The parameter eDQE can usefully identify aspects of system SNR transfer performance where improvements can be made.

References

1. Marshall, N.W., Bosmans, H.: Measurements of system sharpness for two digital breast tomosynthesis systems. Phys. Med. Biol. 57, 7629–7650 (2012)
2. IEC publication, Medical electrical equipment—characteristics of digital x-ray imaging devices: Part 1–2. Determination of the detective quantum efficiency—detectors used in mammography, IEC 62220, International Electrotechnical Commission, Geneva, Switzerland (2007)

3. Samei, E., Ranger, N.T., Mackenzie, A., Honey, I.D., Dobbins, J.T., Ravin, C.E.: Detector or System? Extending the Concept of Detective Quantum Efficiency to Characterize the Performance of Digital Radiographic Imaging Systems. Radiology 249(3), 926–937 (2008)
4. Boone, J.M., Fewell, T.R., Jennings, R.J.: Molybdenum, rhodium, and tungsten anode spectral models using interpolating polynomials with application to mammography. Med. Phys. 24(12), 1863–1874 (1997)
5. Salvagnini, E., Bosmans, H., Struelens, L., Marshall, N.W.: Quantification of scattered radiation in projection mammography: four practical methods compared. Med. Phys. 39(6), 3167–3180 (2012)

Comparison of SNDR, NPWE Model and Human Observer Results for Spherical Densities and Microcalcifications in Real Patient Backgrounds for 2D Digital Mammography and Breast Tomosynthesis

Lesley Cockmartin[*], Nicholas W. Marshall, and Hilde Bosmans

KU Leuven, Department of Imaging and Pathology, Division of Medical Physics and Quality Assessment, Herestraat 49, 3000 Leuven, Belgium
{Lesley.Cockmartin,Nicholas.Marshall,Hilde.Bosmans}@uzleuven.be

Abstract. The development of objective detection performance measures is of great value for both optimization purposes and inter-comparison of different mammographic (2D) or digital breast tomosynthesis (DBT) systems. They would be valuable as an alternative for human observer studies. In this study, we have calculated contrast (C), signal-difference-to-noise ratio (SDNR) and a NPWE model observer (d') for spherical densities and microcalcifications in patient 2D and DBT images. Contrast was higher in 2D compared to DBT reconstructions. In contrary, SDNR values were higher in DBT for the spheres and were comparable between 2D and DBT for the microcalcifications. A comparison between d' and SDNR showed a strong correlation between these two measures for both spheres and microcalcifications in 2D and DBT. Only weak and moderate correlations were found for SDNR and d' versus human confidence scores, indicating that there is room for improvement for the NPWE model observer as a theoretical predictor of human detection performance.

Keywords: digital breast tomosynthesis, digital mammography, signal-difference-to-noise ratio, model observer, human observer study.

1 Introduction

Image quality and performance measures have a crucial role in the acceptance or the optimization of X-ray imaging systems, and this is particularly true for two-dimensional (2D) digital mammography. To date, most measures, such as signal-difference-to-noise ratio (SDNR) and threshold contrast-detail (c-d) detectability, are assessed from test objects with a homogeneous background. In clinical practice, however, detection of lesions is affected by the amount of overlying or surrounding glandular tissue. With the introduction of digital beast tomosynthesis (DBT), the overlying breast tissue is reduced due to the pseudo-3D presentation of the breast. Recent clinical trial studies have shown that this results in a significant improvement for the

---

[*] Corresponding author.

H. Fujita, T. Hara, and C. Muramatsu (Eds.): IWDM 2014, LNCS 8539, pp. 134–141, 2014.
© Springer International Publishing Switzerland 2014

detection of masses in DBT compared to 2D [1], while it is less clear whether DBT offers any improvement (or can match) microcalcification detection achieved in 2D mammography. A more direct, objective parameter that quantifies this difference has not yet been proposed. Much research effort goes into predicting the radiologists' clinical detection performance using model observers that link measured image quality parameters to a detectability index (d'). Comparisons between human and model observer readings have been made for 2D mammography but only limited literature is available for DBT and for real patient backgrounds.

In this study, we will investigate the correlation between SDNR, Fourier-based non-prewhitening with eye filter (NPWE) model observer and human observer detection results for spherical densities and microcalcifications inserted (1) in images of homogenous polymethyl methacrylate (PMMA) and (2) in real patient images for 2D digital mammography and DBT.

2   Methods and Materials

2.1   Image Dataset and Human Observer Study

In order to provide data for a basic validation, images of the quality assurance phantom, Agatha [2] (Leeds Test Objects, UK), were acquired at constant beam quality (W/Rh 29 kV) and increasing tube load (56, 100, 140, 220 and 400 mAs) on a Siemens Inspiration mammography system with tomosynthesis option (Siemens, Erlangen, Germany). This phantom is made of homogeneous PMMA and includes a 5 mm diameter sphere of 70% glandular tissue equivalent material and a microcalcification-like object made of Aluminum with a 0.5 mm diameter.

A dataset for human observer studies was previously created using a hybrid technical-clinical method to insert spherical densities or groups of microcalcifications in patient data [3,4]. The method used 2D and DBT images that had been randomly selected from our patient database.

Attenuation templates of spheres made of 0%, 30% and 50% glandular tissue equivalent material (CIRS, Norfolk VA, USA), with a diameter of 5 mm and embedded in vegetable oil of variable breast equivalent thicknesses, were generated. For the microcalcifications, spheres of calcium carbonate ($CaCO_3$) were taken from the Voxmam phantom (Leeds Test Objects, UK). In this phantom, groups of calcifications are embedded in 1 cm of PMMA and each group consists of five calcifications within a certain diameter range: 354-224, 283-180 and 226-150 μm. The thickness of the PMMA was varied to obtain variable breast equivalent thicknesses. Within these stacks, the Voxmam phantom containing the calcifications was placed at two heights above the detector. To create the templates, projection image(s) with object were divided by the image(s) of the background only. Next, spheres and calcification groups were segmented and this resulted in the final templates. The templates were then multiplied in unprocessed 2D and DBT projection images of patients. Finally, the Opview2 processing was applied to the 2D images while the DBT projections were reconstructed with the clinical standard filtered back projection (FBP) based algorithm (Siemens, Erlangen, Germany). In total, the dataset consisted of 178 2D and DBT images with spheres and of 321 2D and DBT images with microcalcifications. An example of 2D processed and DBT reconstructed hybrid patient images with an inserted sphere and microcalcification group are shown in figure 1.

For the detection study, seven observers scored the absence or presence of the sphere in the center of a highlighted region via a 5-point confidence rating scale (1 = definitely absent, 2 = probably absent, 3 = possibly present, 4 = probably present, 5 = definitely present). For each image, the median confidence score of all 7 observers was used in the further analyses.

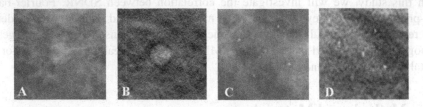

Fig. 1. Example of 2D processed (A, C) and DBT in focus reconstructed (B, D) patient images with inserted spherical density of 30% glandular density equivalence (A, B) and microcalcifications of sizes 283-180 μm (C, D)

2.2   SDNR and Contrast Measurements

2.2.1   Spherical Densities

Signal-difference-to-noise ratio (SDNR) and contrast (C) of the spheres were measured in unprocessed 2D images and DBT in-focus reconstructed planes. For the spheres, mean pixel value (PV) and standard deviation (σ) were measured in a circular region of interest (ROI) with a diameter of 46 pixels. In order to measure the PV and σ of the background with anatomical noise, 18 half overlapping ROIs were drawn at a distance of 23 pixels from the sphere center (Figure 2(a)). The average PV and σ of these 18 ROIs were calculated and used as background value.

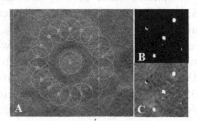

Fig. 2. Example of region of interest selection for SDNR and contrast measurements for spherical inserts and surrounding anatomical background (A) and for microcalcification groups segmented and separated (B) from the local background (C)

2.2.2 Microcalcifications

Peak SDNR and peak contrast of the microcalcifications were calculated in unprocessed 2D images and DBT in-focus reconstructed planes. Each group of calcifications was selected within a squared region of 80 x 80 pixels and segmented by using the function 'find edges' and manual threshold in ImageJ (NIH, USA). In this way, microcalcifications could be distinguished from the background and PV of the microcalcifications and background could be measured individually (Figure 2 (b, c)).

2.3   NPWE Model Observer

The NPWE model observer in equation (1) was used to calculate the detectability index d':

$$d' = \frac{\sqrt{2\pi}C \int_0^\infty |S(f)MTF(f)VTF(f)|^2 f df}{\sqrt{\int_0^\infty |S^2(f)MTF^2(f)VTF^4(f)NPS(f)| f df}} \qquad (1)$$

where C is the contrast measured in the 2D unprocessed and DBT reconstructed images, f is the spatial frequency, MTF(f) is the modulation transfer function, NPS(f) is the noise power spectrum and VTF(f) is the Visual Transfer Function. The VTF follows the version given by Kelly et al [5]. The signal was defined as a 2D Gaussian profile using equation (2) [6]:

$$S(f) = (\exp(-\pi r^2 f))^2 \qquad (2)$$

For the spheres, a radius (r) of 2.5 mm was used while for the microcalcification groups the maximum radius of the calcification size range was chosen. The calculation of d' requires a measurement of detector pre-sampling MTF and NPS. For the NPS, half overlapping records of size 128 x 128 pixels were drawn similarly to the background ROIs for the SDNR calculation of the spherical densities. For the microcalcifications, the NPS was measured in a square of 128 x 128 pixels within the original 2D and DBT patient images before insertion of the microcalcifications but at the same position where the microcalcifications were afterwards inserted. These were input to a 2D NPS calculation with a Hann window applied to each record. The final NPS was the radial (R) average of the ensemble, including the 0° and 90° spatial frequency axes. Normalization of the NPS was performed by dividing by the square of the mean signal. In the case of the DBT reconstructed images, however, axial NPS in both tube-travel (TT) and front-back (FB) directions were measured and no normalization was applied. In-plane MTF was measured in TT and FB directions using a 25 μm W wire at the same height above the detector as where the sphere/calcifications were initially imaged. This resulted in two d' values for DBT images, one for each direction.

3   Results and Discussion

Figure 3 shows the results of SDNR and d' (for both TT and FB directions), calculated in DBT planes of the Agatha phantom for the sphere and calcification at increasing tube load. Taken individually, both SDNR and d' showed a square root dependence with changing tube load (exposure), as expected for objects imaged in x-ray quantum noise (homogeneous background). Plotting SDNR against d' showed a good correlation for these homogeneous background images [7], both increasing with increasing tube load.

Table 1 and 2 summarize the mean PV and σ of C, SDNR, d' and human confidence ratings for the three spherical densities and three microcalcification groups in 2D and DBT patient images. Although contrast was significantly lower in DBT compared to 2D for the spherical densities (p<0.0001), SDNR values were higher in DBT (p=0.005), possibly illustrating the effect of the reduced anatomical noise (reduced signal variation). Also for the microcalcifications, contrast was higher in 2D compared to DBT images (p<0.0001). Then again, SDNR values remained slightly but not significantly higher in 2D (p=0.099). The absolute values of the model observer results cannot be compared between 2D and DBT since neither linearization nor explicit normalization were applied to the NPS calculation in DBT. In the human observer study the presence of the spherical densities was rated with a higher confidence in DBT than in 2D, contrary to the microcalcifications which were better detected in 2D. This indicates that the visibility of calcifications is degraded less by overlapping breast tissue, thus the ability of DBT to reduce this anatomical noise will have less influence on (successful) microcalcification detection. It is also possible that microcalcifications are imaged more faithfully (sharper) in 2D mode compared to DBT.

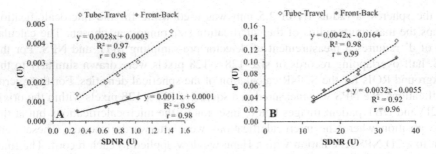

Fig. 3. Correlation of SDNR and d' for DBT reconstructed planes of a 70% glandular tissue equivalent sphere (A) and an Aluminum calcification (B) embedded in 45 mm PMMA acquired with increasing tube load

Figure 4 shows plots of SDNR versus d' values for both imaging modalities and for spheres and microcalcifications separately. SDNR and d' values are normalized against the maximum value for better interpretation and plotting of the data. A strong correlation between SDNR and d' was found in 2D for both spherical densities (r=0.81) and microcalcifications (r=0.78). Also in DBT these correlations remained between SDNR and d' in both tube-travel and front-back direction for spherical densities (r=0.62 and r=0.66 respectively) and microcalcifications (r=0.66 and r=0.64 respectively). This indicates that basic SDNR measurements can already give an indication of detectability d' in DBT reconstructed planes, despite not taking into account the correlations present in signal and noise. For microcalcifications in 2D these results are not surprising since previously published work found that c-d threshold values could be predicted by a NPWE model observer [7]. Another paper has shown that even in structured phantom images for small details in 2D, SDNR and d' behave similarly [8]. More studies with human observers should ultimately lead to a better understanding and a more sophisticated model.

Table 1. Mean values ± σ of C, SDNR, d' and human confidence score for 2D and DBT reconstructed images for each spherical density separately. (NA = not applicable)

Modality	2D			DBT		
Spherical density (%)	50	30	0	50	30	0
C (%)	7.8±3.6	6.8±3.4	5.3±3.9	4.9±1.6	3.7±1.1	2.2±1.4
SDNR	2.1±0.93	1.8±0.85	1.2±0.82	2.6±0.80	2.0±0.69	1.2±0.68
d'(R)	2.0±1.1	1.8±0.94	1.1±0.75	NA	NA	NA
d'(TT)	NA	NA	NA	1.2E-03±0.65	0.91E-03±0.53	0.55E-03±0.42
d'(FB)	NA	NA	NA	0.50E-03±0.25	0.37E-03±0.21	0.22E-03±0.14
Confidence score	4.7±0.84	4.1±1.1	2.5±0.88	5.0±0.0	5.0±0.0	4.2±0.93

Table 2. Mean values ± σ of C, SDNR, d' and human confidence score for 2D and DBT reconstructed images for each microcalcification size group separately. (NA = not applicable, NM = not measured)

Modality	2D			DBT		
Microcalcification size range (µm)	354-224	283-180	226-150	354-224	283-180	226-150
C (%)	20±3.4	17±4.6	11±4.8	11±5.5	7.5±4.6	5.4±3.4
SDNR	4.2±1.6	3.9±1.6	2.4±1.1	5.3±2.2	3.6±2.0	2.1±0.98
d'(R)	8.8±2.7	6.8±2.4	4.0±1.8	NA	NA	NA
d'(TT)	NA	NA	NA	5.2E-03±3.2	3.2E-03±2.3	NM
d'(FB)	NA	NA	NA	5.0E-03±2.9	3.0E-03±2.0	NM
Confidence score	5.0±0.0	4.9±0.29	4.4+1.1	4.9±0.53	4.1±1.4	2.5±1.1

Spearman correlation coefficients for SDNR versus human confidence scores were 0.35 and 0.44 for the spheres and 0.35 and 0.71 for the calcifications for 2D and DBT respectively. In figure 5 model observer results are plotted as boxplots for each confidence score separately, allowing a visualization and comparison of the trend that d' follows versus the human confidence score. Model observer results were overlapping for the different confidence rates in both modalities and for both spheres (Spearman coefficient of 0.39 in 2D and 0.34 in DBT), and calcifications (Spearman coefficient of 0.40 in 2D and 0.25 in DBT), resulting in only weak or moderate correlations between the two measures. However, average d' values for the highest confidence score were higher compared to the d' values for the other confidence ratings in all plots (Figure 5).

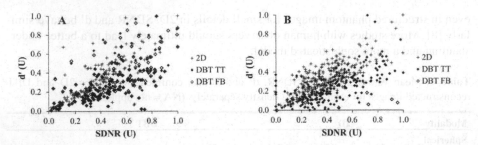

Fig. 4. Graphs illustrating the correlation between SDNR and d' for 2D and DBT (tube-travel and front-back direction) for spheres (A) and microcalcifications (B)

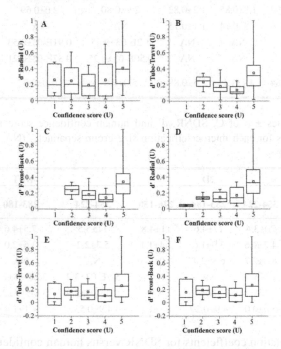

Fig. 5. Boxplots showing minimum and maximum (whiskers), standard deviation (rectangular box) together with mean d' value (square) for each human confidence score for 2D (radial) and DBT (tube-travel and front-back) for spherical densities (A,B,C) and microcalcifications (D,E,F)

Best results were achieved for detectability indices for microcalcifications in 2D with increasing average d' values for increasing confidence score and a small variation in d' for each confidence score separately (Figure 5(d)). In contrast, for spheres d' fails to predict human detection results in 2D images, showing large variations of d' for all scores (Figure 5(a)). It is interesting to note the smaller variation for the spheres in DBT (Figure 5(a) vs (b) and (c)), perhaps consistent with lower structural noise, however correlation with reader score remains low. We attribute this to the relatively low number of spheres with low confidence scores in DBT: even spheres with very limited contrast remained well visible in DBT.

Some limitations are worth emphasizing. First, we are comparing data calculated using 'FOR PROCESSING' for the 2D versus reconstructed data for the DBT results. Second, the linearization of NPS in the calculation can influence model observer results and therefore further work should examine the dynamic range of the reconstructed image, its dependence on image content and its influence on NPS magnitude.

4   Conclusions

We have demonstrated good correlation between NPWE model observer and SDNR values for spheres and microcalcifications in 2D and DBT images of patients. While reasonably good correlation was found between NPWE data and human observer results for microcalcifications in 2D mammography, only weak or moderate correlations were seen for sphere data. This can be partly due to the limitations of the dataset which contains a majority of obvious spheres in DBT at the one side and easily detectable microcalcifications in 2D on the other side. In conclusion, the NPWE model observer described in this paper is a start for the development of a theoretical predictor of human detection performance in real DBT patient images but needs further optimization and databases with a large number of subtle or small lesions.

References

1. Rafferty, E.A., Park, J.M., Philpotts, L.E., et al.: Assessing radiologist performance using combined digital mammography and breast tomosynthesis compared with digital mammography alone: results of a multicenter, multireader trial. Radiology 266(1), 104–113 (2013)
2. Jacobs, J., Marshall, N. W., Cockmartin, L., et al.: Towards an international consensus strategy for periodic quality control of digital breast tomosynthesis systems. In: SPIE Proc. vol. 7622, pp. 7622–15 (2010)
3. Cockmartin, L., Stalmans, D., Zanca, F., et al.: A new hybrid technical-clinical test demonstrates improved low contrast detectability in tomosynthesis when compared to 2D mammography. RSNA (2012)
4. Cockmartin, L., Aerts, G., Zanca, F., et al.: Comparison of microcalcification detection in digital mammography and breast tomosynthesis using a hybrid technical-clinical test method. RSNA (2013)
5. Kelly, D.H.: Motion and vision. II Stabilized spatio-temporal threshold surface. J. Opt. Soc. Am. 69(10), 1340–1349 (1979)
6. Hu, Y.-H., Zhao, W.: The effect of angular dose distribution on the detection of microcalcifications in digital breast tomosynthesis. Med. Phys. 38(5), 2455–2466 (2011)
7. Monnin, P., Marshall, N.W., Bosmans, H., et al.: Image quality assessment in digital mammography: part II. NPWE as a validated alternative for contrast detail analysis. Phys. Med. Biol. 56, 4221–4238 (2011)
8. Salvagnini, E., Bosmans, H., Monnin, P., et al.: The use of detectability indices as a means of automatic exposure control for a digital mammography system. In: Proceedings of SPIE (2011)

Assessing Radiologist Performance and Microcalcifications Visualization Using Combined 3D Rotating Mammogram (RM) and Digital Breast Tomosynthesis (DBT)

Hitomi Tani[1], Nachiko Uchiyama[1], Minoru Machida[1], Mari Kikuchi[1], Yasuaki Arai[1], Kyoichi Otsuka[2], Anna Jerebko[3], Andreas Fieselmann[3], and Thomas Mertelmeier[3]

[1] Department of Radiology, National Cancer Center, Tokyo, Japan
{hittani,nuchiyam,mmachida,markikuc,yaarai}@ncc.go.jp
[2] Siemens Japan K.K., Tokyo, Japan
Kyoichi.otsuka@siemens.com
[3] Siemens AG, Healthcare Sector, Erlangen, Germany
{anna.jerebko,andreas.fieselmann,
thomas.mertelmeier}@siemens.com

Abstract. We evaluated the diagnostic performance of a novel 3D visualization approach (rotating mammogram, RM) in combination with DBT compared with that of FFDM and DBT alone. FFDM, DBT alone and DBT images plus reconstructed RM from 110 breasts (34 cases of breast cancer and 76 normal breasts) were evaluated and rated independently by 6 readers. DBT plus RM demonstrated superior diagnostic accuracy compared to FFDM ($p<0.05$) and a small improvement in performance compared to DBT alone. Visualization of microcalcifications was significantly better on RM than DBT ($p<0.05$) for all 14 microcalcification-dominant cancer lesions. Adjunction of RM to DBT will offer the benefit of increased diagnostic accuracy and contribute to more accurate assessment of DBT alone.

Keywords: Digital Mammography, Tomosynthesis, Rotating Mammogram.

1 Introduction

DBT has been demonstrated to be a promising imaging technique for breast cancer detection. While breast structures are superimposed in 2D FFDM images, the slice images reconstructed from DBT acquisitions have decreased overlap of breast tissue. Compared with 2D mammography, DBT provides an advantage in the detection of breast masses and reduces false positive detections caused by overlapping anatomical structures [1-5]. However, in case of microcalcification-related lesions, 2D mammography shows some advantage compared to DBT [6-7]. On DBT slice images, it is often difficult to assess the overall appearance of clustered microcalcifications and to analyze the morphology of each microcalcification's outline.

H. Fujita, T. Hara, and C. Muramatsu (Eds.): IWDM 2014, LNCS 8539, pp. 142–149, 2014.

In this study, we evaluated a novel 3D visualization approach (rotating mammogram). This approach generates a 3D overview rendering of a reconstructed DBT volume which can be viewed at from different angles. The RM could be used for improved 3D visualization of structures, e.g. microcalcifications, in DBT and could lead to faster DBT reading times. The purpose of this study is to compare the diagnostic accuracy of FFDM and DBT using and not using RM and to determine whether DBT plus RM will contribute to the assessment of breast cancer.

2   Materials and Methods

This study was approved by the IRB at our institute. Clinical image data were acquired by an a-Se FFDM system with a detector pixel pitch of 85μm (MAMMOMAT Inspiration, Siemens AG, Germany; MAMMOMAT Inspiration Tomosynthesis is not commercially available in the U.S.). Two-view DBT (rotation angle interval ±25°) was performed with the same compression pressure as with the FFDM. With one-view DBT, the radiation dose was 1.5 times when compared to one-view FFDM. DBT images were reconstructed by filtered back projection (FBP). The RM reconstruction technique is based on a 3D volume rendering method [8]. Using the reconstructed tomosynthesis volume, new 2D projection images are pre-computed at different angles. The user can interactively change the projection angle when viewing the RM. The RM algorithm contains parameters that control the visualization of microcalcifications and soft tissue. In this study, our settings were optimized for the visualization of microcalcifications, rendering soft tissue almost transparent. FFDM, reconstructed slice image of DBT and RM rendering were reviewed on a dedicated workstation (syngo MammoReport, Siemens AG, Germany).

A total of 110 breasts (55 patients) including 34 breasts with cancer and 76 normal or benign breasts were used. The thirty-four cancers were diagnosed using a core or vacuum-assisted biopsy procedure under ultrasound or stereotactic imaging guidance, and final histopathologic diagnoses were obtained at surgery.

Examinations were interpreted by 6 dedicated breast imaging radiologists with experience varying from 5 to 10 years. All readers were trained and certified in tomosynthesis interpretation. In order to evaluate the effectiveness of RM, observer performance studies were conducted for receiver operating characteristic (ROC) analysis. The 55 patient cases were randomly divided into two groups: group A (containing 28 patients) and group B (containing 27 patients). All readers read all patients. The schedule of the reading workflow for each reader is shown in Fig. 1. At first, FFDM from group A and DBT with and without RM from group B were evaluated. Second, DBT with and without RM from group A and FFDM from group B were evaluated. Each participant completed two reading sessions spaced 4 weeks apart to minimize recall bias.

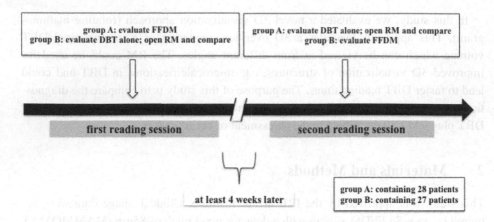

Fig. 1. Schedule of reading workflow for each reader

For observer performance evaluation, two different scales were used to capture each reader's interpretation: modified BI-RADS and percentage probability of malignancy scale (POM: 0-100%, i.e., each reader's subjective assessment of the probability that the breast had malignant foci). The reader-specific area under the curve (AUC) for BI-RADS and POM were analyzed and the average AUCs of all readers were calculated. The visualization of masses and microcalcifications as well as the appearance of noise were also compared and scored separately for each case in DBT and RM on a 4-point scale from 0 to 3 (0, equal or not better; 1, slightly better; 2, better; 3, significantly better). For ROC analysis, the software DBM MRMC version 2.33 [9,10] was used. Differences in observed AUCs and the visualization score of microcalcifications were assessed using a t-test. A p-value < 0.05 was considered statistically significant.

3   Results

Of the 34 malignant cases, 24 lesions were invasive ductal carcinoma, 5 were ductal carcinoma in situ (DCIS), 3 were invasive lobular carcinoma, 1 was mixed of DCIS and lobular carcinoma in situ, and 1 was acinic cell carcinoma. Fourteen malignant lesions were microcalcification-dominant breast cancer and 20 were mass-dominant breast cancer.

Table 1 summarizes the AUCs by each reader and the average of all readers. For the BI-RADS scale, the average AUC for DBT plus RM was 0.907, DBT alone 0.901 and FFDM was 0.793 (Fig.2A). For POM, the average AUC for DBT plus RM was 0.915, DBT alone 0.907 and FFDM was 0.799 (Fig.2B). DBT plus RM demonstrated superior diagnostic accuracy compared with FFDM alone, as shown by significant difference in the average AUC (p<0.05). In terms of average AUC, only a small improvement was seen by DBT plus RM compared to DBT alone. Difference in the average AUC in BI-RADS between DBT plus RM and DBT alone was 0.006 and in POM was 0.008.

Table 1. AUC for each reader and the average of all readers

	BI-RADS scale			POM scale		
	FFDM	DBT	DBT+RM	FFDM	DBT	DBT+RM
Reader 1	0.803	0.880	0.883	0.826	0.887	0.899
Reader 2	0.741	0.857	0.853	0.769	0.875	0.865
Reader 3	0.833	0.911	0.916	0.814	0.916	0.936
Reader 4	0.804	0.955	0.958	0.834	0.967	0.971
Reader 5	0.782	0.953	0.960	0.762	0.951	0.958
Reader 6	0.794	0.853	0.871	0.786	0.844	0.862
Average	0.793	0.901	0.907	0.799	0.907	0.915

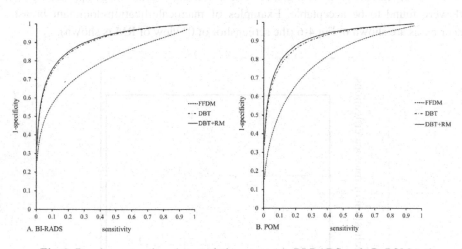

Fig. 2. Receiver operating characteristic curves - A. BI-RADS scale B. POM scale

Regarding BI-RADS scale (dichotomized at category 2 or less vs 3 or greater), summary measures of accuracy are presented in Table 2. The average sensitivity for DBT alone was 0.888, for DBT plus RM was 0.878, and the average specificity for DBT alone was 0.754, for DBT plus RM was 0.781. Equality or little improvement in specificity and positive predictive value (PPV) was seen in all 6 radiologists.

Table 2. Performance in reading study of DBT alone and DBT + RM using BI-RADS scale

| | DBT | | | | | | |
	Reader 1	Reader 2	Reader 3	Reader 4	Reader 5	Reader 6	Average
Sensitivity	0.882	0.853	0.824	0.941	0.971	0.794	0.888
Specificity	0.776	0.750	0.711	0.776	0.737	0.776	0.754
PPV	0.638	0.604	0.560	0.653	0.623	0.614	0.615
NPV	0.937	0.919	0.900	0.967	0.982	0.894	0.933
	DBT+RM						
	Reader 1	Reader 2	Reader 3	Reader 4	Reader 5	Reader 6	Average
Sensitivity	0.882	0.794	0.794	0.941	0.971	0.824	0.878
Specificity	0.829	0.789	0.724	0.789	0.776	0.776	0.781
PPV	0.698	0.628	0.563	0.667	0.660	0.622	0.640
NPV	0.940	0.896	0.887	0.968	0.983	0.908	0.930

For all 14 cancers manifesting as microcalcifications, the visualization was significantly better on RM than DBT ($p<0.05$, Fig. 3). All readers confirmed that RM was useful for analysis of microcalcifications because RM clarified the distribution and extent of microcalcifications at a glance. The noise and overall image appearance of RM were found to be acceptable. Examples of microcalcification-dominant breast cancer cases are shown in Fig.4-6 (the screenshot of 0° view of RM is shown).

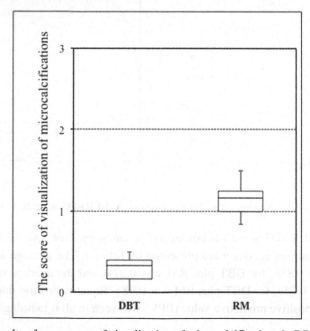

Fig. 3. Results of assessment of visualization of microcalcifications in DBT and RM

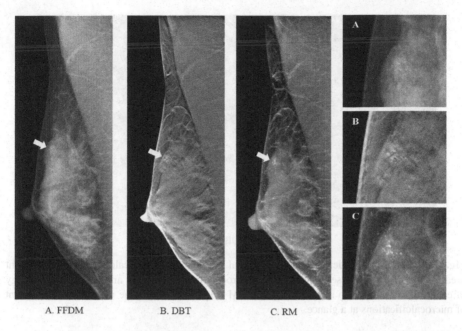

A. FFDM   B. DBT   C. RM

Fig. 4. FFDM (Fig.4A) demonstrated grouped amorphous microcalcifications in the right breast. In DBT (Fig.4B) microcalcifications' outline is blurred. RM (Fig.4C) showed clustered microcalcifications clearly.

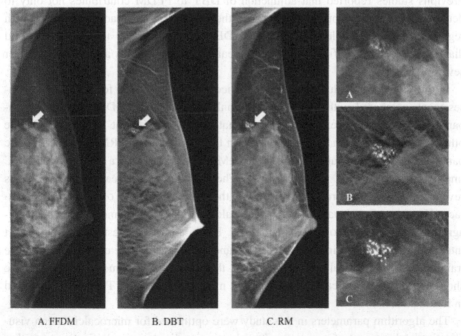

A. FFDM   B. DBT   C. RM

Fig. 5. FFDM (Fig.5A) showed grouped pleomorphic microcalcifications in the left breast. RM (Fig.5C) clarified microcalcification outlines better compared to DBT (Fig.5B).

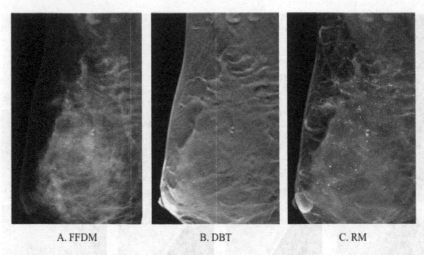

A. FFDM   B. DBT   C. RM

Fig. 6. FFDM (Fig.6A) demonstrated segmental pleomorphic microcalcifications in the right breast. It is difficult to assess the extent of microcalcifications and to analyze the morphology of each microcalcification in DBT (Fig.6B). RM (Fig.6C) clarified the distribution and extent of microcalcifications at a glance.

4   Discussion

Previous studies reported that adjunction of DBT to FFDM contributes not only to detecting the lesions, but also improves the diagnostic accuracy, especially with regard to mass-related lesions. However, DBT can complicate the assessment and diagnosis of microcalcifications when the calcification particles are distributed over several slices.

In this study, we evaluated the performance of DBT plus RM for breast cancer assessment, compared with FFDM or DBT only. The benefit of DBT plus RM compared to FFDM was demonstrated with statistically significant difference. On the other hand, our preliminary results based on this version of the RM with the specific parameter settings indicate that DBT with RM translated to only a small overall AUC improvement compared with only DBT. The analysis of the reader-specific AUCs revealed little reader-to-reader variability in the effect of RM use on interpretive accuracy. However, for visualization of microcalcifications, RM demonstrated better diagnostic performance compared with DBT. Early studies suggested that radiologist interpretation time will increase with DBT and may not improve even with extensive training. If RM was evaluated before DBT, the interpretation time of DBT might be shortened especially in cases manifesting as microcalcifications. This can be assessed in future studies.

The algorithm parameters in this study were optimized for microcalcification visualization. Adjustment of parameters in order to visualize microcalcifications together with masses and soft tissue could further increase the diagnostic usability of the RM.

5   Conclusion

The visualization of microcalcifications was significantly better on RM than DBT. With the RM parameter settings used in this study, the combination of DBT plus RM showed only small improvement compared to that of DBT alone in terms of ROC curve area, sensitivity and specificity. Adjunction of RM to DBT will offer the benefit of increased diagnostic accuracy and contribute to more accurate assessment of DBT alone.

Acknowledgment. This study was supported by Grant-in-Aid for Scientific Research (C) (No.23591810) in Japan. The authors are grateful to Julitta Unland, Shiras Abdurahman, and Frank Dennerlein for their support in this study.

References

1. Gur, D., Abrams, G.S., Chough, D.M., et al.: Digital breast tomosynthesis: observer performance study. AJR 193(2), 586–591 (2009)
2. Good, W.F., Abrams, G.S., Catullo, V.J., et al.: Digital breast tomosynthesis: a pilot observer study. AJR 190(4), 865–869 (2008)
3. Gennaro, G., Toledano, A., di Maggio, C., et al.: Digital breast tomosynthesis versus digital mammography: a clinical performance study. Eur. Radiol. 20(7), 1545–1553 (2010)
4. Skaane, P., Bandos, A.I., Gullien, R., et al.: Comparison of digital mammography alone and digital mammography plus tomosynthesis in a population-based screening program. Radiology 267(1), 47–56 (2013)
5. Svahn, T.M., Chakraborty, D.P., Ikeda, D., Zackrisson, S., Do, Y., Mattson, S.: Andersson I: Breast tomosynthesis and digital mammography: a comparison of diagnostic accuracy. Brit. J. Radiol. 85(1019), e1074–e1082 (2012)
6. Spangler, M.L., Zuley, M.L., Sumkin, J.H., et al.: Detection and classification of calcifications on digital breast tomosynthesis and 2D digital mammography: a comparison. AJR 196(2), 320–324 (2011)
7. Uchiyama, N., et al.: Diagnostic impact of adjunction of digital breast tomosynthesis (DBT) to full field digital mammography (FFDM) and in comparison with full field digital mammography (FFDM). In: Maidment, A.D.A., Bakic, P.R., Gavenonis, S. (eds.) IWDM 2012. LNCS, vol. 7361, pp. 119–126. Springer, Heidelberg (2012)
8. Dennerlein, F., Jerebko, A., Fieselmann, A., Mertelmeier, T.: Efficient synthesis of virtual projections from a tomosynthesis data set using a 2D image processing method. In: Proc. SPIE Medical Imaging 2013: Physics of Medical Imaging, 86680W (2013)
9. Dorfman, D.D., Berbaum, K.S., Metz, C.: Receiver operating characteristic rating analysis: Generalization to the population of readers and patients with the jackknife method. Invest. Radiol. 27(9), 723–731 (1992)
10. Hillis, S.L., Berbaum, K.S., Metz, C.E.: Recent developments in the Dorfman-Berbaum-Metz procedure for multireader ROC study analysis. Acad. Radiol. 15(5), 647–661 (2008)

Digital Breast Tomosynthesis: Image Quality and Dose Saving of the Synthesized Image

Julia Garayoa[1], Irene Hernandez-Giron[2,3], Maria Castillo[3], Julio Valverde[1], and Margarita Chevalier[3]

[1] Servicio de Protección Radiológica, Hospital Universitario Fundación Jiménez Díaz, 28040 Madrid, Spain
garayoa.julia@gmail.com, JValverde@fjd.es
[2] Unitat de Física Médica, Universitat Rovira i Virgili, 43201 Reus, Spain
irene.debroglie@gmail.com
[3] Unidad de Física Médica, Departamento de Radiología, Universidad Complutense de Madrid, 28040 Madrid, Spain
mcastillogar@gmail.com, chevalier@ucm.es

Abstract. In this paper, the impact on image quality and dose reduction related to the use of a synthesized 2D image in digital breast tomosynthesis examinations is analyzed. 2D and 3D images of the TORMAM phantom were acquired at clinical conditions. Syntesized 2D images (C-View) were also obtained. Seven observers scored the detectability and visibility of microcalcification (MC) clusters in both types of images. Low contrast objects were studied measuring contrast-to-noise ratio (CNR) and applying a non-prewhitening matched filter (NPW) model observer. Glandular doses were estimated from a sample of 50 patients. The detectability and visibility of the microcalcification clusters were higher in C-View than in 2D images (50% and 100%, respectively). CNR values were higher for C-View for all contrasts. The NPW got slightly higher detectability values for the lowest contrast details in C-View. We have estimated a dose reduction of 43% by replacing the conventional 2D by the C-View image.

Keywords: Digital breast tomosynthesis, synthetic 2D breast image, glandular dose, image quality, model observer.

1 Introduction

Digital breast tomosynthesis (DBT) is a radiographic technique based on the acquisition of a series of 2D low-dose projections over a limited angular range from which the whole breast volume is reconstructed in 3D slices. These 3D slices have the advantage of reducing tissue superposition which improves lesion detectability particularly in dense breasts [1].

Several clinical studies involving a large number of patients have proved the benefits of this technique especially when DBT is used in combination with digital conventional mammography (2D) [2]. The breast radiation dose involved in this practice (as it was approved by the FDA) approximately doubles the one delivered in 2D conventional mammography [3]. The main motivation to follow this protocol (2D+3D)

H. Fujita, T. Hara, and C. Muramatsu (Eds.): IWDM 2014, LNCS 8539, pp. 150–157, 2014.
© Springer International Publishing Switzerland 2014

arises from radiologists' experience, who find that some lesions, in particular micro-calcification clusters, are easier to detect and more correctly interpreted in conventional 2D images.

Recently, a synthesized 2D image reconstructed from DBT datasets has been introduced in clinical practice to replace the conventional 2D image with the aim of reducing radiation dose [4].

The objective of this work is to evaluate the dose saving and the impact on the image quality of the synthesized image (SI). Few commercialized phantoms with a proper design to assess the image quality of DBT systems are available to date. We selected the TORMAM phantom, traditionally used to evaluate the image quality in 2D mammography. The main reason for this choice is that this phantom has a section with a structured background containing several microcalcification (MC) clusters of different sizes which allow assessing the ability of the SI to show MC and compare with their visibility in the conventional 2D image. Furthermore, the noise structure in the SI of the phantom section with a uniform background can affect the visibility of low contrast (LC) details. The detectability of the LC inserts has been evaluated based on the non-prewhitening matched filter (NPW) model observer [5].

The dose reduction achieved with the replacement of the 2D image by the synthesized image was estimated for a sample of patients.

2   Material and Methods

This work is based on the images obtained with the DBT Hologic Selenia Dimensions (Hologic Inc., Bedford, USA) system, licensed to reconstruct the synthesized 2D image commercialized as C-View. For 2D image acquisition, the system selects W/Rh and W/Ag anode/filter combinations depending on the breast thickness. DBT images are acquired using W/Al and the grid is removed. In both modalities, the tube kilovoltage is selected as a function of compressed breast thickness and the tube loading depends on the breast attenuation. In the tomosynthesis modality the device acquires 15 low-dose projections over 15° (-7.5 - +7.5). Reconstruction is performed using a FBP algorithm obtaining contiguous planes 1 mm thick. 2D and DBT images are acquired within one scan in the same breast compression (COMBO mode). The synthesized image is produced from the reconstructed planes using a Hologic proprietary algorithm [4].

Image quality evaluation was based on the TORMAM phantom (Leeds Test Objects Ltd, Boroughbridge, UK). The middle right of the phantom test plate (15 mm thickness) simulates the appearance of breast tissue (structured background) and it contains 6 microcalcification clusters with sizes of: 354-224, 283-180, 226-150, 177-106, 141-90, 106-93 μm (Fig. 1). The exact location of the MC clusters in the structured background is unknown. The middle left with uniform background contains 18 low contrast objects (3 mm diameter) distributed on six groups. The nominal contrasts of these objects range between 0.5 and 4 (Fig. 2). The test plate was positioned on top of PMMA of 3 cm thickness. Eight phantom images were acquired with the COMBO mode and C-View images were also synthesized. The exposure technical parameters (filter, kVp and mAs) were automatically selected by the automatic exposure control of the system.

The detectability of the MC clusters was evaluated by 7 experienced observers (3 radiologists and 4 medical physicists) who analyzed 8 C-View images and 8 2D images. In both backgrounds (uniform and structured) the observers counted the number of detected MC clusters (0-6) and scored their visibility (0 = Non visible; 1 = Subtle visible cluster; 2 = Highly visible cluster but blurred individual MC; 3 = Highly visible cluster and sharp individual MC). The results were statistically analyzed using a non parametric test for multiple sample comparisons (Kruskal-Wallis with 5% significance level).

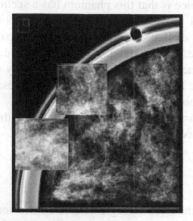 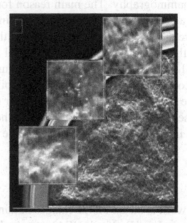

Fig. 1. Microcalcification groups detected in the phantom structured background corresponding to the 2D (on the left) and C-View (on the right) images

Using the uniform background section of the phantom, the contrast to noise ratio (CNR) (eq. 1) was measured using ROIs defined over each low contrast object (dot) and over the background (bg) next to the object:

$$CNR = \frac{MPV_{dot} - MPV_{bg}}{\sigma_{bg}} \tag{1}$$

where MPV is the mean pixel value and σ is the standard deviation. ROI size was adapted to each type of image pixel size (0.0652 mm/px for 2D and 0.1125 mm/px for C-View) to assure the ROI size and location was exactly the same in both sets of images (Fig. 2). An average CNR value was obtained for each of the 18 LC details, taking into account the values obtained for the 3 images available in this test for 2D and C-View, respectively. Additionally, for each of the six nominal contrasts, a mean CNR was calculated.

A non-prewhitening matched model observer (NPW) was used to analyze the dots/bg samples for both sets of images. This model uses a template for each object that is cross-correlated with the dots/bg samples. A high resolution template was created and downsized to fit it to the samples. From the test-statistics, a detectability index d' can be derived, as follows:

$$d' = \frac{\langle T \rangle_1 - \langle T \rangle_2}{\sqrt{\frac{1}{2}\sigma_1^2 + \frac{1}{2}\sigma_2^2}} \qquad (2)$$

where $\langle T \rangle_i$ represents the mean value and σ_i the statistical deviation of the dots/bg samples after correlating them with the template [6]. An average d' was obtained for each nominal contrast following the same procedure as with CNR.

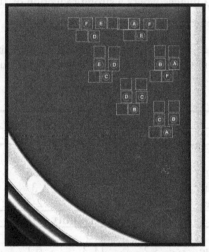

Fig. 2. ROI distribution for the LC objects/background samples for low contrast analysis in the TOR MAM phantom. The nominal contrasts are 4% (A), 3% (B), 2% (C), 1.5% (D), 1% (E) and 0.5% (F).

A sample of 50 patients who underwent COMBO acquisitions for the two common views (CC and MLO) was included to estimate the mean glandular dose (MGD). MGD calculation was performed using the method proposed by Dance [7] for 2D and DBT, respectively:

$$MGD = K\, g c s\, T \qquad (3)$$

where K is the incident air kerma at the upper surface of the breast and g, c and s are the conversion factors of air kerma to glandular dose, respectively. The tomo factor T is included for MGD calculations for DBT modality. All these factors are tabulated as a function of breast thickness, glandularity and X-ray beam quality. Air kerma and half-value layer (HVL) were measured with a 10x5-6M Radcal ionization chamber. High purity aluminum foils were also used for HVL measurements. The exposure technical factors (target, filter, kVp and mAs) and the compressed breast thickness where obtained from the DICOM header of the patient images.

3   Results

Statistically significant differences were found for the detectability and visibility of MC clusters in 2D and C-View images independently of the phantom background (table 1). The detectability (visibility) of the MC in the structured background for the C-View image increased by 50% (100%) compared to the 2D images. The results for the uniform background showed the same detectability values and a slight degradation in visibility (9%) for the C-View images (table 1). As it was expected, the presence of the structured background reduces the detectability and visibility of MC clusters. This is more noticeable for 2D images where a strong reduction of 100% and 267% respectively was found.

Table 1. Summary of the statistics for the scores of detectability and visibility of the microcalcification clusters in the C-View and 2D images for the structured (SB) and uniform (UB) backgrounds

	2D		C-View	
	Detectability (0-6)			
	SB	UB	SB	UB
Average	1.6	4	2.6	3.8
Median	2	4	3	4
Range	1-3	4-4	2-3	3-4
	Visibility (0-18)			
	SB	UB	SB	UB
Average	3.2	11.3	6.1	9.9
Median	3	11	6	10
Range	2-4	10-14	4-7	9-11

C-View offers an average improvement in CNR for all the analyzed details compared to 2D (Fig 3). Some visible artifacts were present in the image, which led to some unexpected values (like one negative CNR for one of the objects). The exact location of some of the objects had to be done approximately as they were hardly visible in the sets of images, especially both upper groups (Fig. 2). The NPW model obtained improved detectability (higher d') with increasing contrast as expected for both 2D and C-View images. Detectability values for some objects were not taken into a count in this calculation as they did not follow this general trend, probably due to artifacts and inexact object location. The model got slightly higher values in C-View compared to 2D images for the lowest contrast objects (0.5 and 1%) (Fig.4). The linear fits of this

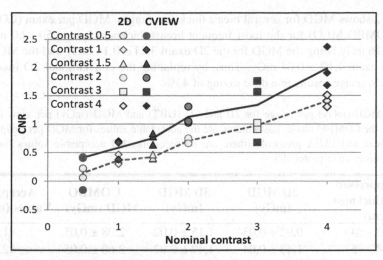

Fig. 3. Contrast-to-noise ratio (CNR) of the LC objects as a function of their nominal contrast. Symbols correspond to average values for each individual object. Lines represent the mean CNR for the details with the same nominal contrast (dash ---2D, −CView).

preliminary results (d' as a function of contrast) showed that the model obtained a higher slope for 2D images than for CView. Further investigation is needed, as it can be seen that the range of d' obtained for each condition was wide, especially for the higher contrasts. This limitation could be overcome with bigger sets of images, as for this study only 3 images per set were available.

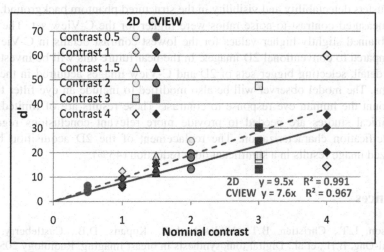

Fig. 4. Detectability index d' obtained with the NPW model observer as a function of the objects nominal contrast. Linear fits are overlaid for the 2D and the CView image sets.

Table 2 shows MGD for several breast thickness ranges. MGD per exam (COMBO CC + COMBO MLO) for the most frequent breast thickness (range 50 - 60 mm) is 7,34 ± 0,16 mGy being the MGD for the 2D exam 3,24 ± 0,14 mGy and the MGD for the tomo exam 4,10 ± 0,04 mGy. Thus, by replacing the conventional 2D image by the C-View image results in a dose saving of 43%.

Table 2. MGD (mGy) per image for 2D and 3D (DBT) and MGD (mGy) per view (CC or MLO) for the COMBO mode. Last column are the acceptable values for MGD per image from the European and IAEA protocols (there are no recommended acceptable values for DBT examinations in these protocols).

Compressed breast thickness (cm)	2D MGD (mGy)	3D MGD (mGy)	COMBO MGD (mGy)	Acceptable Values (mGy)
>3 - ≤4	0,92 ± 0,03	1,15 ± 0,02	2,08 ± 0,05	<1,5
>4 - ≤5	1,13 ± 0,04	1,47 ± 0,02	2,60 ± 0,05	<2,0
>5 - ≤6	1,62 ± 0,07	2,05 ± 0,02	3,67 ± 0,08	<2,5
>6 - ≤7	1,96 ± 0,07	2,76 ± 0,03	4,72 ± 0,08	<3,0
>7 - ≤8	2,29 ± 0,12	3,51 ± 0,04	5,80 ± 0,13	<4,5
>8 - ≤9	2,01 ± 0,01	4,30 ± 0,10	6,31 ± 0,10	<6,5

4   Conclusions

C-View images present superior image quality than 2D images for both microcalcification clusters detectability and visibility in the structured phantom background.

The measured contrast-to-noise ratios were higher for the C-View set. The NPW model obtained slightly higher values for the lowest contrast details in C-View images compared to conventional 2D images. In the near future this will be investigated more in detail, selecting bigger sets of 2D and C-View images acquired in the same conditions. The model observer will be also modified to include an eye filter to take into account the human eye response to contrast. These results are of limited value since clinical studies are needed to provide more relevant conclusions regarding microcalcification characterization. The replacement of the 2D acquisition by the synthesized image results in a significant dose reduction (43%).

References

1. Niklason, L.T., Christian, B.T., Niklason, L.E., Kopans, D.B., Castleberry, D.E., Ophsal-Ong, B.H., et al.: Digital tomosynthesis in breast imaging. Radiology 205, 399–406 (1997)
2. Skaane, P., Bandos, A.I., Gullien, R., Eben, E.B., Ekseth, U., Haakenaasen, U., et al.: Comparison of digital mammography alone and digital mammography plus tomosynthesis in a population-based screening program. Radiology 267, 47–56 (2013)

3. Feng, S.S., Sechopoulos, I.: Clinical digital breast tomosynthesis system: dosimetric characterization. Radiology 263(1), 35–42 (2012)
4. Food and Drug Administration. P080003/S001 Hologic Selenia Dimensions C-View Software Module FDA Panel Pack. Sponsor Executive Summary (2013)
5. Eckstein, M.P., Abbey, C.K., Bochud, F.O.: A practical guide to model observers for visual detection in synthetic and natural noisy images. In: Van Metter, R.L., Beutel, J., Kundel, H.L. (eds.) Handbook of Medical Imaging, vol. 1, pp. 595–628. SPIE-The International Society for Optical Engineering, Washington (2000)
6. Hernandez-Giron, I., Geleijns, J., Calzado, A., Veldkamp, W.J.H.: Automated assessment of low contrast sensitivity for CT systems using a model observer. Med. Phys. 35, S25–S35 (2011)
7. Dance, D.R., Young, K.C., Van Engen, R.E.: Estimation of mean glandular dose for breast tomosynthesis: factors for use with the UK, European and IAEA breast dosimetry protocols. Phys. Med. Biol. 56, 453–470 (2011)

Patient Specific Dose Calculation Using Volumetric Breast Density for Mammography and Tomosynthesis

Christopher E. Tromans[1], Ralph Highnam[1], Oliver Morrish[2], Richard Black[2], Lorraine Tucker[3], Fiona Gilbert[3], and Sir Michael Brady[1]

[1] Volpara Solutions Ltd., Level 6, 86 Victoria Street, Wellington, New Zealand
[2] Cambridge University Hospitals NHS Foundation Trust, Cambridge, United Kingdom
[3] Department of Radiology, University of Cambridge, Cambridge, United Kingdom
chris.tromans@volparasolutions.com

Abstract. Minimising the mean glandular dose (MGD) received by the patient whilst maximising image contrast during mammographic imaging is of paramount importance due to the widespread use of the modality for screening, where subjects are for the most part healthy. The advent of digital mammography brought about a general reduction in MGD, however the introduction of tomosynthesis, particularly when used in combination with conventional projection mammography has the potential for unwanted and often unnecessary MGD increases. We describe a method to calculate the patient-specific MGD using a representation of the patient's volumetric breast density to derive the breast glandularity. This personalises the MGD to the individual woman, rather than assuming a constant value, or one that depends solely on compressed breast thickness. The calculated patient specific MGDs are compared to those reported by the manufacturer for a database of 2D mammograms. Though agreement is generally good for dense breasts, we have found that the MGD is underestimated in fatty breasts. A separate database of 2D mammogram and 3D tomosynthesis acquisitions acquired in "combo" is also analysed. In general, the MGDs are approximately equal for dense (VDG 3 and 4) breasts, but fatty (VDG 1 and 2) breasts exhibited significant differences with tomosynthesis MGDs being higher than mammogram MGDs for these cases.

Keywords: Personalised Patient Mean Glandular Dose, Volumetric Breast Density.

1   Introduction

The breast is among the organs most sensitive to radiation [1], and it is therefore essential to keep x-ray mean glandular dose (MGD) as low as possible, while achieving as diagnostically useful an image as possible, for fear of inducing cancers during mammography and/or tomosynthesis screening. The ACRIN DMIST study summarized the paired screen-film mammography (SFM) and digital mammography (DM) MGDs to over 5000 women, reporting DM as being 22% lower per view, with two-view DM MGDs averaging 3.7 mGy [2]. Subsequently, the introduction both of breast tomosynthesis and of shorter screening intervals for high-risk women

H. Fujita, T. Hara, and C. Muramatsu (Eds.): IWDM 2014, LNCS 8539, pp. 158–165, 2014.
© Springer International Publishing Switzerland 2014

potentially erode this reduction in patient MGD. This in turn has renewed interest in the accurate MGD calculation, tracking, and accountability on an individual patient basis.

A number of different algorithms have been published to estimate of the MGD for any x-ray examination, for example those of Dance et al [3]–[7], Wu et al [8]–[10], and Boone et al [11]. Each of these algorithms embodies slightly different assumptions about the anatomy and the image formation process in the associated Monte-Carlo simulations, for example in the subcutaneous fat surrounding the breast.

A crucial issue arising in breast dosimetry is how to ascertain a key parameter in all MGD calculations, namely the percentage of the breast that contains glandular tissue (the "glandularity"). This has been estimated simply from the compressed breast thickness, or, with even less justification but most commonly, a fixed percentage is assumed for all breasts. In this paper we describe how to use the *Volpara*™ (Matakina, Wellington NZ) volumetric breast density measurement software to estimate the glandularity of each breast from the mammogram, and the MGD calculation method presented by Dance et al [4], to yield a patient-specific MGD. We compare the values calculated by our method with those reported by the manufacturer (as specified in the DICOM header). We also compare results for 2D projection images and 3D tomosynthesis acquisitions in "combo" mode.

2   Materials and Methods

As an illustration of our approach, the method of Dance et al [3]–[7] was selected for calculating MGD, however the approach is equally applicable to other methods in the literature. The method employs a series of multiplicative factors derived from extensive Monte Carlo simulations that are applied to a measure of the incident air kerma upon the upper surface of the breast (the "entrance dose"). In the case of mammography, three factors are used:

(i)   The incident air kerma to MGD conversion factor - this depends on beam quality (measured via the Half Value Layer (HVL)) and the compressed breast thickness;

(ii)   A correction for any difference in breast composition from 50% glandularity – this also depends on the beam quality measured via HVL and compressed breast thickness;

(iii)   A correction for different anode or target materials (which naturally generate different x-ray spectrums).

A further factor is included in the case of tomosynthesis MGD to take consideration of the angle of the x-ray beam.

The Volpara volumetric breast density software quantifies the proportion of the breast occupied by fibroglandular tissue by assessing the difference between the incident photon fluence and that measured by the detector (the output), in terms of the attenuation coefficients of adipose and fibroglandular tissue. Scatter is taken into account. The system is self-calibrating in that an area of the breast image is identified which corresponds to an x-ray beam traversal through entirely fat, the pixel intensity of which is defined as P_{fat}. The P_{fat} point is used as a reference intensity value to facilitate the measure of the thickness of dense tissue d (x, y) at each pixel (x, y). Specifically, the thickness of the dense tissue is computed as:

$$d(x, y) = \frac{\ln\left(\frac{P(x,y)}{P_{fat}}\right)}{\mu_{fat} - \mu_{dense}} \qquad (1)$$

where $P(x, y)$ is the pixel intensity of the raw mammographic image after scatter removal, and μ_{fat} and μ_{dense} are the attenuations of adipose and fibroglandular tissue respectively.

The volumetric breast density is mapped to the breast glandularity according to the assumptions underlying Dance et al's model, in particular: the removal of the subcutaneous fat layer, and the measurement of density in a centralized glandular disk area. **Fig. 1** shows a comparison of Dance's findings and ours as regards relationship between breast thickness and glandularity.

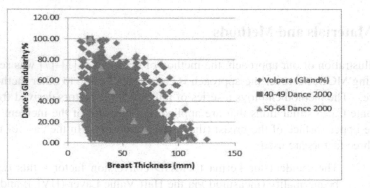

Fig. 1. The relationship between breast thickness and Dance's glandularity as reported by Dance [3], and as found by the density map output from Volpara (blue dots)

Our method has to date been applied to two datasets: 403 2D projection mammogram images acquired on Hologic (Bedford, MA) Selenia equipment (using both Molybdenum and Tungsten targets) in January 2013; and 91 2D-3D image pairs of a distinct set of women, collected on Hologic tomosynthesis equipment operating in "combo" mode. The entrance dose was taken from the DICOM metadata information header, and the HVL was taken from the Volpara output. In the 3D cases, breast density was calculated volumetrically from a single projection image.

3   Results

Fig. 2 shows the relationship between the MGD calculated using the proposed technique including the volumetric breast density derived glandularity, and the MGD reported by the manufacturer in the DICOM header, for the lowest density (fatty) VDG1 (the volumetric correspondent to BIRADS 1) and highest density VDG4 (BIRADS 4).   An underestimation of the MGD in the fatty category may be observed, together with a general trend for higher MGDs in the denser cases, as is to be expected from the greater photon fluences required to give an optimal contrast-to-noise ratio in dense tissue.

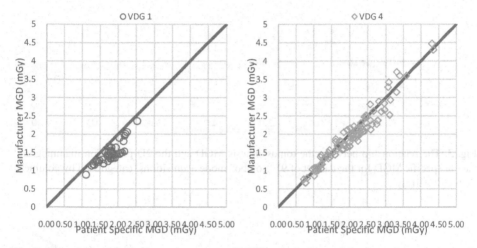

Fig. 2. The relationship between the proposed MGD calculation and the manufacturer reported dose for the dataset of 403 2D projection mammograms

Fig. 3 shows the relationship between the tomosynthesis and mammographic projection acquisitions for the personalised patient MGD using the glandularity derived from the volumetric breast density. The Pearson correlation coefficient between the personalised patient MGDs for tomosynthesis and projection mammography is 0.608.

Fig. 4 shows the same relationship between the two acquisition types, but uses the manufacturer reported MGD included in the DICOM metadata header. The Pearson correlation coefficient in this case being 0.578.

The Pearson correlation coefficient between the personalised patient MGD and the manufacturer reported MGD is 0.970 in the case of projection mammography, and 0.974 for tomosynthesis acquisition.

It may be observed, for both the personalised MGD, and the manufacturer reported MGD, that at lower breast density (specifically VDG 1 and 2) the mammographic MGD is lower than the tomosynthesis MGD, but at higher breast density (VDG 3 and 4) the MGDs are approximately equal (though where a high MGD is delivered tomosynthesis gives the lower MGD).

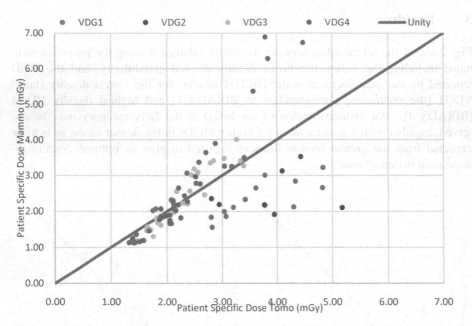

Fig. 3. The relationship between the tomosynthesis MGD and the 2D projection mammogram patient specific MGD for the dataset of 91 "combo" mode acquisitions, categorised by volumetric breast density

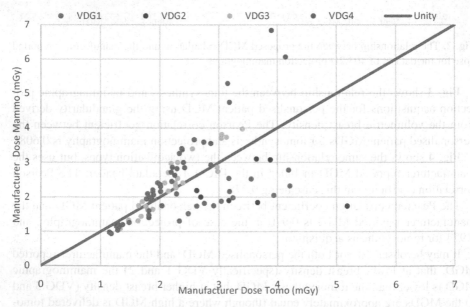

Fig. 4. The relationship between the tomosynthesis MGD and the 2D projection mammogram manufacturer reported MGD from the DICOM metadata for the dataset of 91 "combo" mode acquisitions, categorised by volumetric breast density

4   Discussion

The pertinent question arising from the results in **Fig. 3** and **Fig. 4**, is whether or not the higher tomosynthesis MGD in the case of low density breasts\is a fundamental characteristic of the image formation process, i.e. the relation between the incident photon fluence and the contrast-to-noise characteristics of the detector, or a lack of optimisation in the automatic exposure control (AEC) algorithms. This phenomena has also been observed in a compressible water-oil mixture phantom study presented in the literature by Feng et al [12]. They reported that for a breast with a compressed thickness of 50 cm and a 50% glandularity, a tomosynthesis acquisition resulted in an 8% higher MGD than an project mammogram (1.30 and 1.20 mGy, respectively); whilst for a breast with a compressed thickness of 60 mm and a 14.3% glandularity, tomosynthesis resulted in an 83% higher MGD than the mammogram (2.12 and 1.16 mGy, respectively). The tomosynthesis acquisitions are all acquired using a Tungsten anode, and a 0.7mm thick Aluminium filter, so the only variation in the beam quality selected by the AEC results from the tube voltage (kVp). **Fig. 5** shows a histogram depicting the variations in tube voltage over the four VDG categories. Generally, lower density breasts, are imaged at higher tube voltages.

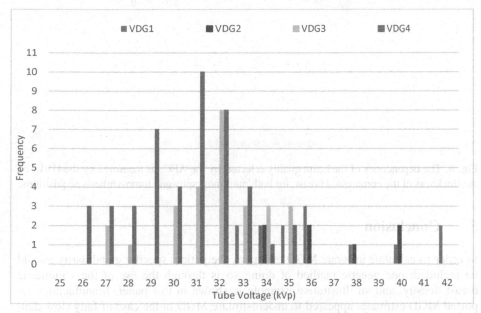

Fig. 5. The variation in tube voltage selected by the AEC for the tomosynthesis acquisitions with volumetric breast density, categorised using VDG

Fig. 6 shows the relationship between the beam quality selected by the AEC (expressed using the HVL), and the compressed breast thickness, for both projection mammography, and tomosynthesis acquisitions. The near linear relationship, with coefficients of determination of almost unity, confirms the AEC is placing considerable emphasis on the compressed breast thickness to select the beam quality. This is to be expected, since the difference in the attenuation coefficients of adipose and fibroglandular tissue are small compared to the significantly different attenuation of air. Therefore the changes in breast density are of secondary effect in terms of the total attenuation of the breast, and hence the incident photon fluence on the detector, compared to a change in compressed breast thickness.

Since superposition leading to feature noise (and hence potential masking) is limited in low density breasts, this raises the question of whether the increased MGD in the tomosynthesis exam is beneficial compared to that of the mammo, since the clinical benefit of the 3D slices in this situation is unclear. Investigating this topic is an area of our future work.

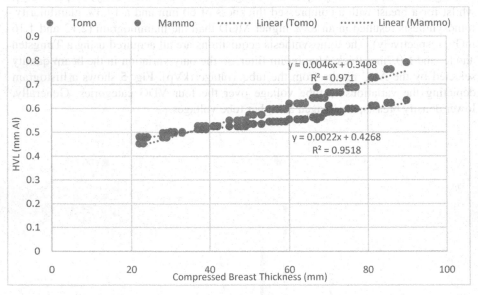

Fig. 6. The dependency of the beam quality selected by the AEC, as measured by the HVL, on the thickness of the compressed breast, for both mammography and tomosynthesis acquisitions.

5   Conclusion

In order to calculate accurate MGD estimates the patient specific glandularity should be included: one generic method of doing so is through the use of the volumetric breast density, and an illustrative example is shown in this paper. Manufacturer reported MGD estimates appeared to underestimate MGD in the case of fatty (low density) breasts in comparison to our calculations, but gave good agreement in the case of dense breasts. When comparing MGD in "combo" mode tomosynthesis/mammography examinations, at lower breast density the mammographic MGD is lower than in tomosynthesis, but at higher density the MGDs are approximately equal. This raises the issue of whether the higher tomosynthesis MGDs for low density breasts with limited to no tissue superposition, and hence unlikely to contain masked malignancies, is beneficial.

References

[1] The 2007 Recommendations of the International Commission on Radiological Protection. ICRP publication 103. Ann. ICRP 37(2-4), 1–332 (January 2007)

[2] Hendrick, R.E., Pisano, E.D., Averbukh, A., Moran, C., Berns, E.A., Yaffe, M.J., Herman, B., Acharyya, S., Gatsonis, C.: Comparison of acquisition parameters and breast dose in digital mammography and screen-film mammography in the American College of Radiology Imaging Network digital mammographic imaging screening trial. AJR. Am. J. Roentgenol. 194(2), 362–369 (2010)

[3] Dance, D.R., Skinner, C.L., Young, K.C., Beckett, J.R., Kotre, C.J.: Additional factors for the estimation of mean glandular breast dose using the UK mammography dosimetry protocol. Phys. Med. Biol. 45(11), 3225 (2000)

[4] Dance, D.R., Young, K.C., van Engen, R.E.: Estimation of mean glandular dose for breast tomosynthesis: factors for use with the UK, European and IAEA breast dosimetry protocols. Phys. Med. Biol. 56(2), 453–471 (2011)

[5] Dance, D.R., Thilander, A.K., Sandborg, M., Skinner, C.L., Castellano, I.A., Carlsson, G.A.: Influence of anode/filter material and tube potential on contrast, signal-to-noise ratio and average absorbed dose in mammography: a Monte Carlo study. Br. J. Radiol. 73(874), 1056–1067 (2000)

[6] Dance, D.R., Young, K.C., van Engen, R.E.: Further factors for the estimation of mean glandular dose using the United Kingdom, European and IAEA breast dosimetry protocols. Phys. Med. Biol. 54(14), 4361–4372 (2009)

[7] Dance, D.R.: Monte Carlo calculation of conversion factors for the estimation of mean glandular breast dose. Phys. Med. Biol. 35(9), 1211–1219 (1990)

[8] Wu, X., Barnes, G.T., Tucker, D.M.: Spectral dependence of glandular tissue dose in screen-film mammography. Radiology 179(1), 143–148 (1991)

[9] Sobol, W.T., Wu, X.: Parametrization of mammography normalized average glandular dose tables. Med. Phys. 24(4), 547–554 (1997)

[10] Wu, X., Gingold, E.L., Barnes, G.T., Tucker, D.M.: Normalized average glandular dose in molybdenum target-rhodium filter and rhodium target-rhodium filter mammography. Radiology 193(1), 83–89 (1994)

[11] Boone, J.M.: Glandular breast dose for monoenergetic and high-energy X-ray beams: Monte Carlo assessment. Radiology 213(1), 23–37 (1999)

[12] Feng, S.S.J., Sechopoulos, I.: Clinical digital breast tomosynthesis system: dosimetric characterization. Radiology 263(1), 35–42 (2012)

Comparative Performance Evaluation of Contrast-Detail in Full Field Digital Mammography (FFDM) Systems Using Ideal (Hotelling) Observer versus Automated CDMAM Analysis

Ioannis Delakis[1,2], Robert Wise[2], Lauren Morris[2], and Eugenia Kulama[2]

[1] Sidra Medical and Research Centre, Doha, Qatar
idelakis@sidra.org
[2] Radiological Sciences Unit, Charing Cross Hospital, Fulham Palace Road, London, United Kingdom
{robert.wise2,lauren.morris,eugenia.kulama}@imperial.nhs.uk

Abstract. The purpose of our work was to evaluate contrast-detail performance for a range of full field digital mammography systems using Hotelling observer SNR analysis and ascertain whether it can be considered an alternative to CDMAM evaluation. Five FFDM systems were evaluated, which differed in generation (age), Automatic Exposure Control (AEC) behaviour, tube/target combination and detector type. Contrast-detail performance was first analysed using CDMAM phantom analysis and then using the Hotelling observer SNR methodology. The Hotelling observer SNR was calculated for input signal originating from gold discs of varying thicknesses and diameters and then used to estimate the threshold gold thicknesses for each diameter as per CDMAM analysis. There were small differences between the two techniques, especially in small diameter details, which can be attributed to structural characteristics of the CDMAM phantom. The Hotelling observer SNR technique showed lower variability than results from CDMAM analysis. Overall, the Hotelling observer SNR methodology showed variations in the FFDM systems performance consistent with previous findings, demonstrating its value as a performance assessment metric.

Keywords: CDMAM, Hotelling Observer, Ideal Observer, image quality.

1 Introduction

The main methodology used to evaluate mammographic image quality in European quality control programmes is based on the analysis of threshold detectability characteristics, using the contrast-detail phantom for mammography (CDMAM) [1-3]. Images acquired using the CDMAM phantom can be analysed either with observer or automated readings. Observer-based readings are affected by intra-observer error, which can compromise the reliability and confidence of the results. In addition, reading CDMAM images can be time consuming, and therefore often not practical for routine assessment of image quality. Although recent work has tried to link automated

H. Fujita, T. Hara, and C. Muramatsu (Eds.): IWDM 2014, LNCS 8539, pp. 166–173, 2014.

readings with human-observer performance, results can be further dependent on structural differences between CDMAM phantoms [3-4].

As an alternative to CDMAM analysis, the ideal-observer methodology can be used to evaluate threshold detectability characteristics of FFDM systems. An ideal observer is a hypothetical device that performs a given task at the optimal level possible, given the available information and any specified constraints. The correlation between ideal observer results and human performance is dependent on the type of ideal observer used. In this study we used the Hotelling ideal observer as it takes into account both first- and second-order statistics of image data to incorporate some of the human observer limitations [5-6]. Previous work has generalised the definition of Hotelling observer to include the effects of focal spot unsharpness, magnification and scattering, and successfully applied the methodology in the evaluation of FFDM systems [7-12]. The purpose of our work was to study the threshold detectability performance for a range of FFDM systems, using both CDMAM and ideal (Hotelling) observer analysis and ascertain whether the ideal observer methodology can offer some advantages over CDMAM evaluation.

2   Materials and Methods

The FFDM systems included in our study are shown in Table 1 and the properties of their detectors are shown in Table 2.

Table 1. List of FFDM systems included in the study

Manufacturer	System Type	Installation	AEC setting
GE Healthcare	Senographe DS	July 2007	Contrast
GE Healthcare	Senograhe Essential	August 2010	Standard
Hologic	Selenia (Mo target)	June 2007	Autofilter
Hologic	Selenia (W target)	March 2011	Autofilter
Hologic	Dimensions	November 2010	Autofilter

Table 2. Detector properties of FFDM systems included in the study

Manufacturer	System Type	Detector Type	Size (cm)	Pixel size (μm)
GE Healthcare	Senographe DS	CsI (indirect)	19x23	100
GE Healthcare	Senographe Essential	CsI (indirect)	24x29	100
Hologic	Selenia (Mo target)	Selenium (direct)	24x29	70
Hologic	Selenia (W target)	Selenium (direct)	24x29	70
Hologic	Dimensions	Selenium (direct)	24x29	70

The FFDM systems differ with respect to generation, detector, tube technology, as well as the behaviour of their Automatic Exposure control (AEC) and the subsequent choice of target/filter combination, tube potential (kVp) and mAs for clinical exposures. The AEC setting used in this work is the same as what is currently applied on each system for breast screening studies of 60mm breast thickness, as prescribed by European and UK evaluation protocols [1], [13]. All FFDM systems had a nominal focal spot of 0.3mm.

2.1   CDMAM Methodology

FFDM systems were evaluated with the CDMAM phantom following the methodology described by EUREF, the European Reference Organisation for Quality Assured Breast Screening and Diagnostic References [1] and the NHS Breast Screening programme [13]. For each of the FFDM systems listed in Table 1, sixteen "for processing" CDMAM images were evaluated using the CDMAM Analyser (version 1.5.5) and CDCOM (version 1.6), software provided by EUREF.

Threshold detectability was also evaluated with five different CDMAM phantoms, currently in use by mammography physics services in London, as shown in Table 3. CDMAM data acquisition and analysis was repeated on the same FFDM system (GE Healthcare, Senograph DS) and results were compared to identify variability across CDMAM phantoms.

Table 3. CDMAM phantoms used in cross-phantom evaluation

CDMAM #	Serial #	Clinical site
1	1013	The Royal Marsden NHS Trust
2	1036	Bart's Health NHS Trust
3	1683	Imperial College Healthcare NHS Trust
4	1227	Mount Vernon Hospital - Hillingdon Hospital NHS Trust
5	1512	Royal Free London NHS Foundation Trust

2.2   Hotelling Observer SNR Methodology

GNNPS and GMTF Data Acquisition. Estimating the Hotelling observer SNR requires calculation of the Generalised Modulation Transfer Function (GMTF), Generalised Normalised Noise Power Spectrum (GNNPS) and their respective Generalised Noise Equivalent Quanta (GNEQ). The steps involved in the calculation of the Modulation Transfer Function (MTF), Normalised Noise Power Spectrum (NNPS) and Noise Equivalent Quanta (NEQ) have been described extensively in previous work, for example by Marshall (2006) [14]. The Generalised definition of MTF includes the effect of detector blur, focal spot unsharpness, magnification and scatter properties of the system [11]. In our work, the GMTF was measured by calculating the MTF on an image acquired by placing a thin (0.2mm), sharp edge of tungsten foil between two slabs of 25mm PMMA, at a slightly oblique angle (1-2°). The Generalised definition of the NNPS includes the effect of scatter on the input signal and was measured by calculating the NNPS of four "for processing" images of 50mm of PMMA, using the same exposure settings as for the CDMAM methodology. By using the GMTF and GNNPS we then calculated the GNEQ as:

$$GNEQ(f_x,f_y) = \frac{GMTF(f_x,f_y)^2}{GNNPS(f_x,f_y)} \tag{1}$$

where f_x and f_y is spatial frequency in x and y directions, respectively.

Hotelling Observer SNR Calculation. The Hotelling observer SNR can be calculated for any given signal. In order to compare results with CDMAM methodology, the signal (ΔS) used in this study is the Fourier transform of golden discs with varying thickness (h) and diameter (r):

$$\Delta S(f,h,r) = \alpha(h) \cdot \frac{\sqrt{3r}}{4f} \cdot J_1 \cdot (2\pi fr) \tag{2}$$

where f is the vectorial sum of f_x and f_y, J_1 is the Bessel function of the first kind and $\alpha(h)$ is the radiographic contrast of gold at thickness h. The attenuation characteristics of gold for each kVp and filter/target combination were based on work published by the National Health Service Breast Screening Programme (NHSBSP) and are different for each kV and spectrum (target/filter) [13]. The SNR for this signal was calculated as an integral of the GNEQ over all spatial frequencies, weighted by the spectrum of the signal ΔS [15]:

$$SNR^2 = \iint_{f_x,f_y} GNEQ\left(f_x,f_y\right) \Delta S(f,h,r)\, df_x\, df_y \tag{3}$$

The SNR calculated for a disc of set diameter and thickness was then compared to a threshold SNR value to determine whether the disc can be considered detected. In order to have a detection task comparable to CDMAM analysis, the threshold SNR was determined on the basis of multiple alternative forced choice (MAFC) analysis, as the CDMAM methodology requires the observer to make a decision on which of four corners the signal is present. Work performed by Burgess (1995) [16] outlines the probability of detection in a MAFC experiment for a given SNR. As typical for 4AFC tests, CDMAM details were considered detected when the probability of detection, based on their Hotelling observer SNR, was equal or higher than 0.625, which is the midway point between 0.25 (random guessing) and 1.00 (perfect response).

Intra-System Reproducibility. In order to compare the short-term reproducibility of CDMAM and Hotelling observer SNR methodologies, the GE Healthcare, Senographe Essential, FFDM system was evaluated at the same time (noon) over a period of five consecutive working days. The mean and standard deviation values of the threshold detectability values were then calculated for results from each methodology.

3   Results and Discussion

Fig. 1 shows the magnitude difference between CDMAM results from each phantom and the overall mean value. The dotted lines in the figure show the average error margin (2sem) expected from CDMAM results at each disc diameter, and indicate that the magnitude difference at small details is equal or greater than the error margin. It is worth noting that CDMAM #3, which is used in subsequent parts of this study, appears to be overestimating threshold detectability, especially for small details, suggesting under-performance of the FFDM system across the range of detail diameters.

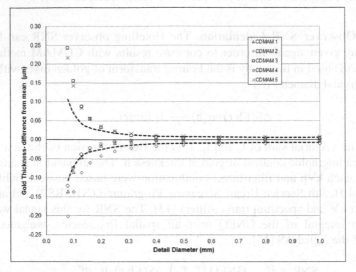

Fig. 1. Magnitude difference of threshold detectability gold thickness results from mean

As shown in Fig. 2, both methodologies indicate that threshold detectability is lower for Selenium compared to CsI detectors, which is consistent with previous work [17] and reflects differences in detector type (direct vs. indirect) and pixel size.

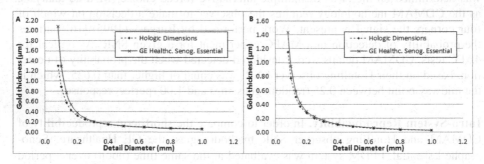

Fig. 2. Threshold detectability results using CDMAM (**A**) and Hotelling observer SNR (**B**) methodologies, for FFDM systems of different detector type

Both methodologies also show an improvement in the performance of new generation FFDM systems, which may be attributed to technological improvements but could also indicate the impact of wear and tear on account of age and workload. As shown in Table 4, the average ratio of threshold detectability for New-to-Old generation FFDM systems tends to be less than unity, indicating the superiority in performance of new compared to older generation FFDM systems. Overall, results show that the Hotelling observer SNR methodology can be a more sensitive performance differentiator.

Table 4. Average ratio of threshold detectability results (New-to-Old FFDM system)

	GE Sen. Essential/ GE Senog. DS	Hologic Selenia (W)/ Hologic Selenia (Mo)	Hologic Dimensions/ Hologic Selenia (Mo)
CDMAM fit to predicted	0.83	0.89	0.99
Hotelling observer	0.89	0.90	0.89

Fig. 3 shows the mean and standard deviation of threshold detectability results using both methodologies on the same FFDM system for five consecutive days. The standard deviation, as indicated by the error bars in Fig. 3, is a measure of the intra-system variability of results from each methodology. On average, there was 7% variation in CDMAM results, reaching 10% for small details (0.08mm diameter). Results using the Hotelling observer SNR methodology were more consistent, with average variation of approximately 1%.

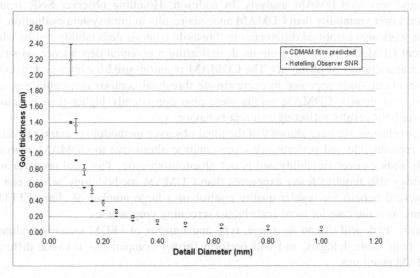

Fig. 3. Mean and standard deviation (error bars) of threshold detectability results using both methodologies on the same FFDM system for five consecutive days

Threshold detectability results using the Hotelling observer SNR methodology were consistently lower than CDMAM results, across all detail diameters and for all FFDM systems, as shown in Table 5. This may reflect the structural characteristics of the CDMAM phantom #3 used in this study, which appears to be overestimating threshold detectability, as previously discussed. The difference between threshold detectability results is higher at small diameter details, which is also consistent with the behaviour of the CDMAM phantom #3, as shown in Fig. 1.

Table 5. Average ratio of threshold detectability results (Hotelling observer-to-CDMAM methodology) for each FFDM system

Manufacturer	System Type	Ratio
GE Healthcare	Senographe DS	0.67
GE Healthcare	Senographe Essential	0.71
Hologic	Selenia (Mo target)	0.83
Hologic	Selenia (W target)	0.85
Hologic	Dimensions	0.74

4   Conclusions

Threshold contrast detectability was evaluated on a number of FFDM systems using both CDMAM and Hotelling observer SNR methodologies. Results showed that the Hotelling observer SNR methodology can be used as a performance metric for FFDM systems, displaying differences with respect to system generation and detector type, in the same way as CDMAM analysis. In addition, Hotelling observer SNR results showed lower variability than CDMAM analysis results in intra-system evaluation.

Our work also identified differences in threshold contrast detectability results when different CDMAM phantoms were used, indicating a potential dependence on structural characteristics of phantoms. The CDMAM phantom used for inter-system comparison in our study appeared to overestimate threshold contrast detectability across all diameter details. CDMAM results were also consistently higher than Hotelling observer SNR results, reflecting a similar behavior.

In conclusion, we have shown that the ideal observer methodology could provide a more reproducible and performance-representative alternative to CDMAM analysis, as it is shows lower variability and is not phantom-specific. The ideal observer methodology also requires fewer exposures than CDMAM methodology, which can be of practical benefit for regular quality control of a large number of clinical FFDM systems, as is the case for large-scale breast screening programmes.

Future work will extend the range, type and number of FFDM systems evaluated using both methodologies, and will perform further comparisons between different CDMAM phantoms.

References

1. Van Engen, R., Young, K., Bosmans, H., Thijssen, H.: The European protocol for the quality control of the physical and technical aspects of mammography screening. Euref, Luxembourg (2006)
2. Young, K., Johnson, B., Bosmans, H., Van Engen, R.: Development of minimum standards for image quality and dose in digital mammography. In: Digital Mammography IWDM 2004, Durham NC, USA (2005)

3. Young, K., Alsager, A., Oduko, J., Bosmans, H., Verbrugge, B., Geerste, T., et al.: Evaluation of software for reading images of the CDMAM test object to assess digital mammography systems. In: Proc. SPIE, vol. 6913, p. 69131C (2008)
4. Young, K.C., Cook, J.J.H., Oduko, J.M., Bosmans, H.: Comparison of software and human observers in reading images of the CDMAM test object to assess digital mammography systems. In: Proc. SPIE, vol. 6142, p. 614206 (2006)
5. Sandrik, J., Wagner, R.: Absolute measures of physical image quality: measurement and application to radiographic magnification 9(4), 540-9 (1982)
6. Barrett, H., Yao, J., Rolland, J., Myers, K.: Model observers for assessment of image quality. Proc. Natl. Acad. Sci. 90(21), 9758–9765 (1993)
7. Kyprianou, I.S.: A method for total x-ray imaging system evaluation. PhD Thesis. University of New York, Buffalo, NY (2004)
8. Kyprianou, I.S., Rudin, S., Bednarek, D., Hoffman, K.: Generalizing the MTF and DQE to include x-ray scatter and focal spot unsharpness: application to a new microangiographic system. Med. Phys. 32(2), 613–626 (2005)
9. Kyprianou, I., Ganguly, A., Rudin, S., Bednarek, D., Gallas, B., Myers, K.: Efficiency of the Human Observer Compared to an Ideal Observer Based on a Generalized NEQ Which Incorporates Scatter and Geometric Unsharpness: Evaluation with a 2AFC Experiment. In: Proc. Soc. Photo. Opt. Instrum. Eng., vol. 5749, pp. 251–262 (2005)
10. Liu, H., Kyprianou, I.S., Badano, A., Myers, K.J., Jennings, R.J., Park, S., et al.: SKE/BKE Task-based methodology for calculating Hotelling observer SNR in mammography. In: Proc. of the SPIE, Medical Imaging, vol. 7258 (2009)
11. Liu, H., Badano, A., Chakrabarti, K., Kaczmarek, R., Kyprianou, I.: Task specific evaluation of clinical full field digital mammography systems using the Fourier definition of the Hotelling observer SNR. In: Proc. of the SPIE, Medical Imaging, vol. 7622 (2010)
12. Liu, H.: Task specific evaluation methodology for clinical Full Field Digital Mammography. PhD Thesis. University of Maryland, College Park (2012)
13. Commissioning and routine testing of Full Field Digital Mammography Systems. NHSBSP Equipment Report 0604. NHS Cancer Screening Programmes, Sheffield. Report No.: version 4 (in press)
14. Marshall, N.: A comparison between objective and subjective image quality measurements for a full field digital mammography system 51(10), 2441–63 (2006)
15. Wagner, R.F., Brown, D.: Unified SNR analysis of medical imaging systems. Phys. Med. Biol. 30, 489–518 (1985)
16. Burgess, A.: Comparison of receiver operating characteristic and forced choice observer performance measurement methods. Medical Physics 22(5), 643 (1995)
17. Review of measurements on full field digital mammography systems. NHSBSP Equipment Report 0901. NHS Cancer Screening Programme (2009)

Mammographic Density Effect on Readers' Performance and Visual Search Pattern

Dana S. AL Mousa, Patrick C. Brennan, Elaine A. Ryan,
and Claudia Mello-Thoms

Department of Medical Imaging and Radiation Sciences, Faculty of Health Sciences,
University of Sydney, Cumberland Campus, East Street, P.O. Box 170, Lidcombe, NSW 2141,
Australia
dalm3874@uni.sydney.edu.au,
{patrick.brennan,elaine.ryan,claudia.mello-thoms}@sydney.edu.au

Abstract. A test set of 150 digital mammograms were examined by 14 radiologists, seven of which underwent eye-position recording. Mammograms were classified into low- and high- density cases, in order to investigate the impact of density on readers' performance and visual search patterns. Lesions overlaying were compared to those outside the dense fibroglandular tissue. Our results suggest that when the lesion was overlaying the fibroglandular tissue, readers' performance significantly improved in high- compared to low- density cases. Also the dense area of breast parenchyma attracted the radiologists' visual attention, in both low- and high- mammographic density cases. When the lesions were outside the dense fibroglandular tissue, no difference was noted in radiologist' performance. In conclusion, dense areas of the breast parenchyma attracted the radiologists' visual attention, in both low- and high density cases, which might improve lesion detection when the malignancy is overlaying the dense parts of the breast tissue.

Keywords: Mammographic breast density, digital mammography, readers' performance, visual search pattern.

1   Introduction

Mammography generates an image that represents the breast tissue including fatty and fibroglandular tissue. The proportion of fibroglandular tissue in relation to the fatty tissue in the breast is called 'mammographic density' [1] . Mammographic density is associated with a 4- to 6-times increased risk for breast cancer in women with high mammographic breast density [2, 3]. The contrast between cancerous lesions and the dense fibroglandular tissue is low; therefore, it is assumed that lesions overlaying the fibroglandular tissue are difficult to be detected.

The evidence with screen-film mammography suggests that increased mammographic density has the potential to decrease sensitivity [4-6] and specificity [7, 8]. In addition, higher density in the film screen era was associated with increased risk of interval cancers [4, 9], as well as increased numbers of large screen-detected tumours

H. Fujita, T. Hara, and C. Muramatsu (Eds.): IWDM 2014, LNCS 8539, pp. 174–180, 2014.

(>15mm) [10-13]. Studies that have compared digital with screen-film mammography have incidentally found that sensitivity may increase marginally in high- (83.6%) compared with low- (68.1%) mammographic breast density cases [14, 15]. The increased performance in high density breasts was also shown by a recent study, were they found that false positive rates were higher in low mammographic density images [16]. However the precise effect of density in the digital era remains under-explored, especially with the availability of post processing tools, potentially allowing better differentiation between dense fibroglandular tissue and cancer. Moreover, the effect of mammographic density on radiologists' searching patterns has not been fully studied, in the sense that it is unclear whether the dense areas of the parenchyma have a distracter or attractor effect for visual attention. If mammographic density impact is fully understood, we will be able to optimize viewing algorithms and design training strategies.

The purpose of this study is to determine the impact of mammographic breast density on radiologists' performance and in their visual search processes, using digitally acquired and displayed mammograms.

2   Methods

Institutional ethical approval was granted, patient consent waived and participated radiologists signed a consent form for their participation. Fourteen radiologists voluntarily participated in this study and seven underwent eye-position recording. From BreastScreen NSW, Australia, a test set of 150 cranio-caudal (CC) digital mammographic cases with a range of mammographic breast densities were selected. All patient identification was removed from the mammograms. The test set included 75 malignancy-free mammograms and 75 cases with 78 biopsy proven malignant lesions. Malignancy-free images were confirmed after two years of follow up. Cancerous lesions had a median diameter of 12 mm (min of 8 mm; max of 20.6 mm). Malignancy containing cases were chosen depending on whether or not the lesion was completely overlaying or whether it was completely outside the fibroglandular tissue. An expert radiologist (who did not participate as a reader in the study), outlined the "true" locations of all malignancies with the help of pathology reports.

Mammographic density was classified according to the Synoptic Breast Imaging Report of the National Breast Cancer Centre (NBCC, now Cancer Australia), endorsed by the Royal Australian and New Zealand College of Radiologists (RANZCR) [17], which is similar to the 4th edition American College of Radiology Breast Imaging Reporting and Data System (BI-RADS) [18]:

1) Low mammographic density cases: RANZCR/NBCC first level (<25% glandular tissue) and second level (25-50%);
2) High mammographic density cases: RANZCR/NBCC third level (51-75% glandular tissue) and fourth level (>75%).

In low mammographic density category, 18 cases had the lesion completely overlaying and 19 cases had it outside the fibroglandular tissue. In high mammographic density cases, 21 and 16 had the lesion completely overlaying and outside the fibroglandular tissue, respectively.

The study included two concurrent phases that were performed in a single viewing session: 1) Visual search and; 2) Reporting and localizing detected cancers. Mammograms were displayed on 5 Mega-pixel medical LCD monitor (EIZO, Japan) driven by SECTRA (Sectra Imtec AB, Sweden) workstations with ATI FirePro V5800 (FIREGL) video cards (Sunnyvale, California). The display was calibrated using Digital Imaging and Communications in Medicine (DICOM) part 14 standard. The observers freely examine each case until they confidently provided an initial impression of the case (namely normal or abnormal). They had full access to standard postprocessing tools, including windowing, zooming and panning. If the case was deemed abnormal, radiologists reported the locations of all malignant masses that they believe to be present, using a mouse-controlled cursor. Their confidence level was also reported on a scale from 1–5, with a higher number indicating increased confidence. Radiologists' performance was evaluated using metrics such as specificity (correct identification of malignancy-free images), location sensitivity (correct localization of true cancers with a confidence score of 3, 4 or 5), and jackknife free-response receiver operating characteristic (JAFROC) figure of metric (FOM).

For a sub-group of participants visual search was recorded using the Mobile Eye XG (MEXG) eye-tracking system (Applied Sciences Laboratories, Bedford, MA, USA) to calculate line-of-gaze by monitoring pupil and corneal reflection. The system has 0.5-1° of visual angle accuracy with 30 Hz frequency for data collection. Radiologists were seated on an average of 60 cm distance from the diagnostic monitor. Fixation was defined by at least three sequential eye-position points within a circle of diameter 0.5° of visual angle with a duration of $\geq$ 100 ms. Using the Applied Science Laboratories ASL Results Plus software, fixation location ((x,y) coordinates) and total fixation duration (in ms) were collected, in 3 areas of interests (AOI): background breast parenchyma, dense areas of breast parenchyma and lesion. An interactive semiautomated thresholding Cumulus algorithm [19] was used to segment the dense areas of the breast parenchyma from the background breast parenchyma.

The following visual search parameters were calculated: 1) Total reading time, 2) Time to first fixate a lesion, 3) Total gaze time in each AOI, per case and 4) Number of hits in each AOI per case.

The impact of mammographic density on the readers' performance and visual search was assessed by comparing low- with high- mammographic density cases using two groupings:

1.   Lesion overlaying the dense fibroglandular tissue;
2.   Lesion outside the dense fibroglandular tissue.

Statistical analyses was performed using the non-parametric Wilcoxon signed-rank test, while visual search was contrasted using the non-parametric Mann-Whitney U test. For all analyses, significance was set at $P < 0.05$.

3   Results

Results are described in two comparisons for the impact of mammographic density on readers' 1) performance and 2) visual search.

3.1   Impact of Mammographic Density on Readers' Performance

Lesion Overlaying the Fibroglandular Tissue. Table 1 shows the readers' performance when lesions are completely overlaying the fibroglandular region. As shown, lower location sensitivity (50.0 vs 59.1) (W=-71, P =0.03) and JAFROC FOM (0.63 vs 0.68) (W=-64, P =0.05) were observed between low- and high- mammographic density cases, respectively.

Table 1. Mammographic density impact on readers' performance: lesion overlaying fibroglandular dense tissue. Median values (IQR) are presented.

Metrics	Low density	High density	P value
Specificity	77.0 (25.68)	76.3 (38.16)	0.41
Location sensitivity	50.0 (20.84)	59.1 (38.64)	0.03
JAFROC	0.63 (0.1)	0.68 (0.13)	0.05

IQR, Inter-quartile Range

Lesion Outside the Fibroglandular Tissue. Table 2 shows the readers' performance when lesions are completely outside the fibroglandular region. No significant changes were found in readers' performance.

Table 2. Mammographic density impact on readers' performance: lesion outside fibroglandular dense tissue. Median values (IQR) are presented.

Metrics	Low density	High density	P value
Specificity	77.0 (25.68)	76.3 (38.16)	0.41
Location sensitivity	65.8 (35.52)	62.5 (39.06)	0.22
JAFROC	0.71 (0.14)	0.72 (0.09)	0.13

IQR, Inter-quartile Range

3.2   Impact of Mammographic Density on Readers' Visual Search

Lesion Overlaying the Fibroglandular Tissue. No significant differences were noted in total reading time and time to first fixate a lesion between high and low mammographic density images when the lesion was overlaying the fibroglandular tissue. As shown in table 3, significant increases in total gaze time (Z= -4.672, P< 0.0001) and number of hits (Z= -5.02, P< 0.0001) were observed on dense areas of the breast parenchyma in high- compared to low-density mammograms.

Table 3. Impact of mammographic density on readers' visual search when lesion overlaid   the fibroglandular tissue Median values (IQR) are presented. Times are shown in seconds.

Parameter	AOI	Low density	High density	P
Total gaze time	Background	4.91 (3.37)	5.17 (3.2)	0.72
	Dense	0.715 (2.48)	1.26 (4.8)	<0.0001
	Lesion	1.76 (5.72)	1.67 (4.68)	0.391
Number of hits per AOI	Background	18 (28.25)	20 (27.71)	0.332
	Dense	3 (9.73)	6 (18.34)	<0.0001
	Lesion	7 (13.5)	6 (11.01)	0.444

IQR, Inter-quartile Range

Lesion Outside the Fibroglandular Tissue. No significant differences were noted in total reading time and time to first fixate a lesion between high and low mammographic density cases when the lesion was outside the fibroglandular tissue. Table 4 presents the comparison between low- and high- mammographic density cases when the lesion was outside the fibroglandular tissue. As presented, total gaze time on dense areas of the breast parenchyma was significantly shorter (Z=-2.95, P =0.003) and the number of hits was lower (Z=-2.628, P =0.009) in low- compared to high-mammographic density images.

Table 4. Impact of mammographic density on readers' visual search when lesion was outside the fibroglandular tissue. Median values (IQR) are presented. Times are shown in seconds.

Parameter	AOI	Low density	High density	P
Total gaze time	Background	4.38 (3.65)	4.64 (3.5)	0.954
	Dense	0.97 (3.93)	1.65 (5.81)	0.003
	Lesion	1.13 (4.57)	1.04 (3.16)	0.265
Number of hits per AOI	Background	18 (3.34)	17 (5.26)	0.993
	Dense	4 (15.95)	7 (22.45)	0.009
	Lesion	4 (13.67)	4 (8.96)	0.387

IQR, Inter-quartile Range

4   Discussion

The evidence with screen-film mammography suggested that lesion detection may decrease with high density breasts. However, with digital mammography it has been conjectured that readers' performance increases in high- compared to low- density cases [14-16]. A better understanding of the precise impact of mammographic density on readers' performance and visual search patterns when reading digital mammograms would present a basis for improving lesion detection.

The results of this study suggest that high mammographic density cases improve the radiologists' performance with regards to location sensitivity and JAFROC FOM, when lesion was overlaying the dense fibroglandular tissue. One potential explanation is the fact that high mammographic density is associated with increased risk of breast cancer; therefore dense areas of breast parenchyma may attract readers' visual attention. In this study radiologists had longer gaze time and higher number of hits on dense area of breast parenchyma, perhaps to look for possible lesions hidden in the dense tissue. This will improve radiologists' performance when examining high mammographic density cases in the digital systems, where high mammographic density resulted in higher mammographic sensitivity [14, 15] and lower false positive rates [16] when compared to low density mammograms. This finding is supported by a recent study [20], where radiologists' performance was significantly higher in high- compared to low- mammographic density cases in terms of sensitivity ($P=0.0174$) and Receiver Operating Characteristic (ROC) area under the curve ($P=0.0001$). When the lesion was outside the dense tissue, readers' performance did not change significantly between high- and low- mammographic density cases, although dense areas of breast parenchyma received longer gaze time. Therefore, post processing tools in digital mammography made lesion detectability easier, perhaps because it allows the separation of targets from the background. Hence, lesions being masked by dense fibroglandular tissue are not a major issue when using digital mammographic units.

In conclusion, the results of this study suggest that dense parenchyma areas attract readers' visual attention, leading to improved performance in high- compared to low- mammographic density images.

References

1. McCormack, V.A., dos Santos Silva, I.: Breast density and parenchymal patterns as markers of breast cancer risk: a meta-analysis. Cancer Epidemiol. Biomarkers Prev. 15, 1159–1169 (2006)
2. Boyd, N.F., Byng, J.W., Jong, R.A., Fishell, E.K., Little, L.E., Miller, A.B., Lockwood, G.A., Tritchler, D.L., Yaffe, M.J.: Quantitative classification of mammographic densities and breast cancer risk: results from the Canadian National Breast Screening Study. J. Natl. Cancer Inst. 87, 670–675 (1995)
3. Byrne, C., Schairer, C., Wolfe, J., Parekh, N., Salane, M., Brinton, L.A., Hoover, R., Haile, R.: Mammographic features and breast cancer risk: effects with time, age, and menopause status. J. Natl. Cancer Inst. 87, 1622–1629 (1995)
4. Mandelson, M.T., Oestreicher, N., Porter, P.L., White, D., Finder, C.A., Taplin, S.H., White, E.: Breast density as a predictor of mammographic detection: comparison of interval- and screen-detected cancers. J. Natl. Cancer Inst. 92, 1081–1087 (2000)
5. Kolb, T.M., Lichy, J., Newhouse, J.H.: Comparison of the performance of screening mammography, physical examination, and breast US and evaluation of factors that influence them: An analysis of 27,825 patient evaluations. Radiology 225, 165–175 (2002)

6. Cawson, J.N., Nickson, C., Amos, A., Hill, G., Whan, A.B., Kavanagh, A.M.: Invasive breast cancers detected by screening mammography: A detailed comparison of computer-aided detection-assisted single reading and double reading. J. Med. Imaging Radiat. Oncol. 53, 442–449 (2009)

7. Leham, C.D., White, E., Peacock, S., Drucker, M.J., Urban, N.: Effect of age and breast density on screening mammograms with false-positive findings. AJR Am. J. Roentgenol. 173, 1651–1655 (1999)

8. Carney, P.A., Miglioretti, D.L., Yankaskas, B.C., Kerlikowske, K., Rosenberg, R., Rutter, C.M., Geller, B.M., Abraham, L.A., Taplin, S.H., Dignan, M., Cutter, G., Ballard-Barbash, R.: Individual and combined effects of age, breast density, and hormone replacement therapy use on the accuracy of screening mammography. Ann. Intern. Med. 138, 168–175 (2003)

9. Ciatto, S., Visioli, C., Paci, E., Zappa, M.: Breast density as a determinant of interval cancer at mammographic screening. Br. J. Cancer 90, 393–396 (2004)

10. Roubidoux, M.A., Bailey, J.E., Wray, L.A., Helvie, M.A.: Invasive cancers detected after breast cancer screening yielded a negative result: relationship of mammographic density to tumor prognostic factors1. Radiology 230, 42–48 (2004)

11. Porter, G.J.R., Evans, A.J., Cornford, E.J., Burrell, H.C., James, J.J., Lee, A.H.S., Chakrabarti, J.: Influence of mammographic parenchymal pattern in screening-detected and interval invasive breast cancers on pathologic features, mammographic features, and patient survival. AJR Am. J. Roentgenol. 188, 676–683 (2007)

12. Kavanagh, A.M., Byrnes, G.B., Nickson, C., Cawson, J.N., Giles, G.G., Hopper, J.L., Gertig, D.M., English, D.R.: Using mammographic density to improve breast cancer screening outcomes. Cancer Epidemiol. Biomarkers Prev. 17, 2818–2824 (2008)

13. Nickson, C., Kavanagh, A.M.: Tumour size at detection according to different measures of mammographic breast density. J. Med. Screen. 16, 140–146 (2009)

14. Pisano, E.D., Hendrick, R.E., Yaffe, M.J., Baum, J.K., Acharyya, S., Cormack, J.B., Hanna, L.A., Conant, E.F., Fajardo, L.L., Bassett, L.W., D'Orsi, C.J., Jong, R.A., Rebner, M., Tosteson, A.N.A., Gatsonis, C.A., Grp, D.I.: Diagnostic accuracy of digital versus film mammography: Exploratory analysis of selected population subgroups in DMIST. Radiology 246, 376–383 (2008)

15. Kerlikowske, K., Hubbard, R.A., Miglioretti, D.L., Geller, B.M., Yankaskas, B.C., Lehman, C.D., Taplin, S.H., Sickles, E.A.: Comparative effectiveness of digital versus film-screen mammography in community practice in the United States: a cohort study. Ann. Intern. Med. 155, 493–502 (2011)

16. Ciatto, S., Houssami, N., Bernardi, D., Caumo, F., Pellegrini, M., Brunelli, S., Tuttobene, P., Bricolo, P., Fantò, C., Valentini, M., Montemezzi, S., Macaskill, P.: Integration of 3D digital mammography with tomosynthesis for population breast-cancer screening (STORM): a prospective comparison study. Lancet Oncol. 14, 583–589 (2013)

17. National Breast Cancer Center.:Synoptic breast imaging report: National Breast Cancer Center (2007), http://canceraustralia.nbocc.org.au/view-document-details/rsig-1-synoptic-breast-imaging-report-update

18. American College of Radiology. American College of Radiology Breast Imaging Reporting and Data System (BI-RADS), 4th ed. American College of Radiology, Reston (2003)

19. Byng, J.W., Boyd, N.F., Fishell, E., Jong, R.A., Yaffe, M.J.: The quantitative analysis of mammographic densities. Phys. Med. Biol. 39, 1629–1638 (1994)

20. Al Mousa, D., Ryan, E., Lee, W., Nickson, C., Pietrzyk, M., Reed, W., Poulos, A., Li, Y., Brennan, P.: The impact of mammographic density and lesion location on detection. In: Proc. SPIE, 86730U-86730U-9 (2013)

Towards a Quantitative Measure of Radiographic Masking by Dense Tissue in Mammography

James G. Mainprize[1], Xinying Wang[1], Mei Ge[1], and Martin J. Yaffe[1,2]

[1] Physical Sciences, Sunnybrook Research Institute, Toronto, Canada
[2] Department of Medical Biophysics, University of Toronto, Toronto, Canada
james.mainprize@sri.utoronto.ca

Abstract. The detection sensitivity of screening mammography is reduced for dense breasts where the appearance of fibroglandular tissue can mask suspicious lesions. A measure of the degree of masking expected for a mammogram could be useful for informing the decision to direct some women to supplemental imaging procedures not affected by density. Here, we present an adaptation of a model observer to estimate the detection task SNR, d_{local}, of a lesion embedded in various portions of the breast to indicate the level of detection difficulty. Rank correlation of mean mammogram d_{local} with density category is $\rho = -0.58$. Correlation of fractional area of mammograms with low $d_{local} < 2$ versus density category is $\rho = 0.61$. This suggests that a metric based on d_{local} may be useful in quantifying masking effects of breast density.

Keywords: Breast density, mammography, sensitivity, masking, detectability.

1 Introduction

Women presenting with mammographically dense breasts have increased risk of developing breast cancer[1, 2]. In addition, screening mammography has been shown to have reduced sensitivity for dense breasts[3]. While there is considerable interest in quantification of mammographic density, little attention has been directed at developing an index that reflects the "difficulty" of interpreting a mammogram related to that density.

The mechanisms of masking by dense tissue are likely related to 1) low contrast between lesion and dense tissue, 2) the increased complexity of the background structures surrounding the lesion, and 3) potentially reduced x-ray fluence behind dense structures. Model observers have been developed that can incorporate each of these parameters and may be useful in identifying images where lesion conspicuity may be compromised by density.

Here, we propose the use of a simple signal-known-exactly, background-known-statistically (SKE/BKS) model observer to create a map of the SNR of a detection task (d') and compare to perceptions of radiologists' difficulty of reading.

2 Methods

A formal model for d' across a full clinical mammogram that matches a radiologist's performance, i.e., incorporating all of the visual scanning behaviours and considering

H. Fujita, T. Hara, and C. Muramatsu (Eds.): IWDM 2014, LNCS 8539, pp. 181–186, 2014.

all of the likely signs of cancer would be extremely difficult to formulate. Here, we will focus on a single task: detection of a simple known lesion shape in a statistically defined background and calculate it over all regions-of-interest (ROI) in the mammogram. This would be equivalent to asking a radiologist to view each ROI extracted from the mammogram, in turn, and attempting to detect a lesion within each ROI without the context of the rest of the mammogram. The process would be repeated for each ROI from the mammogram.

Because we are not calculating the conventional observer SNR in the full mammogram, we propose to use the symbol d_{local} to emphasize that the SNR is calculated only in localized ROIs. As such, d_{local} for a non-prewhitening (NPW) model observer can be calculated from the known system response, (MTF, NPS, etc.) as follows

$$d_{local}{}^2 = \frac{\left[\int T^2(u,v)W^2(u,v)dudv\right]^2}{\int NNPS^2(u,v)T^2(u,v)W^2(u,v)dudv},\tag{1}$$

where (u, v) are spatial frequencies in the x and y direction, $T(u, v)$ is the MTF of the system, $W(u, v)$ is the task function and $NNPS(u, v)$ is the normalized noise power spectrum. In this case, we will consider each ROI as an independent image.

Although we can extract a direct measure of the NNPS from each ROI, we believe that such an approach would lead to d_{local} values with high variability. Instead, a simple model was created to estimate an appropriate NNPS from each ROI. We can estimate the NNPS, building on an approach previously published[4],

$$NNPS_0(\rho) = \frac{\Phi_p + \Phi_s + \Phi_p^2 S_a(\rho)}{(\Phi_p + \Phi_s)^2} = \frac{1}{\Phi_p + \Phi_s} + \frac{S_a(\rho)}{\left(1 + \frac{\Phi_s}{\Phi_p}\right)^2}\tag{2}$$

where ρ is the radial spatial frequency, Φ_p and Φ_s are the absorbed fluences in the detector due to the primary and scattered x-rays respectively. The absorbed fluences include the effects an antiscatter grid (primary and scatter transmissions of T_p=0.66 and T_s=0.15 respectively) and quantum efficiency (η=0.77) was assumed to be the same for both Φ_p and Φ_s. Average primary transmission was estimated from the calculated thickness and volumetric breast density (VBD)[5]. The anatomic noise power spectrum is modeled as an inverse power-law of the form $S_a(f) = K/(1 + \rho/f_0)^\beta$, where K is a scale factor related to the signal difference between fat and fibroglandular tissue, β is the estimated power-law spectrum exponent extracted from the ROI and $f_0 = 0.1$ mm^{-1} to provide a stable equation at low spatial frequencies. Scatter was added to the model using the scatter point spread function from Boone, knowing the thickness and composition of the breast[6]. The MTF of the Senographe 2000D was measured in the horizontal and vertical directions using a slanted-edge method [7]. For simplicity we assumed that the x-ray spectrum was monoenergetic and we ignored added electronic noise. Estimates of the incident fluence were obtained by extracting the imaging technique factors from the DICOM headers.

Finally, to ensure that the NNPS is scaled appropriately to the clinical image, the modeled NNPS is rescaled such that

$$NNPS(u,v) = mNNPS_0(u,v), \qquad (3)$$

and

$$m = \frac{\int_{f_1}^{f_2} NNPS_{\text{meas}}(\rho\cos\theta, \rho\sin\theta)\rho d\rho}{\int_{f_1}^{f_2} NNPS_0(\rho)\rho d\rho}, \qquad (4)$$

where $(f_1, f_2) = (4\ \text{mm}^{-1}, 5\ \text{mm}^{-1})$ denotes the region of the NNPS that is assumed to be dominated by quantum noise rather than the anatomic component and is likely to be relatively stable between measurements.

The model for the NNPS incorporates both the quantum noise effects related to the incident x-ray exposure, the x-ray transmission through the breast and the mammographic texture as modeled by the inverse power law spectrum equation and its β factor. Thus, we have d_{local} that is sensitive to breast density and to the general texture of the mammographic background.

The task assumed here is the detection of a uniform disk of radius R=2.5 mm, whose task function, $W(\rho) = C\, RJ_1(2\pi R\rho)/\rho$, the Fourier transform of a uniform disc and $J_1(\rho)$ is the Bessel function of the first kind, and the object signal difference ('contrast') is assumed to be $C \approx \Delta\mu L$ where $\Delta\mu$ is the difference in linear attenuation between lesion and adipose tissue and $L = 2R$ is the thickness of the simulated lesion.

3   Results

De-identified mammograms (n=138) were selected from a previous study. Images were acquired on a GE Senographe 2000D (GE Healthcare, Chalfont St. Giles, UK) between 2002 and 2003. DICOM for-processing images were used for the density calculation and the subsequent d_{local} calculation. Fig. 1 shows examples of mammograms and the corresponding d_{local} maps generated using Eq. (1). Darker regions of the d_{local} map are those where it is expected to be more difficult to detect lesions. In general, these areas correspond to areas of increased density, although texture clearly plays a role in decreasing detectability as well.

Fig. 2 (left) shows the average d_{local} plotted against the volumetric breast density measured using a volumetric density algorithm, Cumulus V[5]. There is evidence of a trend with very large d_{local} values for the fattiest breasts and decreasing for the highest density categories. The Pearson correlation between $\log_e(d_{\text{local}})$ and VBD was $r=-0.82$. The background texture appears to have a strong impact on d_{local}. As shown in Fig. 2 (right), there appears to be an almost linear relationship between $\log_e(d_{\text{local}})$ and β with a Pearson's correlation of $r=-0.90$.

Fig. 3 (left) shows the average d_{local} for each radiologist-reported density category. The Spearman ranked correlation between d_{local} and BIRADS category is ρ=−0.58. The average d_{local} is not likely to be a reliable indicator of the difficulty of the mammogram. In other words, mammograms with high average d_{local} could still contain very difficult-to-read areas.   To capture this effect, the fractional area of each mammogram that was below an arbitrary threshold of $d_{local}=2$ was also calculated and is presented in Fig. 3 (right). Here, the fattiest breasts have the smallest fractional areas with low d_{local} and the densest breasts generally contain much higher fractions with this characteristic. The ranked correlation between d_{local} and BIRADS category is ρ=0.61. Note however, that the densest category in these analyses is underrepresented and this may bias the results.

(a)   (b)

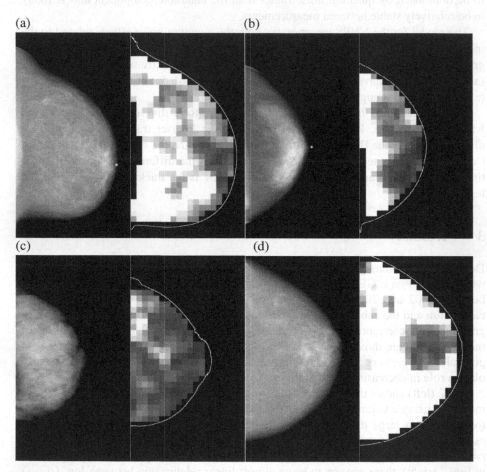

Fig. 1. Examples of mammograms (unprocessed, raw) and their corresponding d_{local} maps. The VBD for the images are (a) 9.1 (b) 17.7 (c) 50.5, and (d) 5.06. The grayscale range for the d_{local} is set between 0 (black) and 4 (white) for all maps.

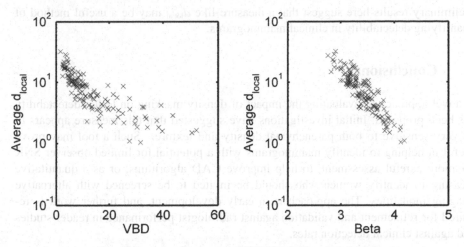

Fig. 2. Average d_{local} versus VBD (%) (left) and β (right)

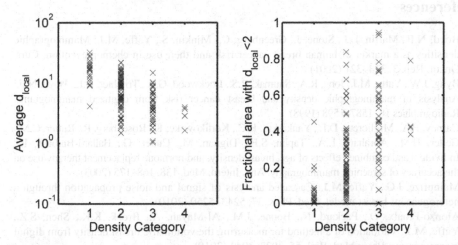

Fig. 3. Average d_{local} (left) and fractional area of the breast that has d_{local} less than a threshold of 2.0 (right) versus BIRADS density category

4   Discussion

The signal propagation model used in this analysis is very simple and does not incorporate several effects, including stochastic blurring in the noise model and added electronic noise. As a result, the scaling factor required to match the model NNPS to the measured NNPS was not close to 1 and highly variable across ROIs (range ~0.01 to ~1.5, mean 0.27). In addition, an isotropic inverse power-law model for the background structure is also crude and lacks several texture features including that of texture directionality, which has been shown in mammograms[8]. Nevertheless, the preliminary results here suggest that a measure like d_{local} may be a useful method of quantifying detectability in clinical mammograms.

5   Conclusions

A novel approach to evaluating the impact of density masking on lesion detectability has been proposed. Initial investigations have suggested that this measure appears to be very sensitive to both parenchymal density and texture. Such a tool may prove useful in helping to identify mammograms with a potential for limited observer SNR for more careful assessment, to help improve CAD algorithms, or as a quantitative measure to identify women who should be invited to be screened with alternative imaging modalities. The approach is in early development, and further work is required for refinement and validation against radiologist performance in reader studies and against clinical detection rates.

References

1. Boyd, N.F., Martin, L.J., Stone, J., Greenberg, C., Minkin, S., Yaffe, M.J.: Mammographic densities as a marker of human breast cancer risk and their use in chemoprevention. Curr. Oncol. Rep. 3, 314–321 (2001)
2. Byng, J.W., Yaffe, M.J., Jong, R.A., Shumak, R.S., Lockwood, G.A., Tritchler, D.L., Boyd, N.F.: Analysis of mammographic density and breast cancer risk from digitized mammograms. Radiographics 18, 1587–1598 (1998)
3. Carney, P.A., Miglioretti, D.L., Yankaskas, B.C., Kerlikowske, K., Rosenberg, R., Rutter, C.M., Geller, B.M., Abraham, L.A., Taplin, S.H., Dignan, M., Cutter, G., Ballard-Barbash, R.: Individual and combined effects of age, breast density, and hormone replacement therapy use on the accuracy of screening mammography. Ann. Intern. Med. 138, 168–175 (2003)
4. Mainprize, J.G., Yaffe, M.J.: Cascaded analysis of signal and noise propagation through a heterogeneous breast model. Med. Phys. 37, 5243–5250 (2010)
5. Alonzo-Proulx, O., Packard, N., Boone, J.M., Al-Mayah, A., Brock, K.K., Shen, S.Z., Yaffe, M.J.: Validation of a method for measuring the volumetric breast density from digital mammograms. Phys. Med. Biol. 55, 3027–3044 (2010)
6. Boone, J.M., Cooper, V.N.: Scatter/primary in mammography: Monte Carlo validation. Med. Phys. 27, 1818–1831 (2000)
7. Samei, E., Flynn, M.J., Reimann, D.A.: A method for measuring the presampled MTF of digital radiographic systems using an edge test device. Med. Phys. 25, 102–113 (1998)
8. Reiser, I., Lee, S., Nishikawa, R.M.: On the orientation of mammographic structure. Med. Phys. 38, 5303–5306 (2011)

Three Dimensional Dose Distribution Comparison of Simple and Complex Acquisition Trajectories in Dedicated Breast CT – A Monte Carlo Study

Jainil P. Shah[1,3], Steve D. Mann[2,3], Randolph L. McKinley[4], and Martin P. Tornai[1,2,3]

[1] Department of Biomedical Engineering, Duke University, Durham, NC 27705
[2] Medical Physics Graduate Program, Duke University Medical Center, Durham, NC 27705
[3] Multi Modality Imaging Lab, Duke University Medical Center, Durham, NC 27710
{jainil.shah,steve.mann,martin.tornai}@duke.edu
[4] ZumaTek, Inc., Research Triangle Park, NC 27709
rmckinley@zumatek.com

Abstract. The purpose of this study was to characterize the three dimensional (3D) x-ray dose distributions in a target scanned with different acquisition trajectories for dedicated breast CT imaging. Monte Carlo simulations were used to evaluate two acquisition trajectories: circular azimuthal (no tilt) and complex sinusoidal (saddle) orbit with $\pm15°$ tilts around a pendant breast. Simulations were performed with tungsten (W) and cerium (Ce) filtration of a W-anode source; the simulated source flux was normalized to the measured exposure of a clinically used W-anode source. A water filled cylindrical phantom, was divided into 1cc voxels, and each voxel was set to track the cumulative energy deposited. Energy deposited per voxel was converted to dose, yielding the 3D distributed dose volumes. Results indicate that the mean absorbed dose at the isocenter of a volume for the un-tilted acquisition is ~10% higher than that from a saddle scan, regardless of filtration used.

Keywords: Breast CT, dosimetry, cone beam CT, Monte Carlo simulations.

1 Introduction

For any clinical imaging system, minimizing the dose delivered to and absorbed by the target volume is important for the patient. The American College of Radiology (ACR) stipulates that 6 mGy is the upper limit of the average absorbed dose from dual-view mammography for a 4.2 cm thick, compressed, 50-50% adipose-glandular breast volume. A few institutions in the USA are investigating pendant breast CT imaging systems [1-12]; however there still exists a dearth of an equivalent dosimetry standard. Therefore, despite the fact that we acquire hundreds of projection images on a cone beam CT system, we adhere to the mammography standard and try to restrict the cumulative absorbed dose by the breast to <6 mGy without compromise to reconstructed image quality. Indeed, the exposure efficiency (SNR^2/exposure) has been shown to be more than a factor of 2 better with certain breast CT systems due to the x-ray beam quality [13,14]. Cumulative absorbed dose for a tomographic scan depends on numerous factors – mean x-ray

H. Fujita, T. Hara, and C. Muramatsu (Eds.): IWDM 2014, LNCS 8539, pp. 187–194, 2014.
© Springer International Publishing Switzerland 2014

beam energy and flux [6,12] mass of the target volume, material composition of the volume [12], etc. Therefore, all these factors have to be taken into consideration for evaluating dose delivered by a breast CT system.

Dose studies have previously been performed on our fixed tilt angle, dedicated breast CT system with a quasi-monochromatic x-ray beam [15]. Both geometric and anthropomorphic phantoms were used and results have shown that the average absorbed doses in the volumes for 100% glandular-equivalent and 100% adipose-equivalent tissue are 4.5 mGy and 3.8 mGy, respectively [15]. Also, other studies have demonstrated the benefit of using complex 3D acquisition trajectories that utilize the system's polar tilting capability [16]. Such trajectories overcome the cone beam under-sampling problem while also promoting imaging further into the breast volume, resulting in more uniformly sampled images. With the inclusion of complex 3D acquisition trajectories in the proposed future iterations of the hybrid breast SPECT-CT system [17], it is imperative to characterize the differences between the dose distribution within a breast volume for a simple azimuthal (fixed tilt) and complex 3D acquisition trajectories.

2   Materials and Methods

The simulation program Monte Carlo N-Particle (MCNP 5.0) [18] was used to perform the dosimetry studies. A fully 3D tilt capable breast CT imaging system [19] consisting of a flat panel detector, tungsten anode x-ray source with a 16 degree anode angle, and a source to image distance (SID) of 70cm was used as the basis for the simulations (Fig 1). The exposure of this system at 49kVp potential and 1.25 mAs technique was measured at the iso-center with an exposure meter and was found to be 4.11 mR. Fig1 shows a schematic of the system set up and illustrates the tilting motions. The simulations only model the x-ray spectra and tilting capabilities based on the system depicted in Fig 1, and do not include a flat panel detector.

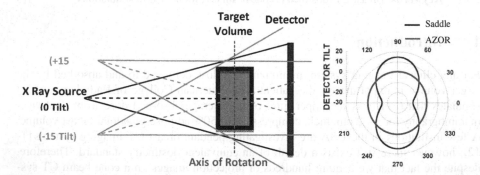

Fig. 1. (LEFT)Schematic showing the geometrical set-up of a tilt capable breast CT system where the source and detector tilt ±15°.GRAY dotted lines represent the central X-ray beam and the vertical BLUE dotted line represents the Axis of rotation of the system. (RIGHT) Polar plot depicting the AZOR and Saddle orbits about a 360 degree azimuthal trajectory path.

X-ray spectra were modeled in the XSPECT simulation package [20], a validated x-ray system simulation program that models the output of an x-ray tube under various operating parameters such as tube potential, anode material, anode angle, and the thickness and composition of absorbing materials in the beam path. Two different spectra, with external Tungsten (W, 0.005cm) and Cerium (Ce, 0.0506cm) filtration were modeled to simulate x-ray beam filtration used on our breast CT system [18]. The flux of the simulated W spectrum was calibrated to match the physically measured exposure (4.11 mR) at the iso-center of the real system.The Ce spectrum was scaled such that the total number of x-ray photons emitted from the source matched that of the W spectrum (60.2 Million/cm^2 at iso-center), to allow for similar noise characteristics on both sets of data. The XSPECT spectra (Fig 2) were used in this simulation as a probability density input model of the x-ray source distribution in MCNP.

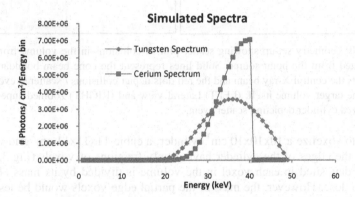

Fig. 2. X-ray spectra simulated from XSPECT using Tungsten and Cerium filters

In MCNP, the X-ray source was modeled as a point source emitting a 32 degree full cone angle towards the target volume. A 10 cm diameter, 10 cm tall, cylindrical phantom was used as the target volume in the modeled CT system (Fig 3). The cylinder was composed of water, a common substitute for glandular tissue in physical phantom studies, and was divided into 1x1x1 cm^3 voxels (Fig 3). 240 projection images were acquired over 360 degrees for each scan. Simulations were performed with 2 different orbits – 1) Azimuthal orbit (AZOR) which is the simple no tilt trajectory around the volume, and 2) Complex 3D (Saddle) orbit including polar tilts (up to ±15°) following a two lobed sinusoidal path around the pendant object (Fig 1, right). Two sets of these simulations were performed for each trajectory: once with the W filter and then again with the Ce filter.

Each cubic voxel of the object was defined as an individual 'detector element' recording the total energy deposited. The elements recorded the deposited energy regardless of interaction type, including photoelectric absorption, Compton and coherent scattering. Fig 3 shows a subset of accumulated histories at a single projection angle from a simulated run with 10,000 incident photons. The MCNP visualization tool depicts scatter events with absolute position (x,y,z, coordinates); however only the cumulative energy deposited in every 1 cm voxel is extracted for the final dose deposition volumes. The energy deposited (MeV) in each individual voxel was divided by the mass of the voxels (1 g), converted to Joules (1 MeV = 1.60218E-13 J), and finally converted to dose (Gy = joules / kg), yielding a voxelized, 3D representation of absorbed dose in a volume.

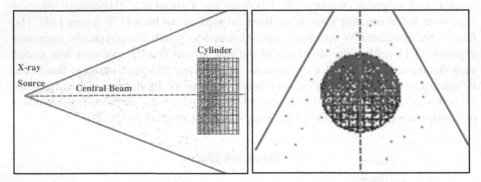

Fig. 3. MCNP geometry set-up showing scatter plot of collisions in the volume from 10,000 photons emitted from the point source. Solid lines represent the cone beam boundary, dotted line represents the central X-ray beam and the red dots depict collisions / scattered events in air and within the target volume itself. (LEFT) Lateral view and (RIGHT) zoomed superior view of the voxelized cylinder depicting scatter events.

In order to voxelize a 10x10x10 cm^3 cylinder, a cubic 11x11x11 cm^3 grid was used resulting in the edges of the cylinder having only fractions of voxels (Fig 3, Right). The energy deposited in each voxel in the volume is divided by its mass (1 gm) to convert it to dose. However, the mass of the partial edge voxels would be less than 1 gm, thereby underestimating the dose in these voxels.

Due to the enormous number of particle interactions (in the target volume as well as in the air at standard temperature and pressure around the object) that occur with 60.2 million incident x-ray photons per projection, our fastest computer (*Intel's* 3rd generation i7 extreme processor 3.7GHz, 12 cores, 24GB RAM) took ~20 minutes per simulation projection, i.e. 80 hours of CPU processing for a 240 projection CT scan, which is about three and a half CPU-days per data set, whereas on an average computer, the simulations took 1 hour per projection, indicating 240 hours or 10 CPU-days per data-set.

3   Results

The average dose values, measured on the central sagittal slice of the volumes, obtained from the simulations compare well with other Monte Carlo studies [6] as well as physical measurements [15,21] and are reported in Table 1. Dose distribution volumes were calculated as described in the previous section (Fig 4), and profiles were plotted near the chest, mid and nipple region of central slices (Fig 5). The profiles clearly illustrate that for the AZOR scan, since the x-ray cone beam is centered on the target volume, the mid region (medial volume) has the highest deposited dose, and that it tapers symmetrically towards the chest (top) and nipple (bottom) as the divergence of the x-rays increases

(Fig 1). For the saddle scan, there are an equal number of projection angles where the central ray of the x-ray cone beam is closer to the chest or nipple regions, yielding a more uniform dose distribution at the edges (sagittal slice on Fig 4). Regardless of the filtration type (W or Ce), the overall distributions and profiles had identical patterns, and only differed in absolute values of the absorbed doses (the minimum values within each simulated volume for each condition are included in Table 1).

The total mean absorbed dose was measured on the central sagittal slice using a 9x9 pixel ROI, ignoring partial edge pixels, for all filtration conditions and trajectories. For the Ce filtered beam, the average dose deposited for an AZOR scan is 9.6% higher than for the saddle scan (Table 1). For the W filtered beam, the average dose deposited for the AZOR scan is 9.8% higher than for the saddle scan. Note the larger standard deviations for the saddle scans. The average dose deposited throughout the entire volume was also measured using a 9x9x9 voxel volume of interest (VOI), continuing to ignore the partial edge voxels. For the Ce filtered case, the average dose deposited was 5.46 mGy for the saddle orbit and 5.50 mGy for the AZOR orbit; whereas for the W filtered case, the average dose throughout the volume was 5.38 mGy for the saddle orbit and 5.43 mGy for AZOR.

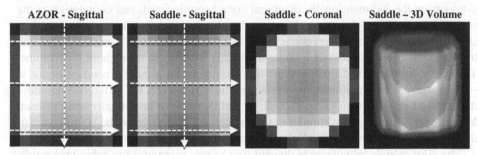

Fig. 4. Cumulative dose map for the Ce filtered case - (LEFT to RIGHT) Sagittal slice through the center of the cylinder depicting the 2D dose map for AZOR orbit, Saddle orbit, Coronal slice through center of Saddle orbit and 3D volume rendered image of dose distribution for Saddle orbit. Dotted lines indicate location and direction of the profile plots (Fig 5). Black indicates lowest dose and white the highest dose.

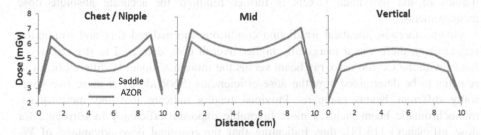

Fig. 5. Plotted dose profiles near the chest, middle and nipple regions of the central sagittal slice of the cylinder for the Ce filtered case (Fig 4). Dose deposited at the edges is considerably higher than the center of the volume. Absorbed dose for the Saddle orbit is consistently lower than the AZOR.

Table 1. Total average and minimum absorbed doses (mGy) measured in the central slice of the cylinder

Condition	Average Central Slice Dose (mGy)	
	Ce	*W*
Saddle		
Average	5.16 ± 0.61	5.05 ± 0.66
Minimum	4.12	3.98
AZOR		
Average	5.21 ± 0.62	5.10 ± 0.68
Minimum	4.09	3.95

4   Discussion and Conclusions

The dose distribution in a target volume was characterized for different acquisition trajectories and various x-ray spectra for dedicated breast CT imaging, using Monte Carlo simulations. For a fixed tilt trajectory (i.e. AZOR), the distribution of tilted x-rays from the 2-dimensionally divergent cone beam is fixed, and cumulative as the source moves around the object. However for the sinusoidally variant trajectory (i.e. saddle), the cone beam divergence is fixed, but the distribution of x-rays changes and therefore the energy deposited is more uniformly distributed throughout the volume. The mean dose absorbed from a scan with a saddle orbit around a pendant breast is ~10% lower than a traditional circular acquisition. However, the difference is within the standard deviations measured (Table 1) and therefore is statistically insignificant. Multiple replications of the simulations are necessary to determine the significance of these results, in addition to physical measurements on a real breast CT system.

The 10cc cylindrical volume is divided into voxels using an 11cc cubic grid resulting in fractional voxels near the edges of the cylinder. Ignoring the fractional voxel from the dose calculations results in a slight underestimation of the average dose deposited in the volume. However, the amount of underestimation is constant across all the different scans and therefore does not affect the inter-comparison made between orbits. Thus one caveat of this set-up is that proper normalization with accurate masses of the individual voxels is further required for accurate absolute dose measurements.

Given otherwise identical irradiation conditions (normalized flux and irradiation trajectories), there was a marginally higher overall dose delivered to the target volumes with the Ce-filtered x-ray beam versus the more traditional W-filtered beam. It remains to be determined how the dose efficiencies (SNR²/dose) of these two spectrally different beams compare. Previous results indicate that the more quasi-monochromatic beam yields a more favorable exposure efficiency (a surrogate for dose efficiency) [13,14], thus indicating that the marginal dose advantage of W-filtration determined here is compensated by a necessarily increased flux (hence dose) in order to yield a similar dose efficiency.

In the future, results of the Monte Carlo simulations will be validated with physical experiments similar to previous measurements [15].

Acknowledgements. This work was funded by the National Cancer Institute of the National Institutes of Health (R01-CA096821 and T32-EB007185). JP Shah is supported by the Jo Rae Wright Fellowship from Duke BME. MP Tornai and RL McKinley are co-founders and shareholders of *ZumaTek*.

References

1. Glick, S.J.: Breast CT. Annu. Rev. Biomed. Eng. (2007)
2. Ning, R., Conover, D., Lu, X., Zhang, Y., Yu, Y., Schffhauer, L., Cullinan, J.: Evaluation of flat panel detector cone beam CT breast imaging with different sizes of breast phantoms. In: 2005 SPIE Medical Imaging Conference, San Diego, CA, pp. 626–636 (2005)
3. McKinley, R.L., Samei, E., Brzymialkiewicz, C.N., Tornai, M.P., Floyd, C.E.: Measurements of an optimized beam for x-ray computed mammotomography. In: 2004 SPIE Medical Imaging Conference, San Diego, CA, pp. 311–319 (2004)
4. McKinley, R.L., Brzymialkiewicz, C.N., Madhav, P., Tornai, M.P.: Investigation of conebeam acquisitions implemented using a novel dedicated mammotomography system with unique arbitrary orbit capability. In: 2005 Proc. SPIE: Phys. Med. Imag., vol. 5745, pp. 609–617 (2005)
5. Tornai, M.P., McKinley, R.L., Brzymialkiewicz, C.N., Madhav, P., Cutler, S.J., Crotty, D.J., Bowsher, J.E., Samei, E., Floyd, C.E.: Design and development of a fully-3D dedicated x-ray computed mammotomography system. In: 2005 Proc. SPIE: Phys. Med. Imag., vol. 5745, pp. 189-197 (2005)
6. Boone, J.M., Nelson, T.R., Lindfors, K.K., Siebert, J.A.: Dedicated breast CT: radiation dose and image quality evaluation. Radiology 221, 657–667 (2001)
7. Boone, J.M., Kwan, A.L.C., Nelson, T.R., Shah, N., Burkett, G., Seibert, J.A., Lindfors, K.K., Ross, G.: Performance assessment of a pendant-geometry CT scanner for breast cancer detection. In: 2005 SPIE Medical Imaging Conference, San Diego, CA, pp. 319–323 (2005)
8. Chen, B., Ning, R.: Cone-beam volume CT mammographic imaging: feasibility study. Med. Phys. 29, 755–770 (2002)
9. Ning, R., Yu, Y., Conover, D.L., Lu, X., He, H., Chen, Z., Schiffhauer, L., Cullinan, J.: Preliminary system characterization of flat-panel-detector-based cone-beam CT for breast imaging. In: 2004 SPIE Med. Imag. Conf., vol. 5368, pp. 292–303 (2004)
10. Vedula, A.A., Glick, S.J.: Computer simulations of CT mammography using a flat panel imager. In: 2003 SPIE Medical Imaging Conference, San Diego, CA, pp. 349–360 (2003)
11. Chen, L., Shaw, C.C., Tu, S., Altunbas, M.C., Wang, T., Lai, C., Liu, X., Kappadath, S.C.: Cone-beam CT breast imaging with a flat panel detector: a simulation study. In: 2005 SPIE Medical Imaging Conference, San Diego, CA, pp. 943–951 (2005)
12. Boone, J.M., Shah, N., Nelson, T.R.: A comprehensive analysis of DgNCT coefficients for pendant-geometry cone-beam breast computed tomography. Med. Phys. 31, 226–235 (2002)
13. McKinley, R.L., Samei, E., Brzymialkiewicz, C.N., Tornai, M.P., Floyd, C.E.: Measurements of an Optimized Beam for X-ray Computed Mammotomography. In: Proc. SPIE: Physics of Medical Imaging, vol. 5389, pp. 311–319 (2004)
14. McKinley, R.L., Tornai, M.P., Samei, E., Bowsher, J.E.: Quasi-Monochromatic Beam Measurements for Dedicated Cone-Beam Mammotomography of an Uncompressed Breast. In: Proc. of 7th International Workshop on Digital Mammography, pp. 56–63. Dovetail Publishing Inc. (2005)

15. Crotty, D.J., Brady, S.L., Jackson, D.C., Toncheva, G.I., Anderson-Evans, C., Yoshizumi, T.T., Tornai, M.P.: Evaluation of the Absorbed Dose to the Breast Using Radiochromic Film in a Dedicated CT Mammotomography System Employing a Quasi-Monchromatic Beam. Med. Phys. 38(6), 3232–3245 (2011)
16. Madhav, P., Crotty, D.J., McKinley, R.L., Tornai, M.P.: Evaluation of tilted cone-beam CT orbits in the development of a dedicated hybrid mammotomography. Phys. Med. Biol. 54(12), 3659 (2009)
17. Shah, J.P., Mann, S.D., McKinley, R.L., Tornai, M.P.: Design of a nested SPECT-CT system with fully suspended CT sub-system for dedicated breast imaging. In: Proc. of SPIE: Medical Imaging (2014)
18. Briesmeister, J.F.: MCNP-A general Monte Carlo code for neutron and photon transport. LA-7396-M (1986)
19. McKinley, R.L., Tornai, M.P., Tuttle, L.A., Steed, D., Kuzmiak, C.M.: Development and initial demonstration of a low-dose dedicated fully 3D breast CT system. In: Maidment, A.D.A., Bakic, P.R., Gavenonis, S. (eds.) IWDM 2012. LNCS, vol. 7361, pp. 442–449. Springer, Heidelberg (2012)
20. XSpect Simulation Toolkit, Henry Ford Health Systems, Detroit, MI
21. McKinley, R.L., Tornai, M.P.: Preliminary investigation of dose for a dedicated mammotomography system. In: Medical Imaging, pp. 614208–614208. International Society for Optics and Photonics (2006)
22. Shah, J.P., Mann, S.D., McKinley, R.L., Tornai, M.P.: Comparison of the Effect of Simple and Complex Acquisition Trajectories on the 2D SPR and 3D Voxelized Differences for Dedicated Breast CT Imaging. In: Proc. of SPIE: Medical Imaging (2014)

Quantitative MRI Phenotyping of Breast Cancer across Molecular Classification Subtypes

Maryellen L. Giger, Hui Li, Li Lan, Hiroyuki Abe, and Gillian M. Newstead

Department of Radiology, The University of Chicago, 5841 South Maryland Avenue,
Chicago, Illinois 60637
m-giger@uchicago.edu

Abstract. The goal of our study was to investigate the potential usefulness of
quantitative MRI analysis (i.e., phenotyping) in characterizing and data mining
the molecular subtypes of breast cancer in order to better understand the difference among HER2, ER, and PR expression, triple negative, and other molecular
classifications. Analyses were performed on 168 biopsy-proven breast cancer
MRI studies acquired between November 2008 and August 2011, on which molecular classification was known. MRI-based phenotyping analysis included:
3D lesion segmentation based on a fuzzy c-means clustering algorithm, computerized feature extraction, leave-one-out linear stepwise feature selection, and
discriminant score estimation using Linear Discriminant Analysis (LDA). The
classification performance between the molecular subtypes of breast cancer was
evaluated using ROC analysis with area under the ROC curve (AUC) as the
figure of merit. AUC values obtained for 26 HER2+ vs. 142 HER2-, 118 ER+
vs. 50 ER-, 93 PR+ vs. 75 PR-, 40 Triple Negative (ER-, PR-, and HER2-) vs.
128 all others are 0.65, 0.70, 0.57, and 0.68, respectively for the combined datasets that included images from both 1.5T and 3T scanners. Contributions to the
classifiers come from the shape, texture, and kinetics of the lesion, triple negative cases exhibiting increased margin variability, distinct kinetics, and increased surface area. Analyzing the datasets within magnet strength substantially improved performances, e.g., the AUC for triple negative vs. all other cancer
subtypes increased from 0.69 (SE=0.05) to 0.88 (SE=0.05). The results from
this study indicate that quantitative MRI analysis shows promise as a means for
high-throughput image-based phenotyping in the discrimination of breast cancer subtypes.

Keywords: Computer-aided diagnosis, Breast MRI, image-based phenotype,
molecular classifications.

1 Introduction

Breast cancer is the most frequently diagnosed cancer and is the second leading cause
of death in women [1]. Dynamic contrast-enhanced magnetic resonance imaging
(DCE-MRI) of the breast has been increasingly used in clinical practice for screening
and diagnostic imaging as well as post-treatment evaluation [2, 3]. MRI in addition to
mammography was recommended for screening of women at high-risk of developing
breast cancer by the American Cancer Society in 2007 [4].

H. Fujita, T. Hara, and C. Muramatsu (Eds.): IWDM 2014, LNCS 8539, pp. 195–200, 2014.
© Springer International Publishing Switzerland 2014

Breast cancer can be classified based on the receptor status (ER, PR, and HER2) traditionally identified by immunohistochemistry. HER2+ breast cancers tend to be more aggressive and have a poorer prognosis than HER2/neu-negative cancers. However, it is not clear whether HER2/neu status is an independent risk factor. ER+ and PR+ cases have lower risks of mortality compared to women with ER- and/or PR-disease. Triple negative cases (HER2-, ER-, PR-) overall do not respond well to treatment, and thus account for a large portion of breast cancer deaths [5].

The goal of our study was to investigate the potential usefulness of quantitative MRI analysis (i.e., phenotyping) in characterizing and data mining the molecular subtypes of breast cancer in order to better understand the difference among HER2, ER, and PR expression, triple negative, and other molecular classifications. Identification of the molecular subtypes of breast tumors is expected to allow for improved prognostic assessment and more effective cancer treatment plans.

2   Materials and Methods

2.1   Database

Breast DCE-MR images used in this study were obtained retrospectively under an IRB-approved protocol at the University of Chicago Medical Center. Table 1 lists the acquisition parameters.

Table 1. Summary of DCE-MR imaging protocols. TR=repetition time, TE=echo time.

	1.5 Tesla DCE-MRI	3 Tesla DEC-MRI
Magnet	1.5 T Philips Achieva	3T Philips Achieva
Number of Coil Channels	16	16
Acquisition Plane	Axial	Axial
Pulse Sequence	3D Gradient Echo (THRIVE)	3D Gradient Echo (THRIVE)
TR/TE (ms)	5.5 / 2.7	5.0 / 2.5
Flip Angle (degrees)	12	10 or 12
Voxel Size (mm^3)	0.74 x 0.74 x 1	0.60 x 0.60 x 0.80
Temporal Resolution	60	70
Number of Post-Contrast	6	5
Fat Suppression (Y or N)	Y	Y
Parallel Imaging (Y or N)	Y	Y

Analyses were performed on 168 biopsy-proven breast cancer MRI studies acquired between November 2008 and August 2011, on which molecular classification was known as listed in Table 2. All cases are invasive ductal carcinoma.

Table 2. Molecularclassifications and distribution of the dataset

	Molecular Classifications and Distribution of the 168 cases	
HER2	HER2-	HER2+
	142	26
ER	ER-	ER+
	50	118
PR	PR-	PR+
	75	93
Triple Negative	Triple Negative	All Others
	40	128

2.2 MRI-Based Phenotyping Analysis

MRI-based phenotyping analysis included several steps: (1) 3D lesion segmentation based on a fuzzy c-means clustering algorithm [6], (2) computerized feature extraction [7-9], leave-one-out linear stepwise feature selection, and discriminant score estimation using Linear Discriminant Analysis (LDA) in a leave-one-out evaluation.

2.3 Performance Evaluation

The classification performance between the molecular subtypes of breast cancer was evaluated using receiver operating characteristic (ROC) analysis [10-12] with area under the ROC curve (AUC) as the figure of merit. The AUC values were calculated to assess the discrimination performance of the individual lesion features/phenotypes as well as the merged lesion signatures in the tasks of distinguishing between HER2+ and HER2-, ER+ and ER , PR+ and PR-, and triple negative and all others.

3 Results

The performance of individual lesion characteristics/phenotypes in terms of AUC value in the task of distinguishing molecular subtypes is shown in Figure 1.

AUC values obtained for 26 HER2+ vs. 142 HER2-, 118 ER+ vs. 50 ER-, 93 PR+ vs. 75 PR-, 40 Triple Negative (ER-, PR-, and HER2-) vs. 128 all others are 0.65, 0.70, 0.57, and 0.68, respectively for the combined datasets that included images from both 1.5T and 3T MR scanners. Contributions to the classifiers come from the shape, texture, and kinetics of the lesion, triple negative cases exhibiting increased margin variability, distinct kinetics, and increased surface area. One example of image-based phenotype arrays showing the color map of individual features and the output from LDA output on ER status is shown in Figure 2.

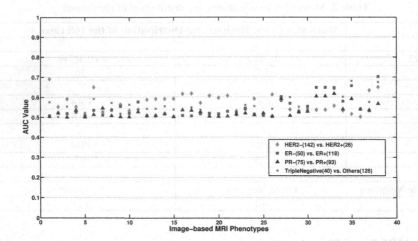

Fig. 1. Lesion features were automatically extracted from dynamic contrast-enhanced breast MRI images (obtained with both 1.5T and 3T scanners) and analyzed on their own as well as merged into lesion signatures for the assessment of molecular classification. Individual lesion features were only weak classifiers, as evidenced by the modest areas under the ROC curve (AUC value). When artificial intelligence was used, however, to merge the features into lesion signatures, performance substantially improved.

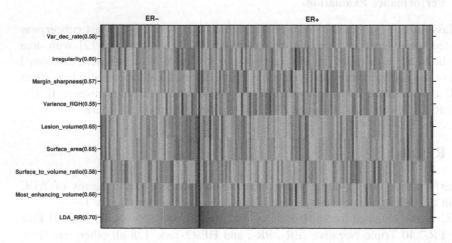

Fig. 2. Image-based phenotype arrays showing the color map of individual features of ER- and ER+ subjects. The individual subjects are ordered based on the output values from the LDA classifier. Values in parentheses corresponded to AUC using image-based phenotypes as decision variables in the task of distinguishing between ER- and ER+ subjects. For each image-based phenotype, red corresponds to high value and green corresponds to low value [13].

Analyzing the datasets within magnet strength substantially improved performances, e.g., the AUC for triple negative vs. all other cancer subtypes increased from 0.69 (SE=0.05) to 0.88 (SE=0.05) as shown in Table 3. This difference in terms of two AUC values is statistically significant with a p-value of 0.0017 (95% Confidence Interval of ΔAUC [-0.3593, -0.0832]). This performance difference within magnet strength needs to be further investigated with a larger dataset.

Table 3. Classification performance in the task of distinguishing triple negative cases from other molecular subtypes within magnet strength

	1.5T	3T
Cases	117	51
Triple Negative Cases	29	11
Others	88	40
Features	AUC	AUC
Size	0.63	0.70
Kinetics	0.61	0.71
Shape	0.56	0.70
Texture	0.56	0.80
Classifier (LDA)	AUC (SE)	AUC (SE)
	0.69(0.05)	0.88 (0.05)

4   Conclusion

The results from this study indicate that quantitative MRI analysis shows promise as a means for high-throughput image-based phenotyping in the discrimination of breast cancer molecular subtypes.

Acknowledgements. This research was supported in parts by USPHS Grants P50-CA125183, NIH S10 RR021039, and P30 CA14599. M.L. Giger is a stockholder in R2 Technology/Hologic, is co-founder and shareholder of Quantitative Insights, shareholder in QView, and receives royalties from Hologic, GE Medical Systems, MEDIAN Technologies, Riverain Medical, Mitsubishi, and Toshiba. It is the University of Chicago Conflict of Interest Policy that investigators disclose publicly actual or potential significant financial interest with would reasonably appear to be directly and significantly affected by the research activities.

References

1. Siegel, R., Naishadham, D., Jemal, A.: Cancer Statistics. CA Cancer J. Clin. 63, 11–30 (2013)
2. Hylton, N.: MR imaging for assessment of breast cancer response to neoadjuvant chemotherapy. Magn. Reson. Imaging Clin. N. Am. 14, 383–389 (2006)
3. Kuhl, C.K., Schild, H.H.: Dynamic image interpretation of MRI of the breast. J. Magn. Reson. Imaging 12, 965–974 (2000)
4. Saslow, D., Boetes, C., Burke, W., Harms, S., Leach, M.O., Lehman, C.D., Morris, E., Pisano, E., Schnall, M., Sener, S., Smith, R.A., Warner, E., Yaffe, M., Andrews, K.S., Russell, C.A.: American Cancer Society guidelines for breast screening with MRI as an adjunct to mammography. CA Cancer J. Clin. 57, 75–89 (2007)
5. Schnitt, S.J.: Classification and prognosis of invasive breast cancer: from morphology to molecular taxonomy. Mod. Pathol. 64, S60–S64 (2010)
6. Chen, W., Giger, M.L., Bick, U.: A fuzzy c-means (FCM)-based approach for computerized segmentation of breast lesions in dynamic contrast-enhanced MR images. Acad. Radiol. 13, 63–72 (2006)
7. Chen, W., Giger, M.L., Lan, L., Bick, U.: Computerized interpretation of breast MRI: investigation of enhancement-variance dynamics. Med. Phys. 31, 1076–1082 (2004)
8. Chen, W., Giger, M.L., Bick, U., Newstead, G.M.: Automatic identification and classification of characteristic kinetic curves of breast lesions on DCE-MRI. Med. Phys. 33, 2878–2887 (2006)
9. Chen, W., Giger, M.L., Li, H., Bick, U., Newstead, G.M.: Volumetric texture analysis of breast lesions on contrast-enhanced magnetic resonance images. Magn. Reson. Med. 58, 562–571 (2007)
10. Metz, C.E.: ROC methodology in radiographic imaging. Invest. Radiol. 21, 720–733 (1986)
11. Metz, C.E.: Some practical issues of experimental design and data analysis in radiological ROC studies. Invest. Radiol. 24, 234–245 (1989)
12. ROC software,
    http://www-radiology.uchicago.edu/krl/roc_soft6.htm
13. Giger, M.L., Li, H., Lan, L.: Visualization of image-based breast cancer tumor signatures. RSNA 2012, 243 (2012)

A Novel Framework for Fat, Glandular Tissue, Pectoral Muscle and Nipple Segmentation in Full Field Digital Mammograms

Xin Chen, Emmanouil Moschidis, Chris Taylor, and Susan M. Astley

Centre for Imaging Sciences, Institute of Population Health,
University of Manchester, Oxford Road, Manchester, M13 9PT, UK

Abstract. Automated segmentation of mammograms is an important initial step in a wide range of applications including breast density and texture analysis and computer aided detection of abnormalities. In this paper, we propose a unified machine learning framework that enables simultaneous segmentation of the breast region, fatty tissue, glandular tissue, pectoral muscle and nipple region in full field digital mammograms. We calculate both a multi-label segmentation mask and a probability map associated with each of the segmented classes. The probability map facilitates interpretation of the segmentation mask prior to further analysis. The method is evaluated using left or right MLO views from 100 women in a 5-fold cross validation manner. Our framework is shown to be robust and accurate, achieving sensitivity/specificity from 82.7% to 98.5% at the equal-error-rate point of the ROC curves and area under the ROC curve values from 0.9220 to 0.9998 for the corresponding segmentations.

Keywords: Mammogram, fat, gland, pectoral muscle, nipple, breast, segmentation, machine learning.

1   Introduction

X-ray mammography is one of the most effective tools for the diagnosis and evaluation of breast cancer. With the advent of Full Field Digital Mammography (FFDM), opportunities have arisen for applications of automated analysis including abnormality detection, breast density estimation and breast cancer risk prediction. A fundamental and crucial step for computer aided diagnosis and detection systems is the accurate segmentation of key anatomic features in the mammograms, including the breast region, fatty tissue, glandular tissue, pectoral muscle and nipple location.

The relationship between area of dense tissue expressed as a percentage of the breast area and risk of developing breast cancer is well established [1]. A semiautomatic tool (CUMULUS) [2] is well recognized for estimation of mammographic breast density (MD), but requires a considerable amount of user interaction and suffers from intra and inter user variability. Automated segmentation of fatty and glandular tissue will enable fully automated MD analysis [3], and also facilitate development of density-adjusted Computer Aided Detection (CAD) tools.

H. Fujita, T. Hara, and C. Muramatsu (Eds.): IWDM 2014, LNCS 8539, pp. 201–208, 2014.
© Springer International Publishing Switzerland 2014

The pectoral muscle region is frequently excluded from the breast area when analyzing density in the Medio-Lateral Oblique (MLO) mammographic view. Automatic segmentation of pectoral muscle has been addressed previously [4], but still remains a difficult problem to be solved robustly. Initial assumption of a straight pectoral muscle line is often used, followed by refinement processes [5]. The nipple is an important anatomic feature which can be used as a reference point for establishing intra- and inter- breast correspondence. A number of nipple detection methods have been proposed [6], which mainly rely on some initial assumption of locations and characteristic along the breast contours. Robust detection of the nipple remains the most challenging problem in mammographic segmentation. For instance, the nipple may lie inside the breast or have very low contrast. Whilst identifying the breast edge is straightforward, estimation of the other features remains challenging due to the variability in appearance of glandular tissue, pectoral muscle and nipple. Such variations occur due both to differences in anatomy and in imaging parameters and practice. Current mammogram segmentation methods are either designed for one or two specific features or are less robust in certain situations [3-6].

To the authors' best knowledge no single system that is able to segment all of the above mentioned anatomic features in a unified framework has previously been described. The contribution of this paper is a novel machine learning framework that enables simultaneous segmentation of the breast region, fatty tissue, glandular tissue, pectoral muscle and nipple in full field digital mammograms. We calculate both a multi-label mask and a probability map associated with each of the segmented classes. The probability map facilitates interpretation of the segmentation mask prior to further analysis. A detailed description of the method and its evaluation are given in the following sections.

2   Method

In machine learning algorithms, image features and their associated labels are learnt from a training data set. When a similar unknown image feeds into the resulting model, pixels of each class in the new image can be estimated according to their corresponding feature descriptors. In [7], the authors described a system that combines the dual-tree complex wavelet transform (DT-CWT) [8] and random forest (RF) [9] classifier for detection and classification of linear structures in mammograms. We have adapted this method and applied it for the purpose of anatomic feature segmentation in mammograms.

The DT-CWT combines the outputs of two discrete transforms, using real wavelets differing in phase by 90 degrees, to form the real and imaginary parts of complex coefficients. It provides a directionally selective representation with approximately shift-invariant coefficient magnitudes and local phase information. In our implementation, the DT-CWT is applied to a 6-level image pyramid. Each level is a down-sampled version of its immediate higher level by a factor of 0.5. Additionally, the DT-CWT is performed at six different orientations ($\pm15°$, $\pm45°$, $\pm75°$) at each pyramid level. The six sub-bands are then multiplied by {i, -i, i, -1, 1, -1} respectively, so that the phase at the centre of the impulse response of each wavelet is zero. Finally, to achieve 180° rotational symmetry, we replace any coefficient with a negative imaginary part with its complex conjugate.

A Random Forest (RF) classification model can be trained using the DT-CWT feature descriptor for each selected pixel and its corresponding class label. A Random Forest is a decision tree based classifier that comprises a set of tree predictors. Each tree in the forest is built from a bootstrap sample of the training data. During the classification stage, an unseen feature descriptor is classified independently by each tree. The binary decision from each tree contributes to a unit vote in the forest. The final confidence (probability) of the classified outcome results from the proportion votes of trees for each class.

In our training stage, MLO view mammograms were segmented into five classes (1: background, 2: fatty tissue, 3: pectoral muscle, 4: glandular tissue, 5: nipple region). The ground truth segmentation was performed by a trained breast radiologist using a semi-automatic software interface (see Fig. 1). For each training image, 500 pixels (experimentally determined) were randomly selected from each of the five classes. To represent the features of each training pixel, the DT-CTW coefficients together with the normalised X-Y coordinates and the logarithm of the mammogram pixel value are used. The feature descriptor for each pixel is a 75-element vector (magnitude and phase of DT-CWT × 6 orientations × 6 levels of image pyramid + 2 normalized x, y coordinates + 1 pixel value). Based on the feature vectors and their corresponding classes from all training images, we trained a RF model (200 trees) for classifying unseen mammograms.

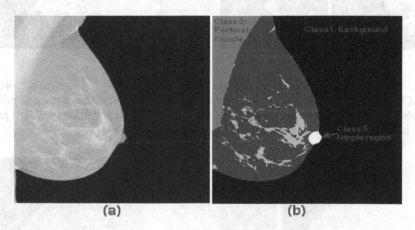

Fig. 1. (a) Logarithm of raw FFDM (b) Ground truth segmentation mask

When an unseen mammogram is analysed, the same method of calculating a feature vector for each pixel is used. By feeding the feature vector into the trained RF classifier, the probability for each pixel of belonging to each of the five classes is obtained. For the input image in Fig. 2 (a), Fig. 2 (b)-(f) present the probability maps (brighter pixels represent higher probabilities) obtained for each of the five classes. Figure 2 (g) is the combined probability map associated with the estimated class labels in Fig. 2 (h). The estimated segmentation mask and associated probability map for a particular difficult example are shown in figure 3. As highlighted in figure 3(c), in this example there are inaccurate estimations of labels in the pectoral muscle region, and although the nipple is not seen in the mammogram its position is nevertheless estimated by our method. The associated probability map (figure 3(b)) shows that the inaccurately classified regions have very low probabilities which reduce the confidence associated with classification to the assigned labels. This smart functionality permits more effective application of the segmentation results in further analysis.

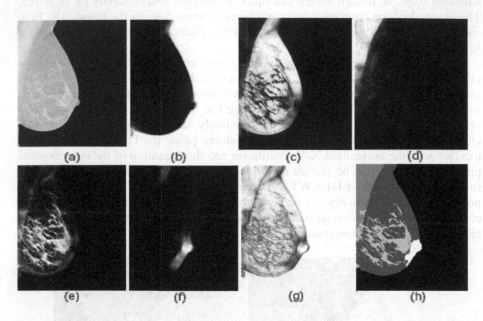

Fig. 2. (a) Input digital mammogram. Outputs from the proposed framework: (b) probability map of background (c) probability map of fatty tissue (d) probability map of pectoral muscle (e) probability map of glandular tissue (f) probability map of nipple region (g) combined probability map (h) label mask. Brighter pixels represent higher probabilities

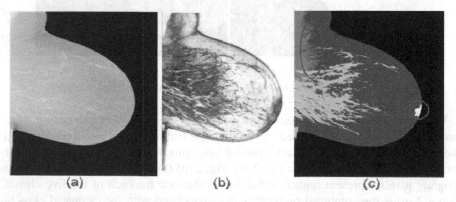

Fig. 3. An example output of the proposed segmentation method: (a) logarithm of the raw FFDM (b) probability map associated with the mask in (c) (c) estimated segmentation mask. Highlighted regions indicate misclassified regions but with low probability values in (b).

3   Evaluations

3.1   Dataset

The dataset used in this study comprised anonymised, randomly selected MLO view images of 50 women without cancer and 50 with cancer from the Nightingale Breast Screening Centre at the University Hospital of South Manchester. The 50 without cancer (referred to as controls) were confirmed by a subsequent normal screening mammogram approximately 3 years later. The 50 cancer mammograms were obtained from the most recent screen-detected unilateral malignant cancers identified, and the contralateral breasts were used for analysis. The ratio of left to right MLO views of the non-cancer images was controlled to match the ratio in the cancer images. All the images had been acquired using GE Senographe Essential mammography systems with a pixel size of 94.1 μm. Raw (unprocessed) FFDM images were pre-processed by applying the logarithm of the original pixel values, and right MLO images were laterally inverted to facilitate analysis. If not mentioned otherwise, all the described evaluation experiments in section 3 were performed in a 5-fold cross validation manner. The dataset was randomly grouped into five subgroups (20 images each, with 10 cancers and 10 controls). Four groups of images were used for training and tested on the remaining group and alternate until all groups are tested.

3.2   ROC Performance

For each of the images tested, the estimated probability maps of each class were obtained and compared with the corresponding ground truth mask. The ground truth masks were obtained as described in section 2. By feeding the estimated probability values and their corresponding ground truth labels, the receiver operating characteristic (ROC) curves for each of the classes are shown in figure 4. Note that, for the breast/background class, all pixels in the image are used as the input to the ROC calculation. For the fatty tissue, glandular tissue, pectoral muscle and nipple classes, only pixels from the breast region are used as the input to the ROC calculation. This is because by taking the background pixels (predominant the image) into account will lower the sensitivities to small error changes in classes with small region (e.g. the nipple region). It is seen from figure 4 that all of the five anatomic features are achieved very good performance. The area under the ROC curve (AUC) values range from 0.9220 to 0.9998, with sensitivity/specificity from 82.7% to 98.5% at the equal-error-rate point of the ROC curves. To test the reliability and repeatability of the system, we repeated the 5-fold cross validation process for five times, each with randomly divided groups. The mean and standard deviation of the AUC values for each class are shown in Table 1. The high mean and low standard deviation of AUC values demonstrated a good repeatability and reliability of the proposed system. It is noteworthy to mention that the nipple region achieved higher AUC values than expected. This is due to the effect discussed earlier, where the nipple region is small compared with the breast region. The majority of pixels in the breast region were correctly classified as not belonging to the nipple region. This makes the ROC calculation less sensitive to errors in the nipple region so we further evaluated our method using the Dice coefficient, which is more sensitive in detecting differences in small regions.

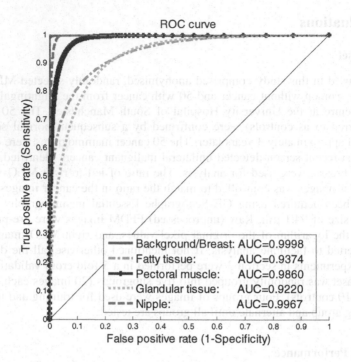

Fig. 4. ROC curves for each of the estimated classes

Table 1. Mean and standard deviation (SD) of AUC values for five random tests of 5-fold cross validation

	Mean of AUC	SD of AUC
Breast	0.9998	0.0000
Fatty tissue	0.9546	0.0243
Pectoral muscle	0.9902	0.0059
Glandular tissue	0.9403	0.0259
Nipple	0.9964	0.0004

3.3   Dice Coefficient

The Dice coefficient (DC) is designed for comparing the similarities of two samples [10]. In our case, the probability map of each class is firstly converted to a binary mask (1-foreground, 0-background) by setting a threshold (T) of the probability value. By overlapping the estimated binary mask with the ground truth mask, the number of pixels of the intersection region of the foreground is calculated, denoted as C. If A and B are the numbers of foreground pixels in the estimated binary mask and ground truth mask respectively, the DC is calculated as $\frac{2C}{A+B}$. The Dice coefficient ranges from 0 to 1, where 1 indicates perfect match and 0 means no overlapping. Hence the DC reflects differences not only in region size but also in location. We present the evaluation results in Fig. 5. The horizontal axis in Fig. 5 is the threshold selected for converting the estimated probability maps to binary masks, ranging from 0 to 1 with step size of 0.01. The vertical axis is the corresponding DC at each threshold level. The circle on each line indicates the best DC of each class, which is listed in the legend of the figure. It is seen from figure 5, the regions of breast, fatty tissue and glandular tissue achieved very good results with DC of greater than 0.9. The DC of glandular tissue and nipple are lower, as the DC is very sensitive to small shifts from the target location, even they are quite close. As with the ROC performance tests, we calculated the DCs for the 5-fold cross validation tests of five randomly sampled groups. The mean and standard deviation of the tests are shown in Table 2, which also demonstrate a high repeatability of the system.

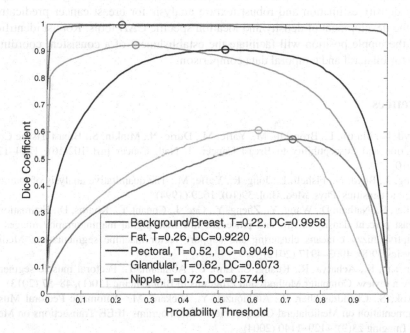

Fig. 5. Dice coefficients (DC) of each class at corresponding probability threshold levels (T)

Table 2. Mean and standard deviation (SD) of Dice coefficients (DC) for five random tests of 5-fold cross validation

	Mean of DC	SD of DC
Breast	0.9958	0.0000
Fatty tissue	0.9224	0.0006
Pectoral muscle	0.9047	0.0001
Glandular tissue	0.6065	0.0011
Nipple	0.5749	0.0007

4   Conclusions and Discussion

We have presented a fully automated and unified framework for simultaneously segmentation of the breast region, fatty tissue, glandular tissue, pectoral muscle and nipple region. With the estimated segmentation mask and associated probability map, the proposed method achieved accurate and robust segmentation, with the area under the ROC curve values range from 0.9220 to 0.9998 for the corresponding segmented features. We also confirmed the evaluation of our method by Dice coefficient (DC) calculation. The DC values of the breast, fatty tissue and pectoral muscle are greater than 0.9, where the DC for glandular and nipple are lower. We also demonstrated the repeatability and reliability of the system by repeated 5-fold cross validations on randomly sampled groups. We foresee this fundamental tool contributing to breast percentage density estimation and robust texture analysis for breast cancer predication, and to the development of density and location specific CAD tools. Robust identification of the nipple position will facilitate the establishment of a consistent coordinate system for bilateral and temporal data comparison.

References

1. Boyd, N., Martin, L., Bronskill, M., Yaffe, M., Duric, N., Minkin, S.: Breast Tissue Composition and Susceptibility to Breast Cancer. J. Natl. Cancer Inst. 102(16), 1224–1237 (2010)
2. Byng, J., Boyd, N., Fishell, E., Jong, R., Yaffe, M.: The quantitative analysis of mammographic densities. Phys. Med. Biol. 39(10), 1629 (1994)
3. Keller, B., Nathan, D., Wang, Y., Zheng, Y., Gee, J., Conant, E., Kontos, D.: Estimation of breast percent density in raw and processed full field digital mammography images via adaptive fuzzy c-means clustering and support vector machine segmentation. Medical Physics 39(8), 4903–4917 (2012)
4. Ganesan, K., Acharya, R., Kuang, C., Lim, C., Abraham, T.: Pectoral muscle segmentation: a review. Computer Methods and Programs in Biomedicine 110(1), 48–57 (2013)
5. Kwok, S., Chandrasekhar, R., Attikiouzel, Y., Rickard, M.: Automatic Pectoral Muscle Segmentation on Mediolateral Oblique View Mammograms. IEEE Transactions on Medical Imaging 23(9), 1129–1140 (2004)
6. Jas, M., Mukhopadhyay, S., Chakraborty, J., Sadhu, A., Khandelwal, N.: A heuristic approach to automated nipple detection in digital mammograms. Journal of Digital Imaging 26(5), 932–940 (2013)
7. Berks, M., Chen, Z., Astley, S., Taylor, C.: Detecting and classifying linear structures in mammograms using random forests. In: 22nd Information Processing in Medical Imaging, pp. 510–524 (2011)
8. Kingsbury, N.: Complex wavelets for shift invariant analysis and filtering of signals. Applied and Computational Harmonic Analysis 10(3), 234–253 (2001)
9. Breiman, L.: Random forests. Machine Learning 45(1), 5–32 (2001)
10. Dice, L.R.: Measures of the Amount of Ecologic Association Between Species. Ecology 26(3), 297–302 (1945)

Texture-Based Breast Cancer Prediction in Full-Field Digital Mammograms Using the Dual-Tree Complex Wavelet Transform and Random Forest Classification

Emmanouil Moschidis, Xin Chen, Chris Taylor, and Susan M. Astley

Centre for Imaging Sciences, Institute of Population Health,
The University of Manchester, Oxford Road, Manchester, M13 9PT, UK

Abstract. In this paper we describe a novel methodology for texture-based breast cancer prediction in full-field digital mammograms. Our method employs the Dual-Tree Complex Wavelet Transform for texture-based image analysis and representation, and Random Forest classification for discriminative learning and breast cancer prediction. We assess the ability of our method to identify women with breast cancer using raw images, processed images and Volpara™ density maps of two case-control datasets. We also investigate whether different regions of the breast exhibit different predictive power with respect to breast cancer. The best results are obtained using the processed images of a case-control dataset consisting of 100 cancers and 300 controls, where we achieve an area under the ROC curve of 0.74 for a texture model based on the whole breast and an equal area under the ROC curve when the most predictive regional model is used.

Keywords: Breast cancer, texture, wavelets, Random Forest, risk, mammogram.

1 Introduction

The reliable identification of women at increased risk of developing breast cancer will pave the way for personalized screening and early intervention [1]. Percentage mammographic density (PD) is an established independent risk factor for breast cancer, and research has also provided evidence that mammographic image texture may contribute differently from PD to breast cancer prediction [2, 3, 4].

Image-based methods related to breast cancer prediction analyze mammograms of controls and cancer-cases prior to diagnosis, and attempt to predict future incidents of cancer. They usually assign a single score corresponding to risk for breast cancer to a set of mammograms through analysis of the entire breast area of each image [2, 3, 4]. However, it is of interest to assess whether different image regions of the breast exhibit different predictive power for breast cancer, since the anatomy of the breast is such that different regions have different tissue composition and organization. It is also important to determine whether methods perform better on the unprocessed (raw) images or on processed versions (often referred to as 'For Presentation' images), since routine storage of raw images is not widespread.

H. Fujita, T. Hara, and C. Muramatsu (Eds.): IWDM 2014, LNCS 8539, pp. 209–216, 2014.

The contributions of this paper address the previously mentioned issues as follows: firstly, we introduce a novel framework for texture-based breast cancer prediction. The framework consists of two stages. In the first stage the Dual-Tree Complex Wavelet Transform (DT-CWT) is employed as means of texture-based analysis and representation of full-field digital mammograms (FFDM). A Random Forest (RF) classifier is then used for discriminative learning and breast cancer risk estimation. Secondly, we assess the framework with respect to its ability to determine the breast cancer status of women on raw images, processed images and Volpara™ density maps (fig. 1). The first two types of images are generated by mammography systems whilst the Volpara™ density maps are normalized images generated by a commercial product [5]. Thirdly, we divide the breast area into six equally sized segments (fig. 1) and assess the predictive ability of our method in each of these regions. Whilst we have evaluated our method on the contralateral breasts of women with and without cancer, it is intended that this approach will eventually be used for risk prediction prior to the development of the disease. In the next sections we elaborate on the different aspects of this work.

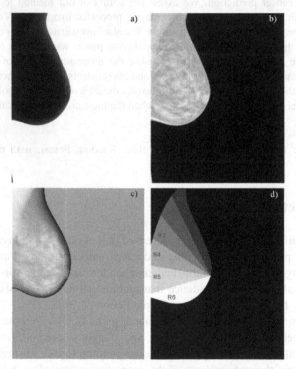

Fig. 1. An example raw image (a), processed image (b) and Volpara™ density map (c) of a control left MLO view, and a schematic depiction of the six segments of the breast evaluated in this work (d)

2   Methods

2.1   Datasets

We use two different case-control datasets. The first dataset consists of 100 mammograms in which a screen detected cancer was present (denoted 'cancer-cases') and 300 screening mammograms without cancer (denoted 'controls'). We refer to this as the 100/300 dataset. In this dataset no matching was performed between cancer-cases and controls. The second dataset consists of 113 cancer-cases and 226 controls; we refer to this as the 113/226 dataset. In this dataset every cancer-case had been age-matched with two controls. There is some overlap between these two datasets, with images from a small number of women appearing in both image sets. All images had previously been anonymized and are FFDM images obtained from the Greater Manchester Breast Screening Service at the Nightingale Breast Centre. All the images had been acquired using GE Senographe Essential mammography systems with a pixel size of 94.1 µm. The cancer-cases were selected randomly from the most recent screen-detected malignant breast cancers identified in the screening database. Interval cancers and mammograms showing bilateral breast cancer were excluded. The controls were selected from a list of women who attended for routine screening on two occasions and did not have cancer. The list was sorted according to the time interval between the two visits. In order to reduce the likelihood that the selected images show any early signs of cancer, the images from the earliest visit were selected. For the 100/300 dataset, the mean age of the cancers and the controls is 60.83 and 58.13 years with a standard deviation of 7.38 and 5.91 years respectively. For the 113/226 dataset, the mean age of both cancers and controls is 59.03 years with a standard deviation of 6.42 for the cancer-cases and 6.40 years for the controls.

For each woman one mediolateral oblique (MLO) view was selected. In all cancer-cases, the contralateral breast was used as a surrogate for the prior mammogram. For the 100/300 dataset, the ratio of left to right MLO views of the controls was controlled to match the cancer-cases. For the 113/226 dataset, the views of the controls were the same as their matching cancer-case. For all images, ground truth masks were generated interactively. These masks exclude the pectoral muscle and divide the breast area into six equally sized regions (fig. 1). The Volpara™ density maps are downscaled by a factor of 3 compared to the resolution of the original input images. In order to allow for the direct comparison of our framework's performance on different type of images, we also downscaled the raw and processed images by a factor of 3 before our experiments took place.

2.2   Dual-Tree Complex Wavelet Transform

In the first stage of our method we employ the DT-CWT as means of texture-based mammographic analysis. Wavelets provide both temporal and spectral information of the events of a signal and are widely used in textured-based image analysis [6]. The DT-CWT enhances the discrete wavelet transform by improving issues related to shift variance and lack of directionality [7]. In this study we perform the DT-CWT in a multi-resolution fashion using an image pyramid. Each level in our pyramid consists of a downscaled version of the image of the immediate lower level by a factor of 0.5. The overall pyramid consists of six different levels with the lowest level being the original image downscaled by a factor of 0.5. For each image in the pyramid the DT-CWT produces real and imaginary responses at six different orientations ($\pm 15°$, $\pm 45°$, $\pm 75°$), thus providing good angular resolution. For each orientation and scale we compute the magnitude and phase of the processed signal. The overall analysis results in a signature that consists of 72 features for each pixel, which are its magnitude and phase DT-CWT coefficients at different scales and orientations computed via efficient interpolation of the pyramid results.

2.3   Random Forest

In the second stage of our method we employ a RF classification scheme to learn the pixel signatures derived from the DT-CWT coefficients of training images of two different classes, cancer cases and controls. RF is an ensemble classifier that consists of decision trees combined via a majority voting scheme [8, 9]. In this study, once the RF models are trained, they are used to classify each pixel signature of a test image into cancer or control. The number of votes of the individual trees represents the confidence of the overall classifier regarding its task. This is considered as a likelihood estimate. For each pixel of a specific breast region of a test image, we record the likelihood estimate for it being a cancer-case pixel. Subsequently, we compute the risk for breast cancer of a test image segment by averaging the likelihood estimates for all pixels of this segment. In order to compute the overall risk of a test image, the risk estimates of the different segments are averaged. However, we also observe how individual segments perform, in order to assess whether a weighted sum approach shows promise as a future research direction.

3   Experiments and Results

We assess the performance of our framework following a 5-fold cross validation approach. For the experiment related to the 100/300 dataset, in each fold 320 images (80 cancers and 240 controls) and 80 images (20 cancers and 60 controls) are used for training and testing respectively. The images used in each fold are selected randomly. For the experiment related to the 113/226 dataset, in the first two folds 273 images (91 cancers and 182 controls) and 66 images (22 cancers and 44 controls) are used for training and testing respectively, whereas in the remaining three folds 270 images (90 cancers and 180 controls) and 69 images (23 cancers and 46 controls) are used for training and testing respectively. In each fold of this experiment the cancer images are selected randomly, whereas the images of the controls are from those matching the cancers.

In this study the RF models consist of 200 trees. Each tree in the forest is trained using a random subset of the initial features. In our experiments each random feature subset consists of 8 features. This is derived from the integer square root of 72, which is the total number of computed DT-CWT coefficients per pixel. These settings are according to published guidelines [8].

For each regional RF model, 5K pixels are used for training. This size of the training sample was selected after several experiments aiming at tuning our algorithm. In these experiments we used gradually increasing sizes of training pixel samples, which varied from 1K to 10K pixels. Our observation was that all RF regional models had reached their plateau in terms of their predictive accuracy when pixel samples consisting of 5K pixels were employed for their training. A sample of this size is drawn from approximately 16% of the pixels that constitute a breast region. The pixels used for training are selected via uniform random sampling. However, in order to allow for the direct comparison of our framework's performance on the three assessed types of images, in all three cases the RF regional models were trained using the same random training pixel samples.

Tables 1 and 2 summarize the area under the ROC curve (AUC) results of our experiments. Overall, our framework achieves the highest AUC when it operates on processed images. The AUC is also higher when raw images are used compared to the AUC obtained when Volpara™ density maps are used. It is noteworthy that in all our experiments our texture-based approach achieves better discrimination between cancers and controls than volumetric percentage density (PD) computed by Volpara™. For the experiment related to the 100/300 dataset, the texture-based model that combines all regional models via averaging achieves an AUC of 0.74 compared to an AUC of 0.50 when PD is used (table 1). Similarly, for the experiment related to the 113/226 dataset, the texture-based model that combines all regional models via averaging achieves an AUC of 0.67 compared to an AUC of 0.50 when PD is used (table 2). The AUC results of our approach are comparable to those reported in the literature when different texture measures are utilized for the same task.

Table 1. Area under ROC curve (AUC) results of the 5-fold cross validation experiment using the 100/300 dataset. The results with an asterisk are statistically significant according to the Mann-Whitney U statistic test ($p<0.05$) and those in bold are the best for each image type. The AUC obtained using PD is 0.50.

Breast region AUC by image type	R1	R2	R3	R4	R5	R6	Total breast area
Raw	0.63*	0.67*	0.70*	**0.71***	0.66*	0.69*	0.70*
Processed	0.71*	0.70*	0.71*	**0.74***	0.69*	0.70*	**0.74***
Volpara™	0.56	**0.61***	0.55	0.52	0.55	0.55	0.59*

Table 2. Area under ROC curve (AUC) results of the 5-fold cross validation experiment using the 113/226 dataset. The results with an asterisk are statistically significant according to the Mann-Whitney U statistic test (p<0.05) and those in bold are the best for each image type. The AUC obtained using PD is 0.50.

AUC by image type \ Breast region	R1	R2	R3	R4	R5	R6	Total breast area
Raw	0.61*	0.64*	**0.65***	0.60*	0.59*	0.62*	0.63*
Processed	0.65*	0.63*	0.64*	0.64*	0.67*	**0.68***	0.67*
Volpara™	0.50	0.60*	0.55	0.57*	**0.65***	0.57*	0.61*

Lastly, in this set of experiments we observe that all regional RF models demonstrate comparable predictive accuracy. The RF regional model that demonstrates the highest predictive performance is different for every different type of image used, and the differences in the AUC between that RF regional model and the remaining RF five regional models are small and potentially within the limits of statistical variation. In an attempt to estimate empirically the variability of our experiments, we performed 10 repetitions of the experiment using the Volpara™ density maps of the 113/226 dataset. The observed 95% confidence intervals (1.96 × standard error) were found to be equal to 0.004 or less. Furthermore, we observe that the texture-based model that combines all regional models via averaging achieves an AUC that is close to the AUC of the RF regional model with the highest predictive performance. Taking also into account the statistical variability, this indicates that averaging all the RF regional models may be the most robust/reliable strategy towards the computation of the overall risk of a test image. Averaging all the RF regional models is in effect the same approach as the one that employs one global RF model trained using samples of pixels drawn from the whole breast area via uniform random sampling.

4   Concluding Remarks

In this paper we introduced a novel framework for texture-based breast cancer prediction. This employs the DT-CWT for texture-based analysis of FFDMs and a RF classifier for discriminative learning and breast cancer prediction. The results presented in this paper demonstrate that our approach exhibits AUC results comparable to results reported in the literature and that it therefore shows promise in tackling the task of texture-based breast cancer prediction. Further validation on different and potentially larger datasets will be able to support this claim with greater confidence in the future.

In addition, we assessed our framework with respect to its ability to determine the breast cancer status of women on different versions of images that are often available in the field of mammography, namely raw images, processed images and Volpara™ density maps. The results of the experiments reported in this paper suggest that our framework operates well on the three types of images. However, it achieves its best performance when operating on processed images. An explanation for the framework's lower performance on Volpara™ density maps could be that the measurements in the peripheral region of the breast in this type of image may be unreliable due to lack of accurate knowledge of compressed breast thickness in the periphery. Due to the random nature of our pixel selection strategy during the construction of the training pixel samples for each breast region, these pixels are also included as candidates. Selection of such pixels may have compromised the learning part of the RF regional models and subsequently their ability to discriminate between cancer and control pixels. It is our intention to investigate this further and assess whether we can improve the performance of our framework when using Volpara™ density maps by excluding pixels close to the periphery of the breast during the construction of the training pixel samples for each breast region.

Furthermore, in this study we used two different case-control datasets, one consisting of 100 cancers and 300 controls with no matching between cancers and controls, and one consisting of 113 cancers and 226 controls with age-matching between cancer and controls. The sizes of the two datasets are similar; therefore the differences in the results could be attributed to the effect of age-matching. Using the 113/226 dataset, we observe worse AUC results when our framework operates on raw and processed, and slightly better AUC results when it operates on Volpara™ density maps, compared to the respective AUC results when the 100/300 dataset is used. The effect of age on the texture-based analysis is of particular interest and deserves further investigation, as age is a strong risk factor for breast cancer. Also, as a woman ages the texture patterns observed in her mammograms will most likely alter, therefore it may not be appropriate to train RF models on images drawn from a certain age group and apply them on images drawn from a different age group. We acknowledge that this potential flaw exists in both experiments presented in this paper. A solution to this is to construct n-fold cross validation experiments, in which the age distribution of the selected images is the same across all folds.

Lastly, we also investigated whether different regions of the breast exhibit different predictive power with respect to breast cancer. The underlying assumption of this hypothesis testing was that the anatomy of the breast is such that different regions have different tissue composition and organization. The reported results suggest that this hypothesis may not hold and that the analysis of pixels drawn randomly from the whole breast area may be the most robust/reliable strategy towards the computation of the overall risk of a test image, as long as the size of the pixel sample is large enough to represent reliably the total breast area. We also have to acknowledge the fact that our approach gives no guarantee that the same sector will correspond to the same anatomical area between the breasts of two images. Also the production of the masks that define the six regions for each image suffers of subjectivity due to its interactive nature. A more robust regional assessment analysis of a mammogram could be based on our scheme combined with image registration or on a coordinate system for mammograms similar to the one described by Brandt et al. in [10]. In the future we also intend to assess whether texture-based analysis of regions consisting predominantly of fatty tissue have different predictive potential with respect to breast cancer from regions consisting of dense tissue. In order to assess this hypothesis, we will utilize our recent segmentation framework presented in Chen et al. [11], which is able to distinguish robustly these two types of tissue.

Acknowledgements. We thank Elaine Harkness and staff at the Nightingale Breast Centre for assisting us with data selection and retrieval. We thank Mike Berks for providing useful comments, insight and code related to the DT-CWT. We would also like to acknowledge the assistance given by IT Services and the use of the Computational Shared Facility at The University of Manchester. We are grateful to Matakina Technology Limited for their support in our use of Volpara™. This work was performed in the ASSURE project, which is supported by the European Union under the 7th Framework Programme for Health Research.

References

1. Evans, D.G.R., Warwick, J., Astley, S.M., Stavrinos, P., Sahin, S., Ingham, S., McBurney, H., Eckersley, B., Harvie, M., Wilson, M., Beetles, U., Warren, R., Hufton, A., Sergeant, J.C., Newman, W.G., Buchan, I., Cuzick, J., Howell, A.: Assessing Individual Breast Cancer Risk within the U.K. National Health Service Breast Screening Program: A New Paradigm for Cancer Prevention. Cancer Prevention Research 5(7), 943–951 (2012)
2. Nielsen, M., Karemore, G., Loog, M., Raundahl, J., Karssemeijer, N., Otten, J.D.M., Karsdal, M.A., Vachon, C.M., Christiansen, C.: A novel and automatic mammographic texture resemblance marker is an independent risk factor for breast cancer. Cancer Epidemiology 35, 381–387 (2011)
3. Manduca, A., Carston, M.J., Heine, J.J., Scott, C.G., Pankratz, V.S., Brandt, K.R., Sellers, T.A., Vachon, C.M., Cerhan, J.R.: Texture Features from Mammographic Images and Risk of Breast Cancer. Cancer Epidemiology Biomarkers and Prevention 18(3), 837–845 (2009)
4. Häberle, L., Wagner, F., Fasching, P.A., Jud, S.M., Heusinger, K., Loehberg, C.R., Hein, A., Bayer, C.M., Hack, C.C., Lux, M.P., Binder, K., Elter, M., Münzenmayer, C., Schultz-Wendtland, R., Adamietz, B.R., Uder, M., Beckmann, M.W., Wittenberg, T.: Characterizing mammographic images by using generic texture features. Breast Cancer Research 14(2), 1–12 (2012)
5. Highnam, R., Brady, S.M., Yaffe, M.J., Karssemeijer, N., Harvey, J.: Robust Breast Composition Measurement - Volpara™. In: Martí, J., Oliver, A., Freixenet, J., Martí, R. (eds.) IWDM 2010. LNCS, vol. 6136, pp. 342–349. Springer, Heidelberg (2010)
6. Gonzalez, R.C., Woods, R.E.: Digital Image Processing, 2nd edn. Prentice Hall (2001)
7. Selesnick, I.W., Baraniuk, R.G., Kingsbury, N.G.: The Dual-Tree Complex Wavelet Transform. IEEE Signal Processing Magazine, 123–151 (2005)
8. Breiman, L.: Random forests. Machine Learning 45(1), 5–32 (2001)
9. Breiman, L.: Bagging predictors. Machine Learning 24(2), 123–140 (1996)
10. Brandt, S.S., Karemore, G., Karssemeijer, N., Nielsen, M.: An anatomically oriented breast coordinate system for mammogram analysis. IEEE Transactions on Medical Imaging 30(10), 1841–1851 (2001)
11. Chen, X., Moschidis, E., Taylor, C., Astley, S.: A Novel Framework for Fat, Glandular Tissue, Pectoral Muscle and Nipple Segmentation in Full-Field Digital Mammograms. In: Fujita, H., Hara, T., Muramatsu, C. (eds.) IWDM 2014. LNCS, vol. 8539, pp. 201–208. Springer, Heidelberg (2014)

Evaluation of a New Design of Contrast-Detail Phantom for Mammography: CDMAM Model 4.0

Celia J. Strudley and Kenneth C. Young

National Coordinating Centre for the Physics of Mammography (NCCPM), Guildford, UK
celia.strudley@nhs.net

Abstract. The standard test object used to assess the imaging performance of digital mammography systems in Europe is the CDMAM model 3.4. The recently released CDMAM model 4.0 differs from the model 3.4 in the layout, number and range of thicknesses of gold contrast details used to assess threshold contrast detail detection. In order to evaluate CDMAM 4.0 we compared its performance with that of the CDMAM 3.4 using several digital mammography systems at various dose levels. We also assessed the reproducibility of the results compared to that of the previous model. CDMAM 4.0 results were comparable to results for CDMAM 3.4 for detail diameters in the range 0.1 to 0.5mm and for the larger detail diameters there were increased differences as would be expected due to the design differences of the CDMAM 4.0. The reproducibility of CDMAM 4.0 results was found to be better than that of CDMAM 3.4 results.

Keywords: CDMAM 3.4, CDMAM 4.0, CDMAM Analysis, threshold contrast detail detection, image quality, digital mammography.

1 Introduction

The standard test object used to assess the imaging performance of digital mammography systems in Europe is the CDMAM model 3.4[1]. The recently released CDMAM model 4.0[2] [1] differs from the model 3.4 in the number and range of thicknesses of the gold contrast details used to assess threshold contrast detail detection. The changes increase the number of details within the critical range for determination of threshold gold thickness relative to the minimum acceptable and achievable standards of image quality defined in the European protocol [2]. The layout of the new phantom also differs from the previous model and incorporates additional high contrast discs which are placed to assist automatic reading software in locating the exact position of the matrix of gold details. Fig. 1 shows images of the two phantoms and Fig. 2 shows the ranges of thickness and diameter of the contrast detail diameters for

---

[1]   UMC St. Radboud, Nijmegen University, Netherlands.
[2]   Artinis, Netherlands.

H. Fujita, T. Hara, and C. Muramatsu (Eds.): IWDM 2014, LNCS 8539, pp. 217–224, 2014.
© Springer International Publishing Switzerland 2014

the two phantoms compared to the threshold gold thickness standards defined in the European protocol. Automated software, CDCOM[3], is commonly used to read CDMAM 3.4 images and this has formed the basis for new software, CDCOM4[4], for reading CDMAM 4.0 images. NCCPM have previously developed CDMAM analysis software to calculate the predicted human threshold gold thickness results using the output from CDCOM for CDMAM 3.4. We have recently upgraded this software so that it now performs the same analysis for CDMAM 4.0.

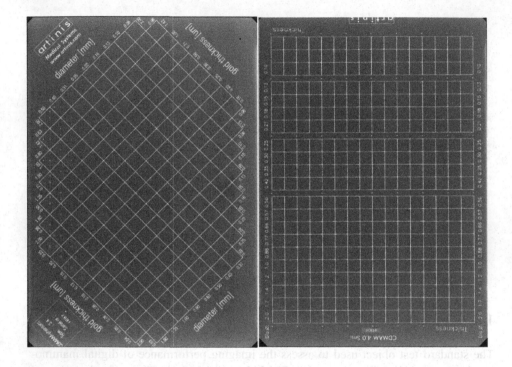

Fig. 1. Mammographic images of the CDCOM 3.4 (left) and CDCOM 4.0 (right)

In order to evaluate CDMAM 4.0 we compared its performance with that of the CDMAM 3.4 by imaging using four digital mammography systems at multiple dose levels. We also assessed the reproducibility of the results compared to that of the previous model.

---

3   www.euref.org
4   Artinis, Netherlands.

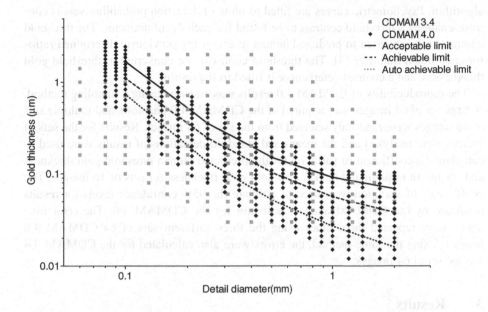

Fig. 2. Comparison of the range of detail diameter and thickness for the two phantoms: Grey and black points show the diameter and thickness of each gold disc in CDMAM 3.4 and CDMAM 4.0 respectively. The threshold gold thickness limits as defined in the European protocol are shown, as well as the threshold gold thickness for automatic reading that corresponds to the achievable level for human reading.

2   Method

A recently manufactured CDMAM 3.4 (serial number 1897) was used to make the comparison with the new CDMAM 4.0 (serial number 4004). Sets of sixteen images of each phantom were acquired following the method described in the European protocol.

Version 1.6 of CDCOM (currently available for download from the EUREF website[5]) was used to read images of the CDMAM 3.4 test object. For the CDMAM 4.0 images, the version of CDCOM4 used was cdcom4_artinis1024.

The results from reading the images of both phantoms were analyzed using our own recently revised CDMAM analysis software, which runs on a Java platform and deals with both phantom designs in an equivalent manner. The method of analysis has been described in detail previously [3]. CDCOM outputs for a set of repeat images are averaged to create a detection probability matrix, which is smoothed using a simple

---

[5] www.euref.com

algorithm. Psychometric curves are fitted to plots of detection probability versus contrast, enabling a threshold contrast to be found for each detail diameter. The threshold contrasts are converted to predicted human results using previously determined ratios for each detail diameter [3]. The threshold contrasts are converted to threshold gold thicknesses, and a contrast detail curve is fitted to the results.

The reproducibility of CDMAM 4.0 results was assessed using a sampling method. A large set of 64 images was acquired of the CDMAM 4.0 phantom, and multiple sets of 16 images were randomly selected from the set of 64 images. Results for the sets of images were analyzed and the means and standard deviations of results were used to calculate the coefficient of variation for the predicted human threshold gold thickness and for the fit to predicted human threshold gold thickness for sets of 16 images. The coefficients of variation were used to estimate the 95% confidence levels for results produced by our CDMAM analysis software for the CDMAM 4.0. The error estimates were repeated three times using the three different sets of 64 CDMAM 4.0 images. Using the same method, the errors were also calculated for the CDMAM 3.4 for one set of 64 images.

3   Results

Threshold gold thickness results for CDMAM 4.0 and 3.4 are shown for each of the systems in Figures 3-6. Results for the systems in terms of the differences between the results for the two phantoms for the four detail diameters which are common to both phantoms are shown in Table 1.

Table 1. Differences between results for CDMAM 4.0 and 3.4 fit to predicted human threshold gold thickness

| | Detail diameter | | | |
System and dose setting	0.1mm	0.25mm	0.5mm	1.0mm
Hologic Dimensions: Double AEC dose	0%	6%	22%	56%
Hologic Dimensions: AEC dose	-1%	6%	18%	53%
Hologic Dimensions: Half AEC dose	1%	10%	13%	17%
Hologic Selenia: AEC dose	18%	13%	15%	34%
GE Essential: AEC dose	11%	7%	7%	22%
GE Essential: Half AEC dose	-13%	-6%	-2%	6%
Fuji Innovality: Double AEC dose	-14%	-8%	-10%	-1%
Fuji Innovality: AEC dose	-18%	-9%	-7%	4%
Fuji Innovality: Half AEC dose	-29%	-9%	-7%	0%
Average	-5%	1%	5%	21%

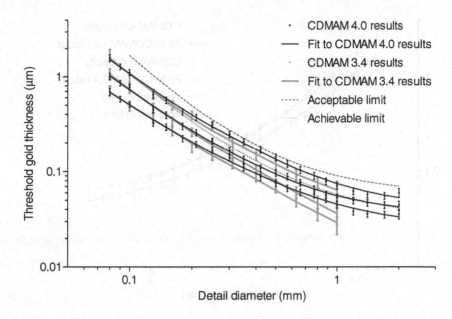

Fig. 3. Comparison of CDMAM 4.0 and CDMAM 3.4 results for images acquired at three different dose levels on Hologic Selenia Dimensions

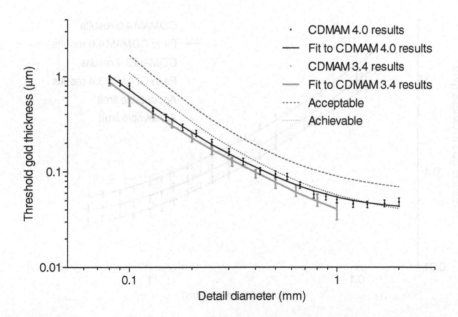

Fig. 4. Comparison of CDMAM 4.0 and CDMAM 3.4 results for images acquired at one dose level on Hologic Selenia

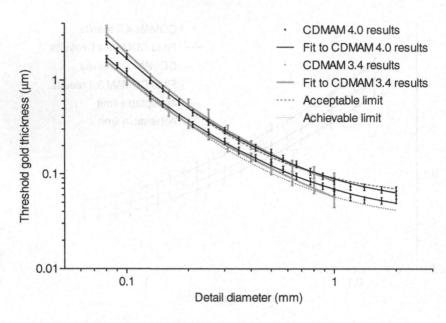

Fig. 5. Comparison of CDMAM 4.0 and CDMAM 3.4 results for images acquired at two different dose levels on GE Senographe Essential

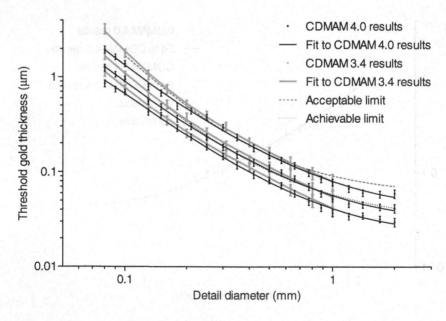

Fig. 6. Comparison of CDMAM 4.0 and CDMAM 3.4 results for images acquired at three different dose levels on Fuji Amulet Innovality

The reproducibility results for sets of 16 images are summarized in Table 2 (unfitted data) and Table 3 (fitted data).

Table 2. Estimated 95% confidence limits on predicted human threshold gold thicknesses for the two CDMAMs

	0.1mm	0.25mm	0.5mm	1.0mm	2.0mm
CDMAM 3.4	±9.8%	±10%	±12%	±20%	-
CDMAM 4.0	±7.0%	±7.0%	±7.9%	±8.0%	±10%

Table 3. Estimated 95% confidence limits on the fit to predicted human threshold gold thicknesses for the two CDMAMs

	0.1mm	0.25mm	0.5mm	1.0mm	2.0mm
CDMAM 3.4	±7.7%	±7.6%	±9.1%	±14%	-
CDMAM 4.0	±5.3%	±4.5%	±4.8%	±4.6%	±8.5%

4   Discussion

In Figures 3-6 and Table 1 it can be seen that there is mostly fair agreement between results for the two phantoms for 0.1mm to 0.5mm details, with the majority of differences between fit to predicted human threshold gold thicknesses being less than 15%, and a maximum difference of 29%. For the larger 1.0mm details, differences in results for the two phantoms are in some cases greater (up to 56%) where image quality significantly exceeds the achievable level. This is as expected because the CDMAM 3.4 does not have sufficiently thin gold thicknesses for the larger details to cover the range of automatic threshold gold thicknesses for better than the achievable level of image quality. Some of the difference in threshold gold thickness results between the two phantoms may be explained by a change in the impact of the heel effect due to the difference in layout of the discs. In the past, inter-phantom variations have been found for the model 3.4 phantom [4], and some differences between the results for the 3.4 and 4.0 are therefore to be expected. A limitation of the evaluation carried out was that only one sample each of the CDMAM 4.0 and CDMAM 3.4 were used.

The reproducibility of CDMAM 4.0 results for predicted human gold thicknesses and for fitted data were found to be better than for CDMAM 3.4.

The results of this evaluation are dependant, not only on the CDMAM phantoms used, but also on the software used to read the images and analyze the results. Our analysis software was designed to carry out equivalent analysis for the two phantoms designs. Since this evaluation, CDCOM4 has undergone further development, and the version of CDCOM4 which we used has been superseded. It will therefore be necessary to repeat the evaluation using the latest version of CDCOM4.

5   Conclusions

The design of the CDMAM 4.0 is an improvement on the design of the CDMAM 3.4, with a range of detail diameters and thicknesses better suited to measuring the imaging performance of good digital mammography systems. For the CDMAM reading and analysis software used, CDMAM 4.0 results were comparable to results for the older CDMAM 3.4 for detail diameters in the range 0.1 to 0.5mm and for the larger detail diameters there were increased differences as would be expected due to the design improvements of the CDMAM 4.0. The reproducibility of CDMAM 4.0 results in terms of fit to predicted gold thickness was also improved.

References

1. Floor-Westerdijk, M.J., Colier, W.N.J.M., van der Burght, R.J.M.: CDMAM Phantom Optimized for Digital Mammography Quality Control by Automatic Image Readout. In: Roa Romero, L.M. (ed.) XIII Mediterranean Conference on Medical and Biological Engineering and Computing 2013. IFMBE Proceedings, vol. 41, pp. 467–470. Springer, Heidelberg (2014)
2. European Commission (EC) 2006 European Guidelines for Quality Assurance in Breast Cancer Screening and Diagnosis, 4th edn. Office for Official Publications of the European Communities, Luxembourg (2006)
3. Young, K.C., Cook, J.J.H., Oduko, J.M., Bosmans, H.: Comparison of software and human observers in reading images of the CDMAM test object to assess digital mammography systems. In: Flynn, M.J., Hsieh, J. (eds.) Proceedings of SPIE Medical Imaging 2006, 614206, pp. 1–13 (2006)
4. Young, K.C., Alsager, A., Oduko, J.M., Bosmans, H., Verbrugge, B., Geertse, T., van Engen, R.: Evaluation of software for reading images of the CDMAM test object to assess digital mammography systems. In: Proceedings of SPIE Medical Imaging 2008, 69131C, pp. 1–11 (2008)

Threshold Target Thickness Calculated Using a Model Observer as a Quality Control Metric for Digital Mammography

Aili K. Bloomquist[1], James G. Mainprize[1], Melissa Hill[1], and Martin J. Yaffe[1,2]

[1] Physical Sciences, Sunnybrook Research Institute, Toronto, Canada
[2] Department of Medical Biophysics, University of Toronto, Toronto, Canada
aili.bloomquist@sri.utoronto.ca

Abstract. Task-based measures estimated by model observers may provide a more clinically relevant and objective way of assessing image quality and system performance for quality control of digital mammography. One approach is to calculate the required threshold thickness (t_t) of a material necessary to render test objects just visible, using the detectability index (d') calculated from measured system parameters and a non-prewhitening observer model incorporating an eye-filter and internal noise (NPWE). Our previous work developed methodology for simply measuring the parameters required to calculate d' and t_t using a NPWE model. Here we test the sensitivity of t_t to changes in image quality by varying entrance exposure and by imaging with and without a grid. Calculated t_t values are compared with those reported by automated analysis of CDMAM (^{TM}) phantom images (CDCOM). Sensitivity to dose changes was seen, and good correlation was achieved between CDCOM and our model.

Keywords: quality control, threshold thickness, noise-equivalent quanta, model observer.

1 Introduction

Conventional quality control (QC) methods for digital mammography are limited by their subjectivity and by not making full use of the digital image data. More objective and analytical measures of system performance such as the detective quantum efficiency are challenging to perform and interpret, lacking a clear connection to clinical image quality. Using task-based measures based on model observers may provide a more clinically relevant and objective way of assessing image quality and system performance for QC of digital mammography systems. One approach is to calculate the required threshold thickness (t_t) of a material necessary to render test objects of varying sizes just visible, using the detectability index (d') calculated from measured system performance parameters and a non-prewhitening observer model incorporating an eye-filter and internal noise (NPWE).

In previous work, we have developed a phantom for measuring the parameters required to calculate d' and t_t for a NPWE model [1]. The eye filter and internal noise parameters were fit empirically to match the results of a 4AFC reader study.

H. Fujita, T. Hara, and C. Muramatsu (Eds.): IWDM 2014, LNCS 8539, pp. 225–230, 2014.

Here we test the sensitivity of threshold thickness to changes in image quality by imaging at different entrance exposures, with and without a grid. The results of the model are compared with the results of automatically analyzing images of the CDMAM phantom (version 3.4, Artinis, St. Walburg 4, 6671 AS Zetten, The Netherlands), acquired under the same conditions using the manufacturer supplied software, CDCOM (v 1.6).

2   Methods

2.1   Model Observer

The detectability index (d') of a detection task is a signal to noise ratio. It can be calculated using a non-prewhitening model observer with eye filter and internal noise as follows [1]:

$$d' = \Delta S \sqrt{\frac{\left(\iint_{u,v} W^2(u,v)MTF^2(u,v)E^2(u,v)dudv\right)^2}{\left(\iint_{u,v} W^2(u,v)NNPS(u,v)MTF^2(u,v)E^4(u,v)dudv + N_i\right)}}, \qquad (1)$$

where W is the task function, MTF' is the adjusted measured system modulation transfer function, $NNPS$ is the measured normalized noise power spectrum, E is a filter intended to model the contrast sensitivity of the human eye, and ΔS is the radiological subject contrast. Here subject contrast is defined as the signal difference between the object and the background. It is believed that a human observer cannot make efficient use of the information degraded by long-tailed PSFs, as in the scatter signal.[2] As a result, the matched filter to mimic the human $MTF'(u,v)E(u,v)W(u,v)$ uses the adjusted system $MTF'(u,v)$ which is the system MTF with removal of the long-tail component that was due to scatter and/or glare. The numerator of equation 1 is the integral of the matched filtered representing the perceived signal present in the image. The denominator consists of two terms, the first being the integral of the matched filter multiplied by the perceived noise in the image and the second is the internal noise of the viewer (N_i). The task function is the Fourier transform of the discs being modeled is described by:

$$W(\rho) = \frac{dJ_1(\pi d\rho)}{2\rho}, \qquad (2)$$

where d is the disc diameter and $J_1(\rho)$ is the Bessel function of the first kind. The eye filter it is taken to be of the form:

$$E(\rho) = \rho^n exp(-c\rho^2), \qquad (3)$$

where ρ is the radial spatial frequency. This assumes a radially symmetric eye filter. The parameters for the eye filter were taken to be $n=0.79$ and $c=2.69$, based on previous work with a 4AFC reader study involving the detection of discs.
The internal noise was assumed to be of the form:

$$N_i = \alpha N + \beta, \qquad (4)$$

where αN is the induced internal noise (proportional to the image noise) and β is an independent internal noise component. The noise parameters were taken from the reader study results to be $\alpha=1.61$ and $\beta=0.35$.

2.2   System Parameters

To measure most of the physical parameters required for the model observer a simple phantom designed for evaluation of the noise equivalent quanta (NEQ) was imaged. This phantom consisted of stacks of 1 cm thick slabs of PMMA to create total thicknesses of 3, 4 or 8cm, a slanted brass edge at a level 2cm above the breast support plate for the measurement of the system modulation transfer function, , and a lead disc, positioned on the top surface of the phantom, for the estimation of the scatter fraction. A uniform region of the phantom was used for the measurement of the noise power spectrum. The measurement of MTF and NPS was done following previously published methodology [3].

For the comparison with CDMAM results, the radiological contrast for the calculation of d' and t_t was determined from signal levels in regions of interest behind and adjacent to the 1 mm diameter gold discs on the CDMAM phantom, over the thickness range of 0.10 to 0.71 μm of gold. The signal difference values from repeated images of the CDMAM phantom were averaged together to reduce variability caused by measuring in the small regions of interest behind the discs. A linear least squares fit between gold thickness and ΔS was then performed.

2.3   Imaging Conditions

Images were acquired on a Senographe Essential (GE Healthcare, Chalfont, St. Giles, UK). The standard technique was chosen to closely match the parameters selected by the automatic exposure control when 3, 4 or 8 cm-thick uniform blocks of PMMA were in the beam and the "CNT" mode (optimized for image contrast) was selected. The technique factors are listed in Table 1. Images were taken at the standard techniques with and without the grid in place. Images were also taken at approximately half and double the standard mAs, with the grid in place, for the 4 cm phantom (63 mAs and 225 mAs) to evaluate the sensitivity of t_t to dose. For each imaging condition, 12 images were taken of both the NEQ phantom and the CDMAM phantom.

Table 1. Technique factors used for imaging of the NEQ and CDMAM phantoms. Techniques indicated with an asterisk (*) were those closest to the technique selected by the AEC, and were used for images with and without grid.

Phantom Thickness (cm)	Anode	Filter	kV	mAs	MGD (mGy)
3*	Mo	Mo	26	63	1.3
4	Mo	Rh	27	63	1.2
4*	Mo	Rh	27	110	2.1
4	Mo	Rh	27	225	4.2
8*	Rh	Rh	31	160	3.0

2.4   Automatically Analysing the CDMAM Images

The images of the CDMAM phantom were automatically analysed to determine the threshold thicknesses of gold using the CDCOM software (v 1.6), as described by Karssemeijer and Thijssen[4].   The 95% confidence intervals (1.96 × the standard error) in the resulting values of t_t were taken from the estimates generated using the Guildford CDMAM Analyzer[1] software, version 1.5.5.

The CDCOM software is known to over-estimate the threshold thicknesses of the different diameter discs compared to human readers.   We attempted to account for this by applying the correction proposed by Young et al.[5], using equation 5

$$T_{predicted} = a[T_{auto}]^m \tag{5}$$

where T_{auto} is the threshold thickness determined by the CDCOM software, $T_{predicted}$ is the predicted threshold thickness seen by human readers and a and m are fitted parameters.   For this work we used the published parameters, a= 1.192 and m = 0.880.

3   Results and Discussion

Preliminary results for different entrance exposures and imaging with and without the grid are shown in Figure 1, where threshold thickness is plotted against disc diameter. Calculated values of t_t from measurements using 12 separate repeated images of the parameter measurement phantom showed good repeatability with an average coefficient of variation (COV) of 0.01% and a maximum COV of 2.43%.   Qualitatively the values of t_t calculated through the model and using CDCOM track as expected when the dose is changed. When the grid is removed, no change in t_t is seen with either method for 3 and 4 cm thick phantoms, while for the 8 cm thick phantom a modest decrease in threshold thickness is seen when using a grid, which is consistent with recent reports in the literature[6].   The modeled t_t values are plotted versus the corrected results of running the CDCOM software on images of the CDMAM phantom in Figure 2. A linear least squares fit between the two approaches gives a Pearson's correlation coefficient of 0.92, showing good correlation, however, even with the applied correction to make the results match a set of human readers, CDCOM reports higher performance compared to our model, with a lower value of t_t. The discrepancy between the two approaches requires further investigation to better determine the relationships with human observer performance.   It may be that the parameters used in our model need adjustment for use with the greater range of disc diameters present in the CDMAM phantom.   The reader study used to establish the parameters used discs ranging from 0.625 to 2.5 mm, while the CDMAM phantom diameters range from 0.06 to 2.0 mm.

---

[1]   http://www.euref.org/downloads?download=41:cdmam-analyser-version-1.5.5

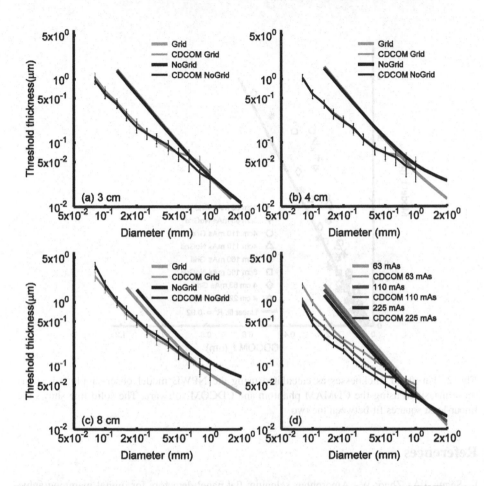

Fig. 1. Threshold thicknesses for different disc diameters, as measured using the NPWE model and CDCOM software.(a), (b) and (c) show system behaviour with and without a grid for the different phantom thicknesses while (d) shows the effect of varying the entrance exposure for the 4 cm thick phantom with the grid in place. The error-bars shown for the CDCOM measurements are 2x the estimated standard error, as reported by the CDMAM analyser software.

In future work, the measurement phantom will be modified to include gold discs of different thicknesses to directly measure subject contrast in a single image. The sensitivity of t_t to other imaging conditions will be tested, including varying beam quality, and using an air gap with and without a grid. The model will also be further validated with a human reader study on the mammography system used here. The greater simplicity of the measurements with this technique than CDMAM, the ability to extend the model to more realistic imaging targets than discs and its potential to predict clinical image quality encourages further work. In the future we plan to incorporate more anatomic-like backgrounds and other shapes and discrimination tasks.

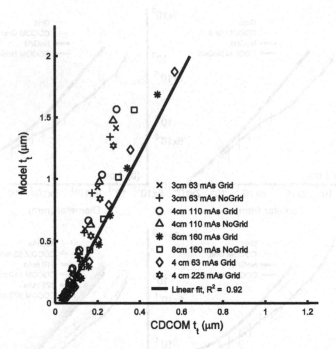

Fig. 2. Threshold thicknesses as calculated using the NPWE model observer plotted versus those measured using the CDMAM phantom and CDCOM software. The solid line shows the linear-least squares fit between the two.

References

1. Segui, J.A., Zhao, W.: Amorphous selenium flat panel detectors for digital mammography: Validation of a NPWE model observer with CDMAM observer performance experiments. Med. Phys. 33, 3711 (2006)
2. Rolland, J.P., Barrett, H., Seeley, G.: Ideal versus human observer for long-tailed point spread functions: does deconvolution help? Phys. Med. Biol. 36, 1091–1109 (1991)
3. Bloomquist, A.K., Mainprize, J.G., Mawdsley, G.E., Yaffe, M.J.: Method of measuring NEQ as a quality control metric for digital mammography. Med. Phys. 41, 031905 (2014)
4. Karssemeijer, N., Thijssen, M.A.O.: Determination of contrast-detail curves of mammography systems by automated image analysis. In: Doi, K. (ed.) Proceedings of the 3rd International Workshop on Digital Mammography, pp. 155–160. Elsevier, Chicago (1996)
5. Young, K.C., Alsager, A., Oduko, J.M., Bosmans, H., Verbrugge, B., Geertse, T., van Engen, R.: Evaluation of software for reading images of the CDMAM test object to assess digital mammography systems. In: Hsieh, J., Sameh, E. (eds.) Proc. SPIE, vol. 6913, p. 69131C (2008)
6. Salvagnini, E., Bosmans, H., Struelens, L., Marshall, N.W.: Effective detective quantum efficiency for two mammography systems: Measurement and comparison against established metrics. Med. Phys. 40, 101916 (2013)

Contrast-Enhanced Digital Mammography Lesion Morphology and a Phantom for Performance Evaluation

Melissa L. Hill[1,2,*], Aili K. Bloomquist[1], Sam Z. Shen[1], James G. Mainprize[1],
Ann-Katherine Carton[3], Sylvie Saab-Puong[3], Serge Muller[3], Clarisse Dromain[4],
and Martin J. Yaffe[1,2]

[1] Physical Sciences, Sunnybrook Research Institute, Toronto, Canada
[2] Department of Medical Biophysics, University of Toronto, Toronto, Canada
[3] GE Healthcare, Buc, France
[4] Department of Radiology, Institut Gustave Roussy, Villejuif, France
melissa.hill.sri@gmail.com

Abstract. Contrast-enhanced digital mammography (CEDM), promises to improve diagnostic accuracy as an adjunct to mammography, especially for women with dense breasts. Here we review 98 enhancing lesions from a previously published dual-energy CEDM study of 120 women to identify enhancing lesion morphologies and to characterize their sizes and margins as detected in CEDM. We have designed a phantom based on these clinical data that incorporates realistic enhancing lesion morphologies for CEDM evaluation. The phantom includes elements of four lesion types observed in CEDM, which broadly follow analogous categories developed from the MRI Breast Imaging, Reporting and Data System (BI-RADS) lexicon. This phantom uses solid iodinated plastic features with accurate iodine concentrations for detection sensitivity experiments. We believe that comparisons of the lesion morphologies through quantitative metrics and reader studies will be useful to test lesion classification and discrimination tasks that can contribute to CEDM performance evaluation.

Keywords: CEDM dual-energy mammography iodine morphology phantom.

1 Introduction

Contrast-enhanced digital mammography promises to be a cost-effective and accurate alternative to breast MRI to assess hypervascularized tissues that may be related to tumour angiogenesis [1, 2]. One approach to CEDM is a dual-energy (DE) technique, where an iodinated contrast agent is administered intravenously and then a pair of low-energy (LE) and high-energy (HE) mammograms are acquired with mean x-ray beam energies below and above the iodine K-edge [3]. The LE and HE images are combined in a manner to cancel the appearance of normal breast tissue and to reveal regions of increased iodine uptake. Currently, there are no standardized classifications for radiologists reporting on CEDM tumour morphology, and relatively few published

---

* Corresponding author.

H. Fujita, T. Hara, and C. Muramatsu (Eds.): IWDM 2014, LNCS 8539, pp. 231–238, 2014.
© Springer International Publishing Switzerland 2014

observations of lesion enhancement types. Investigators have generally relied on the MRI BI-RADS lexicon to provide guidance on classifications for enhancing lesions in CEDM [1, 2, 4]. In this work, we review enhancing lesion morphologies observed by Dromain *et al.* in a DE CEDM clinical pilot study of 120 women who were recalled from screening with unresolved findings after mammography and ultrasound [4]. The shape, margin appearance and extent of the enhancing regions were analyzed.

Typically discs or spheres are used as physics test objects for CEDM [5]. These simplified lesions may not represent the characteristics of real enhancing lesions such as the margin appearance, and consequently may not assess the frequency content important for diagnostic detection and discrimination tasks. Thus, the clinical characteristics of enhancing lesions on CEDM evaluated in this work as used to design a physical phantom with corresponding simulated lesions. We present a novel description of a CEDM morphology phantom with iodinated features, and perform preliminary detection sensitivity testing of these inserts under clinical imaging conditions.

2   Methods

2.1   CEDM Lesion Morphology

In the original clinical study [4], eight separate categories were used to classify the morphology of enhancing lesions. These categories included focus < 5 mm, focal mass, focal zone, regional, multiple regional, linear, ductal or segmental, and diffuse. In the present work these categories were pared down to three main types to be more consistent with those defined in the MRI BI-RADS lexicon and based on experience from the clinical study [6]. Some of the previous categories were combined to update the CEDM morphology lexicon as: 1) focal mass (focus < 5 mm, focal mass, focal zone); 2) regional (regional, multiple regional, and diffuse) and; 3) ductal or segmental (linear, and ductal or segmental). The numbers of malignant and benign lesions in each category were determined to get an indication of the morphology type prevalence, and their positive predictive values (PPV) in this diagnostic population.

The margin appearance and lesion maximum extent were evaluated by Dr. Dromain in the original study, with the margins classified as smooth, irregular and spiculated. The frequency of margin appearance and lesion extent for each enhancing lesion type were studied here to refine the enhancement morphology characteristics.

2.2   Phantom

Using a series of simplified shapes, phantoms with iodinated features at realistic concentration were developed to represent enhancing CEDM lesion morphologies. The margin characteristics, internal enhancement, and lesion sizes were designed to be consistent with those observed in the clinic and to present a representative visual test.

For this first-generation morphology phantom, two margin types, smooth and spiculated, and two types of internal enhancement, homogeneous and rim, were selected for phantom testing. Rim enhancement refers to the appearance of enhancing lesions when a highly vascularized region surrounds a necrotic core, which was not reported in the Dromain *et al.* dataset, but is commonly seen on breast MRI [7], and has been previously reported in CEDM [8]. Based on the observed margin types and their maximum extents, lesion diameters of 5 and 10 mm were specified for the outer diameters of central masses in each of smooth and rim morphologies. Rim thicknesses of about 1 to 2 mm are expected from breast MRI and histology observations. This was simulated by creating a shell of iodinated material of 2 mm thickness around a central core without iodine. Finally, a linear enhancement morphology was designed to represent ducts with 1, 2 and 3 mm diameters, with the smallest diameter also presenting a test for spicule identification. Schematics of the morphology designs are shown for one half of each phantom type in Fig. 1. In each case, two mirrored phantom sections, each 1 cm thick and with hemisphere or half-cylinder iodinated inserts, were stacked to compose a 2 cm thick phantom with three-dimensional (3D) features.

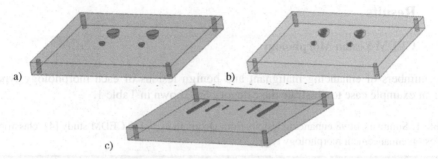

Fig. 1. CEDM morphology phantom schematics for: (a) smooth mass; (b) rim enhancement; and (c) ductal/segmental and spiculated. Morphologies (a) and (b) have 5 and 10 mm central masses, and (c) has 1, 2, and 3 mm diameter cylinders. Each schematic shows a 1 cm thick half of a two-part phantom, that together compose a 2 cm thick phantom with 3D features.

Iodinated features were created by hollowing out epoxy sections to form a mould into which uncured iodinated epoxy could be poured. The iodinated epoxy was made using a procedure previously developed to have good 3D uniformity and concentration accuracy [9]. Iodine concentrations of 1 and 2 mg/mL were used for the central masses, with cylinder concentrations selected to be 6 and 10 mg/mL, near a subjective detectability threshold determined for a 4 cm thick, 50% fibroglandular, 50% adipose breast. Attenuation measurements were made to verify iodine concentrations using iodinated samples cured in spectrophotometer cuvettes (cat.# 67.738, Sarstedt, Montreal QC, Canada). The samples were irradiated using a microfocus x-ray tube, and detection was performed using a CdTe spectrometer (Amptek, Bedford MA, USA), with corrections applied for K-fluorescence, charge trapping and pile-up [10, 11].

2.3   Detection Sensitivity

A feature detection sensitivity test was performed by imaging each morphology phantom stacked with 2, 4 and 6 cm poly(methyl methacrylate) (PMMA) to simulate a range of breast thicknesses and compositions. Images were acquired with a commercial DE CEDM system (Senobright® and Senographe® Essential, GE Healthcare,

Chalfont St. Giles, UK) using automatic exposure control (AEC)-selected technique factors. DE image decomposition was performed using an algorithm packaged with the system [12].

Lesion detection was quantified in terms of the signal-difference-to-noise ratio (SDNR) measured in DE decomposed CEDM phantom images. Regions of interest (ROI) for SDNR measurement were manually placed in a central region of the iodinated features to determine the average signal and an ROI in the adjacent surrounding background to determine the average background intensity. For consistency, the same signal and background ROI were used for each measurement of a particular morphology phantom combined with a given thickness of PMMA. Noise was defined as the standard deviation of the image pixel intensities within background ROI.

3   Results

3.1   CEDM Lesion Morphology

The numbers of enhancing malignant and benign lesions of each morphology type, and an example case to illustrate the category are shown in Table 1.

Table 1. Summary of 98 enhancing lesions from Dromain *et al.* DE CEDM study [4], classified by lesion enhancement morphology type

Enhancement morphology (#)	Cancer	Benign	Example Lesion LE DE
Focus / focal mass (89)	65	24	
Regional (6)	3	3	
Ductal / segmental (3)	3	0	

Given that mass enhancement was the most commonly observed morphology type, there was a large enough sample to study the characteristics of these enhancing regions further. Margin appearance was identified based on 3 types: smooth, irregular, and spiculated. Fig. 2 shows frequency histograms of the enhancing mass lesion margin types and maximum extents. The average maximum extent of all enhancing masses was 15 ± 11 mm (range 4 to 65 mm), with similar size distributions between cancers and benign lesions.

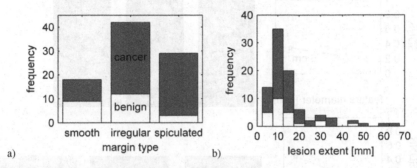

Fig. 2. Enhancing mass characteristics on DE CEDM by; (a) margin type; (b) and maximum extent for cancerous (shaded) and benign lesions

3.2   Phantom Evaluation

Example DE decomposed images of each phantom type and an example CEDM clinical case with corresponding enhancement morphology are shown in Fig. 3.

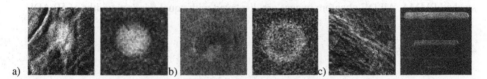

Fig. 3. (a) to (c) Examples of clinically observed lesions in CEDM images are on the left and a DE CEDM image of the corresponding phantom is on the right for: (a) smooth mass; (b) rim (single-energy CEDM clinical image); and (c) ductal/segmental enhancement morphologies. All phantom images show a 2 cm thick phantom acquired with an AEC-selected technique.

The SDNR measured from DE decomposed phantom images versus the iodinated feature outer diameters are plotted for each combination of the 2 cm morphology phantoms, as imaged with 2, 4 or 6 cm blocks PMMA placed on top of the phantoms in Fig. 4(a), (e) and (i). To illustrate the relative change in the detectability of the morphology inserts that the SDNR values represent, the DE CEDM images of the inserts are also shown in Fig. 4 for each imaging condition. All example DE decomposed iodinated insert images are displayed at the same window width of 50 ADU and a constant level relative to the image background signal intensity.

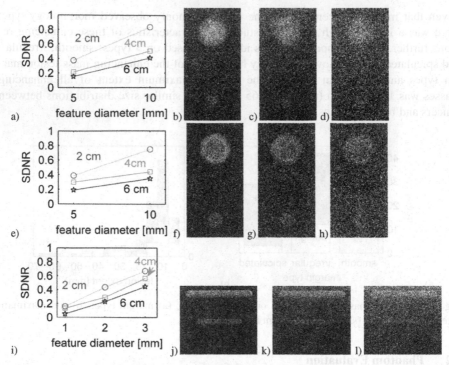

Fig. 4. (a) to (d) 1 mg/mL smooth mass; (e) to (h) 2 mg/mL rim; and (i) to (l) 10 mg/mL ductal/segmental and spiculated enhancement morphologies. The plots in (a), (e) and (i) show SDNR versus feature outer diameter with 2 (O), 4 (□), and 6 cm (★) PMMA stacked on the 2 cm phantom. Phantom images shown with 2 cm (b, f, j), 4 cm (c, g, k) and 6 cm (d, h, l) stacked PMMA. All DE phantom images are displayed with equal window widths of 50 ADU.

4   Discussion

In a review of 98 enhancing lesions in 120 clinical CEDM cases, 89 enhancing lesions (91%) were found to be of a mass-like morphology, with a PPV of 72% for malignancy. Most of these enhancing mass lesions had irregular (47%) or spiculated (33%) margins. Although mass-like lesions were most common in this study population, we recognize that the sample size is small, especially for benign lesions, and larger studies are needed to have adequate statistics to make strong conclusions about CEDM morphology frequency. Also, the clinical protocol and imaging techniques applied likely play important roles in determining the observed morphologies. For example, it is possible that the imaging system was not sensitive to enhancement from very small features such as spicules or ducts, and regions that may have otherwise expressed these types of enhancement morphologies may have been missed. Therefore, it is one of the goals of this study to develop a morphology phantom that can be used to study such system sensitivity to lesion morphology.

Using the results of the clinical morphology review as a guide for phantom design, we incorporated iodinated features to cover the typical lesion enhancement shapes. Towards testing system detectability limits for these morphologies, the feature sizes and iodine concentrations were carefully selected to present both an 'easy' test with an average clinically observed size and iodine concentration (e.g., 10 mm diameter and 2 mg/mL iodine), and a difficult test (e.g., 5 mm diameter and 1 mg/mL iodine).

The SDNR measurements demonstrated that quantitative analysis of the morphology features can be useful to guide morphology-based detection limits. For example, the DE images in Fig. 4(j) to (l) illustrate that the cylinder conspicuity correlates with SDNR plotted in Fig. 4(i), with a subjective detection cutoff of about 0.3. It is encouraging that this same SDNR detectability threshold of about 0.3 appears to also apply to the smooth mass and rim enhancement morphologies since this threshold should be independent of the lesion characteristics. However, although the absolute values of the SDNR are roughly equivalent between the different morphologies presented in Fig. 4, each of the morphology phantoms analyzed has a different iodine concentration. While it is reasonable that a tumour with a large amount of angiogenesis around its rim could have a higher iodine concentration within the rim (i.e., 2 mg/mL) than that throughout a comparable solid smooth mass (i.e., 1 mg/mL), a very high iodine concentration of 10 mg/mL is required for similar detection of the small linear features. Such a high iodine concentration may not be physiological, and suggests that the CEDM system is likely limited for the visualization of the ductal/segmental and spiculated morphologies. This finding may at least partly explain the low number of lesions with ductal/segmental enhancement in Table 1. One hypothesis to explain the comparatively high numbers of enhancing masses with spiculations is that the conventional mammogram, read in combination with the CEDM, influenced the radiologist's interpretation of the margin appearance on CEDM. It is also possible that spicules appeared to be visible on CEDM due to motion artifact in the images.

5   Conclusions

A review of a DE CEDM clinical study with 98 enhancing lesions over 120 cases was carried out to characterize the morphology of these enhancing lesions. Common lesion shapes, margins and extents of enhancement were identified. These features were used to guide the design of a morphology phantom that can be used to test system detection limits of these enhancement morphologies. This type of sensitivity testing can be used to improve system performance and guide radiologist morphology interpretation through an understanding of the system limitations.

Apart from the assessments of lesion detectability considered here, these phantoms could be used to test classification and discrimination tasks for a comprehensive CEDM performance evaluation. Also, their 3D nature allows for a comparison with CE breast tomosynthesis/CT. In future work we suggest the use of a metric that accounts for lesion spatial frequency content in a comprehensive manner, such as a detectability index, where the margin appearance has greater importance than in SDNR. The iodinated features could also be revised to test different tasks such as diameter discrimination, with linear features of the same length at different diameters, rather than discrimination between identical shapes at difference scales. In addition, a human reader study is important to calibrate detectability limits.

Acknowledgements. The authors wish to thank Jacqueline Craig, David Green, Gordon Mawdsley, and Mayan Murray for their assistance with this project.

References

1. Fallenberg, E.M., Dromain, C., Diekmann, F., Engelken, F., Krohn, M., Singh, J.M., Ingold-Heppner, B., Winzer, K.J., Bick, U., Renz, D.M.: Contrast-enhanced spectral mammography versus MRI: Initial results in the detection of breast cancer and assessment of tumour size. Eur. Radiol. (2013)
2. Jochelson, M.S., Dershaw, D.D., Sung, J.S., Heerdt, A.S., Thornton, C., Moskowitz, C.S., Ferrara, J., Morris, E.A.: Bilateral Contrast-enhanced Dual-Energy Digital Mammography: Feasibility and Comparison with Conventional Digital Mammography and MR Imaging in Women with Known Breast Carcinoma. Radiology 266, 743–751 (2013)
3. Lewin, J.M., Isaacs, P.K., Vance, V., Larke, F.J.: Dual-energy contrast-enhanced digital subtraction mammography: feasibility. Radiology 229, 261–268 (2003)
4. Dromain, C., Thibault, F., Muller, S., Rimareix, F., Delaloge, S., Tardivon, A., Balleyguier, C.: Dual-energy contrast-enhanced digital mammography: initial clinical results. Eur. Radiol. 21, 565–574 (2011)
5. Leithner, R., Knogler, T., Homolka, P.: Development and production of a prototype iodine contrast phantom for CEDEM. Phys. Med. Biol. 35, N25–N35 (2013)
6. Liberman, L., Morris, E.A., Lee, M.J.-Y., Kaplan, J.B., LaTrenta, L.R., Menell, J.H., Abramson, A.F., Dashnaw, S.M., Ballon, D.J., Dershaw, D.D.: Breast lesions detected on MR imaging: features and positive predictive value. Am. J. Roentgenol. 179, 171–178 (2002)
7. Macura, K.J., Ouwerkerk, R., Jacobs, M.A., Bluemke, D.A.: Patterns of enhancement on breast MR images: interpretation and imaging pitfalls. Radiographics 26, 1719–1734 (2006)
8. Jong, R.A., Yaffe, M.J., Skarpathiotakis, M., Shumak, R.S., Danjoux, N.M., Gunesekara, A.: Contrast-enhanced digital mammography: initial clinical experience. Radiology 228, 842–850 (2003)
9. Hill, M.L., Mainprize, J.G., Mawdsley, G.E., Yaffe, M.J.: A solid iodinated phantom material for use in tomographic x-ray imaging. Med. Phys. 36, 4409–4420 (2009)
10. Mainprize, J.G., Hunt, D.C., Yaffe, M.J.: Direct conversion detectors: The effect of incomplete charge collection on detective quantum efficiency. Med. Phys. 29, 976 (2002)
11. Miyajima, S., Imagawa, K., Matsumoto, M.: CdZnTe detector in diagnostic x-ray spectroscopy. Med. Phys. 29, 1421 (2002)
12. Puong, S., Bouchevreau, X., Patoureaux, F., Iordache, R., Muller, S.: Dual-energy contrast enhanced digital mammography using a new approach for breast tissue canceling. In: Proc. SPIE. vol. 6510, 65102H (2007)

Stability of Volumetric Tissue Composition Measured in Serial Screening Mammograms

Katharina Holland[1], Michiel Kallenberg[2], Ritse Mann[1],
Carla van Gils[3], and Nico Karssemeijer[1]

[1] Radboud university medical center, PO Box 9101, 6500 HB Nijmegen,
The Netherlands
[2] Matakina Technology, 86 Victoria Street, Wellington 6011, New Zealand
[3] University Medical Center Utrecht, PO Box 85500, 3508 GA Utrecht,
The Netherlands

Abstract. The purpose of this study is to investigate the categorization and variation of serial mammogram pairs in dense and non-dense classes. When introducing density based stratified screening, the differences in density between screening rounds should be as small as possible to prevent women and clinicians losing confidence in the stratification scheme. A total of 8843 mammogram pairs (current and prior, mean screening interval 22.65 months) were categorized in dense and non-dense cases based on percent density and volume of glandular tissue. The reproducibility of the categories (prior to current) was tested with simple kappa statistics and the causes for a category change were investigated.

When comparing two examinations, the majority of pairs remained in the same category, with $\kappa= 0.783$ and $\kappa = 0.696$ based on percent density and glandular tissue volume respectively. For most women, glandular tissue volume and percent density decreases with age. However in 3.2% (4.6%) of the pairs an examination was classified as non-dense followed by dense based on percent density (glandular tissue volume). Natural circumstances can lead to a change in category, for example glandular tissue volume decreases with age, or increases with the use of HRT. However a higher reproducibility in categorization in dense and not-dense classes based on automatic breast density calculations was found, than reported in the literature based on visual assessment. The reproducibility was higher when using percent density for classification.

Keywords: Digital mammography, volumetric breast density, temporal change.

1 Introduction

An association between breast density and breast cancer risk is well established[1,2]. Several studies show that the risk of developing breast cancer is 1.8-6.0 times higher for women with dense breasts than for women in the lowest density category[4,5]. The most common breast density reporting method

H. Fujita, T. Hara, and C. Muramatsu (Eds.): IWDM 2014, LNCS 8539, pp. 239–244, 2014.
© Springer International Publishing Switzerland 2014

uses the four density categories of the Breast Imaging Reporting and Data System (BI-RADS)[6]: (1) almost entirely fat (2) scattered fibroglandular densities (3) heterogeneously dense and (4) extremely dense.

Several clinics offer women with dense breasts, which is BI-RADS category 3+4, additional screening with (automatic 3D) ultrasound. It is important to have a consistent, objective and reproducible measurement of breast density to determine an unambiguous classification and to maintain the confidence of the women and clinicians in the stratification process. The BI-RADS categories are not suited for this, as several studies show a high inter and intra reader variability[7]. The temporal aspect of classification is important, as it may make women insecure if additional screening is offered in an irregular pattern.

To objectively investigate the variations we calculated percent density: glandular tissue volume over breast volume. Each examination was categorized into dense or non-dense classes based on glandular tissue volume or percent density.

2   Material

Screening mammograms from the Dutch Breast Cancer Screening Program, Bevolkingsonderzoek Midden-West were used. The full field digital mammograms (FFDM) with a pixel size of 70 μm were acquired on a Hologic Selenia system for the period 2006-2008. All women with two digital examinations and available Volpara score (VolparaAlgorithm 1.5b, Matakina) were included. For mammograms with breasts implants or if the breast did not fit on the detector, no Volpara score was available. This resulted in 8844 mammogram pairs. Women in the Netherlands aged 50-75 receive a biennial invitation for breast cancer screening, the average screening interval in our case sample is 22.65 $\pm$ 1.89 months. After the introduction of the first FFDM system at the screening center in 2003, women who came for their first screening were given a higher priority for digital screening than older women. Women who started with digital screening continued with FFDM, so no film mammograms are available for them, thus more FFDM data is available for women aged 60 or under.

3   Methods

For all images, breast volume, volume of glandular tissue, and percent density were calculated with Volpara including tilt correction. Volpara averages results obtained for available images to come to a single score.

All examinations were categorized in dense and non-dense using the Volpara density grade (VDG). VDG is a four point scale analogous to the BI-RADS categories and based on percent density[8]. Studies with a VDG one and two classification were categorized as non-dense; studies with a VDG three and four as dense.

To find a threshold for the division into dense and non-dense classes using glandular tissue volume, we required that the percentage of studies categorized as dense was the same as for percent density.

Density assessment at both screenings was analyzed using simple kappa statistics. For women with a dense categorized current examination, while the previous one was categorized as non-dense, the change of breast and glandular tissue volume, and percent density was analyzed using box plots.

We performed subgroup analysis for different age groups, depending on age at prior screening. The groups were: age <55, 55-59, 60-64, 65-69, and age ≥70.

4   Results

The categorization of all studies into dense and non-dense classes based on percent density is presented in Table 1a. The second screening is represented by the columns, the previous study is given per row. Most women have two studies categorized as non-dense (57.8%). Both examinations are labeled as dense in 32.1% of the pairs. The kappa value is 0.783 (0.679-0.796 95% CI). The well-known decrease in density is visible, the percentage of pairs with two dense examinations decreases with age.

Table 1b shows the categorization into dense and non-dense classes based on glandular tissue volume. For most age groups, the percentage of pairs with both examination in the same category is less than compared with the categorization based on percent density, a kappa of 0.696 (0.680-0.712 95% CI) was calculated. The number of pairs with one dense and one non-dense examination increased compared with percent density.

Fig. 1 compares the subgroup 'non-dense → dense' to all pairs. The difference in breast and glandular tissue volume, and percent density is given as percentage of the prior screening, eg (V2-V1)/V1 with V1 and V2 the breast volume at the prior and current screening respectively. On average, breast volume did not change between two screenings. The glandular tissue volume decrease with subsequent screening causes a decrease in percent density. Using percent density, it can be observed that a density increase can be caused by an increase of glandular tissue volume and a decrease of the measured breast volume. When using glandular tissue volume to classify in dense and non-dense classes, women showed an increase in both breast and glandular tissue volume.

5   Conclusion and Discussion

In this study, we demonstrated a high reproducibility of breast classification in dense and non-dense classes in two serial examinations. 89.7% of the mammogram pairs remained in the same category. In 3.2% of the pairs, a percent density increase led to a change from the non-dense to dense category. When using glandular tissue volume to classify in dense and non-dense classes, less pairs had the same category: 4.6% of the pairs have a non-dense prior and a current dense mammogram. On average, the breast volume and glandular tissue volume increased in these pairs. This might be caused by inaccuracy of the breast thickness measurement reported in the dicom header of the images, a property used by Volpara. As the breast thickness inaccuracy effects the breast and the glandular tissue volume in the same way, the effect is less strong on percent density.

We compared our results to visual density grading by radiologists using results by Spayne[9]. In the study, 34 radiologists interpreted between 119 and 1033 film mammogram pairs in a total of 11755 women. The screening interval of these pairs was between 3 and 24 month. When summarizing the cases with BIRADS 1 and 2, and 3 and 4 to non-dense and dense categories respectively, 7.1% of the pairs have a prior categorized as non-dense with a dense current. A higher reproducibility is observed using an automatic breast density estimate than with using visual assessment by an radiologist.

Volpara provides us with a 4 point density scale, while in this paper a binary classification is used for the analysis. This indicates a loss of information. However for breast density stratified screening or additional screening with ultrasound, a binary categorization in dense and non-dense classes is necessary as the advice is either positive or negative for an additional examination. Here we suppose that breast density itself is the basis for the stratification and we investigated the temporal consistency. Though a change in density could be used as additional factor in the stratification process. Then the 4 point scale or percent breast density should be used instead of the binary classification.

Table 1. Number of pairs (%) categorized in non-dense and dense for the different age groups. The second column gives the number of current non-dense examinations, the third column the current dense examinations. The categories are percent density (a) or glandular tissue volume (b) based.

| | | (a) current | | | (b) current | |
age		non-dense	dense		non-dense	dense
all pairs	non-dense	5109 (57.8)	280 (3.2)	non-dense	4928 (55.7)	408 (4.6)
	dense	618 (7.0)	2836 (32.1)	dense	851 (9.6)	2656 (30.0)
< 55	non-dense	1781 (46.0)	100 (2.6)	non-dense	1953 (50.5)	180 (4.7)
	dense	308 (8.0)	1680 (43.4)	dense	391 (10.1)	1345 (34.8)
55 – 59	non-dense	1280 (59.4)	65 (3.0)	non-dense	1200 (55.7)	108 (5.0)
	dense	167 (7.7)	643 (29.8)	dense	203 (9.4)	644 (29.9)
60 – 64	non-dense	890 (67.3)	65 (4.9)	non-dense	782 (59.1)	58 (4.3)
	dense	75 (5.7)	293 (22.1)	dense	115 (8.7)	368 (27.8)
65 – 69	non-dense	823 (76.1)	33 (3.0)	non-dense	694 (64.1)	44 (4.1)
	dense	50 (4.6)	176 (16.3)	dense	107 (9.9)	237 (21.9)
≥ 70	non-dense	335 (80.9)	17 (4.1)	non-dense	299 (72.2)	18 (4.3)
	dense	18 (4.3)	44 (10.6)	dense	35 (8.5)	62 (15.0)

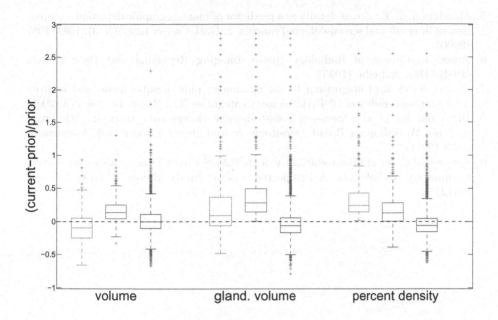

Fig. 1. Change in breast and glandular tissue volume, and percent density as percentage of the quantity at the prior screening, for the subset where the category changed from non-dense to dense based on percent density (left/red) and glandular tissue volume (middle/blue), and the full data set (right/black).

Acknowledgements. The research leading to these results has received funding from the European Union's Seventh Framework Programme FP7 under grant agreement no 306088.

Special thanks to Bevolkingsonderzoek Midden-West for providing the images and Ralph Highnam at Volpara for providing access to the Volpara Software.

References

1. Wolfe, L.N.: Risk for breast cancer development determined by mammographic parenchymal pattern. Cancer 37, 2486–2492 (1976)
2. van Gils, C.H., et al.: Changes in mammographic breast density and concomitant changes in breast cancer risk. Eur. J. Cancer Prev. 8(6), 509–515 (1999)
3. McCormack, V.A., et al.: Breast density and parenchymal patterns as markers of breast cancer risk: A meta-analysis. Cancer Epidemiol. Biomarkers Prev. 15, 1159 (2006)
4. Boyd, N.F.: Quantitative classification of mammographic densities and breast cancer risk: results from the Canadian National Breast Screening Study. J. Natl. Cancer Inst. 87(9), 670–675 (1995)

5. Mandelson, M.T.: Breast density as a predictor of mammographic detection: comparison of interval- and screen-detected cancers. J. Natl. Cancer Inst. 92(13), 1081–1087 (2000)
6. American College of Radiology Breast Imaging Reporting and Data System (BI-RADS), 2nd edn. (1995)
7. Ciatto, S., et al.: Categorising breast mammographic density: intra- and interobserver reproducibility of BI-RADS density categories. The Breast 14, 269–275 (2005)
8. Highnam, R., et al.: Assessing breast density change over time. In: 5th International Workshop on Breast Densitometry and Breast Cancer Risk Assessment, p. 38 (2011)
9. Spayne, M.C., et al.: Reproducibility of BI-RADS Breast Density Measures Among Community Radiologists: A Prospective Cohort Study. Breast J. 18(4), 326–333 (2012)

Breast Density Classification Based on Volumetric Glandularity Measured by Spectral Mammography

Henrik Johansson, Miriam von Tiedemann, and Björn Cederström

Philips Women's Healthcare,
Smidesvägen 5, 171 41 Solna, Sweden
henrik.johansson@philips.com

Abstract. Observations of significant variability in radiologists' classification of breast density signals the need for objective classification methods. In this study, we develop a model for a radiologist's BI-RADS classification based on the volumetric glandularity image measured by spectral mammography and a reader study where ten MQSA certified radiologists assigned BI-RADS scores to 300 screening cases. Several combinations of features such as area glandularity based on a certain volumetric glandularity threshold, breast thickness and the spread of glandular tissue were tested as linear classifier parameters. Logistic regression was used to optimize the parameters and cross-validation to assess the agreement with the radiologists' majority vote, regarded as truth. We show a clear indication that the automatic classification algorithm performs on par with or better than the average individual radiologist.

Keywords: breast density, spectral imaging, glandularity, classification.

1 Introduction

It is well established that breast density, i.e. the amount of fibroglandular tissue in the breast, is directly correlated to the risk of developing breast cancer [1,2], and to the diagnostic accuracy of mammography [3,4]. Quantifying breast density shows great promise in clinical decision support, e.g. in individualizing screening programs. The most common way of quantifying breast density is by subjective assessment by a radiologist according to the ACR BI-RADS breast composition categories [5]. However, a significant observer variability has been seen, indicating uncertain reproducibility [6,7].

In this study, we aim to develop an objective model of a radiologist's BI-RADS classification, using spectral breast density measurement on a commercially available photon counting mammography system [8], extraction of features from a volumetric glandularity image and a linear classifier. The model is based on the results of a reader study where ten MQSA certified radiologists assigned BI-RADS scores to 300 screening cases.

H. Fujita, T. Hara, and C. Muramatsu (Eds.): IWDM 2014, LNCS 8539, pp. 245–250, 2014.

2 Materials and Methods

2.1 Measuring Volumetric Glandularity

For the spectral mammography system, detected photons are binned according to their energy, into a low energy and a high energy bin. Obtaining the volumetric density from spectral x-ray projection data corresponds approximately to solving the following equation:

$$I_{\text{bin}} = \int_{E_1}^{E_2} \nu(E)S_0(E)\exp[-\mu_{\text{tissue}}(E,g) \times t_{\text{breast}}]dE, \tag{1}$$

where I_{bin} is the photon count in the energy bin defined by the threshold energies E_1 and E_2, ν is the quantum efficiency, S_0 is the incident spectral density, and t_{breast} is the thickness of the traversed breast tissue of glandularity g.

For most natural body constituents at mammographic x-ray energies, x-ray attenuation is dominated by only two interaction effects: photoelectric absorption and scattering processes. The x-ray attenuation depends on density and atomic number, resulting in a unique attenuation energy dependence per material. This makes it possible to represent the attenuation of one material with a linear combination of any two reference materials according to:

$$\mu_{\text{tissue}}(E) \times t_{\text{breast}} = t_1\mu_1(E) + t_2\mu_2(E). \tag{2}$$

By inserting Eq. 2 into Eq. 1, and given the known attenuations of the reference materials (μ_1, μ_2), and given that we know the incident flux, we can solve the system of equations for t_1 and t_2. Suitable reference materials for breast density measurement are adipose and fibroglandular tissue.

2.2 Clinical Data and BI-RADS Classification

A reader study was performed where ten MQSA certified radiologists assigned BI-RADS breast composition scores to 300 screening cases. A number of conditions had to be fulfilled for spectral breast density measurements to be performed, including a compression height between 20 and 110 mm and requirements on the mammography system configuration and validity of calibration data. The conditions were met by 289 of the 300 examinations.

We define a "true" BI-RADS score for a case as the majority vote, which was calculated as the mode (the most frequent value) of the radiologists' scores. As figure of merit we use fraction of agreement, f_a, i.e. the fraction of cases where the majority vote equals the individual score. To assess the performance of individual radiologists, the majority vote was calculated without the contribution from the individual radiologist to avoid bias. The mean f_a between the radiologists was 0.75 ± 0.03 (1 SD).

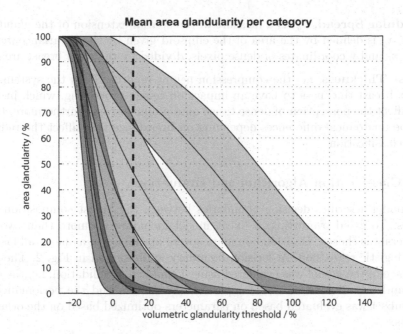

Fig. 1. Area glandularity as a function of glandularity threshold for different BI-RADS categories. The dashed line indicates a threshold optimal for a one-parameter model based solely on area glandularity.

2.3   Indicators of BI-RADS Classification

With this study we aim to develop a few-parameter model of a radiologist's BI-RADS classification. From the ACR definition of the BI-RADS breast composition categories we expect the classification to correlate to the relative amount and spatial structure of dense tissue as observed on a mammogram. The spectral breast density measurement results in images with pixel values of volumetric breast glandularity and breast thickness, from which further parameters can be derived. The following parameters were investigated in this study.

Volumetric Glandularity, g_v, is a measure of the relative amount of dense tissue in terms of volume.

Area Glandularity, g_a, is a measure of the relative amount of dense tissue in terms of area. Based on a volumetric glandularity threshold, pixels are classified as dense or non-dense. g_a is then defined as the ratio of dense area to total breast area. From a previous investigation we know that a glandularity threshold of 11% is close to optimal for a one-parameter model based solely on area glandularity. Here, we have also found optimal glandularity thresholds for a two-parameter model based solely on area glandularity, resulting in threshold values of 2% and 33%. Fig. 1 shows area glandularity as a function of glandularity threshold for different BI-RADS categories. The observed optimum was quite broad and threshold values in the range 0 – 5% and 30 – 36% yielded similar performance.

Glandular Spread, σ_g, is a measure of the spatial extension of the glandular tissue. σ_g is defined by the area of the ellipsoid given by the covariance matrix of the x- and y-coordinates of dense pixels, divided by the total breast area.

Breast Thickness, i.e. the compression height reported from the system. We expect breast thickness to have an impact on image processing, which in turn may affect the perception of dense tissue on a mammogram. Furthermore, there may be anatomical differences depending on breast size that affect the radiologist's classification.

2.4 Classification Algorithm and Evaluation

The model describes decision boundaries between the breast composition categories. To avoid overfitting, a linear model including no more than two parameters was chosen. Decision boundaries were optimized in a one-vs-all fashion using logistic regression. A decision boundary is illustrated in Fig. 2. The performance of the model was evaluated using 12-fold cross validation, i.e. the data was randomly divided into 12 complementary subsets and the perfomance on each subset was evaluated based on parameters optimized based on the other 11 subsets.

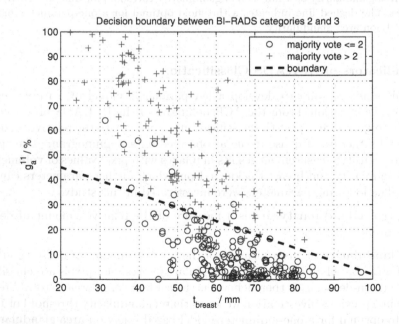

Fig. 2. Decision boundary between BI-RADS categories 2 and 3, based on area glandularity and breast thickness. Here, optimization was performed on the full dataset for illustrative purposes.

3   Results

The outcome from the cross-validation for four different parameter sets is shown in Fig. 3. We omitted the combination of volumetric glandularity and area glandulatity, as this only marginally improved the performance compared to area glandularity alone. The uncertainty of the expectation value of f_a is computed as the standard deviation of the subset results divided by the square root of the number of subsets, and a $\pm 1\sigma$ confidence interval is given, as well as indicated by the shadowed regions in the graphs.

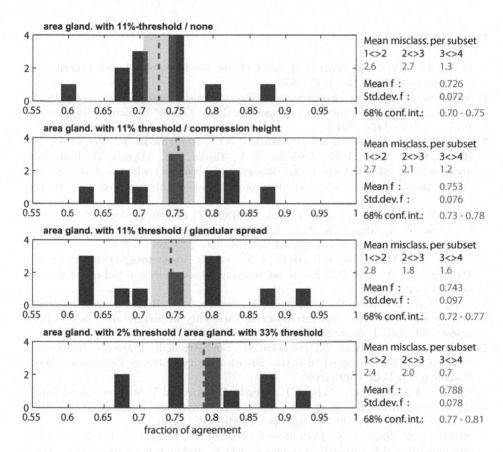

Fig. 3. Cross-validation results for the four sets of classification parameters. The 68% confidence interval on the estimated fraction of agreement is indicated by the shaded area.

4   Conclusions

Based on a dataset with 289 screening cases scored by ten MQSA certified radiologists, we have evaluated the performance of four one- or two-parameter models describing a radiologist's BI-RADS classification. Evaluating more complex models would require a larger dataset. The parameter area glandularity is shown to be a particularly good indicator, and performance is improved further by inclusion of an additional parameter. The best result is obtained by using two area glandularity parameters with different thresholds, for which the fraction of agreement was 77–81%. This is higher than reported for a method based on volumetric glandularity assessed by non-spectral means [9]. There is a clear indication that the performance of the investigated automatic classification method is better than the mean performance of individual radiologists.

References

1. Wolfe, J.N.: Breast patterns as an index of risk for developing breast cancer. Am. J. Roentgenol. 126, 1130–1137 (1976)
2. McCormack, V.A., dos Santos Silva, I.: Breast density and parenchymal patterns as markers of breast cancer risk: a meta-analysis. Cancer Epidemiol. Biomarkers Prev. 15, 1159–1169 (2006)
3. Carney, P.A., Miglioretti, D.L., Yankaskas, B.C., Kerlikowske, K., Rosenberg, R., Rutter, C.M., Geller, B.M., Abraham, L.A., Taplin, S.H., Dignan, M.: Individual and combined effects of age, breast density, and hormone replacement therapy use on the accuracy of screening mammography. Annals of Internal Medicine 138, 168 (2003)
4. Boyd, N.F., Guo, H., Martin, L.J., Sun, L., Stone, J., Fishell, E., Jong, R.A., Hislop, G., Chiarelli, A., Minkin, S., Yaffe, M.J.: Mammographic density and the risk and detection of breast cancer. New Engl. J. Med. 356, 227–236 (2007)
5. D'Orsi, C.J., Mendelson, E.B., Ikeda, D.M., et al.: Breast Imaging Reporting and Data System: ACR BI-RADS - Breast Imaging Atlas. American College of Radiology, Reston (2003)
6. Berg, W.A., Campassi, C., Langenberg, P., Sexton, M.J.: Breast imaging reporting and data system: inter- and intraobserver variability in feature analysis and final assessment. Am. J. Roentgenol. 174, 1769–1777 (2000)
7. Nicholson, B.T., LoRusso, A.P., Smolkin, M., Bovbjerg, V.E., Petroni, G.R., Harvey, J.A.: Accuracy of Assigned BI-RADS Breast Density Category Definitions. Acad. Radiology 13, 1143–1149 (2006)
8. Gooßen, A., Heese, H.S., Erhard, K., Norell, B.: Spectral Volumetric Glandularity Assessment. In: Maidment, A.D.A., Bakic, P.R., Gavenonis, S. (eds.) IWDM 2012. LNCS, vol. 7361, pp. 529–536. Springer, Heidelberg (2012)
9. Highnam, R., Sauber, N., Destounis, S., Harvey, J., McDonald, D.: Breast Density into Clinical Practice. In: Maidment, A.D.A., Bakic, P.R., Gavenonis, S. (eds.) IWDM 2012. LNCS, vol. 7361, pp. 466–473. Springer, Heidelberg (2012)

Is Volumetric Breast Density Related to Body Mass Index, Body Fat Mass, Waist-Hip Ratio, Age and Ethnicity for Malaysian Women?

Norhasnah Zakariyah[1], Kwan-Hoong Ng[1], Susie Lau[1], Kartini Rahmat[1],
Farhana Fadzli[1], and Nur Aishah Mohd Taib[2]

[1] Department of Biomedical Imaging and University of Malaya Research Imaging Centre,
Faculty of Medicine, University of Malaya, Kuala Lumpur, Malaysia
[2] Department of Surgery, Faculty of Medicine, University of Malaya, Kuala Lumpur, Malaysia
ngkh@um.edu.my

Abstract. Previous studies have shown that breast cancer has been linked to breast density as well as obesity. We aim to investigate the relationships between body mass index (BMI), body fat mass (BFM), waist-hip ratio (WHR), age and ethnicity with volumetric breast density (VBD) among Malaysian women. In this context, VBD is defined as the ratio of fibroglandular tissue volume to total breast volume. We collected anthropomorphic and body composition data for 2457 subjects undergoing mammographic examination at the University of Malaya Medical Centre, Kuala Lumpur. The data included weight, height, BMI and BFM which were measured with a body composition analyzer. We also measured waist and hip circumferences for 500 of these subjects. A VBD assessment system (Volpara) was used to analyze mammograms. Our results showed that VBD is not significantly correlated with BMI ($r^2 = 0.17$), BFM ($r^2 = 0.19$), WHR ($r^2 = 0.11$). We also noted that VBD is highest among Malaysian women below 40 years old. VBD is highest for Chinese (mean = 11.3%), followed by Malay (mean = 10.1%) and Indian (mean = 9.4%). In conclusion, VBD is dependent on age and ethnicity (ANOVA, $p<0.05$) but not on BMI, BFM and WHR.

Keywords: Body fat mass, body mass index, breast cancer, volumetric breast density, mammography, obesity, waist-hip ratio.

1 Introduction

Previous studies have shown that breast cancer has been linked to obesity [1,2] and also to breast density [3,4,5]. Researchers had reported that there is an inverse relationship between obesity and breast cancer for premenopausal women. However, they stated that there is an increased risk of developing postmenopausal breast cancer among obese women [6]. Two studies on breast density among the three major ethnic groups in Malaysia (Chinese, Malay and Indian) had been published [7,8]. In this study, we investigated the relationships between body mass index (BMI), body fat mass (BFM), waist-hip ratio (WHR), age and ethnicity with volumetric breast density (VBD).

H. Fujita, T. Hara, and C. Muramatsu (Eds.): IWDM 2014, LNCS 8539, pp. 251–256, 2014.
© Springer International Publishing Switzerland 2014

2   Methodology

2.1   Subjects

There were 2457 subjects involved in this study. They comprised of women who underwent mammographic examinations at the University of Malaya Medical Centre (UMMC), Kuala Lumpur, either for first time or subsequent examinations.

2.2   Data Collection

Height, weight, BMI and BFM from these subjects were collected using a body composition analyzer (Tanita Corporation, Japan). The waist and hip circumferences to derive WHR were also measured for 500 of these subjects.

2.3   Image Processing

Raw mammographic images were acquired from two clinical mammography systems (GE Essential and Siemens Novation) installed at the UMMC. The images were then analyzed using a VBD assessment system (Volpara 1.4.3, Matakina Technology, New Zealand) to obtain VBD values for all the subjects who underwent mammographic examinations. The VBD estimated by Volpara is expressed as the ratio of volume of fibroglandular tissue in the breast to the total volume of the breast, in percentage (%) [9].

2.4   Volumetric Breast Density Measurement

Volpara, the VBD assessment system, is based on a "relative physics" model given by the equation below [9,10,11].

$$h_d(x, y) = \frac{\ln\left(P(x, y)/P_{fat}\right)}{\mu_{fat} - \mu_{dense}}$$

An area of the breast that corresponds to an entirely fatty tissue is set as a reference level (P_{fat}) to compute the thickness of the dense tissue (h_d) at each pixel (x,y). The pixel value (P) is assumed to be linearly related to the energy imparted to the x-ray detector. μ_{fat} and μ_{dense} are the effective x-ray linear attenuation coefficients for fatty and dense tissues respectively. The volume of dense tissue is computed by integrating $h_d(x,y)$ over the entire digital mammographic image, whereas the volume of the breast is the product of the area of the breast and the compressed breast thickness. The VBD is the ratio of volume of the dense tissue to volume of the breast [9,10,11].

2.5   Data Analysis

All the data collected were analyzed using a statistical package (SPSS V16.0). Univariate analysis was used to investigate the relationships between BMI, BFM, WHR, age and ethnicity with VBD.

3   Results and Discussion

Table 1. Demographic, anthropomorphic and body composition data for the three ethnic groups studied. The values are presented as (mean ± s.d.)

		Chinese (n = 1247)		Malay (n = 652)		Indian (n = 558)
Age (year)		58 ± 9.2		53 ± 9.0		56 ± 9.6
Body Fat Mass (kg)		20.4 ± 7.6		26.4 ± 9.3		26.9 ± 9.2
VBD (%)		11.3 ± 5.7		10.1 ± 5.2		9.4 ± 4.8
BMI (kg/m²)						
Underweight (< 18.5)	(n = 84)	17.3 ± 0.9	(n = 13)	17.3 ± 1.0	(n = 14)	17.2 ± 1.2
Normal (18.5 - 24.9)	(n = 738)	22.0 ± 1.7	(n = 204)	22.6 ± 1.7	(n = 185)	22.8 ± 1.6
Overweight (25.0 - 29.9)	(n = 331)	26.9 ± 1.3	(n = 270)	27.3 ± 1.4	(n = 238)	27.3 ± 1.4
Obese (≥ 30)	(n = 94)	32.6 ± 2.7	(n = 165)	33.6 ± 3.4	(n = 121)	34.0 ± 3.4

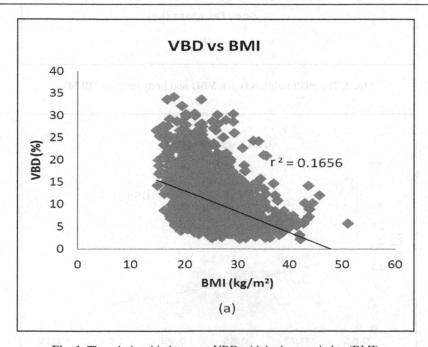

Fig. 1. The relationship between VBD with body mass index (BMI)

Table 1 summarizes the measured data for the subjects involved in this study. They consist of women from three ethnic groups, namely Chinese (50.8%), Malay (26.5%)

and Indian (22.7%). The mean age for these women is 58 ± 9.2 yrs. There are small differences in BMI between the three ethnic groups. Indian women have the highest BFM (26.9 kg) followed by Malay (26.4 kg) and Chinese (20.4 kg). For VBD, Chinese women have the densest breast (11.3%) followed by Malay (10.1%) and Indian (9.4%).

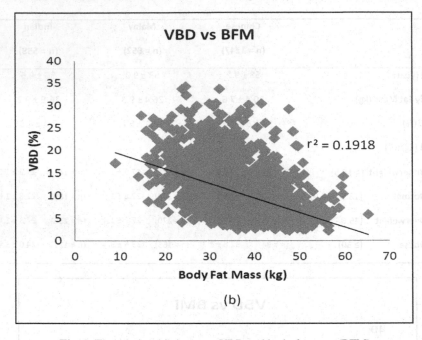

Fig. 2. The relationship between VBD and body fat mass (BFM)

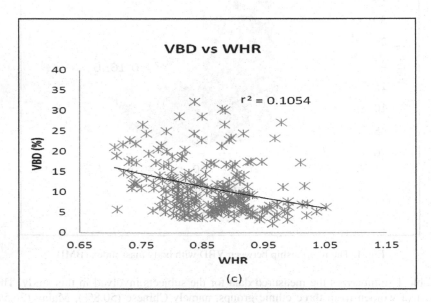

Fig. 3. The relationship between VBD with waist-hip ratio (WHR)

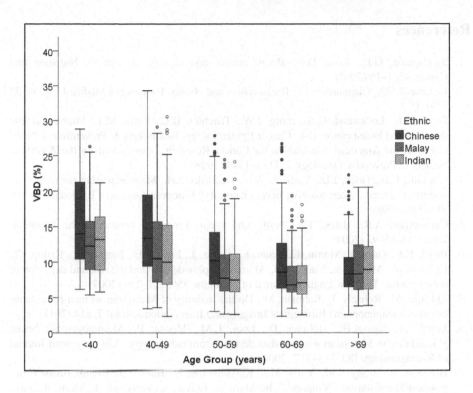

Fig. 4. Boxplot of VBD with respect to age group for Chinese, Malay and Indian

We observed that VBD is not correlated with BMI (Fig. 1), BFM (Fig. 2) and WHR (Fig. 3). Statistical analysis of data also showed that the VBD is not significantly related to BMI (r^2 = 0.17), BFM (r^2 = 0.19) and WHR (r^2 = 0.11). We noted that VBD decreases with age (Fig. 4). We also observed that VBD is highest for Chinese (mean VBD = 11.3%), followed by Malay (mean VBD = 10.1%) and Indian (mean VBD = 9.4%) in Malaysia. The current finding is in agreement with the studies by Zulfiqar *et al.* [7] and Jamal *et al.* [8] which reported that Chinese women have the highest breast density among the three ethnic groups.

In conclusion, there is no correlation between VBD with BMI, BFM and WHR on the Malaysian women whom we studied, nevertheless VBD is significantly dependent on age and ethnicity respectively (ANOVA, p<0.05 for both parameters). Further study using multivariate analysis would be able to elucidate further the complex relationships between VBD and anthropomorphic as well as body composition parameters.

Acknowledgments. This study was supported by the High Impact Research Grant, UM.C/625/1/HIR/MOHE/06, from the Ministry of Higher Education, Malaysia.

References

1. Stephenson, G.D., Rose, D.P.: Breast cancer and obesity: an update. Nutrition and Cancer 45, 1–16 (2003)
2. La Guardia, M., Giammanco, M.: Breast cancer and obesity. Panminerva Medica 43, 123–133 (2001)
3. Boyd, N.F., Lockwood, G.A., Byng, J.W., Tritchler, D.L., Yaffe, M.J.: Mammographic densities and breast cancer risk. Cancer Epidemiology, Biomarkers & Prevention: a Publication of the American Association for Cancer Research, cosponsored by the American Society of Preventive Oncology 7, 1133–1144 (1998)
4. van Gils, C.H., Otten, J.D., Verbeek, A.L., Hendriks, J.H.: Mammographic breast density and risk of breast cancer: masking bias or causality? European Journal of Epidemiology 14, 315–320 (1998)
5. Carmichael, A.R., Bates, T.: Obesity and breast cancer: a review of the literature. Breast 13, 85–92 (2004)
6. Boyd, N.F., Guo, H., Martin, L.J., Sun, L., Stone, J., Fishell, E., Jong, R.A., Hislop, G., Chiarelli, A., Minkin, S., Yaffe, M.J.: Mammographic density and the risk and detection of breast cancer. The New England Journal of Medicine 356, 227–236 (2007)
7. Zulfiqar, M., Rohazly, I., Rahmah, M.: Do the majority of Malaysian women have dense breasts on mammogram? Biomedical Imaging and Intervention Journal 7, e14 (2011)
8. Jamal, N., Ng, K.H., McLean, D., Looi, L.M., Moosa, F.: Mammographic breast glandularity in Malaysian women: data derived from radiography. AJR American Journal of Roentgenology 182, 713–717 (2004)
9. Highnam, R., Brady, S.M., Yaffe, M.J., Karssemeijer, N., Harvey, J.: Robust Breast Composition Measurement - Volpara™. In: Martí, J., Oliver, A., Freixenet, J., Martí, R. (eds.) IWDM 2010. LNCS, vol. 6136, pp. 342–349. Springer, Heidelberg (2010)
10. Highnam, R., Brady, M., Shepstone, B.: A representation for mammographic image processing. Medical Image Analysis 1, 1–18 (1996)
11. van Engeland, S., Snoeren, P.R., Huisman, H., Boetes, C., Karssemeijer, N.: Volumetric breast density estimation from full-field digital mammograms. IEEE Transactions on Medical Imaging 25, 273–282 (2006)

Automated Volumetric Breast Density Derived by Statistical Model Approach

Serghei Malkov[1], Amir Pasha Mahmoudzadeh[1], Karla Kerlikowske[2], and John Shepherd[1]

[1] Dept. of Radiology & Biomedical Imaging, Univ. of California at San Francisco
{Serghei.Malkov,AmirPasha.Mahmoudzadeh,John.Shepherd}@ucsf.edu
[2] Depts. of Medicine and Epidemiology and Biostatistics, Univ. of California at San Francisco
Karla.Kerlikowske@ucsf.edu

Abstract. Interest is growing in the developing automated breast density measures because of its strong association with breast cancer risk. Although a number of automated methods to quantify mammographic and volumetric density appeared, they still have issues with accuracy and reproducibility; there is demand for developing new accurate and automated breast density estimation techniques. The purpose of this paper is to design and to test a new approach for automatically quantifying true volumetric fibroglandular tissue volumes from clinical screening full-field digital mammograms.

The approach consists in building a statistical model using a training set of digital mammograms with known measures of percent fibroglandular tissue volume, breast volume and fibroglandular tissue volume calculated by phantom based calibration method. To derive these measures, we follow the standard procedure in machine learning: feature generation, feature selection, regression classification of outputs, final model building and testing.

The correlation of features to known volumetric breast volumes was analyzed. In addition, the performance of models created from different groups of features were studied. By building a statistical model with 28 degrees of freedom, we achieved an $R^2=0.83$ between the predicted and measured volumetric breast densities for the testing set of 2000 mammograms which were independent of the training set of 2000 images.

Keywords: Volumetric breast density, mammographic features, statistical model, regression.

1 Introduction

Interest is growing in the developing automated breast density measures because of its strong association with breast cancer risk. Although a number of automated methods to quantify mammographic and volumetric density appeared they still have issues with accuracy and reproducibily, and there is a demand to developing new accurate and automated breast density estimation thechniques. The purpose of this paper is to design and to test new approach for automatically quantifying true volumetric fibroglandular tissue volumes from clinical screening full-field digital mammograms.

H. Fujita, T. Hara, and C. Muramatsu (Eds.): IWDM 2014, LNCS 8539, pp. 257–264, 2014.

The measure of dense breast tissue volume from mammograms has been shown to be a strong risk factor for breast cancer. There are several approaches to automatically estimate planimetric mammographic and true volumetric breast densities. We could classify them as in-image phantom based calibration [1-3], prior calibration [4,5], physical image formation model [6,7], image processing adaptive thresholding [8-12], and statistical model building [13,14] approaches.

Recently, single energy absorptiometry (SXA) - an automated method for quantifying fibroglandular tissue volume has been developed [1]. It demonstrated good accuracy and precision for a broad range of breast thicknesses, paddle tilt angles, and percent fibroglandular tissie volume (%FGV) values. The method uses a breast tissue-equivalent phantom in the unused portion of the mammogram as a reference to estimate breast composition. To perform quality control monitoring and cross-validation between sites and machines a new modified calibration approach for the SXA method [15] was developed. It provides stable thickness measurements and grayscale to density pixel conversion and different machine and sites cross-validation. The cross-calibration is achieved by quality control monitoring with specially designed calibration phantom to control thickness and grey-scale conversion stability by the phantom weekly scanning. Thus, quality control allowed us to derive accurate and precise %FGV estimates measured during long period of time for mammography machines of different centers and manufacturers. Clinicaly, acquiring a calibrated SXA image is difficult because of SXA phantom. Thus, we introduced a novel method to automatically quantify volumetric fibroglandular tissue volumes from clinical screening full-field digital mammograms without usage of the SXA phantom. The new high throughput automated approach for volumetric breast density estimation proposed in this paper combines volumetric density measures derived by the SXA method and statistical model building technique based on image parameters extracted from the mammogram. Thus, we can achieve automatic volumetric breast density estimation from digital mammograms not using the SXA phantom.

2   Methods

Our approach consists in building statistical model using training set of digital mammograms with known measures of percent fibroglandular tissie volume, breast volume and fibroglandular tissie volumes (FGV) measured by SXA. To derive predicted   %FGV we followed the standard classification/regression procedure in machine learning: feature generation, feature selection, regression classification of outputs and final model building and testing.

2.1   Datasets

The training and testing sets were created to build and to test the models. To create training set we used 2000 full field digital mammograms from the San Francisco Mammography Registry with known volumetric breast density measures. The mammograms in this study were obtained during 2.5 period of time on 3 Hologic Selenia machines at California Pacific Medical Center, San Francisco. The %FGV, FGV and breast volumes were calculated by the phantom based calibration method

[1]. Moreover, weekly recalibration was applied to realize quality assurance procedure using weekly scans of specially designed quality assurance phantom. All images that contained implants were excluded from analysis. The training and testing sets consisted of randomly selected mammograms representing %FGV from 0% to 100%.

2.2   Feature Generation

The following several groups of mammographic morphological and texture features (number = 45) were calculated.

The first-order features are calculated from the histogram of pixel grey values in the images. They included image standard deviation, skewness, kurtosis, balance [16, 17].

The second-order features considered spatial relationships between pixel intensities were derived from two matrixes: grey-level co-occurrence matrix (GLCM) and neighbourhood gray-tone difference matrix (NGTDM). The Energy, Enthropy, Dissimilarity, Contrast, Homogeneity, Correlation, Mean and Variance were estimated from the GLCM matrix. And Coarseness, Contrast, Complexity, Strength and Busyness were extracted from the NGTDM matrix [16-18].

By using Fourier Transform (FT) operation to images we estimated the following features in frequency domain: root mean square (FT_RMS), first (FT_FMP) second moments (FT_SMP) of power spectrum, and fractal dimension (FD) from power spectrum exponent (FT_FD) [16].

A set of FD and FD-like features such as FD with threshold at X% of the total contrast, FD_TH_X where X = 5, 10, 15....85, FD of the standard deviation (FD_Sigma), intercept of the plot of the standard deviation of the high frequency image as a function of the size the kernel (CD_Yint), slope of the plot of the standard deviation of the high frequency image as a function of the size the kernel (CD_Slope), standard deviation of the mean value of the breast pixels rows (HZ_PROJ), FD of the surface of the breast considering the gray value represent the height (FD_CALDWELL), and FD from morphological image operations (FD_Minkowski) [19, 20]. As a result of edge frequency analysis mean gradient parameter was created [16].

Another group of features were extracted from DICOM image file headers. We used the following DICOM tags characterized physical conditions and parameters of x-ray image formation such as mAs, kVp, DetectorTemperature, EntranceDoseInm-Gy, ExposureTime, HalfValuelayer, force, BodyPartThickness, image file size (or paddle type), and filter/target combination.

In addition, a group of image breast regions of interest (ROI) such as the breast area, width of image (nipple to chest wall) and height of image (top to bottom) was obtained from images using global threshold segmentation and skin detection algorithm.

We considered that by combining these parameters and features together we would be able to maximally boost the performance of the final model and to predict efficiently %FGV.

2.3   Statistics

The linear regression method was used to build statistical model. The SAS proc glmselect with different options was used. The forward selection and backward elimination, stepwise selection and elimination, ten-fold cross-validation, and LASSO (least absolute shrinkage and selection operator) selection methods with different stop criteria were investigated to build the optimal model matched number of features selected and average error of prediction achieved. The Schwarz Bayesian information, Akaike's information, predicted residual sum of squares statistics (PRESS), and adjusted R-square statistic criteria were monitored.

3   Results

A %FGV frequency distribution of the training set of 2000 mammograms is shown at Fig. 1. It is characterized by the following parameters: mean = 32.8%, median = 27.8%, standard deviation = 18.3, minimum = 1.2%, maximum = 99.8%. The Table 1 represent linear correlation coefficients between features and %FGV, FGV and breast volume. The features under investigation were found to correlate highly and moderately to breast %FGV, dense tissue and actual volumes (see Table 1). The highest Pearson correlation coefficients were equal 0.96 and 0.94 for relationship between actual breast volume, and the breast area and Fourier FT_RMS parameter, respectively. The high correlation to %FGV demonstrates all three groups: mammographic features, DICOM header parameters, and ROI image parameters. The correlation with r around 0.55-0.6 showed kVp, breast thickness, height of breast ROI, mean of gradient, CD_Slope, and FT_FD. The highest Pearson correlation coefficients to dense tissue volumes demonstrated two mammographic features, and r values were 0.61 and 0.69 for CD_Yint and FT_RMS features respectively.

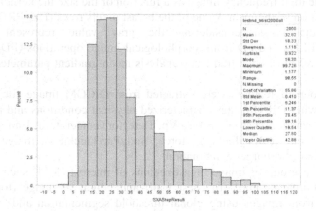

Fig. 1. %FGV frequency distribution of 2000 mammogram training set

The models outputs of different groups of features such as 45 mammographic features, 10 physical parameters from DICOM, 3 breast ROI parameters, and all 58 features together presented at Table 2. The models were created using 10-fold cross validation for different feature groups. The selection stopped at a local minimum of the cross validation PRESS. As one seen the mammographic features and DICOM header parameter groups showed the same association with %FGV equal 0.68 but the latter group needs only 6 features in comparison with 20 features of the former groups. The breast ROI image parameters demonstrate $r^2 = 0.36$ association with %FGV using two features. By adding groups together we managed to increase adjusted r^2 value to 0.84 using 58 features.

Table 1. Correlation coefficents between features and %FGV, FGV and breast volume

NAME	%FGV	Volume	FGV
%FGV	1.0000	-0.4867	0.2476
Volume	-0.4867	1.0000	0.5655
FGV	0.2476	0.5655	1.0000
mAs	0.5105	-0.1181	0.3558
kVp	-0.5901	0.6433	0.2794
Entrance Dose In mGy	0.1378	0.1537	0.4332
Exposure Time	0.5015	-0.0918	0.3670
Half Value Layer	-0.3864	0.4749	0.1953
Force	-0.2128	0.3491	0.1850
Body Part Thickness	-0.5635	0.6615	0.3111
Technique_id	-0.3167	0.5100	0.1893
breast area	-0.4413	0.9641	0.5793
ROI_width	-0.4158	0.9140	0.5814
ROI height	-0.5928	0.8462	0.4355
FD_TH_75	-0.523	0.348	-0.184
FD_RMS	-0.210	0.426	0.329
CD_Yint	-0.466	0.860	0.608
CD_Slope	0.551	-0.560	-0.143
FD_CALDWELL	-0.292	0.392	0.147
GLCM_Enthropy	0.311	-0.417	-0.061
GLCM_Dissimilarity	0.470	-0.742	-0.452
GLCM_Contrast	0.349	-0.639	-0.463
GLCM_Homogeneity	-0.500	0.744	0.419
GLCM_Correlation	-0.275	0.555	0.429
GLCM_Mean	-0.248	0.601	0.418
NGTDM_Coarseness	0.280	-0.349	-0.268
NGTDM_Strength	0.294	-0.405	-0.145
Mean_Gradient	0.543	-0.641	-0.143
FT_RMS	-0.376	0.945	0.688
FT_FMP	0.429	-0.758	-0.521
FT_SMP	0.387	-0.639	-0.460
FT_FD	0.581	-0.574	-0.110

In addition to the cross-validation method we tested the final model using two independent training and testing sets. Fig. 2 demonstrates progression of average squared errors for %FGV while adding the new features in the order of their contribution performance. The linear regression model with stepwise selection method and significance level selection criterion was used. We applied a set of entry and stay significance levels from 0.00001 to 0.1. The optimal entry and stay significance levels had value 0.001. It provides a trade-off between a number of features in the model and prediction efficiency, and it could prevent the model from using highly interactive features.

Table 2. Feature selection with 10-fold cross validation for different feature groups. Selection stopped at a local minimum of the cross validation PRESS.

Groups	Number	R_square	Number selected
Mammographic features	45	0.68	20
DICOM header parameters	10	0.68	6
ROI image parameters	3	0.36	2
All features together	58	0.84	36

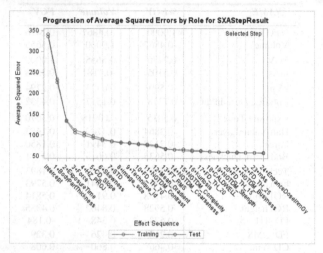

Fig. 2. Progression of Average Squared Errors by Role for %FGV

By building a statistical model with 28 degrees of freedom, we achieved an $R^2=0.83$ between the predicted and measured volumetric breast densities for the testing set of 2000 mammograms which were independent of the training set of 2000 images. The progression dependence is characterized by continuously decreasing of average square errors, with a fast drop at the beginning and slow monotonous downward trend for the rest of features. The sets follow the same trend but the errors of the testing set are a little bit higher than ones for the training set. We consider that obtained correlation between the predicted and measured volumetric breast densities is good enouph for clinical studies. We noted that the study presented in Tables and Figures relied on the same manufacture (Hologic); in addition, these results are not representative of all types of manufacture machines. Perhaps other conclusions would be obtained by the use of different manufacture machines. Further exploring and testing of this approach for different centers and manufacturers are required.

4   Conclusions

We applied statistical model approach for automated volumetric breast density estimation. The models combined different groups of features such as mammographic features, DICOM header parameters, and ROI image parameters were analyzed. By building a statistical model with 28 degrees of freedom, we achieved an $R^2=0.83$ between the predicted and measured volumetric breast densities for the testing set of 2000 mammograms which were independent of the training set of 2000 images. Further exploring and testing of this approach is warranted. There are several ways to expand on this paper. One way is to use different machines and manufactures, i.e., GE and Philips. Another way would be to improve the calibration method [15] to increase %FGV accuracy.

References

1. Malkov, S., Wang, J., Kerlikowske, K., Cummings, S., Shepherd, J.A.: Single x-ray absorptiometry method for the quantitative mammographic measure of fibroglandular tissue volume. Medical Physics 36(12), 5525–5536 (2009)
2. Pawluczyk, O., Augustine, B.J., Yaffe, M.J., Rico, D., Yang, J., Mawdsley, G.E., Boyd, N.F.: A volumetric method for estimation of breast density on digitized screen-film mammograms. Med. Phys. 30(3), 352–364 (2003)
3. Diffey, J., Hufton, A., Astley, S.M.: A new step-wedge for the volumetric measurement of mammographic density. In: Astley, S.M., Brady, M., Rose, C., Zwiggelaar, R. (eds.) IWDM 2006. LNCS, vol. 4046, pp. 1–9. Springer, Heidelberg (2006)
4. Kaufhold, J., Thomas, J.A., Eberhard, J.W., Galbo, C.E., Trotter, D.E.: A calibration approach to glandular tissue composition estimation in digital mammography. Med. Phys. 29(8), 1867–1880 (2002)
5. Heine, J.J., Cao, K., Rollison, D.E.: Calibrated measures for breast density estimation. Acad. Radiol. 18, 547–555 (2011)
6. Highnam, R., Pan, X., Warren, R., Jeffreys, M., Davey Smith, G., Brady, M.: Breast composition measurements using retrospective standard mammogram form (SMF). Phys. Med. Biol. 5111, 2695–2713 (2006)
7. van Engeland, S., Snoeren, P.R., Huisman, H., Boetes, C., Karssemeijer, N.: Volumetric breast density estimation from fullfield digital mammograms. IEEE Trans. Med. Imaging 25(3), 273–282 (2006)
8. Zhou, C., Chan, H., Petrick, N., Helvie, M.A., Goodsitt, M.M., Sahiner, B., Hadjiiski, L.M.: Computerized image analysis: Estimation of breast density on mammograms. Med. Phys. 28(6), 1056–1069 (2001)
9. Kallenberg, M.G., Lokate, M., van Gils, C.H., Karssemeijer, N.: Automatic breast density segmentation: an integration of different approaches. Phys. Med. Biol. 56(9), 2715–2729 (2011)
10. Kim, Y., Kim, C., Kim, J.: Automated Estimation of Breast Density on Mammogram using Combined Information of Histogram Statistics and Boundary Gradients. In: Proc. of SPIE, vol. 7624, p. 76242F-1 (2010)
11. Keller, B.M., Nathan, D.L., Wang, Y., Zheng, Y., Gee, J.C., Conant, E.F., Kontos, D.: Estimation of breast percent density in raw and processed full field digital mammography images via adaptive fuzzy c-means clustering and support vector machine segmentation. Med. Phys. 39(8), 4903–4917 (2012)
12. Saidin, N., Mat Sakim, H.A., Ngah, U.K., Shuaib, I.L.: Computer Aided Detection of Breast Density and Mass, and Visualization of Other Breast Anatomical Regions on Mammograms Using Graph Cuts. Computational and Mathematical Methods in Medicine 2013, Article ID 205384, 13 pages (2013)

13. Heine, J.J., Velthuizen, R.P.: A statistical methodology for mammographic density detection. Med. Phys. 27, 2644–2651 (2000)
14. Li, J., Szekely, L., Eriksson, L., Heddson, B., Sundbom, A., Czene, K., Hall, P., Humphreys, K.: High-throughput mammographic-density measurement: a tool for risk prediction of breast cancer. Breast Cancer Research 14(4), R114 (2012)
15. Malkov, S., Wang, J., Duewer, F., Shepherd, J.A.: A Calibration Approach for Single-Energy X-ray Absorptiometry Method to Provide Absolute Breast Tissue Composition Accuracy for the Long Term. In: Maidment, A.D.A., Bakic, P.R., Gavenonis, S. (eds.) IWDM 2012. LNCS, vol. 7361, pp. 769–774. Springer, Heidelberg (2012)
16. Li, H., Giger, M.L., Olopade, O., Margolis, A., Lan, L., Chinander, M.: Computerized Texture Analysis of Mammographic Parenchymal Patterns of Digitized Mammograms. Acad. Radiol. 12, 863–873 (2005)
17. Castella, C., Kinkel, K., Eckstein, M.P., Sottas, P., Verdun, F., Bochud, F.: Semiautomatic Mammographic Parenchymal Patterns Classification Using Multiple Statistical Features. Acad. Radiol. 14, 1486–1499 (2007)
18. Haralick, R., Shanmugan, K., Dinstein, I.: Textural Features for Image Classification. IEEE Trans. Syst., Man Cybernet 3, 610–621 (1973)
19. Caldwell, C.B., Stapleton, S.J., Holdsworth, D.W., Jong, R.A., Weiser, W.J., Cooke, G., Yaffe, M.J.: Characterisation of mammographic parenchymal pattern by fractal dimension. Phys. Med. Biol. 35, 235–247 (1990)
20. Boone, J.M., Lindfors, K.K., Beatty, C.S., Seibert, J.A.: A breast density index for digital mammograms based on radiologists' ranking. J. Digit. Imaging 11, 101–115 (1998)

Volumetric Breast Density and Radiographic Parameters

Jennifer Khan-Perez[1], Elaine Harkness[2,3,4,*], Claire Mercer[3], Megan Bydder[3],
Jamie Sergeant[2,5,6], Julie Morris[4,7], Anthony Maxwell[2,3,4,8], Catherine Rylance[3],
and Susan M. Astley[2,3,4,8]

[1] Manchester Medical School, University of Manchester, Stopford Building, Oxford Road,
Manchester, M13 9PT
[2] Centre for Imaging Sciences, Institute of Population Health, University of Manchester,
Stopford Building, Oxford Road, Manchester, M13 9PT
Elaine.F.Harkness@manchester.ac.uk
[3] Genesis Breast Cancer Prevention Centre,
University Hospital of South Manchester NHS Trust,
Wythenshawe, Manchester M23 9LT, UK
[4] The University of Manchester, Manchester Academic Health Science Centre,
University Hospital of South Manchester NHS Foundation Trust,
Wythenshawe, Manchester M23 9LT, UK.
[5] Arthritis Research UK Centre for Epidemiology, Institute of Inflammation and Repair,
Faculty of Medical and Human Sciences, Manchester Academic Health Science Centre,
University of Manchester, Oxford Road, Manchester M13 9PT
[6] NIHR Manchester Musculoskeletal Biomedical Research Unit,
Central Manchester NHS Foundation Trust,
Manchester Academic Health Science Centre
[7] Centre for Biostatistics, Institute of Population Health,
University of Manchester, Oxford Road, Manchester, M13 9PT
[8] Manchester Breast Centre, Manchester Cancer Research Centre,
University of Manchester, Christie Hospital, Withington,
Manchester, M20 4BX, UK

Abstract. The detection of breast cancer relies on high-quality images from digital mammography. Optimal levels of compression force are unknown, and UK national guidelines recommend forces of less than 200N. However, large variations in compression forces exist and may be influenced by the mammography practitioner and the breast size and pain threshold of the patient. This study examined the relationship between breast density and compression force. Women attending for routine breast screening and who had a mammogram taken by the same practitioner on the same equipment were included in the study (n=211). Volumetric density measurements were obtained using Volpara™ and details on imaging parameters were obtained from the DICOM headers. There was a strong, positive correlation between compression force and fibroglandular tissue. There was also evidence of a significant positive association between compression force and breast volume which was independent of the volume of fibroglandular tissue present.

---

* Corresponding author.

H. Fujita, T. Hara, and C. Muramatsu (Eds.): IWDM 2014, LNCS 8539, pp. 265–272, 2014.
© Springer International Publishing Switzerland 2014

1   Introduction

The production of high-quality images during mammography is necessary for the adequate detection of breast cancer. Breast compression is used to enhance mammographic image quality by immobilising the breast and reducing superimposition of overlying breast tissue. It also reduces the radiation dose by reducing breast thickness [1]. There is conflicting opinion related to the optimum level of compression force that should be applied [1]. The UK National Health Service Breast Screening Programme guidelines recommend a compression force of less than 200 N [2], however the level actually applied depends on a number of factors including practitioner technique [3] and the pain threshold of the patient.

Breast density has been shown to be one of the strongest risk factors for breast cancer [4,5], but high breast density may also make it more difficult to detect cancer due to masking [6]. It has been hypothesised that higher compression forces applied to dense breasts may lead to less superimposition of tissue and to better visualisation of lesions [7].

The aim of this study was to examine the relationship between breast density and compression force. Furthermore, the study aimed to look at the relationship between these measurements and radiation dose, and fibroglandular and breast volume.

2   Methods

A sample of 211 women who had been invited for routine mammographic screening in Greater Manchester, UK and had agreed to take part in the PROCAS (Predicting Risk Of Cancer At Screening) study were included in the current study. Women taking part in PROCAS attend routine NHS breast cancer screening and provide additional information in relation to family history, hormonal and lifestyle factors by completing a 2-page questionnaire which they bring with them to their screening appointment [8].

The women included in this study all had a full-field digital screening mammogram taken by a single practitioner on the same equipment. The practitioner had over 13 years of experience, and the mammograms were taken between July 2012 and October 2012. One woman was excluded from the study because the compression force recorded was invalid (0 N). There were no other exclusion criteria, and data were not corrected for any other risk factors. Volumetric breast density (VBD %), fibroglandular volume (cm^3) and breast volume (cm^3) were calculated using Volpara^{TM} 1.4.0 [9]. Details of imaging parameters (compression force (N), breast thickness (mm) and estimated dose (dGy)) were extracted from the information recorded in the DICOM headers at the time of image acquistion.

Relationships were tested for statistical significance using Spearman's Rank Order coefficient. Linear regression was used to examine the relationships between compression force, breast thickness and radiation dose with fibroglandular and breast volumes. All analysis was performed using SPSS version 20.0.

3   Results

Compression force

There was a significant negative correlation between compression force and volumetric breast density for the left (LCC) and right crano-caudal (RCC) views (r=-0.22 and -0.32 respectively) i.e. the compression force applied was lower in those with larger volumetric breast density (p<0.01). There was no association with compression force and volumetric breast density for the medio-lateral oblique views (LMLO or RMLO) (Table 1). Fibroglandular and breast volume were both significantly correlated with compression force for all four mammographic views, indicating larger forces were applied for larger breasts; but also, for breasts with higher fibroglandular volumes (Table 1). Figure 1 shows the relationship between compression force (recorded to the nearest 10N) and fibroglandular volume for the LCC view.

Table 1. Correlations between compression force and volumetric breast density (VBD), fibroglandular and breast volume for each mammographic view (* p<0.05, ** p<0.01)

	View	VBD	Fibroglandular volume	Breast Volume
Compression	RMLO	-0.078	0.169*	0.193*
	LMLO	-0.106	0.196*	0.226**
Force	RCC	-0.317**	0.333**	0.526**
	LCC	-0.224**	0.244**	0.377**

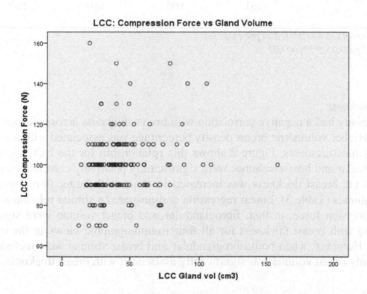

Fig. 1. Compression force versus fibroglandular volume in the LCC view

In univariate linear regression fibroglandular and breast volume were significantly associated with compression force for all mammographic views (p<0.01). However, when fibroglandular and breast volume were both included in the model, only breast volume was significantly associated with compression force for three of the four mammographic views (Table 2). Fibroglandular and breast volume were significantly correlated across all four views (correlations between r=0.57 and 0.66).

Table 2. Regression results for compression force (standard deviations from the mean)

	RMLO	LMLO	RCC	LCC
Constant	99.9	96.2	86.8	88.3
	(2.70)***	(3.18)***	(2.38)***	(2.82)***
Fibroglandular volume	0.051	0.095	-0.002	0.024
	(0.059)	(0.065)	(0.051)	(0.063)
Breast volume	0.005	0.007	0.017	0.014
	(0.003)*	(0.003)***	(0.003)***	(0.003)***
R-squared	0.061	0.121	0.242	0.140
Adjusted R-squared	0.049	0.110	0.232	0.129
N	161	160	160	160

Standard errors are reported in parentheses
*p<0.1, **p<0.05, ***p<0.01

Breast thickness
Breast density had a negative correlation with breast thickness across all four views (p < 0.01). Higher volumetric breast density percentage was associated with lower breast thickness measurements. Figure 2 shows this relationship for the LCC view. Larger fibroglandular and breast volumes were significantly positively correlated with breast thickness i.e. breast thickness was increased in those with larger fibroglandular and breast volumes (Table 3). Linear regression demonstrated a similar relationship to that for compression force, in that, fibroglandular and breast volume were significantly associated with breast thickness for all four mammographic views in the univariate analysis. However, when both fibroglandular and breast volume were included in the model, only breast volume was significantly associated with breast thickness.

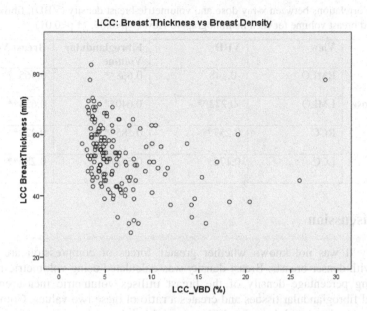

Fig. 2. Breast thickness versus volumetric breast density in the LCC view

Table 3. Correlations between breast thickness and volumetric breast density (VBD), fibroglandular and breast volume for each mammographic view (* p<0.05, ** p<0.01)

	View	VBD	Fibroglandular Volume	Breast Volume
Breast	RMLO	-0.622**	0.505**	0.822**
	LMLO	-0.615**	0.551**	0.836**
Thickness	RCC	-0.470**	0.340**	0.637**
	LCC	-0.441**	0.394**	0.643**

X-ray dose

There was a negative correlation between x-ray dose and volumetric breast density for the MLO views, but positive significant correlations for CC views. There was also a positive correlation for fibroglandular and breast volumes and x-ray dose for all four views (Table 4). Again in the univariate linear regression both breast and fibroglandular volume were significantly associated with x-ray exposure, however when both breast and fibroglandular volume were included in the regression model, both variables were independent predictors of radiation dose for three of the four mammographic views. For the LCC view, only fibroglandular volume was an independent predictor of radiation dose.

Table 4. Correlations between x-ray dose and volumetric breast density (VBD), fibroglandular volume and breast volume for each mammographic view (* p<0.05, ** p<0.01)

	View	VBD	Fibroglandular Volume	Breast Volume
	RMLO	-0.148	0.668**	0.565**
X-ray Dose	LMLO	-0.272**	0.640**	0.624**
	RCC	0.257**	0.585**	0.229**
	LCC	0.172*	0.553**	0.286**

4   Discussion

Previously it was not known whether greater forces of compression are used in women with denser breasts. Breast density was calculated using volumetric methods. Calculating percentage density of the breast utilises volumetric measurements of breast and fibroglandular tissues and creates a ratio of these two values. Compression force was correlated with breast and fibroglandular volume, but negatively associated with volumetric breast density. As the breast volume increases so too does compression force, but since breast volume is also correlated with fibroglandular volume, and fibroglandular volume also increases but not to the same extent, the overall percentage of volumetric breast density decreases.

The other results confirmed the earlier hypotheses, in that strong, positive correlations were found between higher compression forces and fibroglandular and breast volumes. This was also true for larger fibroglandular and breast volumes, and breast thickness and mean X-ray dose. These values signify that larger breasts and breasts with abundant fibroglandular tissue will require higher X-ray doses, despite using greater forces to reduce their comparatively-larger compressed breast thicknesses. Linear regression analysis was employed to determine whether the association between the size of a breast and greater compression forces were due to greater fibroglandular volumes. However, fibroglandular volume was not found to be an independent predictor of compression force when breast volume was added to the regression model, suggesting that breast volume drives the relationship with compression force.   A similar relationship was found for breast thickness.

X-ray dose demonstrated associations with VBD for all four mammographic views which were inconsistent, however the correlations with fibroglandular volume tended to be much stronger than those for breast volume for the CC views. In linear regression with both breast and fibroglandular volume included in the model both variables were found to be independent predictors of x-ray dose for three of the four mammographic views.

Women included in this study were a sample of women seen by one practitioner with thirteen years of experience.   The practitioner was blind to the nature of the study.   However, whether the sample was representative of the screening population more generally and whether the current findings would be replicated for other practitioners is not known.   In addition, it would be of interest to look at the relationship between compression force and density measures after adjusting for other known breast cancer risk factors such as age, BMI, menopausal status and HRT use. Age has been found to be correlated with increased compressibility of the breast [10]. It is believed that this is due to a reduction in breast density and a greater proportion of fatty tissue, thus lowering the amount of force required for optimal breast compression. Therefore the amount by which a breast is compressed not only changes with the machine used, the mammographic view and the operator, but also with time.

5   Conclusions

Greater densities may influence image quality if breast thickness is not reduced [5,11], which also has implications for the X-ray dose [12,13] to the breast. Greater forces applied, however, may lead to a negative and painful experience and impact on screening attendance rates [10,14].

Our results show that there was evidence of a significant positive association between compression force and breast thickness with breast volume which is independent of the volume of fibroglandular tissue present.

A more objective process where compression force is tailored to an accurate representation of the composition of a breast is needed. Current methods involve either visual or automated systems which utilise different parameters for evaluating the internal structures of a breast, resulting in differences in measured breast density.

Acknowledgements. We acknowledge the support of the National Institute for Health Research (NIHR) and the Genesis Prevention Appeal for their funding of the PROCAS study. We would like to thank the women who agreed to take part in the study and the study staff for recruitment and data collection. We also thank Matakina Technology Limited for providing Volpara^{TM}. This paper presents independent research funded by the National Institute for Health Research (NIHR) under its Programme Grants for Applied Research programme (reference number RP-PG-0707-10031: "Improvement in risk prediction, early detection and prevention of breast cancer"). The views expressed are those of the author(s) and not necessarily those of the NHS, the NIHR, or the Department of Health.

References

1. Mercer, C.E., Hogg, P., Lawson, R., et al.: Practitioner compression force variability in mammography: a preliminary study. Br. J. Radiol. (2013), doi:10.1259/bjr.20110596
2. National Quality Assurance Coordinating Group for Radiography. Quality Assurance Guidelines for Mammography Including Radiographic Quality. NHSBSP Publication No 63 (April 2006)
3. Huang, Z., Hankinson, S.E., Colditz, G.A., et al.: Dual Effects of Weight and Weight Gain on Breast Cancer Risk. JAMA 278(17), 1407–1411 (1997)
4. Wolfe, J.N.: Breast patterns as an index of risk for developing breast cancer. Am. J. Roentgenol. 126, 1130–1139 (1976)

5. McCormack, V.A., Silva, D.S.: Breast Density and Parenchymal Patterns as Markers of Breast Cancer Risk: a Meta-Analysis. Cancer Epidemiol. Biomarkers Prev. 15(6), 1159–1169 (2006)
6. Assi, V., Warwick, J., Cuzick, J., Duffy, S.W.: Clinical and epidemiological issues in mammographic density. Nat. Rev. Clin Oncol. 9, 33–40 (2012), doi:10.1038/nrclinonc.2011.173.
7. Dustler, M., Anderson, I., Brorson, H., et al.: Breast Compression in mammography: pressure distribution patterns. Acta. Radiol. 53, 973–980 (2012)
8. Evans, G.: PROCAS study (2011), http://www.uhsm.nhs.uk/research/Pages/PROCASstudy.aspx (June 16, 2013)
9. Volpara Density (2013), http://www.volparadensity.com/
10. Poulos, A., McLean, D., Rickard, M., et al.: Breast Compression in Mammography: how much is enough? Australian Radiology 47, 121–126 (2003)
11. Helvie, M.A., Chan, H.P., Adler, D.D., Boyd, P.G.: Breast Thickness in Routine Mammograms: effect on image quality and radiation dose. American J. of Roentgenology 163, 1371–1374 (1994)
12. Nelson, H.D., Tyne, K., Naik, A., et al.: Screening for Breast Cancer: an update for the US Preventive Services Task Force. Ann. Intern. Med. 151(10), 727–737 (2009)
13. Ronckers, C.M., Erdman, C.A., Land, C.E.: Radiation and Breast Cancer: A Review of Current Evidence. Breast Cancer Res. 7(1), 21–32 (2005)
14. Nimmo, L.J., Alston, L.A.C., McFayden, A.: The Influence of HRT on Technical Recall on the UK Breast Screening Programme: are pain, compression force, and compressed breast thickness contributing factors? Clinical Radiology 62, 439–446 (2007)

The Relationship of Volumetric Breast Density to Socio-Economic Status in a Screening Population

Louisa Samuels[1], Elaine Harkness[2,3,4,*], Susan M. Astley[2,3,4,9],
Anthony Maxwell[2,3,4,9], Jamie Sergeant[2,5,6], Julie Morris[4,7], Mary Wilson[3],
Paula Stavrinos[3,4], D. Gareth Evans[1,3,4,8], Tony Howell[3,4,9], and Megan Bydder[3]

[1] Manchester Medical School, University of Manchester, Stopford Building, Oxford Road,
Manchester, M13 9PT
[2] Centre for Imaging Sciences, Institute of Population Health, University of Manchester,
Stopford Building, Oxford Road, Manchester, M13 9PT
Elaine.F.Harkness@manchester.ac.uk
[3] Genesis Breast Cancer Prevention Centre, University Hospital of South Manchester NHS
Trust, Wythenshawe, Manchester M23 9LT, UK
Megan.Bydder@uhsm.nhs.uk
[4] The University of Manchester, Manchester Academic Health Science Centre, University Hospital of South Manchester NHS Foundation Trust, Wythenshawe, Manchester M23 9LT, UK
[5] Arthritis Research UK Centre for Epidemiology, Institute of Inflammation and Repair, Faculty
of Medical and Human Sciences, Manchester Academic Health Science Centre, University of
Manchester, Oxford Road, Manchester M13 9PT
[6] NIHR Manchester Musculoskeletal Biomedical Research Unit, Central Manchester NHS
Foundation Trust, Manchester Academic Health Science Centre
[7] Centre for Biostatistics, Institute of Population Health, University of Manchester, Oxford
Road, Manchester, M13 9PT
[8] Manchester Centre for Genomic Medicine, Central Manchester Foundation Trust, St. Mary's
Hospital, Oxford Road, Manchester M13 9WL, UK
[9] Manchester Breast Centre, Manchester Cancer Research Centre, University of Manchester,
Christie Hospital, Withington, Manchester, M20 4BX, UK

Abstract. Breast cancer incidence has previously been shown to be greater in women of higher socio-economic status (SES), although the picture is complex due to variations in breast cancer risk factors. We have investigated the relationship between one of the strongest risk factors, breast density, with SES in a population of 6398 post- and peri-menopausal women. Volumetric breast density was measured using Quantra™ and Volpara™, and SES was based on the Index of Multiple Deprivation (IMD) associated with each woman's postcode. The mean IMD score was 26.39 (SD 16.7). Our results show a weak but significant association between SES and volumetric breast density; women from more deprived areas have slightly less dense breasts. After controlling for age, BMI and HRT use the relationship remained significant for density measured by Volpara™ (gradient -0.01, p <0.005) but not Quantra™ (gradient -0.007, p=0.07).

---

* Corresponding author.

H. Fujita, T. Hara, and C. Muramatsu (Eds.): IWDM 2014, LNCS 8539, pp. 273–281, 2014.
© Springer International Publishing Switzerland 2014

Keywords: digital, mammogram, volumetric breast density, socio-economic status.

1   Introduction

Breast cancer incidence has been shown to be associated with higher socioeconomic status (SES) [1-3]. The relationship between higher SES and breast cancer risk factors has been explored in a number of studies and it is still contentious whether the perceived SES gradient in breast cancer incidence is independent of established breast cancer risk factors [1-3].

Heck et al. found that after controlling for several known breast cancer risk factors, the relationship between breast cancer risk and higher education levels became non-significant, confirming that the higher incidence seen among well-educated women is likely to be attributable to established breast cancer risk factors [1].   Higher levels of education and higher SES have been shown to be associated with later age of primiparity and low total parity, both established breast cancer risk factors [4,5]. However, a strong positive association between SES and breast cancer risk persists after adjustments for fertility, marital status, education and late primiparity [6]. HRT use, which is both a breast cancer risk factor and a cause of increased breast density [7], has also been shown to be significantly higher among women of higher SES [8]. In addition, high BMI is associated with lower breast density and women in developed societies are more likely to be obese [9]. Furthermore, women of higher SES are more likely to attend routine breast screening which may lead to better detection rates [10].

Despite the evidence for the relationship between SES and breast cancer risk, there is a gap in the literature regarding the relationship between SES and breast density. Educational level is inversely associated with breast density among premenopausal women but not postmenopausal women [11]. In premenopausal women breast density was negatively associated with SES, however this was mainly attributable to BMI [12]. Given changes in breast density following the menopause, it is important to establish the relationship in peri-and post-menopausal women using a more comprehensive marker of SES.

This study aimed to investigate the relationship between SES and volumetric breast density in peri- and postmenopausal women.

2   Methodology

The Predicting Risk of Cancer At Screening (PROCAS) study was used to obtain information on breast density and other breast cancer risk factors from approximately 50,000 women in Greater Manchester, UK. Women attending routine breast screening are invited to participate in the study and for those that consent to take part information on a number of breast cancer risk factors are collected via a questionnaire [13]. Premenopausal women were excluded from the study as were women with missing postcode, age or density data. Only women with a BMI value within the range 16-65 were included.

Mammographic breast density measurements were performed on the screening mammograms of eligible women using two fully-automated volumetric methods (Quantra[TM] version 1. 3 [14] and Volpara[TM] version 1.4.0 [15]) to assess the volumetric percentage of fibroglandular tissue in the breast. To be included in the study women had to have breast density measurements for both Quantra[TM] and Volpara[TM]. Quantra[TM] data provides an average volumetric density measurement per breast and an overall average for breast density for each woman that was used in the study. Volpara[TM] provides a volumetric breast density measurement for each mammographic view of each breast (CC and MLO). The average was calculated from these four values.

SES for each patient was based on the Index of Multiple Deprivation (IMD) associated with their postcode [16]. The IMD is a single score created using information from the UK National Census which combines several indicators of deprivation: income, employment, health, education, crime, access to services and living environment. A high IMD score correlates to high levels of deprivation i.e. a low SES. The scale ranges from 0 (no deprivation) to 100 (most deprived) and is a continuous measure of relative deprivation with no single cut off point defining a deprived or affluent area [16].

3   Analysis

Descriptive analyses were performed to assess the characteristics of the sample. Pearson correlations were calculated to establish the existence of a relationship between IMD and breast density and to estimate the degree of association between the variables. Linear regression models were used to assess the dependence of breast density on IMD. Similar models were used to assess the effect of potential confounders (age, BMI or HRT use).

As the sample size was so large, disproportionately strong significance can be attributed to relationships. Furthermore, the use of continuous variables on large samples can mask relationships. For this reason, breast density measurements were divided into categories so the average IMD for women with different breast densities could be computed. Volpara[TM] density grades (VDG) exist to correlate Volpara[TM] density scores with the Breast Imaging Reporting and Data System (BI-RADS) density category (BIRADS 1: <4.5% Volpara[TM]; BIRADS 2: 4.5 - 7.5% Volpara[TM]; BIRADS 3: 7.6 - 15.5% Volpara[TM]; BIRADS 4: >15.5% Volpara[TM]) [17]. A similar categorisation is not available for Quantra[TM] and thus categories were based on quintiles.

4   Results

A total of 6398 women were included in the sample. The average age was 60.3 years and ranged from 46 to 74 (Table 1). The majority were white (92%) and the average IMD score was 26.39 (SD 16.7), ranging 2.96 to 81.58.

Data on body mass index were available for 5965 women. The average BMI was 27.9 kg/m^2 (SD 5.5), and ranged from 17.1 kg/m^2 to 61.1 kg/m^2). Approximately 40% (n=2577) of women were taking HRT.   Average breast density as measured by Quantra^{TM} was 15.2% (SD: 5.4, range: 6-50) compared to 6.6% as measured by Volpara^{TM} (SD: 3.5, range: 1.9-29.2%). The Pearson correlation coefficient for average breast density between Quantra^{TM} and Volpara^{TM} was 0.88.

Table 1. Descriptive analysis of the women in the sample

		Mean	SD	Minimum	Maximum	Number
Age		60.3	6.4	46	74	6398
IMD		26.39	16.7	2.9	81.5	6398
BMI		27.87	5.53	17.1	61.1	5965
Density	Quantra^{TM}	15.17	5.35	6	50	6398
	Volpara^{TM}	6.59	3.5	1.8	29.2	6398

The Pearson Correlation coefficient between IMD and density was -0.11 for Volpara^{TM} (Figure 1) and -0.067 for Quantra^{TM} (Figure 2). When displayed as scatter plots the absence of a strong correlation between IMD and breast density is clear, regardless of the measurement technique used.

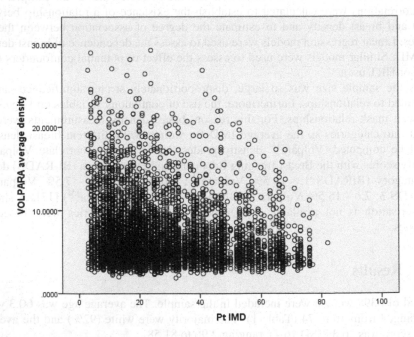

Fig. 1. Relationship between IMD and breast density for Volpara^{TM}

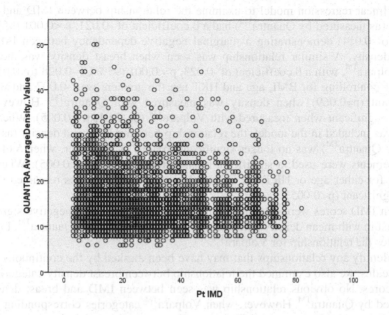

Fig. 2. Relationship between IMD and breast density for Quantra[TM]

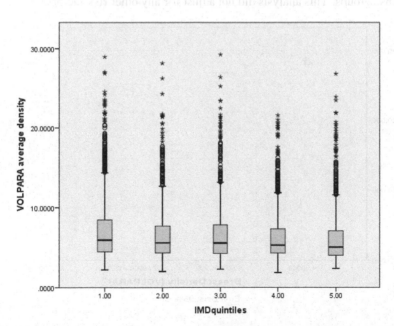

Fig. 3. Box plots of Volpara[TM] average density by IMD score categorised into quintiles

The linear regression model to examine the relationship between IMD and breast density (as measured by Quantra™) had a β coefficient of -0.021, p <0.001 (95% CI - 0.029 to -0.014) demonstrating a marginal negative dependency between IMD and breast density. A similar relationship was seen when breast density was measured with Volpara™, with a β coefficient of -0.023, p <0.001 (95% CI -0.028 to -0.012).

After controlling for BMI, age and HRT use the gradient was -0.007 and was not significant (p=0.069) when density was measured with Quantra™. However, remained significant when measured with Volpara™ (β=-0.01, p <0.005). When BMI alone was included in the model, the relationship between IMD and density (as measured by Quantra™) was no longer significant (p=0.077). However, when Volpara™ measurements were used, a significant relationship remained (p<0.005). When controlling for either age or HRT use independently, the relationships remained statistically significant (p<0.005).

When IMD scores were categorised into quintiles, there was a negative significant relationship with mean density when measured by Volpara™ and Quantra™. Figure 3 illustrates the relationship for Volpara™.

To identify any relationships that may have been masked by the continuous nature of the scales, we also examined the relationship between breast density categories and IMD scores. No obvious relationship was seen between IMD and breast density as measured by Quantra™. However, when Volpara™ categories corresponding to BI-RADS were used the average IMD scores decreased with increasing breast density (Figure 4), with a difference of 7.4 between the average IMD score for the most and least dense groups. This analysis did not adjust for any other risk factors.

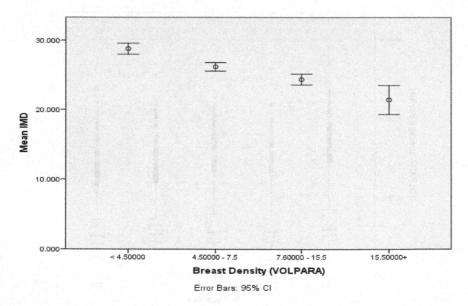

Fig. 4. Graph showing negative trend in the mean IMD for women with different categories of breast density

5   Discussion

Our results show a weak association between SES and volumetric breast density in peri- and post-menopausal women, with women from more deprived areas having slightly less dense breasts. This association persisted after after controlling for age, BMI and HRT use for Volpara^{TM}. By contrast, for Quantra^{TM} the relationship remained significant after controlling for age or HRT use, however further adjustment for BMI rendered the relationship non-significant, suggesting that the association between SES and breast density may be primarily explained by a higher mean BMI in women with a lower SES. This reflects the results found by Aitken et al. [12]. This could be an artefact of the data or it may be due to differences between the two systems; one may be more accurate and therefore more sensitive to slight associations. Volpara^{TM} differs from Quantra^{TM} in that it adjusts for skin volume when assessing the volume of the breast. This may impact on the findings and warrants further investigation.

The current study did not adjust for differences in parity. Age at first pregnancy, number of full term births and pregnancy are associated with both breast cancer risk and SES. Differences in parity and breast feeding are cited as responsible for at least some of the disparities in breast cancer incidence seen between affluent and developing countries and the same may be true between affluent and deprived societies within individual countries.

One limitation of this study is the measurement used to assess SES. The use of IMD is a generally accepted method in health research, but only considers community level SES, rather than individual factors. Furthermore women who attend screening, and who agree to take part in health research studies, are generally more likely to be from the less deprived areas of the population [18]. Women in the current study had a wide range of IMD scores, however the mean was relatively low suggesting that the sample may not be representative of the population as a whole. A potential area for further research would be to make efforts to recruit women from deprived backgrounds to obtain a sample which is representative of the entire population. If evidence suggests that women from a higher SES have denser breasts, these women would be at a higher risk of both developing breast cancer and of having a breast cancer missed at screening due to masking. This may have clinical significance when tailoring breast screening programmes to the risk of individual women.

It may also be interesting to repeat this analysis using an absolute measure of dense tissue volume within the breast, rather than the percentage breast density. By measuring only the volume of dense tissue within the breast and therefore removing the measurement of fatty tissue, it would be possible to eliminate the confounding effect that BMI has on the results and may reveal a direct relationship between SES and actual quantity of dense tissue.

6   Conclusion

This study suggests that there is weak but significant relationship between volumetric breast density and SES as measured by IMD. It is likely that established SES gradients in breast cancer risk are a result of other SES related factors, primarily BMI, rather than mammographic breast density.

The study found a difference between the results obtained using density data from the two respective volumetric density techniques, Quantra™ and Volpara™. This may be an artefact of the data however, and further work is required to assess their reliability and accuracy.

Acknowledgements. We acknowledge the support of the National Institute for Health Research (NIHR) and the Genesis Prevention Appeal for their funding of the PROCAS study. We would like to thank the women who agreed to take part in the study, the radiographers involved in the Greater Manchester Breast Screening Programme and the study staff for recruitment and data collection,. We also thank Hologic Inc. for providing Quantra™ and Matakina Technology Limited for providing Volpara™. This paper presents independent research funded by the National Institute for Health Research (NIHR) under its Programme Grants for Applied Research programme (reference number RP-PG-0707-10031: "Improvement in risk prediction, early detection and prevention of breast cancer"). The views expressed are those of the author(s) and not necessarily those of the NHS, the NIHR, or the Department of Health.

References

1. Heck, K.E., Pamuk, E.R.: Explaining the relation between education and postmenopausal breast cancer. American Journal of Epidemiology 145(4), 366–372 (1997)
2. Braaten, T., Weiderpass, E., Kumle, M., Adami, H.O., Lund, E.: Education and risk of breast cancer in the Norwegian-Swedish women's lifestyle and health cohort study. International Journal of Cancer 110(4), 579–583 (2004)
3. Robert, S.A., Trentham-Dietz, A., Hampton, J.M., McElroy, J.A., Newcomb, P.A., Remington, P.L.: Socioeconomic risk factors for breast cancer: distinguishing individual- and community-level effects. Epidemiology 15(4), 442–450 (2004)
4. Brambilla, D.J., McKinlay, S.M.: A prospective study of factors affecting age at menopause. Journal of Clinical Epidemiology 42(11), 1031–1039 (1989)
5. Rindfuss, R.R., Morgan, S.P., Offutt, K.: Education and the changing age pattern of American fertility: 1963–1989. Demography 33(3), 277–290 (1996)
6. Liu, L., Deapen, D., Bernstein, L.: Socioeconomic status and cancers of the female breast and reproductive organs: a comparison across racial/ethnic populations in Los Angeles County, California (United States). Cancer Causes & Control 9(4), 369–380 (1998)
7. Kaufman, Z., Garstin, W., Hayes, R., Michell, M., Baum, M.: The mammographic parenchymal patterns of women on hormonal replacement therapy. Clinical Radiology 43(6), 389–392 (1991)
8. Egeland, G.M., Matthews, K.A., Kuller, L.H., Kelsey, S.: Characteristics of noncontraceptive hormone users. Preventive Medicine 17(4), 403–411 (1988)
9. Sobal, J., Stunkard, A.J.: Socioeconomic status and obesity: a review of the literature. Psychological Bulletin 105(2), 260–275 (1989)
10. Moser, K., Patnick, J., Beral, V.: Inequalities in reported use of breast and cervical screening in Great Britain: Analysis of cross sectional survey data. British Medical Journal 338, b. 2025 (2009)

11. Vachon, C.M., Kuni, C.C., Anderson, K., Anderson, V.E., Sellers, T.A.: Association of mammographically defined percent breast density with epidemiologic risk factors for breast cancer (United States). Cancer Causes & Control 11(7), 653–662 (2000)
12. Aitken, Z., Walker, K., Stegeman, B., Wark, P., Moss, S., McCormack, V., et al.: Mammographic density and markers of socioeconomic status: a cross-sectional study. BMC Cancer 10(1), 35 (2010)
13. Evans, G.: PROCAS study (2011),
    http://www.uhsm.nhs.uk/research/Pages/PROCASstudy.aspx (June 16, 2013)
14. Hologic- Quantra Volumetric Assessment (2012),
    http://www.hologic.com/en/breast-screening/volumetric-assessment/
15. Volpara Density (2013), http://www.volparadensity.com/
16. Department for Communities and Local Government. English indices of deprivation. Online: GOV.UK (2012),
    https://www.gov.uk/government/organisations/department-for-communities-and-local-government/series/english-indices-of-deprivation (cited June 02, 2013)
17. Sauber, N., Chan, A., Highnam, R.: BI-RADS breast density classification - an international standard? In: EPOS, European Society of Radiology, Online: European Society of Radiology (2013)
18. Gross, C.P., Filardo, G., Mayne, S.T., Krumholz, H.M.: The impact of socioeconomic status and race on trial participation for older women with breast cancer. Cancer 103(3), 483–491 (2005)

Use of Volumetric Breast Density Measures for the Prediction of Weight and Body Mass Index

Elizabeth O. Donovan[1], Jamie Sergeant[2,3], Elaine Harkness[4,5,6], Julie Morris[7], Mary Wilson[4], Yit Lim[4,5], Paula Stavrinos[4], Anthony Howell[4,8], D. Gareth Evans[4,8], Caroline Boggis[4], and Susan M. Astley[4,5,6,8]

[1] Manchester Medical School, University of Manchester, Oxford Road, Manchester, M13 9PT, UK
[2] Arthritis Research UK Centre for Epidemiology, Institute of Inflammation and Repair, Faculty of Medical and Human Sciences, Manchester Academic Health Science Centre, University of Manchester, Oxford Road, Manchester M13 9PT, UK
[3] NIHR Manchester Musculoskeletal Biomedical Research Unit, Central Manchester NHS Foundation Trust, Manchester Academic Health Science Centre, Manchester, UK
[4] Nightingale Centre and Genesis Prevention Centre, University Hospital of South Manchester, Manchester M23 9LT, UK
[5] Centre for Imaging Sciences, Institute of Population Health, Faculty of Medical and Human Sciences, Manchester Academic Health Science Centre, University of Manchester, Oxford Road, Manchester M13 9PT, UK
[6] The University of Manchester, Manchester Academic Health Science Centre, University Hospital of South Manchester NHS Foundation Trust, Wythenshawe, Manchester M23 9LT, UK
[7] Department of Medical Statistics, University Hospital of South Manchester, Manchester M23 9LT, UK
[8] Manchester Breast Centre, Manchester Cancer Research Centre, University of Manchester, Christie Hospital, Withington, Manchester, M20 4BX, UK
sue.astley@manchester.ac.uk

Abstract. Body Mass Index (BMI) is an important confounding factor for breast density assessment, particularly where a relative measure (percentage density) is used. Since height and weight are not routinely collected at screening, we investigated the relationship between breast and fat volumes computed by Quantra™ and Volpara™ and weight/BMI in 6898 women for whom self-reported values are available. A significant positive correlation was found between breast volume and fat volume with both weight and BMI. BMI and Volpara™ average fat volume showed the strongest positive relationship (r = 0.728, p<0.001). Using these results we predicted weight and BMI for a separate group of women; these showed moderate intraclass correlation (ICC) agreement with self-reported weight and BMI. The strongest relationship was with weight predicted using Quantra™ average fat volume (ICC = 0.634, CI = 0.573-0.689, p<0.001), however our results suggest that it is not possible to accurately predict individuals' weight and BMI from volumetric breast density measures.

Keywords: Body Mass Index, breast density, mammogram, weight, breast volume, fat volume.

H. Fujita, T. Hara, and C. Muramatsu (Eds.): IWDM 2014, LNCS 8539, pp. 282–289, 2014.
© Springer International Publishing Switzerland 2014

1   Introduction and Aims

Mammographic density is one of the strongest modifiable risk factors for breast cancer [1]. It is usually reported as a relative measure, describing the proportion of the breast area or volume occupied by radio-dense tissue. However, there is evidence that when women gain weight, they gain breast fat [2]. This results in a decrease in percentage breast density and hence a decrease in the apparent risk of developing breast cancer despite the gain in weight conferring an actual increase in risk for postmenopausal women. Similarly, loss of weight (which is beneficial in terms of breast cancer risk) leads to an increase in percentage density and apparent risk. For this reason, breast density measurements made for the purpose of assessing cancer risk are often corrected for Body Mass Index (BMI) or weight as well as age[3,4].

As weight is not routinely recorded at mammographic screening, and the weight of many women changes between screens, it would be advantageous to find a surrogate measure that could be used to correct relative density measures. It has been proposed that the breast volume or fat volume computed by commercial breast density software could be used in this way [5]. The aim of this research is to evaluate whether this would be appropriate.

2   Method

Data for women recruited to the Predicting Risk Of Cancer At Screening (PROCAS) study were obtained for this analysis. Women in PROCAS complete a questionnaire giving personal information including height, weight and clothes size at the time of screening, and their digital screening mammograms were analysed with Quantra^{TM} (Version 1.3; Hologic Inc.) and Volpara^{TM} (Version 1.3.1; Mātakina International Ltd.) to provide volumetric breast density data. Quantra^{TM} output total breast volume and dense tissue volume for both breasts, combining data from craniocaudal (CC) and mediolateral oblique (MLO) views. A single average total breast volume was calculated for each case. The fat volume was obtained by subtracting the dense tissue volume from the total breast volume. A single average fat volume measurement was obtained in each case. Volpara^{TM} gave measures of average breast volume and average fat volume from both left and right breast. It also provided average total breast volume and average fat volume for each case.

Women were excluded if they had had a previous breast cancer or tissue biopsy; if essential data were missing or invalid; or if their recorded clothes size was unrealistic for their calculated BMI. We thus analysed a sample of 7398 records out of which 500 randomly selected records were set aside for evaluation purposes leaving a sample population of 6898 records. Weight ranged from 36kg to 172kg and BMI from 15.17 to 62.38, with 95.7% declaring themselves to be White British or Irish.

To test the significance of a possible association between weight or BMI and the volumetric breast measures Pearson correlation was used. This was run as a two-tailed test and a correlation co-efficient (r) > 0.4 was taken as a positive correlation between two variables. Due to the large population size, an additional criterion of r>0.7 was used to indicate a significant association, in this instance the correlation squared (r^2) is 0.49 which would indicate that almost half of the variation in 'true' BMI (or weight) between women could be explained by the prediction model.

Linear regression was used to produce predictive models for weight and BMI from the sample population; these models were applied to the test set data in order to predict weight and BMI for these 500 women. Predicted values were then compared with self-reported weight and BMI values and analysed by calculating intraclass correlation.

Finally, to increase the data available for testing, the predictive models were applied to the entire data set available and histograms plotted to show the differences between self reported and calculated weights and BMIs.

3   Results

All volumetric breast measurements showed a positive correlation with either weight or BMI (Table 1). Figure 1 shows an example plot for weight *vs* Volpara™ breast volume. In general the points on the graphs become more scattered with increasing volumetric measurements, suggesting that predictive models may perform better for women of lower weight /BMI.

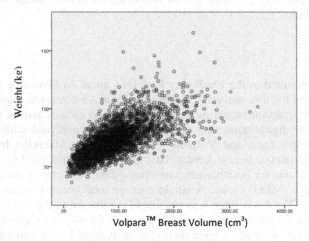

Fig. 1. Self-reported weight plotted against breast volume measured by Volpara™

Table 1. Correlations between density measures and self-reported weight and BMI in the sample population

Breast Density measure	Weight or BMI	Co-efficient Value	p value
Quantra™ Breast Volume	Weight	0.688	<0.001
Quantra™ Fat Volume	Weight	0.695	<0.001
Volpara™ Breast Volume	Weight	0.709	<0.001
Volpara™ Fat Volume	Weight	0.712	<0.001
Quantra™ Breast Volume	BMI	0.701	<0.001
Quantra™ Fat Volume	BMI	0.710	<0.001
Volpara™ Breast Volume	BMI	0.724	<0.001
Volpara™ Fat Volume	BMI	0.728	<0.001

Regression lines were plotted for the sample population of 6898 women, and for data from a separate group of women; an example is shown in figure 2. These graphs show a discrepancy between the two respective regression lines.

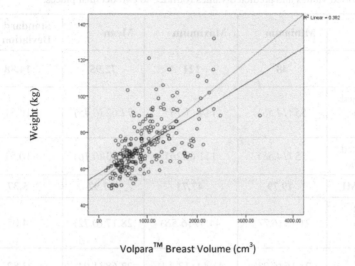

Volpara^{TM} Breast Volume (cm³)

Fig. 2. A pairwise scatterplot of Volpara^{TM} breast volume measurements and self-reported weight from a separate group of 237 women with the regression line (steeper gradient, depicted in red) and the corresponding regression line (depicted in black) from the sample population

For illustration of the application of a prediction model, the self-reported and predicted values for the minimum, maximum and mean self-reported weights and BMIs in a separate group of women were obtained and are presented for Quantra^{TM} in table 2 and for Volpara^{TM} in table 3.

Intraclass correlation (ICC) was used to assess agreement between predicted and self-reported values. For all predicted values, the ICCs indicated moderate agreement. For weight, the ICC ranged between 0.609 - 0.634. The lowest ICC agreement was obtained when using the values predicted using Volpara^{TM} breast volume data where the ICC = 0.609 (CI = 0.522 – 0.683, $p < 0.001$). The highest ICC agreement was obtained when using the values predicted using Quantra^{TM} fat volume data, where the ICC = 0.634 (CI = 0.573 – 0.689, $p < 0.001$).

For BMI the ICC ranged between 0.594 - 0.629. This indicates a slightly weaker agreement between these predicted values and self-reported values than for weight. The lowest ICC agreement between self-reported and predicted values was obtained with values predicted using Volpara^{TM} breast volume data where the ICC = 0.594 (CI = 0.505 – 0.671, $p < 0.001$). The highest ICC was the same for two of the sets of predicted values analysed against self-reported values, the values predicted using Quantra^{TM} breast volume data and those predicted using Quantra^{TM} fat volume data where the ICC = 0.629 (CI = 0.567 – 0.685, $p < 0.001$).

Table 2. Self-reported and predicted weight and BMI in a separate group of 408 women. The predicted values were obtained using the appropriate regression formula obtained from Quantra™ measurements in the sample population. Bracketed values are percentage difference between self-reported values and predicted values rounded to two decimal places.

Variable	Minimum	Maximum	Mean	Standard Deviation
Self-reported weight	**48**	**121**	**72.95**	**14.88**
Weight predicted from breast volume	55 (*14.58*)	114 (*5.78*)	72.62 (*0.45*)	10.31
Weight predicted from fat volume	55 (*14.58*)	111 (*8.26*)	72.83 (*0.16*)	10.51
Calculated BMI	**19.79**	**47.71**	**27.97**	**5.37**
BMI predicted from breast volume	21.13 (*6.77*)	44.57 (*6.58*)	28.17 (0.72)	4.05
BMI predicted from fat volume	21.16 (*6.92*)	41.44 (13.14)	27.68 (1.04)	3.82

Table 3. Self-reported and predicted weight and BMI in a separate group of 237 women. The predicted values were obtained using the appropriate regression formula obtained from Volpara™ measurements in the sample population. Bracketed values are percentage difference between self-reported values and predicted values rounded to two decimal places.

Variable	Minimum	Maximum	Mean	Standard Deviation
Self-reported weight	**49**	**132**	**72.90**	**13.85**
Weight predicted from Breast Volume	56 (14.29)	125 (5.30)	73.32 (0.58)	11.47
Weight predicted from Fat Volume	56 (14.29)	123 (6.82)	72.94 (0.05)	11.31
Calculated BMI	**19.49**	**53.15**	**27.96**	**5.45**
BMI predicted from Breast Volume	21.37 (9.64)	46.58 (12.36)	27.80 (0.57)	4.17
BMI predicted from Fat Volume	21.35 (9.54)	45.98 (13.49)	27.66 (1.07)	4.11

Frequency histograms showing the difference between actual (self-reported) and predicted weight and BMI values and those calculated by applying the predictive models to the entire dataset are shown in figure 3.

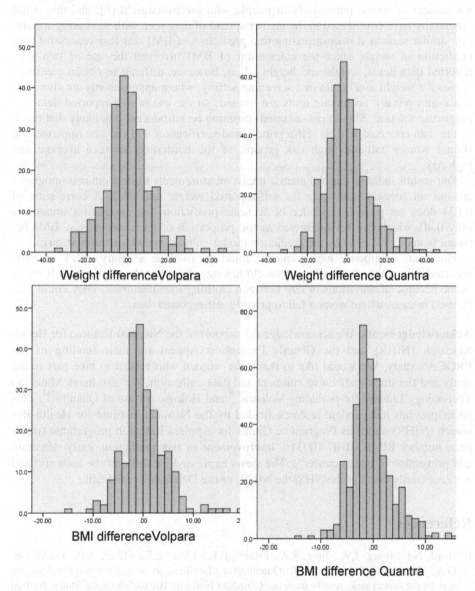

Fig. 3. Frequency histograms showing the difference between actual (self reported) and predicted weight (top row) and BMI (bottom row) for all data using models based on VolparaTM (left column) and QuantraTM (right column)

4   Conclusions and Discussion

One of the limitations of this work is that we have assessed the volumetric measures against self-reported, rather than measured, values. It is known that self-reported data are subject to errors, particularly in people who are overweight [6], and this could potentially have contributed to the greater spread of data seen with increasing weight. For similar reasons it is unsurprising that prediction of BMI was less successful than prediction of weight since the calculation of BMI involved the use of two self-reported data items, weight and height. It is, however, difficult to obtain measured values for weight and height in a screening setting, where appointments are short and space and privacy on mobile units are limited, so the use of self-reported data is a pragmatic solution. Should risk-adapted screening be introduced, it is likely that much of the data collected will be self-reported, and verification will only be implemented should women fall into high risk groups, or the borderline between average and high risk.

Our results indicate that volumetric breast measurements made from mammograms are not an adequate surrogate for self-reported weight and BMI. A correlation of 0.634 does not provide evidence of accurate prediction (the correlation squared is only 0.40, which can be interpreted as the proportion of variation in 'true' BMI between women explained by the prediction model – this is not a large proportion).

However, volumetric measurements could be used as a sanity check on self-reported data, rather than asking about clothes size, for example, which is itself error-prone because of variations in size between clothing manufacturers. They could also be used in cases where women fail to provide self-reported data.

Acknowledgements. We acknowledge the support of the National Institute for Health Research (NIHR) and the Genesis Prevention Appeal for their funding of the PROCAS study. We would like to thank the women who agreed to take part in the study and the study staff for recruitment and data collection. We also thank Matakina Technology Limited for providing Volpara^{TM} and Hologic for use of Quantra^{TM}. This paper presents independent research funded by the National Institute for Health Research (NIHR) under its Programme Grants for Applied Research programme (reference number RP-PG-0707-10031: "Improvement in risk prediction, early detection and prevention of breast cancer"). The views expressed are those of the author(s) and not necessarily those of the NHS, the NIHR, or the Department of Health.

References

1. Boyd, N.F., Byng, J.W., Jong, R.A., Fishell, E.K., Little, L.E., Miller, A.B., Lockwood, G.A., Tritchler, D.L., Yaffe, M.J.: Quantitative classification of mammographic densities and breast cancer risk: results from the Canadian National Breast Screening Study. Journal of the National Cancer Institute 87(9), 670–675 (1995)
2. Patel, H.G., et al.: Automated Breast Tissue Measurement of Women at Increased Risk of Breast Cancer. In: Astley, S.M., Brady, M., Rose, C., Zwiggelaar, R. (eds.) IWDM 2006. LNCS, vol. 4046, pp. 131–136. Springer, Heidelberg (2006)

3. Rutter, C.M., Mandelson, M.T., Laya, M.B., Taplin, S.: Changes in breast density associated with initiation, discontinuation, and continuing use of hormone replacement therapy. Jama 285(2), 171–176 (2001)
4. Nutine, L., Sergeant, J.C., Morris, J., Stavrinos, P., Evans, D.G., Howell, T., Boggis, C., Wilson, M., Barr, N., Astley, S.M.: Volumetric and area-based measures of mammographic density in women with and without cancer. In: Maidment, A.D.A., Bakic, P.R., Gavenonis, S. (eds.) IWDM 2012. LNCS, vol. 7361, pp. 589–595. Springer, Heidelberg (2012)
5. Ellison-Loschmann, L., McKenzie, F., Highnam, R., Cave, A., Walker, J., Jeffreys, M.: Age and Ethnic Differences in Volumetric Breast Density in New Zealand Women: A Cross-Sectional Study. PloS one 8(7), e70217 (2013)
6. Rowland, M.L.: Self-reported weight and height. The American Journal of Clinical Nutrition 52(6), 1125–1133 (1990)

Mammographic Density and Breast Cancer Characteristics

Kathy Ren[1], Elaine Harkness[2,3,4], Caroline Boggis[2], Soujanya Gadde[2],
Mary Wilson[2], Yit Lim[2,3], Jamie Sergeant[3,5,6], Sigrid Whiteside[7],
Julie Morris[7], and Susan M. Astley[2,3,4,8]

[1] Manchester Medical School, University of Manchester, Oxford Road, Manchester, M13 9PT,
UK
[2] Nightingale Centre and Genesis Prevention Centre, University Hospital of South Manchester,
Manchester M23 9LT, UK
[3] Centre for Imaging Sciences, Institute of Population Health, Faculty of Medical and Human
Sciences, Manchester Academic Health Science Centre, University of Manchester, Oxford
Road, Manchester M13 9PT, UK
[4] The University of Manchester, Manchester Academic Health Science Centre, University
Hospital of South Manchester NHS Foundation Trust, Wythenshawe, Manchester M23 9LT,
UK
[5] Arthritis Research UK Centre for Epidemiology, Institute of Inflammation and Repair, Faculty
of Medical and Human Sciences, Manchester Academic Health Science Centre, University of
Manchester, Oxford Road, Manchester M13 9PT, UK
[6] NIHR Manchester Musculoskeletal Biomedical Research Unit, Central Manchester NHS
Foundation Trust, Manchester Academic Health Science Centre, Manchester, UK
[7] Department of Medical Statistics, University Hospital of South Manchester, Manchester M23
9LT, UK
[8] Manchester Breast Centre, Manchester Cancer Research Centre, University of Manchester,
Christie Hospital, Withington, Manchester, M20 4BX, UK
sue.astley@manchester.ac.uk

Abstract. The aim of this research is to investigate, in a screening population,
the relationship between mammographic density and tumour characteristics
including size, invasiveness and mammographic features. Mammograms of 105
women with screen detected breast cancer were analysed; 111 lesions were
identified. Volumetric density measurements were obtained using Quanta™ and
Volpara™. Histological information was extracted from the screening database
and radiological features were assessed by two expert breast radiologists.
Statistical analysis was performed using Mann-Whitney U test and Spearman's
rank order correlation. The median percentage density by Volpara™ of women
with invasive cancers was significantly higher than those with DCIS (6.5 *vs* 5.0,
p =0.046). Similar results were replicated in the Quantra™ measurements,
however the results were not statistically significant (17 *vs* 16, p = 0.19).
Further analysis showed a significant positive association between whole
tumour size and volumetric density for invasive lesions. Architectural distortion
was the only mammographic feature associated with a significant difference in
percentage density.

H. Fujita, T. Hara, and C. Muramatsu (Eds.): IWDM 2014, LNCS 8539, pp. 290–297, 2014.
© Springer International Publishing Switzerland 2014

Keywords: Screening, mammogram, cancer, volumetric breast density, invasive, DCIS, distortion.

1   Introduction

1.1   Breast Density

Breast density, measured as the proportion of the breast occupied by radiodense fibroglandular tissue, is an important risk factor for breast cancer, with women with relatively large proportions of fibroglandular tissue at greatly increased risk compared with those with predominantly fatty breasts [1]. High breast density has also been shown to adversely affect cancer detection in mammograms, and has been related to an increased risk of recurrence after treatment [2,3]. The majority of studies using breast density have involved subjective assessments, with or without assistance from software that allows the user to manipulate a threshold on the mammogram's grey levels to select regions of density [4]. These measures are usually relative (expressing the proportion of dense tissue relative to the overall size of the breast) and area-based. Recent technological developments, and especially the advent of Full Field Digital Mammography (FFDM), have resulted in commercially available software that automatically calculates volumetric breast density from digital mammograms [5,6], paving the way for more robust studies of the relationship between breast density and other factors. These methods also permit measurement of the absolute volumes of dense and fatty tissue rather than relative measures. In this paper we investigate the relationship between volumetric breast density and the characteristics of screen-detected cancers.

1.2   Breast Cancer

Breast cancers can be classified according to the site of origin (e.g. lobular, ductal) and the level of invasiveness (invasive versus non invasive).

Ductal carcinoma in situ (DCIS) is a type of non-invasive breast cancer where the malignant cells have not proliferated beyond the basement membrane. It is considered to be a precursor of invasive carcinoma and must be treated appropriately. DCIS can be classified according to its architectural structure (e.g. cribriform, papillary, etc), tumour grade and the presence of comedo necrosis (associated with poorer prognosis). It is usually asymptomatic, presenting as clustered microcalcifications on screening mammograms. Lobular carcinoma in situ (LCIS) is similar to DCIS, but originates in breast lobules rather than ducts. It does not behave like DCIS, as it does not become cancerous if left untreated.

In invasive breast cancer (primary or secondary), the malignant cells have infiltrated the tissues beyond the basement membrane of the duct or lobule. Once this has spread beyond the breast tissues and the ipsi-lateral lymph nodes, it is termed metastatic breast cancer.

Suspicious breast lesions are usually evaluated using the 'triple assessment' method. This consists of clinical examination, followed by imaging (e.g. mammography, ultrasound) and image guided biopsies (e.g. fine needle aspiration, core needle biopsy). This method can reliably discriminate malignant masses from benign ones.

2   Aims

The aims of this work are to determine, in screen detected mammograms, if larger tumours are found in denser breasts, and whether the lesions detected in denser breasts are more invasive.

3   Method

A total of 105 consecutive women with screen detected cancer, for whom density had been measured by two volumetric breast density methods, were identified from a UK National Health Service Breast Screening Programme database. Prevalent round cancers were excluded, and all the women included had previously been screened by mammography approximately 3 years before detection of cancer. Since 2 of the women had 3 identified lesions and 2 further women had 2 separate lesions, 111 lesions were included in the analysis

Two experienced radiologists assessed the mammographic features found on the mammograms. All suspicious lesions were classified into five categories: spiculated mass; ill defined mass; microcalcifications; architectural distortion; and asymmetrical density. Along with the mammographic features, further information regarding the size of the tumours was also collected from histology reports recorded in the national screening database. All data were anonymised.

Breast density was measured by Quantra™ version 1.3 from Hologic and Volpara™ software version 1.4.0 from Matakina; the volumetric percentage density per breast was used in subsequent analyses. As the data were not normally distributed, Spearman's rank-order correlation coefficient was calculated to assess the relationship between volumetric density and the tumour size. Comparison of density in invasive and non-invasive cancers was undertaken using the Mann- Whitney U test.

4   Results

Table 1 shows the frequencies of lesion characteristics in the study population; the majority of lesions were invasive, and the most common sign of abnormality was microcalcifications. Table 2 shows median percentage volumetric breast density in invasive and non-invasive cancers; density was significantly higher when assessed with Volpara™, and the density distributions are illustrated in Figure 1.

Table 1. Characteristics of lesions in the dataset

Characteristics of lesion	Left Breast	Right Breast	Total
Ill defined mass	13	8	21
Spiculated Mass	13	16	29
Microcalcifications	24	20	44
Asymmetric density	11	11	22
Architectural distortion	8	4	12
Invasive cancers	42	35	77
DCIS	22	12	34
Total	64	47	111

Table 2. Median contralateral breast density of women with invasive and non-invasive unilateral screen detected cancers

	Density (Quantra™)	Density (Volpara™)
Invasive	17	6.5
Non-invasive	16	5.0
P value	0.189	0.046

Table 3. Correlation between density measure and whole tumour size for invasive and in situ tumours

	Spearman's rank correlation coefficient (rho coefficient)	p value
Invasive tumours		
Quantra™	0.284	0.013
Volpara™	0.355	0.002
In Situ tumours		
Quantra™	-0.114	0.523
Volpara™	-0.036	0.841
All tumours		
Quantra™	0.100	0.296
Volpara™	0.160	0.093

Table 3 shows the Spearman rank correlations for the whole tumour size *vs* density for the invasive (significant positive association) and in situ cancers (negative but non-significant) separately, and for all tumours. No significant correlation was found between tumour size and mammographic density in the contralateral breast for either density method for invasive cancers or for DCIS.

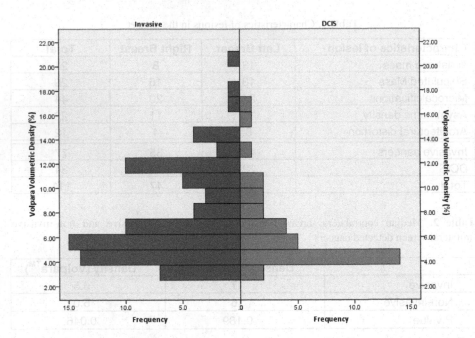

Fig. 1. Volpara™ density distribution for invasive cancers (blue, left hand side) and non-invasive cancers (green, right hand side)

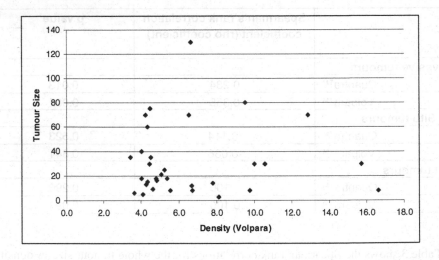

Fig. 2. Whole tumour size (mm) *vs* volumetric breast density for in situ cancers

Figures 2 and 3 show whole tumour size *vs* breast density for in situ and invasive lesions respectively.

Figures 4 and 5 depict the difference in density between the affected and unaffected breast; the differences were obtained by subtracting the volumetric breast density in the normal breast from the volumetric breast density in the breast containing the lesion or lesions. Results from Quantra™ are presented, but those from Volpara™ yield a similar pattern of results. The range of Quantra™ breast density values for all images was 9-48 with the lowest density being in an image showing cancer and the highest in a normal breast. The maximum difference in density between the two breasts was 8 percentage points, and the largest differences were found in mammograms containing microcalcification.

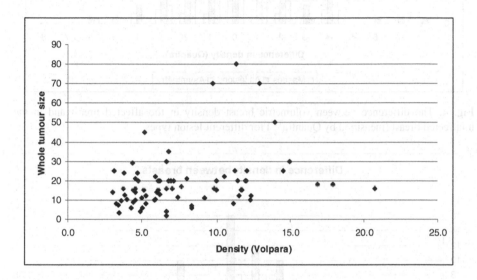

Fig. 3. Whole tumour size (mm) *vs* volumetric breast density for invasive cancers

Comparing those cancer cases with a particular sign of abnormality with those without, the only sign in which significantly higher breast density was found was architectural distortion (p=0.002 for density measured with Quantra™ and p=0.007 for density measured by Volpara™).

5   Discussion

Previous studies have shown a positive link between percentage density and tumour size. Our results were consistent with this in that the relationship for invasive lesions was positive. Such an association could be attributed to the masking effects of dense glandular tissue so lesions are not detected during earlier screening mammograms. However, we did not observe a similar relationship for in situ breast cancer.

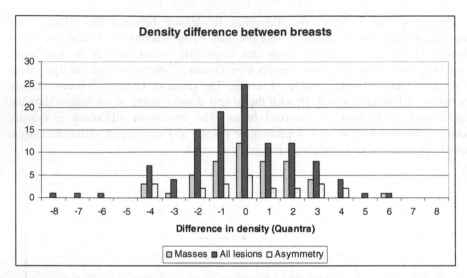

Fig. 4. The difference between volumetric breast density in the affected breast and in the unaffected breast (measured by Quantra™) for different lesion types

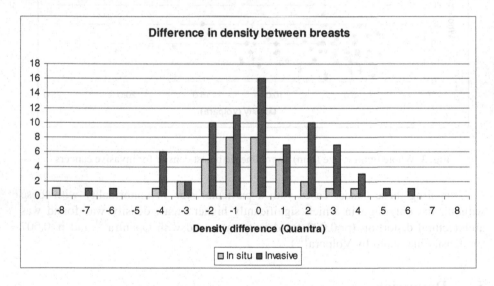

Fig. 5. The difference between volumetric breast density in the affected breast and in the unaffected breast (measured by Quantra™) for invasive and in situ lesions

In this study, density difference between the affected and unaffected breasts showed a similar pattern for invasive and in situ cancers and did not show a systematic increase in density in the affected breast. The larger differences were not due to asymmetries, but tended to be in breasts in which there was microcalcification. This merits further investigation of the degree of microcalcification and the density of the breast.

Breasts containing architectural distortion had significantly higher density to those without, possibly reflecting the more extensive nature of the sign.

The mean percentage density of the invasive cancer group was significantly higher than DCIS group. This is consistent with an association between dense glandular tissues and high concentrations of insulin like growth factor (IGF-1), which may promote cellular activity and growth, resulting in tumours of a more invasive nature.

References

1. Boyd, N.F., Byng, J.W., Jong, R.A., Fishell, E.K., Little, L.E., Miller, A.B., Lockwood, G.A., Tritchler, D.L., Yaffe, M.J.: Quantitative classification of mammographic densities and breast cancer risk: results from the Canadian National Breast Screening Study. Journal of the National Cancer Institute 87(9), 670–675 (1995)
2. Kerlikowske, K., Grady, D., Barclay, J., Sickles, E.A., Ernster, V.: Effect of age, breast density, and family history on the sensitivity of first screening mammography. Jama 276(1), 33–38 (1996)
3. Maskarinec, G., Woolcott, C.G., Kolonel, L.N.: Mammographic density as a predictor of breast cancer outcome. Future Oncology 6(3), 351–354 (2010)
4. Boyd, N.F., Byng, J.W., Jong, R.A., Fishell, E.K., Little, L.E., Miller, A.B., Lockwood, G.A., Tritchler, D.L., Yaffe, M.J.: Quantitative classification of mammographic densities and breast cancer risk: results from the Canadian National Breast Screening Study. J. Natl. Cancer Inst. 87, 670–675 (1995)
5. http://volparasolutions.com/
6. http://www.hologic.com/en/breast-screening/volumetric-assessment/

Managing Tiled Images in Breast Density Measurements

Jennifer Harvey[1,*], Olivier Alonzo[2], Gordon Mawdsley[2],
Taghreed Alshafeiy[3], Ralph Highnam[4], and Martin Yaffe[2]

[1] Department of Radiology, University of Virginia, Charlottesville, Virginia, United States
jharvey@virginia.edu
[2] Department of Physical Sciences, Sunnybrook Health Sciences Center, Toronto, Ontario,
Canada
{oliviera,Gord.Mawdsley,martin.yaffe}@sri.utoronto.ca
[3] Suez Canal University, Suez, Egypt
taghreedi.alshafeiy@gmail.com
[4] Volpara Solutions, Wellington, New Zealand
ralph.highnam@volparasolutions.com

Abstract. Tiled images are sometimes obtained for women with large breasts, which is a limitation of receptor size. In this retrospective HIPAA compliant study, automated breast density measurements for tiled images are compared with full MLO and CC views. Women with tiled views between July and December 2007 followed by full views within 15 months were included. Volumetric breast density (VBD) for tiled MLO views had very good correlation with full views (r = 0.88), while correlation between tiled and full CC views was poor (r = 0.31). VBD for all women requiring tiled CC views was low (<10%). In conclusion, VBD measured from a tiled MLO view is a reasonable substitute for a full MLO measure. Attributable risk of breast density for women requiring tiled CC views may be sufficiently low compared other factors such as high body mass index.

Keywords: Breast density, Mammography, Measures, Risk Models.

1 Introduction

Mammographic breast density is an important risk factor for breast cancer. Women with high mammographic breast density are at 4-fold higher risk for breast cancer compared with women with fatty breasts [1-2]. Incorporation of breast density into a breast cancer risk model may improve accuracy of risk assessment. For optimal use in a risk model, the measurement of mammographic breast density must be automated, accurate, and reproducible.

The accuracy of a measurement depends upon both the validity and reproducibility of the measure. A recent study has found high correlation between the percent breast density obtained using an automated volumetric measurement from mammography (Volpara, Volpara Solutions, Wellington, NZ) and breast magnetic resonance imaging (MRI)

---

* Corresponding author.

H. Fujita, T. Hara, and C. Muramatsu (Eds.): IWDM 2014, LNCS 8539, pp. 298–303, 2014.

[3]. Typically, the measurements from all craniocaudal (CC) and mediolateral oblique (MLO) views are averaged together. However, images without a complete skin line cannot be analyzed using this software. This can occur when multiple projections are obtained due to large breast size relative to the size of the imaging receptor.

Digital mammography receptors vary in size from 19 x 23 cm to 24 x 30 cm. Women with small to average sized breasts will typically have two views of each breast for a screening mammogram; craniocaudal (CC) and mediolateral oblique (MLO) views. However, many large breasts cannot be completely imaged on a small receptor. These women may require two or three images to completely visualize the breast tissue for each projection. Measuring breast density on these tiled images may or may not reflect density measures that would be obtained using a single image of the same breast using a larger detector. The goal of this study is to evaluate if the volumetric breast density (VBD) of tiled MLO or CC images may reasonably approximate the VBD of the full view.

2   Methods

This retrospective study was HIPAA compliant and approved by our Institutional Review Board. A waiver of consent was granted.

We performed a retrospective review of women who underwent mammography on a small image receptor between July and December 2007 at our screening facility to identify women with tiled images. The primary screening site at one author institution (JAH) added a large receptor mammography machine in 2008. Women with either tiled CC or MLO images on a small receptor followed by a single projection image on a large receptor within 15 months were included in the study. Women with a full view obtained greater than 15 months later were excluded as there may be other reasons for changes in breast density such as normal involution.

Breast density was measured on tiled and single projection images using a validated automated measurement software program (Volpara, Volpara Solutions, Wellington, NZ). Briefly, Volpara applies an advanced method to identify a fatty reference point, such that there is less dependence upon accuracy of the compressed breast thickness readout [4].

Pearson correlation coefficients were obtained for each dataset, comparing results for tiled versus full views.

3   Results

Over 1800 women underwent screening mammography on the small image receptor machine between July and December 2007. Of these, only eight women with 15 breasts had tiled MLO views followed by a single projection MLO view on a large receptor within 15 months (Figure 1). Likewise, only seven women with 14 breasts underwent tiled CC views followed by a single projection CC view on a large receptor within 15 months (Figure 2). Two of these patients were excluded; automated density readings could not be obtained as a skin line was not detectable on the images, leaving five patients with tiled CC views for analysis.

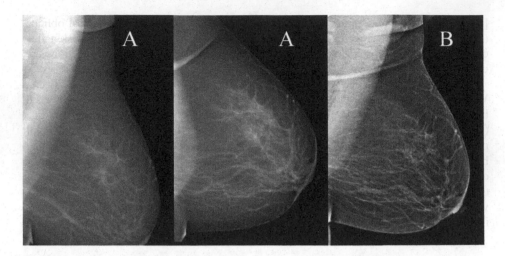

Fig. 1. Tiled MLO views were required to completely image the left breast on the first study (A), but could be completely imaged in one view on the second study (B)

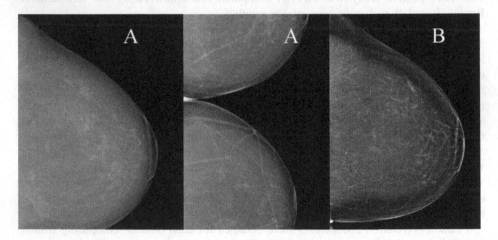

Fig. 2. On the first study (A), the medial left breast was not imaged on the receptor, so a cleavage view was obtained. The entire breast was imaged completely on the larger receptor used on the second study (B).

For the MLO views, VBD for tiled views ranged from 2.0 to 18.9% (mean 6.0%, while VBD for full views ranged from 2.5 to 17.2% (mean 5.9%). Only one patient had a VBD of greater than 10%. Correlation between tiled and full VBD was very good (r = 0.88) (Figure 3). Body mass index (BMI) for these patients ranged from 24.2 to 37.8 (mean 30.0); one patient was normal weight, three patients were overweight, and four patients were obese.

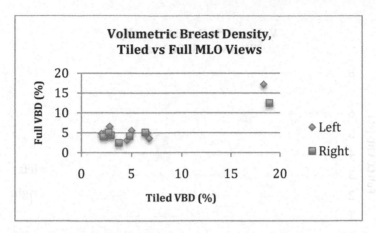

Fig. 3. Automated volumetric breast density of tiled versus full mammographic view for the left and right MLO views. Correlation is very good (r = 0.88).

As expected, total volume of the breast was lower for tiled views (range 725-1772 cm³, mean 1336 cm³) than full MLO views (range 856-2299 cm³, mean 1656 cm³) (Figure 4). The correlation is only good (r = 0.71).

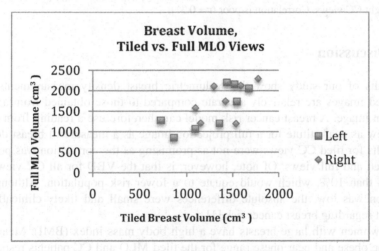

Fig. 4. Automated breast volume of tiled versus full mammographic view for the left and right MLO views. Correlation is good (r = 0.71), but lower than for VBD.

For the CC views, VBD for tiled views (range 4.0-10.1%, mean 6.9%) was similar to full CC views (range 1.9-7.6%, mean 4.5%). However, the correlation was poor (r = 0.31) (figure 5). Total breast volume results for tiled CC views (range 657-1846 cm³, mean 1129 cm³) were similar to results for full CC views (range 856-2123 cm³, mean 1262 cm³). Correlation for total breast volume was very good for tiled compared with full CC views (r = 0.83). BMI for these patients ranged from 23.5 to 37.8 (mean 29.3); one patient was normal weight, two were overweight, and two were obese.

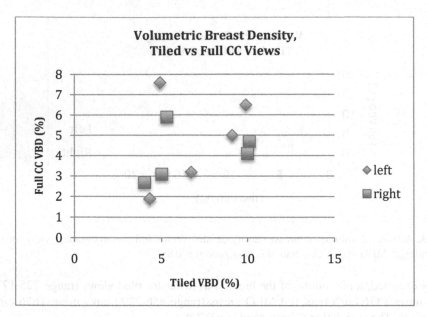

Fig. 5. Automated volumetric breast density of tiled versus full mammographic view for the left and right CC views. Correlation is poor (r = 0.31).

4   Discussion

The results of our study show that volumetric breast density measurements from MLO tiled images are relatively accurate compared to those obtained from a single projection image. A breast cancer risk model can therefore use a reading from a tiled MLO view as a substitute for a full projection image as a measure of breast density. The results for tiled CC views were not as promising as the correlation was poor between tiled and full views. Of note, however, is that the VBD for all CC views was low, less than 10%, which would equate to a lower risk population. Although the correlation was low, the absolute differences were small and likely clinically less important regarding breast cancer risk [1].

Most women with large breasts have a high body mass index (BMI). Mean BMI was in the obese and near obese range for the tiled MLO and CC patients respectively. Obesity increases the amount of fat in the breasts resulting in a lower percent breast density. Our study shows that the percent density for most women with large breasts is reasonably reflected with a low value using either a single tiled view or a full single projection view. Therefore, the use of an automated density measurement from a single tiled view is an acceptable alternative for inclusion in a breast cancer risk assessment model.

Incorporation of breast density into a breast cancer risk model must include adjustment for BMI [5]. Obesity, like breast density, is also an independent breast cancer risk factor [5]. Fatty tissue has high levels of aromatase, an enzyme that converts steroids to estrogens. Although women with a high BMI typically have a low percent breast density, their breast cancer risk may be more significantly driven by their obesity. Because BMI and breast density are independent breast cancer risk factors that can influence each other, the breast cancer risk associated with breast density must be adjusted for BMI.

Our study has limitations. Although the review included a large number of women, only a small number met inclusion criteria, which is a major limitation of our study. A prospective study with a larger number of women may be helpful to confirm these results. A second limitation is the use of only one type of automated density software.

In summary, our study shows that an automated measurement of breast density using a single tiled MLO image may be an adequate reflection of the density obtained from a full mammographic image. The use of VBD from a tiled CC view may not correlate as well with VBD obtained using the full CC view. However, this may be less important given the overall low density of women requiring the use of tiled views. Breast cancer risk for these women may be driven more significantly by high BMI than dense breast tissue.

References

1. Boyd, N.F., Guo, H., Martin, L.J., Sun, L., Stone, J., Fishell, E., Jong, R.A., Hislop, G., Chiarelli, A., Minkin, S., Yaffe, M.J.: Mammographic Density and the Risk and Detection of Breast Cancer. N. Engl. J. Med. 356, 227–236 (2007)
2. Harvey, J.A., Bovbjerg, V.E.: Quantitative assessment of mammographic breast density: Relationship with breast cancer risk. Radiol. 230, 29–41 (2004)
3. Gubern-Merida, A., Kallenberg, M., Platel, B., Mann, R.M., Marti, R., Karssemeijer, N.: Volumetric Breast Density Estimation from Full-Field Digital Mammograms: A Validation Study. PLoS One 9, e85952 (2014)
4. Highnam, R., Brady, S.M., Yaffe, M.J., Karssemeijer, N., Harvey, J.: Robust Breast Composition Measurement - Volpara™. In: Martí, J., Oliver, A., Freixenet, J., Martí, R. (eds.) IWDM 2010. LNCS, vol. 6136, pp. 342–349. Springer, Heidelberg (2010)
5. Lam, P.B., Vacek, P.M., Geller, B.M., Muss, H.B.: The association of increased weight, body mass index, and tissue density with the risk of breast carcinoma in Vermont. Cancer 89, 369–375 (2000)

Reliability of Breast Density Estimation in Follow-Up Mammograms: Repeatability and Reproducibility of a Fully Automated Areal Percent Density Method

Youngwoo Kim[1] and Jong Hyo Kim[2,*]

[1] Interdisciplinary Program of Radiation Applied Life Science,
Seoul National University College of Medicine, Seoul, Republic of Korea
ywkim09@snu.ac.kr
[2] Department of Transdisciplinary Studies, Seoul National University,
Suwon, Republic of Korea
kimjhyo@snu.ac.kr

Abstract. The aim of this study is to evaluate the reliability of the mammographic density estimations in follow-up examinations as measured by using a fully automated density estimation tool in terms of reproducibility and temporal stability. In our previous study, we have developed the fully automated mammographic density estimation method named as SIGMAM, which is based on the prior statistics of mammograms integrated into a novel level set scheme driven by a population-based tissue probability map (PTPM). This scheme was designed to capture the implicit knowledge of experts' visual systems in which the learned knowledge was modeled as the PTPM, which was shown to provide relatively high correlation coefficient of 0.93 with experts' estimations in a single equipment study (Senographe 2000D, GE). In this study, we evaluate the reliability of our SIGMAM method in follow-up mammogram examinations with respect to temporal stability and reproducibility. For evaluation of temporal stability, we selected 170 pairs of CC-view mammograms of 170 female patients taken with the same equipment (Senographe 2000D, GE) within one year from the breast cancer screening database in our institute. On the other hand, we collected pairs of mammograms taken with switched equipment: switched from GE (Senographe DS or Essential) to Hologic (Selenia). In total, 53 pairs of CC-view mammograms from 38 female patients taken within one or two months regarding the menstrual cycle were established as a dataset for reproducibility validation. The correlation coefficient of density estimates in temporal stability mammograms was 0.92, while that of the reproducibility mammograms was 0.87. In conclusion, our SIGMAM method showed relatively high reliability in both reproducibility and temporal stability.

Keywords: CAD, level set, prior knowledge, density, estimation, evaluation.

---

* Corresponding author.

H. Fujita, T. Hara, and C. Muramatsu (Eds.): IWDM 2014, LNCS 8539, pp. 304–311, 2014.
© Springer International Publishing Switzerland 2014

1   Introduction

Mammographic breast density (MBD) refers to the proportion of glandular tissues within the breast area, which has been regarded as a strong biomarker for breast cancer since the pioneering report by Wolfe [1], and Boyd *et al.* showed that higher mammographic density increases the risk of the breast cancer [2]. Accumulated studies also revealed that MBD can be utilized as an effective surrogate for monitoring all stages of patient care with breast cancer: the screening of breast cancer as a risk factor [3], the monitoring of treatments [4,5], and the prediction of recurrence for breast cancer [6]. Despite its effective role in aforementioned procedures, to date, MBD has been qualitatively measured in accordance with the Breast Imaging Reporting and Data System (BI-RADS) that requires experts' visual assessment assigning mammograms into one of four categories with 25% interval [7]. Alternatively, an interactive thresholding technique has been widely used for clinical studies to measure the MBD quantitatively [8], but it still requires experts' intervention so as to determine two thresholds for breast and dense area which is time consuming and results in inter- and intra-rater variation. Accordingly, fully automated measurement of MBD is desirable for studies regarding the relation between MBD and breast cancer risk as well as the retrospective examination of patients using large population database. To this end, we have developed a fully automated MBD estimation method, which is based on the prior statistics of mammograms integrated into a novel level set scheme driven by a population-based tissue probability map (PTPM). This scheme was designed to capture the implicit knowledge of experts' visual systems where the learned knowledge was modeled as the PTPM.

In this paper, we briefly introduce the PTPM-driven level set method for the fully automated MBD assessments, specifically focusing on the evaluation of the method in terms of temporal stability and reproducibility. For the evaluation of the temporal stability, we utilized the mammograms from same patient taken within one year from the breast cancer screening database, and a pair of mammograms taken with different equipment were used for the evaluation of reproducibility.

2   Database

This study received institutional review board (IRB) approval from Seoul National University Hospital for the study of fully automated mammographic density estimation and its association with breast cancer, and we collected full-field digital mammograms (FFDMs) taken from various equipment: Senographe 2000D, DS, and Essential by GE; and Selenia by Hologic. The FFDMs from Senographe 2000D, DS, and Essential have a resolution of 100 μm/pixel and a pixel matrix 2294 × 1914. They were post-processed using Premium View (GE Healthcare) software, which produced adaptive histogram equalized 12-bit gray-level images, whereas FFDMs from Selenia have a resolution of 70 μm/pixel and a pixel matrix 3328 × 2560 were post-processed using AWS (Hologic) software version 3.1. In this study, patients with prior breast cancer surgery or with any abnormal findings (i.e., micro-calcifications, mass, or implant) were excluded.

3 PTPM-Driven Level Set Method for Fully Automated MBD Assessments

The key notion of the PTPM-driven level set method is to utilize the nature of mammograms in that dense regions (i.e., fibroglandular tissues) tend to have higher intensity and heterogeneity than fatty regions (i.e., adipose tissues). These intrinsic information were trained as prior statistics: mean and standard deviation of dense and fatty regions. The trained prior statistics were modeled as PTPM, which cooperated with the imaging feature of a given mammogram so that the prior statistics serve as global information while the imaging features give local information.

In order to construct the PTPM, we first extracted the prior statistics from mammograms where the boundary between dense and fatty region was drawn by radiologists. The statistics were calculated in circular region of interests (ROIs) of 1cm in diameter as shown in Fig. 1.

The extracted statistics were mean intensity, μ, and standard deviation, σ, inside each ROI obtained. The offset mean and standard deviation were computed after the alignment of the histogram since the intensity distribution of mammograms is varied, so the intensity value of α percent of the maximum intensity of the histogram was subtracted from whole pixel intensities in the breast area so that the intensity distribution of a given mammogram is normalized. With means and standard deviations from each ROI in mammograms, 2D scatter plot of statistical samples were obtained as shown in Fig. 2.

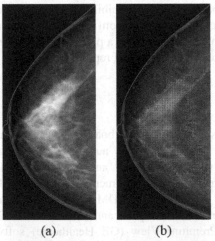

(a)   (b)

Fig. 1. ROI selection for extracting regional statistics in a mammogram: (a) an experts' interactive thresholding for separating fatty and dense regions in which the boundary between two regions are shown as a color overlay of red solid contour, (b) the selection of ROIs within dense and fatty regions with red and green circles, respectively, determined by the expert.

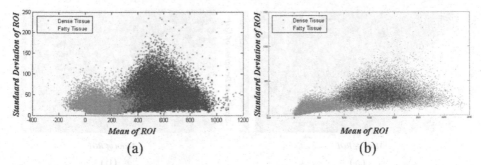

Fig. 2. 2D scatter plots of the extracted regional statistics from mammograms taken with (a) Senographe 2000D, GE and (b) Selenia, Hologic

The dense and fatty regions were determined if an ROI contains more than 95 percent of dense and fatty tissues. By using the statistical samples, the probability density functions (PDFs) of dense and fatty region were generated by non-parametric probability estimation method (i.e., *Parzen* windows). Based on the PDFs shown in Fig. 3, we obtained the class probability as follows:

$$P_D(\mu,\sigma) = \frac{p_d(\mu,\sigma)}{p_d(\mu,\sigma) + p_f(\mu,\sigma)} \quad (1)$$

$$P_F(\mu,\sigma) = 1 - P_D(\mu,\sigma) \quad (2)$$

The energy functional that is minimized when the initial contour reaches the desired boundary between dense and fatty region was defined to integrate the class probability shown in Fig. 4 and regional features from the given mammogram. The defined energy functional is as below:

$$E(\phi(x),\mu_i,\mu_o) = E_{prior}(\phi(x)) + E_{image}(\phi(x),\mu_i,\mu_o) \quad (3)$$

$$E_{prior}(\phi(x)) = -\int_\Omega \log P_D(x) H(\phi(x)) dx - \int_\Omega \log P_F(x)(1 - H(\phi(x))) dx \quad (4)$$

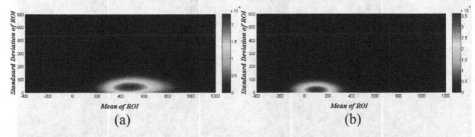

Fig. 3. Estimated PDFs of (a) dense region, $p_d(\mu,\sigma)$, and (b) fatty region, $p_f(\mu,\sigma)$

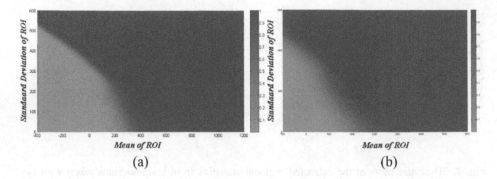

(a)   (b)

Fig. 4. The PTPMs of mammograms taken with (a) Senographe 2000D, GE and (b) Selenia, Hologic obtained from the extracted regional statistics modeled by non-parametric probability density function estimation

$$
E_{image}\left(\phi(x),\mu_i,\mu_o\right) = \int_{\Omega}\left|\nabla H\left(\phi(x)\right)\right|dx
$$
$$
+ \int_{\Omega}\left(f(x)-\mu_i\right)^2 H\left(\phi(x)\right)dx + \int_{\Omega}\left(f(x)-\mu_o\right)^2\left(1-H\left(\phi(x)\right)\right)dx \tag{5}
$$

where μ_i and μ_o are the mean of inside and outside of the current contour, respectively, $\phi(x)$ is an intrinsic signed distance function, $H(\cdot)$ is a characteristic function, and Ω is a set of pixels inside of the breast region. The energy of regional features in (5) was proposed by Chen et al. that is minimized when the contrast between inside and outside of the contour is maximized [9]. Finally, using Euler-Lagrange equation in (9), the motion equation of the contour was obtained as in (10).

$$
\frac{\partial\phi(x)}{\partial t} = -\frac{\partial E\left(\phi(x),\mu_i,\mu_o\right)}{\partial\phi(x)} \tag{6}
$$

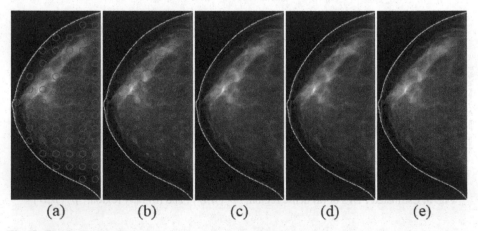

(a)   (b)   (c)   (d)   (e)

Fig. 5. The evolution of the initial contours approaching the desired boundary between dense and fatty region at (a) initial, (b) 5, (c) 10, (d) 30, and final iterations, respectively

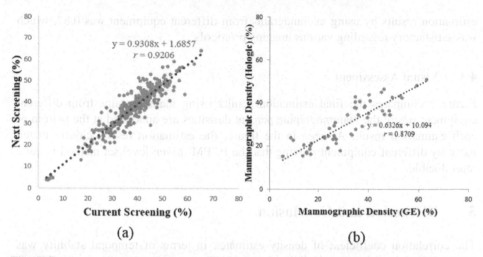

Fig. 6. 2D scatter plots of (a) retrospective and (b) reproducible estimations by PTPM-driven level set scheme. The correlation coefficients are displayed near the trend line drawn as red dotted lines with linear equations.

$$\frac{\partial \phi(x)}{\partial t} = \delta(\phi(x)) \left[div\left(\frac{\nabla \phi(x)}{|\nabla \phi(x)|} \right) - \left(f(x) - \mu_i \right)^2 + \left(f(x) - \mu_o \right)^2 + \log \frac{P_F(x)}{P_D(x)} \right] \quad (7)$$

Figure 5 shows an example of the evolution of the initial contours by using the motion equation (10).

4   Experimental Results

4.1   Temporal Stability

For the evaluation of temporal stability, 170 pairs of CC-view mammograms of 170 female patients were selected taken with the same equipment (Senographe 2000D) with one year interval. In Fig. 6(a), the 2D scatter plot of the retrospective estimations by PTPM-driven level set scheme is shown, in which the trend line is drawn as red dotted line with linear equation. As a result, the correlation coefficient between current screenings and next screenings was 0.92.

4.2   Reproducibility

In order to validate the reproducibility with respect to various equipment, we established the database of mammogram pairs taken with switched equipment: switched from GE (Senographe DS or Essential) to Hologic (Selenia). In total, 53 pairs of CC-view mammograms from 38 female patients taken within one or two months regarding the menstrual cycle. As shown in Fig. 6(b), the correlation coefficient between estimation results by using mammograms from different equipment was 0.87, which was satisfactory regarding various imaging protocols.

4.3 Visual Assessment

Figure 7 compares the final estimation results using mammograms from different equipment where the mammographic percent densities are annotated at the bottom of each estimation result. As seen in the figure, the estimation results closely match those by different equipment proving that the PTPM-driven level set method is quite reproducible.

5 Discussion and Conclusion

The correlation coefficient of density estimates in terms of temporal stability was 0.92, while that of the reproducibility was 0.87. These results showed that the PTPM-driven level set method can be a reliable tool for applying to retrospective clinical studies relating the MBD to breast cancer risk with large databases regardless of equipment. As a future work, we will establish a larger database of paired mammograms taken with different equipment of same patient for studies investigating the factors influencing the reproducibility of MBD between equipment and potential improvements of reproducibility.

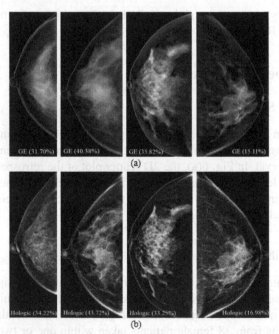

Fig. 7. A comparison of estimations between mammograms from (a) GE and (b) Hologic devices. The boundaries between fatty and dense regions are drawn with red solid lines where percent mammographic densities are annotated below.

Acknowledgement. The research was supported by the Converging Research Center Program through the Ministry of Science, ICT and Future Planning, Korea (2013K000423).

References

1. Wolfe, J.N.: Breast Patterns as an Index of Risk for Developing Breast Cancer. Am. J. Roentgenol. 126, 1130–1139 (1976)
2. Boyd, N.F., Guo, H., Martin, L.J., Sun, L.M., Stone, J., Fishell, E., Jong, R.A., Hislop, G., Chiarelli, A., Minkin, S., Yaffe, M.J.: Mammographic density and the risk and detection of breast cancer. N. Engl. J. Med. 356, 227–236 (2007)
3. Harvey, J.A., Bovbjerg, V.E.: Quantitative assessment of mammographic breast density: Relationship with breast cancer risk. Radiology 230, 29–41 (2004)
4. Lundstrom, E., Wilczek, B., von Palffy, Z., Soderqvist, G., von Schoultz, B.: Mammographic breast density during hormone replacement therapy: Differences according to treatment. Am. J. Obstet. Gynecol. 181, 348–352 (1999)
5. Habel, L.A., Capra, A.M., Achacoso, N.S., Janga, A., Acton, L., Puligandla, B., Quesenberry, C.P.: Mammographic Density and Risk of Second Breast Cancer after Ductal Carcinoma in situ. Cancer Epidem. Biomar. 19, 2488–2495 (2010)
6. Cil, T., Fishell, E., Hanna, W., Sun, P., Rawlinson, E., Narod, S.A., McCready, D.R.: Mammographic Density and the Risk of Breast Cancer Recurrence After Breast-Conserving Surgery. Cancer 115, 5780–5787 (2009)
7. D'Orsi, C.J.: American College of Radiology., American College of Radiology. BI-RADS Committee.: Illustrated breast imaging reporting and data system (illustrated BI-RADS). American College of Radiology, Reston (1998)
8. Byng, J.W., Boyd, N.F., Fishell, E., Jong, R.A., Yaffe, M.J.: The Quantitative-Analysis of Mammographic Densities. Phys. Med. Biol. 39, 1629–1638 (1994)
9. Chan, T.F., Vese, L.A.: Active contours without edges. IEEE T. Image Process. 10, 266–277 (2001)

Usefulness of a Combination DBT (Digital Breast Tomosynthesis) and Automated Volume Analysis of Dynamic Contrast-Enhanced Breast (DCEB) MRI in Evaluation of Response to Neoadjuvant Chemotherapy (NAC)

Nachiko Uchiyama[1], Takayuki Kinoshita[2], Takashi Hojo[2], Sota Asaga[2], Minoru Machida[1], Hitomi Tani[1], Mari Kikuchi[1], Yasuaki Arai[1], and Kyoichi Otsuka[3]

[1] National Cancer Center, Department of Radiology, Tokyo, Japan
{nuchiyam,mmachida,hittani, markikuc,yaarai}@ncc.go.jp
[2] National Cancer Center, Department of Breast Surgery, Tokyo, Japan
{takinosh,tahojo, soasaga}@ncc.go.jp
[3] Siemens Japan K.K., Tokyo, Japan
Kyoichi.otsuka@siemens.com

Abstract. We evaluated the usefulness of DBT and automated volume analysis with DCEB MRI to assess its potential role in estimating viable tumor volume in pre-and pos-t NAC images in response to treatment in comparison with FFDM and US. Twenty women having 21 lesions, in total were recruited for this study. The diagnostic procedures were performed within one month prior to surgery. FFDM, DBT, US and DCEB MRI were performed on each of the patients before and after NAC. The imaging data was analyzed by a medical workstation dedicated to breast MRI imaging. Utilizing the dynamic contrast images from 1st to 4th phase, volume statistics with VOI (volume of interest) and the volume was automatically calculated and evaluated as to the efficacy of NAC. DBT has the advantage of providing macroscopic pathological fidings in total without utitiling contrast medium. On the other hand, DCEB MRI has the advantage of providing numerical and detailed vascularity details of viable areas. In accordance with the results, a combination of DBT and automated volume analysis of DCEB MRI will contribute to more accurate diagnosis in the assessment of pathological response to NAC.

Keywords: DBT, MRI, Breast, Automated Volume Analysis.

1 Introduction

Digital breast tomosynthesis (DBT) has been only recently applied clinically. The diagnostic advantages in comparison to mammography have been reported on, including the fact that the slice images can be evaluated because tomosynthesis decreases the overlap in breast tissue. DCEB MRI provided a more accurate assessment of tumor extent with respect to pathological findings in cases of breast cancer. Although

H. Fujita, T. Hara, and C. Muramatsu (Eds.): IWDM 2014, LNCS 8539, pp. 312–319, 2014.
© Springer International Publishing Switzerland 2014

the results supported the usefulness of measurement by 2D MRI in improving the estimation of out of frame tumor size, this measurement does not evaluate actual volume of viable lesions after NAC. This is because shrinkage of the mass lesion, including fibrotic change after NAC, makes it difficult to evaluate the viable lesion by 2D MRI images only. According to the background in this study, we evaluated the usefulness of DBT and automated volume analysis with DCEB MRI to assess its potential role in estimating viable tumor volume in pre- and post- NAC images in response to treatment in comparison with FFDM (Full Field Digital Mammography) and US.

2   Methods and Materials

Twenty women (ages 29-64, mean age, 47.3 years old) having 21 lesions in total were recruited for this study. Pathological diagnosis was confirmed by Core Needle Biopsy (CNB). Pathological subtypes were Invasive Ductal Carcinoma, Sci (n=10: 47.6%); Invasive Ductal Carcinoma, Sol-Tub or Pap-Tub (n=8: 38.1%); Invasive Ductal Carcinoma, Apocrine (n=1: 4.8%); Invasive Lobular Carcinoma (n=1: 4.8%), and Invasive Micropapillary Carcinoma (n=1: 4.8%). The clinical stages of the patients before NAC were II or III. All patients underwent surgery based on their response to NAC. Residual tumor size estimated by diagnostic imaging was compared with the residual tumor size determined by surgical pathology. The diagnostic procedures were performed within one month prior to surgery. FFDM, DBT, US and DCEB MRI were performed on each of the patients before and after NAC. The diagnostic procedures were performed within one month prior to surgery. Breast MRI was performed with a 3-Tesla system. The four phase dynamic contrast enhanced images were taken with an intravenous injection of 0.1mmol of Gd-DTPA/Kg of body weight. The post-processing procedures of the 2D slice images included multiplanar reconstruction (MPR) by slices and the construction of maximum intensity projection (MIP) images. These images were evaluated by one radiologist and three breast surgeons before the operation. The imaging data was analyzed using a medical workstation dedicated to breast MRI imaging. Utilizing the dynamic contrast images from 1st to 4th phases, the time intensity curve of wash-in and wash-out was automatically determined. The patterns of enhancement were classified into the initial phase (slow, medium, and rapid) and the delayed phase (persistent, plateau, and wash-out). In addition, we measured the positive enhancement integral (PEI). PEI calculates the areas under the enhancement curve over the entire time sequence. It was evaluating by color overlay maps (Type 1:<100 Arbitrary Units (AU), Type 2: 500AU>Type2 >100 AU, and Type 3: >500 AU). In addition, for reference, not only the clinical target lesion, but also normal breasts were evaluated for background. Referring to the color maps of PEI, the viable lesions (Type 2 or Type 3) were traced as VOI (volume of interest) and the volume was automatically calculated and evaluated as to the efficacy of NAC.

Volume statistics with VOI analyzed wash-in and wash-out rates of the pixels within the sphere utilizing the 2nd and 3rd dynamic images (Fig.1).

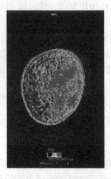

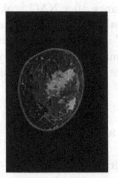

Fig. 1. a. PEI Image   **Fig. 1.** b 2D Coronal Image

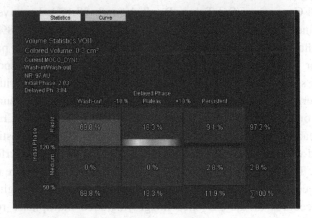

Fig. 1. c. VOI Analysis

The clinical response to NAC was classified into the following categories, based on the "response evaluation criteria in solid tumors" (RECIST) using the measurements obtained with the following different imaging methods: 1) Complete Response (CR), no clinical evidence of residual tumor; 2) Partial Response (PR), reduction in size of the tumor by more than 30%; 3) Non-Responders , Stable disease (SD), reduction in size of the tumor by less than 30%; 4) Progressive disease (PD), increase in size of tumor or presence of new lesions. Pathological response to NAC was classified into four categories: Grade 0 (No Response), Grade 1 (Slight Response), Grade 2 (Fair Response), and Grade 3 (Complete Response).

3   Results and Discussion

Pathological responses of the lesions to NAC were Grade 1 or Grade 2 (n=17), and Grade 3 (n=4). FFDM findings only of pathological Grade 3 (n=4) were diagnosed as clinical CR (n=2/4, 50.0%) and clinical PR (n=2/4, 50.0%). DBT findings were diagnosed as clinical CR (n=2/4, 50.0%) and clinical PR (n=2/4, 50.0%). US findings were diagnosed as clinical CR (n=1/4, 25.0%) and clinical PR (n=3/4, 75.0%). 2D MRI findings were diagnosed as clinical CR (n=2/4, 50.0%) and clinical PR (n=2/4, 50.0%). Among pathological Grade 1 and Grade 2 lesions (n=17), 16 lesions were evaluated as clinical PR and one lesion was evaluated as SD by FFDM, DBT, and 2D MRI. Fifteen lesions were evaluated as clinical PR and 2 lesions were evaluated as SD by US (Table 1). In addition, regarding the evaluation of residual tumor size, its size was over-estimated in one lesion (n=1/17, 5.9%) or under-estimated in six lesions (n=6/17, 35.3%) by FFDM. By US, it was over-estimated in two lesions (n=2/17, 11.8%) or under-estimated in three lesions (n=3/17, 17.6%). By DBT, it was over-estimated in only two lesions (n=2/17, 11.8%). By 2D MRI findings, the viable area was over-estimated in one lesion (n=1/17, 5.9%) or under-estimated in six lesions (n=6/17, 35.3%), when only 2D MRI findings were used.

Table 1. Comparison of NAC Response by Diagnostic Evaluation and Pathological Evaluation

Pathological Response	FFDM	US	(n=21)
Grade 1 or 2 (n=17)	*PR (n=16/17, 94.1%)	PR (n=15/17, 88.2%)	
	SD (n=1/17, 5.9%)	SD (n=2/17, 11.8 %)	
Grade 3 (n=4)	CR (n=2/4, 50.0%)	CR (n=1/4, 25.0%)	
	PR (n=2/4, 50.0%)	PR (n=3/4, 75.0%)	

Pathological Response	DBT	MRI	(n=21)
Grade 1 or 2 (n=17)	PR (n=16/17, 94.1%)	PR (n=16/17, 94.1%)	
	SD (n=1/17, 5.9%)	SD (n=1/17, 5.9 %)	
Grade 3 (n=4)	CR (n=2/4, 50.0%)	CR (n=2/4, 50.0%)	
	PR (n=2/4, 50.0%)	PR (n=2/4, 50.0%)	

Table 1. * The clinical response to chemotherapy was classified in accordance with RECIST

According to the PEI with color overlay maps, the residual viable areas were shown as Type 2 or Type 3, corresponding to pathological Grade1or Grade 2 and the non-residual viable areas were shown as Type1, corresponding to pathological Grade 3 or the same pattern as the normal background breasts. There was no discrepancy with the results of pathological response. In addition, compared to pathological response, volume analysis with VOI referring to PEI with color mapping made a more accurate diagnosis compared to the reference to 2D MRI images only. Colored volume analysis will be able to qualify the volume of viable area. Distribution of the enhancement pattern will be able to provide a detailed vascularity pattern in the viable area (Fig.3-4).

4   Conclusion

DBT has the advantage of providing macroscopic pathological fidings in total without utitiling contrast medium. On the other hand, DCEB MRI has the advantage of providing numerical and detailed vascularity details of viable areas. In accordance with the results, a combination of DBT and automated volume analysis of DCEB MRI will contribute to more accurate diagnosis in the assessment of pathological response to NAC.

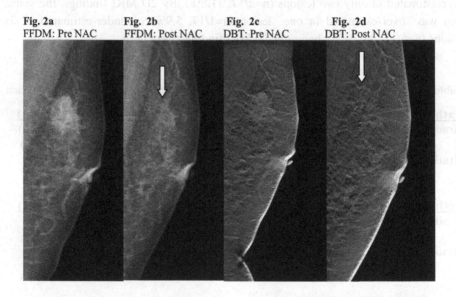

| Fig. 2a | Fig. 2b | Fig. 2c | Fig. 2d |
| FFDM: Pre NAC | FFDM: Post NAC | DBT: Pre NAC | DBT: Post NAC |

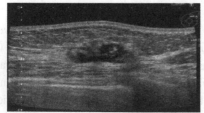
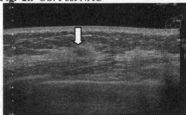

Fig. 2e. US: Pre NAC   Fig. 2f. US: Post NAC

Fig. 2g. MRI Coronal Image: Pre NAC

Fig. 2h. MRI Coronal Image: Post NAC

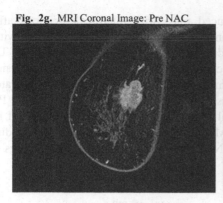

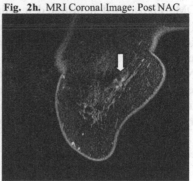

Fig. 2. Case 1: Pathological Grade 3

Fig. 3a. Saggital Image

Fig. 3b. PEI Image

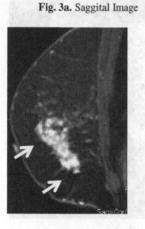

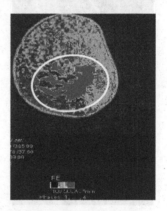

Fig. 3c.VOI Analysis

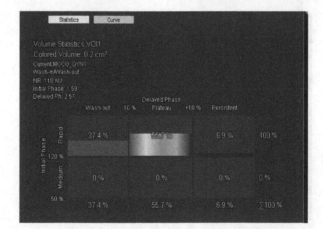

Fig. 3. Case 2: Pathological Grade 2a: Pre NAC

FFDM (Fig.2a-b) demonstrated a reduced mass with micro-calcifications after NAC (white arrow). DBT (Fig.2c-d) demonstrated microcalcifications with scar without core density inside of the corresponding lesion after NAC (white arrow). US (Fig.2e-f) demonstrated a reduced hypo-echoic mass as a suspicious residual lesion after NAC (white arrow). The coronal Image of CE-MRI (Fig.2g-h) demonstrated small enhanced nodules as a suspicious residual lesion after NAC (white arrow). Pathological diagnosis demonstrated residual DCIS corresponding to the enhanced lesions by CE- MRI. In accordance with MMG, US and 2D MRI findings, residual lesion was suspected and the efficacy of NAC was underestimared. The findings of DBT corresponded to pathological results.

Fig. 4a. Saggital Image   **Fig. 4b.** PEI Image

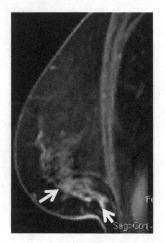
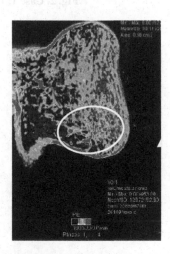

Fig. 4c. VOI Analysis

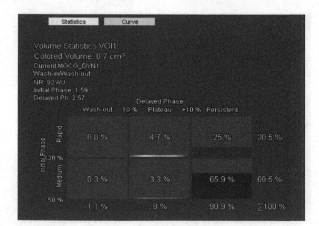

Fig. 4. Case 2: Pathological Grade 2a: Post NAC

MRI saggital image (Fig. 3a, Fig. 4a) demonstrated a reduced mass after NAC (white arrow). The pathological grade was Grade 2a and the size of residual lesion was ILC, 110x44mm. The residul lesion size was underestimated by 2D MRI. On the other hand, PEI image and VOI statistics demonstrated that larger residual area (white circle: Fig. 4b) and 65.9% area suggested non-viable area and others suggested viable area (white arrow: Fig. 4c).The findings of PEI image and VOI analysis corresponded to pathological results more acculately in comparison with 2D MRI images.

Acknowledgment. This study was supported by Grant-in-Aid for Scientific Research (C) (No. 23591810) in Japan.

References

1. Demartini, W.B., Lehman, C.D., Peacock, S., Russell, M.T.: Computer-aided detection applied to breast MRI: assessment of CAD-generated enhancement and tumor sizes in breast cancers before and after neoadjuvant chemotherapy. Acad. Radiol. 12(7), 806–814 (2005)
2. Takeda, K., Kanao, S., Okada, T., Kataoka, M., Ueno, T., Toi, M., Ishiguro, H., Mikami, Y., Togashi, K.: Assessment of CAD-generated tumor volumes measured using MRI in breast cancers before and after neoadjuvant chemotherapy. Eur. J. Radiol. 81(10), 2627–2631 (2012)
3. Baltzer, P.A., Freiberg, C., Beger, S., Vag, T., Dietzel, M., Herzog, A.B., Gajda, M., Camara, O., Kaiser, W.: Clinical MR-mammography: are computer-assisted methods superior to visual or manual measurements for curve type analysis? A systematic approach. Acad. Radiol. 16(9), 1070–1076 (2009)
4. Levman, J.E., Causer, P., Warner, E., Martel, A.L.: Effect of the enhancement threshold on the computer-aided detection of breast cancer using MRI. Acad. Radiol. 16(9), 1064–1069 (2009)

Clinical Efficacy of Novel Image Processing Techniques in the Framework of Filtered Back Projection (FBP) with Digital Breast Tomosynthesis (DBT)

Nachiko Uchiyama[1], Minoru Machida[1], Hitomi Tani[1], Mari Kikuchi[1],
Yasuaki Arai[1], Kyoichi Otsuka[2], Andreas Fieselmann[3], Anna Jerebko[3],
and Thomas Mertelmeier[3]

[1] National Cancer Center, Department of Radiology, Tokyo, Japan
{nuchiyam,mmachida,hittani,markikuc,yaarai}@ncc.go.jp
[2] Siemens Japan K.K., Tokyo, Japan
kyoichi.ostuka@siemens.com
[3] Siemens AG, Healthcare Sector, Erlangen, Germany
{andreas.fieselmann,anna.jerebko,
thomas.mertelmeier}@siemens.com

Abstract. Digital breast tomosynthesis (DBT) slices are reconstructed from projections acquired within a limited angular range. Out-of-plane artifacts are inevitable in reconstructed DBT images. In this study, we evaluated novel image processing techniques in the framework of filtered backprojection (FBP) and compared the results with reconstruction using a previously used FBP method. The novel FBP reconstruction has an adapted filter kernel, uses unbinned projections, performs an adaptive collapsing scheme and statistical artifact reduction, and applies iterative filtering in the image domain. Fifty-four image pairs were evaluated by three experienced radiologists. The images were compared on a 7-point scale (-3, -2, -1, 0, +1, +2, and +3) according to the following five categories: (1) visibility of noise, (2) diagnostic certainty regarding masses, (3) diagnostic certainty regarding microcalcifications, (4) visibility of structures in the pectoral muscle, and (5) overall image quality. The results showed a statistically significant superiority of the novel FBP reconstruction in comparison with standard FBP ($p < 0.05$). In particular, the improvement of the diagnostic certainty related to microcalcifications with the novel FBP is noteworthy.

Keywords: Tomosynthesis, Image Processing, DBT, FBP.

1 Introduction

Digital breast tomosynthesis (DBT) provides an advantage in detection of breast masses compared to 2D mammography since it allows to separate the tissue layers and to noticeably reduce occlusions caused by overlapping anatomical structures (1-6). The 3D representation of the breast is reconstructed from projections acquired only within a limited angular range. Because of this acquisition procedure out-of-plane artifacts are inevitable in reconstructed DBT images.

H. Fujita, T. Hara, and C. Muramatsu (Eds.): IWDM 2014, LNCS 8539, pp. 320–326, 2014.
© Springer International Publishing Switzerland 2014

There are many algorithms designed to reduce these kinds of artifacts (7).

Metal artifact reduction methods coming from CT are often based on segmenting the metal objects in the sinogram or in projection images and removing them before the reconstruction by interpolation of neighboring values (8). Such methods are of very limited use in DBT, where artifacts are caused mainly by the missing data of the tomosynthesis acquisition and originate around dense tissue, masses or calcifications. It is not feasible to detect and remove these in the low dose projections.

One of the state-of-the-art artifact reduction methods specific to tomosynthesis is the slice thickness filter which is used in FBP reconstructions (9). The slice thickness filter is a low-pass filter which reduces the frequency response in z-direction. It allows maintaining constant slice thickness and limits the out-of-plane artifacts but reduces the sharpness of high frequency features in the projections with high angle of incidence. Other methods suggest using statistical outlier detection tests during back projection to further reduce artifacts (10, 11).

Optimization of FBP for DBT reconstruction to reduce artifacts and improve image quality is an ongoing research topic. In this work, we evaluated a novel image processing technique within the framework of FBP. We compared it with standard FBP reconstruction regarding image quality and diagnostic certainty utilizing clinical images.

2   Methods and Materials

The clinical data sets were acquired with a DBT system (MAMMOMAT Inspiration, Siemens, Germany; MAMMOMAT Inspiration Tomosynthesis is not commercially available in the U.S.). The images were reconstructed into 2 mm thick slices having 1mm overlap with high in-plane resolution of 0.085 mm × 0.085 mm. For each patient, CC and MLO views were taken for diagnosis. With one-view DBT, the radiation dose, utilizing the ACR phantom 156, was 1.80mGy. The image reconstruction technique was based on FBP. The previously employed FBP reconstruction that we here call standard FBP reconstruction used a filter kernel that was dominated by the ramp filter for small spatial frequencies for tomosynthesis image reconstruction (Fig. 1a).

The novel FBP reconstruction has an adapted filter kernel which preserves more of the lower frequencies and provides a different image impression. In addition, the images were reconstructed from unbinned projections at high z-resolution, and a subsequent adaptive collapsing scheme to generate thicker slices was applied. A statistical artifact reduction was used to mitigate out-of-plane artifacts (11). In addition, iterative filtering in image space was employed to suppress noise (Fig. 1b). A more detailed description of the image processing algorithms together with a phantom-based evaluation is provided in (12). Note that in this work we focus on a clinical evaluation of the novel reconstruction.

Fifty-four females who had been recalled for further diagnosis were enrolled in this study. The clinical study had been approved by the ethics committee. Informed consent was obtained from all patients. The study population is characterized as follows. The mean age of the women was 51.0 years old (25.0 to 79.0 years old). The findings with FFDM and DBT of the cases in this study were masses (n=27; 50.0%) and microcalcifications (n=28; 51.9%). The breast density was rated as ACR 1 (n=7; 13.0%), ACR 2 (n=20; 37.0%), ACR 3 (n=20; 37.0%), and ACR 4 (n=7; 13.0%) with FFDM (Table 1). Table 2 shows the distribution of the microcalcification-related and mass-related lesions with respect to two breast density categories (ACR 1 or ACR 2 versus ACR 3 or ACR 4).

The image pairs (two-view standard FBP vs. two-view novel FBP) were evaluated by three radiologists, each of them having more than five years of experience of interpreting mammograms. In a blinded side-by-side reading of the image pairs, the radiologists compared the images on a 7-point scale (-3, -2, -1, 0, +1, +2, and +3) and evaluated according to the following five categories: 1. visibility of noise, 2. diagnostic certainty: mass, 3. diagnostic certainty: microcalcifications, 4. visibility of structures in the pectoral muscle, and 5. overall image quality. The p-values corresponding to the paired t-test were analyzed by SPSS Statistics 17.0 (IBM, USA). The significance level was 0.05.

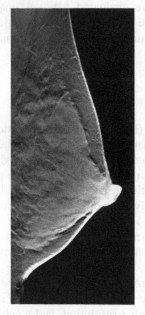   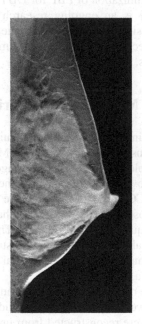

Fig. 1a. Standard FBP reconstruction   **Fig. 1b.** Novel FBP reconstruction

Table 1. Distribution of breast density patterns

Breast Density Patterns	n=54
ACR 1	7 (13.0%)
ACR 2	20 (37.0%)
ACR 3	20 (37.0%)
ACR 4	7 (13.0%)

Table 2. Number of lesions according to breast density patterns

	Breast Density Patterns	
	ACR 1 or ACR 2	ACR 3 or ACR 4
Microcalcifications (n=28)	13 (46.4%)	15 (53.6%)
Masses (n=27)	17 (63.0%)	10 (37.0%)

3   Results and Discussion

The results from the reading study are shown in Table 3. Positive mean values indicate that the novel FBP reconstruction was preferred in comparison with standard FBP. The p-values corresponding to a paired t-test show a statistically significant superiority of the novel FBP reconstruction in comparison with standard FBP for all categories ($p < 0.05$).

Table 3. Results for the reading study comparing image pairs consisting of the novel FBP reconstruction and standard FBP on the 7-point scale

Category	n	Mean Value & SD	p-value
1. Visibility of noise	54	0.488±0.724	$p < 0.001$
2. Diagnostic certainty: Mass	27	0.222±0.612	$p < 0.05$
3. Diagnostic certainty: Microcalcifications	28	0.560±0.782	$p < 0.001$
4. Visibility of structures in the pectoral muscle	54	0.245±0.973	$p < 0.05$
5. Overall image quality	54	0.346±0.775	$p < 0.001$

Results from category 1 (visibility of noise) and category 3 (diagnostic certainty regarding microcalcifications) demonstrated higher mean values compared to other categories. The improvement can be attributed to the reconstruction from unbinned projections at high z-resolution, the statistical artifact reduction, and the iterative filtering. Those reconstruction techniques that are part of the novel FBP method generally result in microcalcifications being visualized clearer and less noisy compared to standard FBP. The results suggest that the novel image processing technique contributed to the reduction of out-of plane artifacts, especially caused by calcifications.

We also investigated if the ratings of the readers for the lesions with masses depended on the breast density pattern. For these cases, no dependency with respect to the breast density pattern was found. On the other hand, for the lesions with microcalcifications, the novel FBP demonstrated lower values in two out of 28 (8.7%) lesions

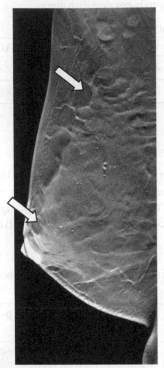

Fig. 2a. Case1: Standard FBP reconstruction

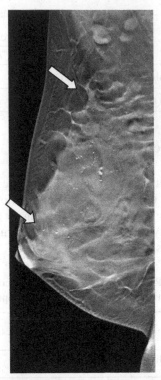

Fig. 3a. Case1: Novel FBP reconstruction

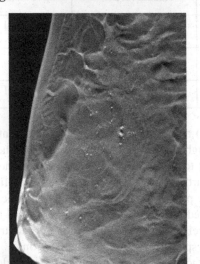

Fig. 2b. Case 1: Standard FBP reconstruction

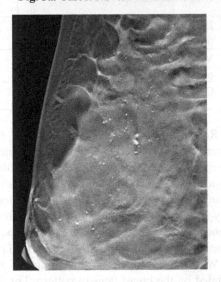

Fig. 3b. Case 1: Novel FBP reconstruction

Fig. 2-3. In case 1 with breast density ACR 3, the novel FBP reconstruction provided a better visualization of microcalcifications (arrow)

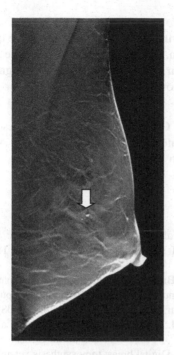

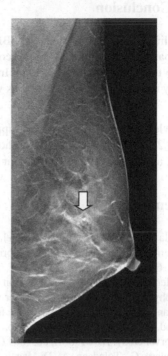

Fig. 4a. Case 2: Standard FBP reconstruction   **Fig. 5a.** Case 2: Novel FBP reconstruction

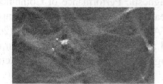

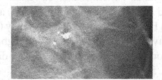

Fig. 4b. Case 2: Standard FBP reconstruction   **Fig. 5b.** Case 2: Novel FBP reconstruction

Fig. 4-5. In case 2 with breast density ACR 1, the standard FBP reconstruction provided a better visualization of microcalcifications (arrow). In two of the 28 cases having microcalcifications-related lesions the visualization was rated better in standard FBP.

which were rated as ACR 1 or ACR 2. All lesions with the new FBP that were rated as ACR 3 or ACR 4 demonstrated higher values in comparison with the standard FBP (Fig. 2-3). According to our preliminary results, the new FBP might demonstrate lower values among relatively fatty breast patterns. The findings showed that the adapted filter kernel made evaluation of microcalcifications more difficult because of decreased density contrast between dense breast tissue and fat compared to cases with relatively dense breast patterns (Fig. 4-5).

4   Conclusion

In our clinical evaluation, the novel FBP reconstruction resulted in better image quality compared to the standard FBP reconstruction. The improvements could be attributed to the change in the algorithm. In particular, the improvement of the diagnostic certainty related to microcalcifications with the novel FBP is noteworthy.

Acknowledgment. This study was supported by Grant-in-Aid for Scientific Research (C) (No.23591810) in Japan. The authors are grateful to Julitta Unland, Shiras Abdurahman, and Frank Dennerlein for their support in this study.

References

1. Poplack, S.P., Tosteson, T.D., Kogel, C.A., et al.: Digital breast tomosynthesis: initial experience in 98 women with abnormal digital screening mammography. AJR 189(3), 616–623 (2007)
2. Andersson, I., Ikeda, D.M., Zackrisson, S., et al.: Breast tomosynthesis and digital mammography: a comparison of breast cancer visibility and BIRADS classification in a population of cancers with subtle mammographic findings. Eur. Radiol. 18(12), 2817–2825 (2008)
3. Good, W.F., Abrams, G.S., Catullo, V.J., et al.: Digital breast tomosynthesis: a pilot observer study. AJR 190(4), 865–869 (2008)
4. Gennaro, G., Toledano, A., Di Maggio, C., et al.: Digital breast tomosynthesis versus digital mammography: a clinical performance study. Eur. Radiol. 20(7), 1545–1553 (2010)
5. Uchiyama, N., Kinoshita, T., Akashi, S., et al.: Diagnostic Performance of Combined Full Field Digital Mammography (FFDM) and Digital Breast Tomosynthesis (DBT) in comparison with Full Field Digital Mammography (FFDM). In: CARS 2011, pp. 32–33. Springer (2011)
6. Förnvik, D., Zackrisson, S., Ljungberg, O., et al.: Breast tomosynthesis: Accuracy of tumor measurement compared with digital mammography and ultrasonography. Acta. Radiol. 51(3), 240–247 (2010)
7. Dobbins, J.T., Godfrey, D.J.: Digital x-ray tomosynthesis: current state of the art and clinical potential. Phys. Med. Biol. 106, R65–R106 (2003)
8. Rinkel, J., Dillon, W.P., Funk, T., Gould, R., Prevrhal, S.: Computed tomographic metal artifact reduction for the detection and quantitation of small features near large metallic implants: a comparison of published methods. J. Comput. Assist. Tomogr. 32(4), 621–629 (2008)
9. Mertelmeier, T., Orman, J., Haerer, W., et al.: Optimizing filtered backprojection reconstruction for a breast tomosynthesis prototype device. In: Proc. SPIE Medical Imaging 2006, vol. 6142, p. 61420F (2006)
10. Wu, T., Moore, R.H., Kopans, D.B.: Voting strategy for artifact reduction in digital breast tomosynthesis. Medical Physics 33, 24612471 (2006)
11. Abdurahman, S., Jerebko, A., Mertelmeier, T., Lasser, T., Navab, N.: Out-of-Plane Artifact Reduction in Tomosynthesis Based on Regression Modeling and Outlier Detection. In: Maidment, A.D.A., Bakic, P.R., Gavenonis, S. (eds.) IWDM 2012. LNCS, vol. 7361, pp. 729–736. Springer, Heidelberg (2012)
12. Abdurahman, S., Dennerlein, F., Jerebko, A., Fieselmann, A., Mertelmeier, T.: Optimizing high resolution reconstruction. In: Digital Breast Tomosynthesis using Filtered Back Projection. accepted at IWDM 2014 (2014)

A Revisit on Correlation between Tabár and Birads Based Risk Assessment Schemes with Full Field Digital Mammography

Wenda He[1], Minnie Kibiro[2], Arne Juette[2],
Erika R.E. Denton[2], and Reyer Zwiggelaar[1]

[1] Department of Computer Science,
Aberystwyth University, Aberystwyth, SY23 3DB, UK
{weh,rrz}@aber.ac.uk
[2] Department of Radiology,
Norfolk & Norwich University Hospital, Norwich, NR4 7UY, UK
{minnie.kibiro,arne.juette,erika.denton}@nnuh.nhs.uk

Abstract. Mammographic risk assessment is used to determine the probability of a woman developing breast cancer and it plays an important role in the early detection and disease prevention within screening mammography. Tabár and Birads are two fundamentally different risk schemes, one is assessed based on mixtures of breast parenchyma and the other one is assessed based on the percentage of dense breast tissue. This paper presents findings on the correlation between these two mammographic risk assessment schemes; aspects with respect to reader experience and related inter reader variability were also investigated. As a follow up (revisit) investigation to a previously published paper, the new results have shown a strong correlation between Tabár and Birads with the highest Spearman's correlation coefficient > 0.92 and $\kappa = 0.86\%$ (almost perfect agreement). The statistical results vary with readers' mammographic reading experience, which also indicated subtle information such as that some mixture of breast parenchma (Tabár specific mammographic building blocks) may be more likely to cause inter reader variability.

Keywords: Tabár, Birads, risk assessment, digital mammography.

1 Introduction

Breast cancer has been considered a major health problem and is the commonest cancer in the UK and across Europe [1]. It is estimated that between one in eight and one in twelve women will develop breast cancer during their lifetime [2]. Recent statistics indicate a rise in breast cancer incident rates in certain segments of the population [3], and the disease development is not fully understood [4]. From a disease prevention point of view, early detection through breast screening programmes is by far the most effective way to tackle breast cancer [4]. Computer aided detection/diagnosis (CAD) systems play a vital role in aiding radiologists

H. Fujita, T. Hara, and C. Muramatsu (Eds.): IWDM 2014, LNCS 8539, pp. 327–333, 2014.

to achieve breast cancer prevention and early intervention, leading to a rise in the number of diagnosed cases and people surviving, after a 5 year cancer treatment period [3].

Within screening mammography, the likelihood of a woman developing breast cancer can be determined through mammoraphic risk assessment [5]. Tabár [6] and Birads (American College of Radiology's Breast Imaging Reporting and Data System) [7] are two fundamentally different risk assessment schemes, one is assessed based on mixtures of breast parenchyma and the other one is assessed based on the percentage of dense breast tissue. It should be noted that currently Birads is widely used through North America and Europe, and unlike the UK five-point based scoring system [8]. It should be noted that the aforementioned risk assessment schemes are image based, which have not fully integrated into non-image based models (e.g. the Gail [9] and the Tyrer-Cuzick model [10]) which focus on patient-specific and enviromental aspects (e.g. family history, diet and genetic markers) [4].

Tabár _et al._ proposed a model based on mixtures of four mammographic building blocks representing the normal breast anatomy, covering nodular, linear, homogeneous and radiolucent tissue [6]; see Fig. 1 for examples. Nodular densities

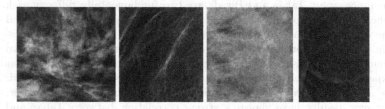

Fig. 1. Example mammographic building blocks, from left to right: nodular, linear structure, homogeneous and radiolucent

mainly correspond to Terminal Ductal Lobular Units (TDLU); linear densities correspond to either ducts, fibrous tissue or blood vessels; homogeneous-structureless densities correspond to fibrous tissue; radiolucent areas are related to adipose fatty tissue. Strongly influenced by Wolfe's original work [11], Tabár _et al._ divided mammograms based on parenchymal patterns into five risk classes [6]. Each risk class has a distribution pattern of the four mammographic building blocks (i.e. [nodular%, linear%, homogeneous%, radiolucent%]); patterns I to V represent low to high mammographic risk: pattern I is composed as [25%, 15%, 35%, 25%]; pattern II is composed as [2%, 14%, 2%, 82%]; pattern III is similar in composition to pattern II, except that the retroareolar prominent ducts are often associated with periductal fibrosis; whilst in pattern II such an association occurs less frequent; pattern IV is composed as [49%, 19%, 15%, 17%]; whilst pattern V is composed as [2%, 2%, 89%, 7%]; see Fig. 2 for examples. Note that in pattern IV the relative proportion of the four building blocks can vary due to involution, which is a process of tissue changes (e.g. total fatty replacement)

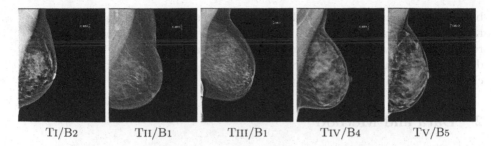

Tı/B2   Tıı/B1   Tııı/B1   Tıv/B4   Tv/B5

Fig. 2. Example mammographic images with Tabár ('T') risk classifications from low to high, and their equivalent according to the Birads ('B') scheme

that is highly individual and can be caused by hormone replacement or pregnancy. This regression also happens in pattern I, leading for pattern I to change to either Pattern II or III [6].

Birads was developed to standardise mammography reporting and reduce confusion in breast imaging interpretations. It is used as a quality assurance tool which covers the significant relationship between increased breast density and decreased mammographic sensitivity in detecting cancer [12]. Each mammography report starts with a breast density description which is used to inform the clinician about possible effect of the sensitivity of the examination due to the mammographic density of the patient [13]. Mammographic breast composition is categorised into four classes: Birads 1, the breast is almost entirely fat ($< 25\%$ glandular); Birads 2, the breast has scattered fibroglandular densities ($25\% - 50\%$); Birads 3, the breast consists of heterogeneously dense breast tissue ($51\% - 75\%$); and Birads 4, the breast is extremely dense ($> 75\%$ glandular); see Fig. 3 for examples.

Muhimmah *et al.* [14] used the MIAS database which contains digitised mammograms and established a strong correlation (Spearman's correlation coefficient > 0.9) between Wolf, Boyd and Birads based classification, but their correlation with Tabár based classification are less clear (Spearman's correlation coefficient < 0.5). This paper is a follow up study to [14] with a focus on the correlation

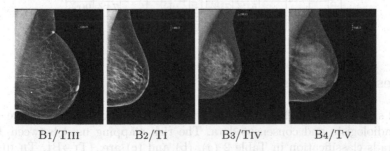

B1/Tııı   B2/Tı   B3/Tıv   B4/Tv

Fig. 3. Example mammographic images with Birads ('B') risk classifications from low to high, and their equivalent according to the Tabár ('T') scheme

between Tabár and Birads based classification, using full field digital mammography. In addition, aspects with respect to reader experience and related inter reader variability were also investigated. The reader is referred to [14] for the details of the study on the correlation between Wolf, Boyd and Birads based classification, using digitised mammograms.

2   Data and Method

The dataset consists of 360 'for presentation' mammographic images processed for optimal visual appearance to radiologists. Three radiologists participated in an independent mammographic risk classification process evaluation, and have different mammogram reading experience at junior (J), expert (E) and consultant (C) levels. Here, we consider a mammogram reader's experience from 0 to 3 years is junior, 3 to 10 years is expert and over 10 years is consultant. A consensus (S) ground true was generated based on J, E, and C; in the case of a tied (mutually exclusive) rating, a weighting mechanism was imposed to assign weights 1.0, 1.5 and 2.0 to J, E and C, respectively. It should be noted that the reader experience categorisation used is for the evaluation purpose; in clinical practice, there is no clear agreement to the categorisation. Table 1 shows inter reader variability; the classification discrepancies in Tabár are more or less the same amongst the radiologists; whilst in Birads, the discrepancies are lower between the consultant and expert radiologists (i.e. C-E), moderate between the expert and junior radiologists (i.e. E-J), and relatively higher between the junior and consultant radiologists (i.e. J-C). Cohen's Kappa (κ) and Spearman's correlation coefficient were used to investigate the correlation between Tabár and Birads based classification, including individual vs. individual, individual vs. consensus.

Table 1. Inter reader variability (agreement) for Tabár (left) and Birads (right) classification schemes

	Reader	E	C	S		Reader	E	C	S
		Tabár					**Birads**		
Tabár J		58%	58%	77%	Birads	J	65%	59%	75%
Tabár E			51%	71%	Birads	E		74%	90%
Tabár C				81%	Birads	C			85%

3   Results and Discussion

Table 2 shows Tabár and Birads classification agreement matrices between the three radiologists and consensus data. The risk mapping used between Tabár and Birads classification in Table 2 (a), (b) and (c) are: ($T_I{\rightarrow}B_1$, $T_{II/III}{\rightarrow}B_2$, $T_{IV}{\rightarrow}B_3$, $T_V{\rightarrow}B_4$), ($T_{II}{\rightarrow}B_1$, $T_{III}{\rightarrow}B_2$, $T_{IV}{\rightarrow}B_3$, $T_V{\rightarrow}B_4$), and ($T_{II/III}{\rightarrow}B_1$, $T_I{\rightarrow}B_2$, $T_{IV}{\rightarrow}B_3$, $T_V{\rightarrow}B_4$), respectively. The results shown in Table 2 (b) were used as a direct comparison with [14], in which the agreement were calculated between the two schemes with Tabár I left out. Note that the tissue compositions for Tabár II and III are the same as described in Tabár scheme. The results shown in Table 2 (a) were based on the assumption that for a similar mammographic appearance, Tabár and Birads have similar perception of breast risk, despite the quantification methods used to measure the risk are fundamentally different. However, the agreement calculated based on the mapping tells otherwise, as the vast majority of the TI are B2, and TII/TIII are spread across B1. If only considering the three radiologists' results (excluding the consensus data), the derived average agreement between such a risk mapping is 61%; this is 10% improvement when compared to the results in [14]; which may indicate that by using digital mammography with improved contrast and texture appearances, the inter reader variability is noticeably reduced. The results shown in Table 2 (c) were based on swapping the risk mapping between TI and TII/TIII to B2 and B1, respectively. Such a mapping shows on average higher correlation between Tabár and Birads based classification, which indicates that for a similar mammographic appearance, Tabár has a different perception to Birads in low breast risk (i.e. TI, TII/III, B1 and B2). According to the results in Table 2 (c), the highest agreement is 92% (Spearman's correlation coefficient > 0.9, $\kappa = 0.86$ almost perfect agreement) for the consultant radiologist; the lowest agreement is 52% (Spearman's correlation coefficient > 0.8, $\kappa = 0.29$ fair agreement) for the junior radiologist; the highest and lowest inter reader agreement are 77% and 63%, respectively. Table 3 (a-1,2) and (b-1,2) are the original confusion matrices and confusion matrices with the risk mapping according to Table 2 (c), for the consultant (i.e. C(Tabár) vs. C(Birads)) and junior (i.e. J(Tabár) vs. J(Birads)) radiologists, respectively. When comparing these four tables, the results indicate that to a less experienced radiologist the confusion may occur more often between TI, TII/TIII, B1 and B2. This confusion may be caused due to that low risk Tabár I consists of 25% nodular (e.g. TDLU) and 35% homogeneous (e.g. fibroglandular) tissue, and both may appear as high intensity dense tissue on mammograms; whilst the proportion of these two types of tissue is close to the tissue composition for Birads 2, where the breast has $25\% - 50\%$ scattered fibroglandular densities. From clinical practice point of view, density based mammographic risk classification is now widely used in clinical environment, and Tabár based mammographic risk classification may be less practised amongst less experienced radiologists.

4   Conclusions

The correlation is much stronger between Tabár and Birads based classification when the risks are mapped as Tabár II/III, I, IV, V to Birads 1, 2, 3, 4. Inter reader variability is reduced; this may partially due to sharper image quality offered by digital mammography. Readers' mammographic reading experience can be linked to the correctness in assessing low breast risk when using Tabár scheme. To our knowledge, this is the first time a direct strong correlation is

Table 2. Inter reader variability (agreement); Tabár vs. Birads with different risk mappings

	Reader	Birads				Birads				Birads			
		J	E	C	S	J	E	C	S	J	E	C	S
Tabár	J	39%	28%	22%	32%	83%	67%	60%	74%	52%	67%	75%	69%
	E	34%	23%	17%	23%	77%	61%	50%	61%	63%	66%	65%	66%
	C	22%	17%	25%	20%	55%	43%	51%	51%	64%	77%	**92%**	86%
	S	28%	18%	21%	20%	79%	61%	61%	68%	64%	76%	86%	83%
		(a)				(b)				(c)			

Table 3. The original and merged confusion matrices for the highest and lowest agreement between Tabár and Birads, according to the risk mapping in Table 2 (c). Table 4 shows the corresponding results based on Tabár and Birads low and high risk classes.

(a-1)

Tabár	Birads			
	1	2	3	4
I	24	121	2	0
II	44	0	0	0
III	102	2	0	0
IV	0	0	41	4
V	0	0	0	20

(a-2)

Tabár	Birads			
	1	2	3	4
II/III	146	2	0	0
I	24	121	2	0
IV	0	0	41	4
V	0	0	0	20

(b-1)

Tabár	Birads			
	1	2	3	4
I	0	19	77	0
II	83	3	0	0
III	31	82	9	0
IV	0	0	52	4
V	0	0	0	0

(b-2)

Tabár	Birads			
	1	2	3	4
II/III	114	85	9	0
I	0	19	77	0
IV	0	0	52	4
V	0	0	0	0

Table 4. The corresponding confusion matrices for the highest and lowest agreement based on the low and high risk classes between Tabár and Birads, and according to the risk mapping in Table 2 (c). Note that Tabár I, II and III are low risk classes, Tabár IV and V are high risk classes; whilst Birads 1 and 2 are low risk classes, Birads 3 and 4 are high risk classes. The agreement between Tabár and Birads for the consultant and junior radiologist are 99% and 76%, respectively.

(a)

Tabár		Birads	
		Low	High
	Low	293	2
	High	0	65

(b)

Tabár		Birads	
		Low	High
	Low	218	86
	High	0	56

established between Tabár and Birads based classification, which can be a useful knowledge in computer aided mammographic risk assessment.

References

1. Cancer statistics registrations, England, 2011. MB1(42) (June 2013)
2. Mukhtar, T.K., Yeates, D.R., Goldacre, M.J.: Breast cancer mortality trends in England and the assessment of the effectiveness of mammography screening: population-based study. Journal of the Royal Society of Medicine 6, 234–242 (2013)
3. DeSantis, C., Ma, J., Bryan, L., Jemal, A.: Breast cancer statistics. CA: A Cancer Journal for Clinicians (2013)
4. Eccles, S.A., et al.: Critical research gaps and translational priorities for the successful prevention and treatment of breast cancer. Breast Cancer Research 15(R92) (2013)
5. Colin, C., Prince, V., Valette, P.J.: Can mammographic assessments lead to consider density as a risk factor for breast cancer? European Journal of Radiology 82(3), 404–411 (2013)
6. Tabár, L., Tot, T., Dean, P.B.: Breast Cancer: The Art and Science of Early Detection With Mamography: Perception, Interpretation, Histopatholigic Correlation, 1st edn. Georg Thieme Verlag (December 2004)
7. American College of Radiology. Breast Imaging Reporting and Data System BI-RADS, 4th edn. American College of Radiology, Reston (2004)
8. Tzias, D., George, S., Wilkinson, L., Mehta, R.: Quantification of breast cancer risk based on the UK five-point classification system. Breast Cancer Research 13:S4 (November 2011)
9. Gail, M.H., Brinton, L.A., Byar, D.P., Corle, D.K., Green, S.B., Schairer, C., Mulvihill, J.J.: Projecting individualized probabilities of developing breast cancer for white females who are being examined annually. Journal of the National Cancer Institute 81(24), 1879–1886 (1989)
10. Tyrer, J., Duffy, S.W., Cuzick, J.: A breast cancer prediction model incorporating familial and personal risk factors. Statistics in Medicine 23, 1111–1130 (2004)
11. Wolfe, J.N.: Breast patterns as an index of risk for developing breast cancer. American Journal of Roentgenology 126(6), 1130–1137 (1976)
12. Sickles, E.A.: Wolfe mammographic parenchymal patterns and breast cancer risk. American Journal of Roentgenology 188(2), 301–303 (2007)
13. Gram, I.T., Bremnes, Y., Ursin, G., Maskarinec, G., Bjurstam, N., Lund, E.: Percentage density, Wolfe's and Tabár's mammographic patterns: agreement and association with risk factors for breast cancer. Breast Cancer Research 7, 854–861 (2005)
14. Muhimmah, I., Oliver, A., Denton, E.R.E., Pont, J., Pérez, E., Zwiggelaar, R.: Comparison between Wolfe, Boyd, BI-RADS and Tabár based mammographic risk assessment. In: Astley, S.M., Brady, M., Rose, C., Zwiggelaar, R. (eds.) IWDM 2006. LNCS, vol. 4046, pp. 407–415. Springer, Heidelberg (2006)

Predicting Triple-Negative Breast Cancer and Axillary Lymph Node Metastasis Using Diagnostic MRI

Jeff Wang[1], Fumi Kato[2], Kohsuke Kudo[2], Hiroko Yamashita[3], and Hiroki Shirato[1]

[1] Department of Radiation Medicine, Hokkaido University Graduate School of Medicine
[2] Department of Diagnostic and Interventional Radiology, Hokkaido University Hospital
[3] Department of Breast Surgery, Hokkaido University Hospital
[1-3] Sapporo, Japan
jeff.wang@pop.med.hokudai.ac.jp

Abstract. Early classification of breast cancers by molecular subtype allows for expeditious characterization of the disease and selection of appropriate treatment options. This ability is especially a concern for "triple-negative" cancers, which lack expression of the three cell surface receptors that most breast cancer hormonal therapies target, tend to be the most aggressive/metastatic compared to other subtypes, have lymph node involvement at diagnoses, and have relatively poor prognoses. In this study, we aim to develop predictive models using Dynamic Contrast-Enhanced (DCE) MRI-extracted features to identify triple-negative cancers and axillary lymph node metastasis at the time of diagnostic imaging. Using only morphological, pharmacokinetic, densitometric, statistical, textural, and textural kinetic features obtained from DCE-MRI, we were able to classify 91.3% of 69 lesions correctly for triple-negative status with a sensitivity of 55.6%, a specificity of 96.7, and an AUC of 0.889; 71.6% of lesions correctly for lymph node metastasis with a sensitivity of 50.0%, a specificity of 82.2%, and an AUC of 0.677.

Keywords: Breast cancer, molecular subtypes, triple-negative, axillary lymph node, metastasis, Dynamic Contrast-Enhanced MRI, imaging biomarkers, texture, textural kinetics, classification.

1 Introduction

Prognosis and treatment regimens of breast cancers differ based on molecular subtype. So called "triple-negative" breast cancers (TN), which do not exhibit estrogen (ER), progesterone (PgR), nor human epidermal growth factor receptor 2 (HER2) receptors on their cell surface are especially difficult to treat since the disease cannot benefit from receptor-specific therapies. TN tumors are generally larger in size, of higher grade, have lymph node involvement at diagnosis, and are more aggressive [1]. For these reasons, it is of significant interest to identify patients who fall into this category as early as possible. As less than 30% of patients with metastatic TN breast cancer survive 5 years [2], it is of even greater priority to identify those with disease further complicated by metastasis.

H. Fujita, T. Hara, and C. Muramatsu (Eds.): IWDM 2014, LNCS 8539, pp. 334–340, 2014.
© Springer International Publishing Switzerland 2014

The purpose of this study is to develop models to predict TN cancers and axillary lymph node metastasis of breast cancer using features obtained from dynamic contrast-enhanced (DCE) MR imaging before surgery.

2   Methods

2.1   Subjects

This retrospective study included 64 women, presenting mass lesions pathologically proven as invasive carcinoma, who underwent 3.0T breast DCE-MRI before their surgical procedure between February 2012 and March 2013. Two of the subjects presented 2 unilateral lesions and 3 presented bilateral lesions. Of the 69 lesions total, 58 were characterized as invasive ductal carcinoma, 4 as invasive lobular carcinoma, and 7 as other. Ages of women included ranged from 40 to 79, averaging 60.

The following health features of subjects were included in the analysis: age, height, weight, body mass index (BMI), age at menarche, days since last menstrual period, and parity status.

2.2   Imaging

MRI. All subjects were imaged using one 3.0T Philips Achieva TX system with a 7-channel breast coil while lying in the prone position. Gadolinium-enhanced fat-suppressed 3-D T1-weighted images were acquired bilaterally in the axial plane using a protocol capturing four time points: one immediately before contrast agent injection (t1), two early phase (t2 and t3, at 1 and 2 minutes after injection respectively), and one late phase (t4, at 6 minutes after injection). Between t3 and t4, a high-resolution fat-suppressed 3-D T1-weighted image was also acquired unilaterally of the diseased side breast in the sagittal plane.

Radiologist Review. A board-certified radiologist specializing in breast imaging with 13 years of experience reviewed all cases. Both DCE-MRI and high resolution sagittal imaging were used. Morphology of the mass (shape, margin, internal enhancement characteristics), kinetics (initial rise, delayed phase), and associated findings for nipple and skin were evaluated for each lesion according to Breast Imaging Reporting and Data Systems (BI-RADS) MRI and included in the analysis. Mass size, lesion laterality, additional findings (necrosis, degeneration, cystic formation in mass), findings of ductal spread (status, morphology, distribution), axillary lymphadenopathy suspicion, and size of axillary lymph node were also evaluated and included.

2.3   Image Processing

All image processing was performed using custom MATLAB R2012b (MathWorks, Inc., Natick, United States) software.

Tissue Compartment Segmentation. Segmentation of the affected breast's tissue into four compartments was performed from the image at t3. Breast segmentation was performed by automatic detection of the skin edge and semi-automatic delineation of the chest wall in every slice. Lesion segmentation was performed semi-automatically using a grey-level intensity threshold region-growing method seeded by the user. Parenchyma and adipose tissue segmentation was performed automatically using a Fuzzy C-means clustering technique within the region previously identified as breast. Each voxel of the breast compartment, except that identified as lesion, was clustered using a fuzzy membership function into either parenchyma or adipose tissue cluster by similar grey-level intensity.

Pharmacokinetic Modeling. Pharmacokinetic modeling based on signal intensity change over time was performed on each image. The following parameters were calculated for each voxel designated as breast tissue, resulting in 10 parameter maps: rate in, mean rate in, peak time, max rate, rate out, percent enhancement, signal enhancement ratio, initial area under the enhancement curve (iAUC) at 1 minute, iAUC at 2 minutes, and iAUC at 6 minutes.

Features. The four tissue compartments' regions of interest obtained from t3 were duplicated onto the t1, t2, and t4 image maps and also onto each of the 10 pharmacokinetic parameter maps. Features were calculated from either the tissue compartments themselves or from each combination of the compartments and 14 maps (56 regions of interest total), including morphological, densitometric, first-order statistical, second-order statistical, and textural kinetic measures.

Three morphological features were calculated of the tissue compartments: volume, surface area, and compactness.

One breast tissue density feature was calculated from the tissue compartments: percent fibroglandular volume. Associated volumes of breast tissue compartments (fibroglandular/parenchyma and adipose volume themselves), commonly labeled density features, are also included, having been calculated in morphological analysis step above.

Twelve first-order statistical features were calculated of each region of interest: mean, median, mode, minimum, maximum, standard deviation, variance, skewness, kurtosis, sum, range, and interquartile range. Twelve second-order statistical features, also known as Haralick texture features [3] or grey-level co-occurrence texture features, were calculated at 4 voxel offset distances (48 total) of each region of interest: energy, contrast, correlation, variance, homogeneity, sum mean, entropy, maximum probability, inertia, cluster shade, cluster prominence, and inverse difference. Each second-order statistical feature calculated was averaged across voxel offsetting in 26 directions of 3-D space.

Textural kinetic modeling [4] based on feature value change over time was performed on each statistical feature (12 first-order + 48 second-order) using the same 10 parameters calculated in pharmacokinetic modeling above, only per region of interest instead of per voxel.

In all, 5776 features were calculated from image processing.

2.4   Pathology Findings

Expression of ER, PgR, and HER2 receptors was examined by immunohistochemistry in specimens. Axillary lymph node metastasis was determined by sentinel lymph node biopsy or axillary lymph node dissection.

2.5   Predictive Modeling

All modeling was performed using Waikato Environment for Knowledge Analysis 3.6.9 [5] (University of Waikato, Hamilton, New Zealand).

Class Definition. Two models were created. Cases were classified as TN if the lesion lacked expression of ER, PgR, and HER2, else they were classified as non-triple-negative (non-TN). Cases were also classified by using results of lymph node pathology findings as metastatic or non-metastatic. Nine lesions were found to be TN and 60 were found to be non-TN. Twenty two exhibited axillary lymph node metastasis, while 45 did not. In 2 subjects, metastasis status was not known.

Classification. Supervised learning of class was performed on the two models described above. A logistic regression classifier with restricted maximum likelihood regularization was used [6]. Generalization performance of classifiers were estimated by use of 10-fold randomized and stratified cross-validation [7] where performance metrics were averaged over the folds.

Feature Reduction. As the number of imaging features was quite large, feature reduction was performed within cross-validation folds of each model. A Subset evaluation method was used on each of the 10 training subsamples defined by cross-validation, which evaluated feature subsets found by backtracking-augmented greedy hill-climbing against accuracy in predicting the class in the corresponding validation subsamples also by logistic regression with regularization.

Performance Metrics. Classification performance was quantified using four metrics: accuracy, sensitivity, specificity, and area under the receiver operating characteristic curve (AUC). The latter three measures were computed relative to the minority classes TN and metastatic.

3   Results

On average, 2.6 features survived feature reduction per fold in the TN status model's cross-validation tests. The features found as most significant predictors of TN status were: standard deviation of the parenchyma's pharmacokinetic rate in (Figure 1, left), mass shape, and kurtosis of the lesion's pharmacokinetic rate in.

On average, 6.4 features survived feature reduction per fold in the lymph node metastasis model's cross-validation tests. The features found as most significant predictors of lymph node metastasis were: max rate of the parenchyma's minimum value textural kinetics (Figure 1, right), max probability of the lesion's pharmacokinetic max rate with an 8-voxel offset, morphology of ductal spread, max probability of the lesion at t4 with an 8-voxel offset, minimum of the adipose's pharmacokinetic iAUC130, correlation of the lesion's pharmacokinetic rate in with a 2-voxel offset, kurtosis of the lesion at t2, correlation of the breast compartment's pharmacokinetic rate out with a 2-voxel offset, and mass internal enhancement characteristics.

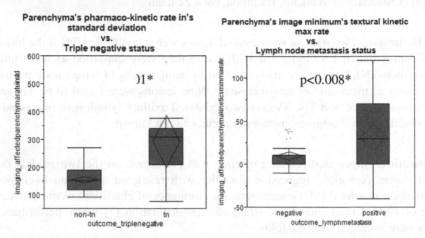

Fig. 1. Examples of a significant first-order statistical feature in the TN model (left) and a significant textural kinetics feature (derived from a second-order statistical feature) in the metastasis model (right). *by Wilcoxon signed-rank test

Performance metrics are summarized below in Table 1. With the first logistic regression model learned, we were able to classify 91.3% of the breast cancers in this data set correctly for TN status with a sensitivity of 55.6%, a specificity of 96.7%, and an AUC of 0.889. The lymph node metastasis model learned was able to classify 71.6% of the breast cancers with a sensitivity of 50.0%, a specificity of 82.2%, and an AUC of 0.677.

Table 1. Summary of classification performance metrics

Model	Accuracy	Sensitivity	Specificity	AUC
Triple negative	91.3%	55.6%	96.7%	0.889
Lymph node metastasis	71.6%	50.0%	82.2%	0.677

4   Discussion

With the numerous options for treatment that have become available, development of a method able to predict triple-negative and lymph node metastatic breast cancer early would be helpful in the selection of care. Much effort is being taken toward customization of healthcare toward personalized medicine and such a tool would benefit the cause. Of course, were such a prediction tool not only non-invasive, but also automated, it would be of even greater clinical value. As detailed in the results section above, nearly all of the features surviving feature reduction in this study were products of image processing. So while the developments here did not go as far as fully automating the predictive classifiers learned, it is our aim to do so in the future with continued investigation of the value of these and other imaging biomarkers in their ability to predict outcomes of breast cancer.

Also of particular interest from the findings above, is one of the surviving features of the TN model - the "standard deviation of the parenchyma's pharmacokinetic rate in". It is worth noting this feature again for further discussion as it is essentially equivalent to the heterogeneity of the new imaging biomarker being heavily researched as "background parenchymal enhancement" for its relationship to breast cancer risk and MRI diagnostic performance [8]–[10]. We show here that it also has predictive value in breast cancer subtyping.

5   Conclusion

We have developed models using diagnostic DCE-MRI-extracted features able to predict TN status at the time of diagnostic image examination with great accuracy and discriminative ability, and able to predict axillary lymph node metastasis with notable accuracy and discriminative ability.

References

1. Voduc, K.D., Cheang, M.C.U., Tyldesley, S., Gelmon, K., Nielsen, T.O., Kennecke, H.: Breast cancer subtypes and the risk of local and regional relapse. Journal of Clinical Oncology 28(10), 1684–1691 (2010)
2. Liedtke, C., Mazouni, C., Hess, K.: Response to neoadjuvant therapy and long-term survival in patients with triple-negative breast cancer. Journal of Clinical Oncology (2008)
3. Haralick, R.: Textural features for image classification. IEEE Transactions on Systems, Man, and Cybernetics (1973)
4. Agner, S.C., Soman, S., Libfeld, E., McDonald, M., Thomas, K., Englander, S., Rosen, M.A., Chin, D., Nosher, J., Madabhushi, A.: Textural kinetics: A novel dynamic contrast-enhanced (DCE)-MRI feature for breast lesion classification. Journal of Digital Imaging 24(3), 446–463 (2011)
5. Hall, M., Frank, E., Holmes, G.: The WEKA data mining software: An update. ACM SIGKDD Explorations 11(1), 10–18 (2009)
6. Le Cessie, S., van Houwelingen, J.: Ridge estimators in logistic regression. Applied Statistics (1992)
7. Hastie, T., Tibshirani, R., Friedman, J.: The Elements of Statistical Learning: Data Mining, Inference, and Prediction (2001)

8. King, V., Brooks, J., Bernstein, J., Reiner, A.: Background Parenchymal Enhancement at Breast MR Imaging and Breast Cancer Risk. Radiology 260(1) (2011)
9. Giger, M.L., Karssemeijer, N., Schnabel, J.A.: Breast image analysis for risk assessment, detection, diagnosis, and treatment of cancer. The Annual Reviews of Biomedical Engineering 15, 327–357 (2013)
10. DeMartini, W.B., Liu, F., Peacock, S., Eby, P.R., Gutierrez, R.L., Lehman, C.D.: Background parenchymal enhancement on breast MRI: impact on diagnostic performance. American Journal of Roentgenology 198(4), W373–W380 (2012)

Understanding the Role of Correct Lesion Assessment in Radiologists' Reporting of Breast Cancer

Claudia Mello-Thoms[1], Phuong Dung Trieu[1], Mohammed A. Rawashdeh[1], Kriscia Tapia[1], Warwick B. Lee[2], and Patrick C. Brennan[1]

[1] Department of Medical Imaging and Radiation Sciences, Faculty of Health Sciences, University of Sydney, Cumberland Campus, East Street, P.O. Box 170, Lidcombe, NSW 2141, Australia
[2] BreastScreen NSW, Cancer Institute NSW, Australia
{claudia.mello-thoms,phuong.trieu, kriscia.tapia,patrick.brennan}@sydney.edu.au, mraw2971@uni.sydney.edu.au, Warwick.Lee_ext@cancerinstitute.org.au

Abstract. Despite the innovations in breast imaging technology, the miss rates of breast cancers at mammography screening have remained stable, ranging from 10-30% per year. While many factors have been linked to radiologist performance (such as volume of cases read, years of experience reading mammograms), little is known about the relationship between the cancers correctly reported by the radiologists and the characteristics of the background and the malignant lesion. In this study we have used the BREAST platform to allow 92 radiologists to read a case set of 60 digital mammograms, of which 20 depicted cancer. Readers were divided in 4 groups, obtained from the quartiles of the median localization sensitivity performance. Median location sensitivity for all readers was 0.71 (IQR=0.21). Statistically significant differences were observed among the groups in correctly reporting several types of lesion; for example, stellate masses were correctly reported only 37.5% by the poorest performers (median location sensitivity < 0.5), vs 88.9% by the top performers (median location sensitivity $\geq$ 0.92, z=-3.317, P=0.0017). When compared to top performers, the poorest performers had more difficulty reporting smaller lesions (<10mm) (40.9% vs 90.9% from top performers, z=-3.354, P=0.0008). Results suggest a link between the types of lesions more often missed by radiologists and their median location sensitivity.

Keywords: Digital mammography, radiologist performance, lesion characteristics, lesion assessment, missed cancers.

1 Introduction

According to the GLOBOCAN, 3.3 million women died from cancer worldwide in 2008, and from these, the greatest proportion lost their lives to breast cancer, which claimed 14% of all these deaths [1]. Despite the great advances in breast imaging technology, with screening programs migrating from a film-based environment to a

H. Fujita, T. Hara, and C. Muramatsu (Eds.): IWDM 2014, LNCS 8539, pp. 341–347, 2014.
© Springer International Publishing Switzerland 2014

digital environment, no reduction has been observed in the rates of cancers missed, which have remained steady between 10-30% per year [2]. At first it was hypothesized that these unreported lesions did not attract the radiologists' visual attention, but eye-position studies have shown that up to 70% of these cancers do attract the radiologists' gaze [3], often for as long as the lesions that are correctly reported [4]. Hence, the issue with missed cancers is not one of detection, but one of perception and decision making. In this domain, the literature is full of studies reporting high variability rates not only among radiologists but also within radiologists [5-7] and this variability has often been suggested as the main underlying cause behind detected but unreported malignancies.

However, very little is known about the relationship between missed (or reported) lesion characteristics and radiologist performance. This is what we set out to explore in this study.

2   Methods

Institutional ethical approval was granted for this study. In addition, patient consent waived and participating radiologists signed a consent form before case reading. Ninety two radiologists who currently report breast images in Australia and New Zealand voluntarily agreed to participate in this study. Radiologists provided some demographic information, such as their age, number of years reading mammograms and number of mammograms read per year, prior to the data collection. Data was collected at the 2011 Royal Australian and New Zealand College of Radiologists Breast Imaging Group meeting in Hobart, AU.

Two Eizo Radiforce GS510 (21.3 inches) monochrome high- class LCD diagnostic monitors were used to display the images. On average, radiologists sat 40 cm away from the displays, in a reading room where the average ambient light ranged from 20-30 lux.

The Breast Screen Reader Assessment Strategy (BREAST) platform was used in this study. BREAST allows for online reading of digital case sets, lesion location marking, and reporting of confidence in lesion malignancy. The radiologists' task was to detect and report breast lesions. They were allowed to digitally manipulate the images (such as panning, zooming). Upon detecting a lesion, radiologists used a mouse-controlled cursor to digitally mark the lesion's location on the image. They also assigned a confidence score to their mark, where 2 = benign lesion and 3-5 represented malignancy, with a higher value indicating higher confidence. If they thought the case was normal, they just used the mouse to click on "next case", and a confidence score of 1 (=normal) was automatically assigned to the case. This classification is based on the grading system for mammographic lesions endorsed by the Royal Australian and New Zealand College of Radiology [8].

Albeit the radiologists did not report lesion or background characteristics, all marked lesions were contrasted with those contained in the "truth table", which was generated using additional imaging and pathology reports, for characterization. These characteristics were chosen according to the Synoptic Breast Imaging Report of the National Breast Cancer Centre (NBCC, now Cancer Australia), endorsed by the Royal Australian and New Zealand College of Radiologists (RANZCR), which is similar to the 4th edition American College of Radiology Breast Imaging Reporting and Data System (BI-RADS).

Background characteristics used consisted of breast density, which was categorized as

    i.   Scattered fibroglandular density;

    ii.   Heterogeneously dense;

    iii.   Extremely dense.

True lesions correctly localized (as well as those not reported by the readers) were characterized according to:

    i.   *Lesion Type*:

         a. cluster of calcifications;

         b. stellate mass;

         c. spiculated mass.

    ii.   *Lesion Margin*:

         a. spiculated;

         b. indistinct;

         c. stellate.

    iii.   *Lesion Shape*:

         a. irregular;

         b. architectural distortion;

         c. round/oval.

    iv.   *Lesion Size*:

         a. <10mm;

         b. $10mm \leq size < 20mm$;

         c. $\geq 20mm$.

In this way, false alarms on normal or abnormal cases were not included in the analysis of lesion characterization, as no characteristics could be attributed to these reports.

No restrictions were imposed on reading time, and clinical history for each case was not provided to the radiologists. Moreover, information on the proportion of normal/abnormal cases in the set was also not provided.

Data Analysis

Radiologists' performance was calculated using location sensitivity, sensitivity and specificity. Radiologists were divided into 4 groups according median group location sensitivity:

    i.   First Quartile (1st QTL): location sensitivity < 0.5

    ii.   Second Quartile (2nd QTL): $0.5 \leq$ location sensitivity < 0.71

    iii.   Third Quartile (3rd QTL): $0.71 \leq$ location sensitivity < 0.92

    iv.   Fourth Quartile (4th QTL): location sensitivity ≥ 0.92.

According to this criterion, radiologists in the First Quartile were the poorest performers whereas those in the Fourth Quartile were the best performers.

Correlation between performance level (quartile) and demographic data was calculated. Kruskall-Wallis test was used to determine statistically significant differences among the 4 groups. The non-parametric Mann-Whitney U-test was used to determine whether significant differences existed between poorest (1st quartile) and best (4th) performers, as well as between radiologists in the 2nd and 3rd quartiles. For all tests, statistical significance was set at $P<0.05$.

3   Results

Median location sensitivity for the entire group was 0.71 (Inter-Quartile Range = IQR = 0.21). Table 1 shows the radiologists' demographic data, per quartile.

As shown, most radiologists' performance fell either into the 2nd (33 radiologists) or 3rd (45) quartiles, with fewer radiologists performing either poorly (only 8 readers in the 1st quartile) or displaying outstanding performance (6 readers). These radiologists read the largest mean number of mammograms per year (6300), as opposed to the poorest performers, who read the lowest number (3750). This difference, however, was not statistically significant ($z=-0.801$, $P=0.4231$). Radiologists in the 1st quartile had a median location sensitivity of 0.440, which significantly contrasted from 0.940 for those in the 4th quartile ($z=-3.416$, $P=0.0006$). Conversely, they had higher median specificity (0.855) when contrasted to those in the 4th quartile (0.690) ($z=-2.228$, $P=0.0259$).

Comparisons between radiologists in the 2nd and 3rd quartiles suggested significant differences for location sensitivity ($z=-7.761$, $P<0.0001$) and for specificity ($z=-2.006$, $P=0.0449$).

Correlation analysis showed no significant relationships between the quartile the radiologist was assigned to and either (i) the number of years reading mammograms ($z=0.301$, $P=0.764$) or (ii) the number of mammograms read per year ($z=0.696$, $P=0.487$). Specificity, however, was significantly correlated to quartile assignment ($z=-2.456$, $P=0.014$), with lower performers showing higher specificity.

Table 1. Demographic data per quartile

	1st QTL	2nd QTL	3rd QTL	4th QTL
Number of radiologists	8	33	45	6
Mean number of years reading mammograms	6.875	13.000	9.044	15.833
Mean number of mammograms/year	3750	4924	4729	6300
Median location sensitivity	0.440	0.580	0.790	0.940
Median Specificity	0.855	0.800	0.730	0.690

Table 2. Assessment of mean percent correct responses accorgin to breast density, per quartile. All values given as percentages

	1st QTL	2nd QTL	3rd QTL	4th QTL
Heterogeneously dense	32.3	53.3	77.9	90.3
Extremely Dense	55.0	73.3	85.7	96.7
Scattered fibroglandular density	41.7	57.6	73.2	94.4

Table 2 shows the mean percent correct responses, per quartile, according to breast density.

Kruskall-Wallis test showed significant differences among the 4 groups for all density types (heterogeneously dense, H=63.587, P<0.0001; extremely dense, H=28.751, P<0.0001; scattered fibroglandular density, H=39.137, P<0.0001). As shown in Table 2, higher performers were more likely to correctly report cancer than lower performers in all density types: heterogeneously dense (z=-3.367, P=0.0008), extremely dense (z=-3.381, P=0.0007) and scattered fibroglandular (z=-3.405, P=0.0007) tissue. Comparisons were also significant between readers in 2nd and 3rd quartile for heterogeneously dense (z=-6.993, P<0.0001), extremely dense (z=-3.810, P=0.0001) and scattered fibroglandular (z=-4.347, P<0.0001) tissue.

Table 3. Assessment of mean correct responses according to lesion characterization, per quartile. All values given as percentages.

		1st QTL	2nd QTL	3rd QTL	4th QTL
Lesion Type	**Cluster**	25.0	36.4	63.8	77.8
	Stellate	37.5	59.6	81.2	88.9
	Spiculated	48.9	69.1	80.4	95.5
Lesion Margin	**Spiculated**	50.0	64.0	84.0	93.8
	Indistinct	34.6	55.0	73.6	94.9
	Stellate	37.5	59.6	81.2	88.9
Lesion Shape	**Irregular**	41.7	66.2	81.2	95.8
	Architectural distortion	50.0	65.2	87.5	91.7
	Round/oval	33.3	38.4	62.3	100
Lesion Size	**< 10mm**	40.9	59.8	75.9	90.9
	10mm ≤ size < 20mm	37.5	55.6	76.8	88.9
	≥ 20mm	43.8	60.6	84.2	100

Correlation analysis showed significant relationship between the quartile the radiologist was assigned to and their correct response rates in backgrounds of different densities, for (i) heterogeneously dense (z=11.385, P<0.0001), extremely dense (z=6.684, P<0.0001) and scattered fibroglandular (z=7.942, P<0.0001) tissue.

Finally, Table 3 shows the mean percent correct responses for different lesion characteristics. Kruskall-Wallis test showed significant differences in mean correct responses according to lesion characteristics amongst the 4 radiologist groups for all characteristics listed in the table. For all tests, P<0.0001.

Contrasting the poorest performers (1st quartile) with the best performers (4th quartile) yielded significant differences in mean correct responses for all lesion characterization metrics used (P<0.05). Similar results were obtained for the comparison between 2nd and 3rd quartile radiologists.

Correlation analyses showed significant relationships (P<0.0001) between mean correct responses according to all lesion characterization measures used and the quartile the radiologist was assigned to.

4   Discussion

Although variability in the performance of radiologists reading screening mammograms has been well documented (for example, see [5-7]), the actual factors influencing reader performance are not well understood. Some factors have been repeatedly reported as influencing reading outcome, such as number of years reading mammograms and number of mammograms read per year [9,10], with a general agreement that more years reading and more mammograms read per year lead to better reader performance (as measured by the area under the Receiver Operating Characteristic curve). However, the relationship between the correctness of the radiologists' responses and both the background characteristics and the cancer characteristics has not been properly investigated, and it is the objective of this study.

Our data suggested that the poorest performers (radiologists whose median location sensitivity was less than 0.5) only correctly reported 25% of the microcalcification clusters, 37.5% of the stellate masses and 48.9% of the spiculated masses. This is in stark contrast with the top performers (median location sensitivity $\geq$ 0.92), who reported 77.8% of the clusters, 88.9% of the stellate and 95.5% of the spiculated masses. Moreover, lesions with indistinct margins were only reported correctly 34.6% of the time by the poorest performers, vs. 94.9% by the top radiologists. Similar staggering differences were observed for the other lesion types.

These results suggest that not only the poorest performers but also the radiologists in the 2nd QTL (with location sensitivity greater than 0.5 but less than the median for the entire group, which was 0.71) had difficulties reporting certain lesion types, with microcalcification clusters and stellate masses being the least frequently correctly identified (36.4% and 59.6%, respectively). Round masses or those with indistinct margins did not fare well either (being correctly reported by this group of radiologists only 38.4% and 55%, respectively), when contrasted with a correct report rate of 100% and 94.9%, respectively, for the best performers.

Interestingly, the best performing radiologists (4th quartile, with median location sensitivity of 0.94) had the lowest median specificity (0.690), whereas the poorest performers (1st quartile, with median location sensitivity of 0.440) had the best specificity (0.855). This trade-off between experience/sensitivity and specificity is in agreement with previous reports [11].

Our study had several limitations, amongst them the small number of cases used. In addition, radiologists were not given any clinical/history information on the cases, and this has been shown to significantly affect their performance when reading mammograms [12], which limits the generalizability of our conclusions. Finally, we divided the radiologists in a non-standard way using the groups' median location sensitivity. Certainly use of different criterion to group the radiologists would have led to different conclusions for this study.

In summary, our data suggests that background and lesion characteristics are significant components of variability in radiologist performance when reading digital mammograms. Hence, perhaps a way to improve reader performance in this task would be to gear radiologist training to perceptual identification of the types of lesions shown herein (and in the assessment of breast screening programs) to be the most challenging for them to correctly report.

References

1. GLOBOCAN Cancer Statistics on (2012), http://globocan.iarc.fr/Pages/fact_sheets_cancer.aspx (accessed March 4, 2014)
2. Martin, J.E., Moskowitz, M., Milbrath, J.R.: Breast cancers missed by mammography. AJR American Journal of Roentgenology 132, 737–758 (1979)
3. Nodine, C.F., et al.: Nature of expertise in searching mammograms for breast masses. Academic Radiology 3, 1000–1006 (1996)
4. Mello-Thoms, C., et al.: Effects of lesion conspicuity on visual search in mammogram reading. Academic Radiology 12, 830–840 (2005)
5. Beam, C.A., Layde, P.M., Sullivan, D.C.: Variability in the interpretation of screening mammograms by US radiologists: Finding from a national sample. Archives of Internal Medicine 156, 209–213 (1996)
6. Elmore, J.G., et al.: Variability in radiologists' interpretation of mammograms. New England Journal of Medicine 331, 1493–1499 (1994)
7. Soh, P.B., et al.: Assessing reader performance in radiology, An imperfect science: Lessons from breast screening. Clinical Radiology 67, 623–628 (2012)
8. http://canceraustralia.gov.au/sites/default/files/publications/big-1-breast-imaging-guide_504af02b4e80c.pdf (accessed on March 9, 2014)
9. Reed, W.M., et al.: Malignancy detection in digital mammograms: Important reader characteristics and required case numbers. Academic Radiology 17, 1409–1413 (2010)
10. Rawashdeh, M.A., et al.: Markers of good performance in mammography depend on number of annual readings. Radiology 269, 61–67 (2013)
11. Haneuse, S., et al.: Mammographic interpretive volume and diagnostic mammogram interpretation performance in community practice. Radiology 262, 69–79 (2012)
12. Carney, P.A., et al.: Use of clinical history affects accuracy of interpretive performance of screening mammography. Journal of Clinical Epidemiology 65, 219–230 (2012)

Realistic Simulation of Breast Tissue Microstructure in Software Anthropomorphic Phantoms

Predrag R. Bakic,[1] David D. Pokrajac,[2]
Raffaele De Caro,[3] and Andrew D.A. Maidment[1]

[1] Dept. of Radiology, University of Pennsylvania, Philadelphia, PA, USA
[2] Computer and Information Sciences Dept., Delaware State University, Dover, DE, USA
[3] Dept. of Human Anatomy and Physiology, University of Padova, Italy
Predrag.Bakic@uphs.upenn.edu

Abstract. Software anthropomorphic breast phantoms have been used in virtual clinical trials for preclinical validation of breast imaging systems. Virtual trial quality depends largely on the realism of the simulated breast anatomy. Our phantom design has been focused on the simulation of large-scale and meso-scale anatomical structures, including the breast outline, skin, and matrix of Cooper's ligaments and tissue compartments. Realism of such a design has been confirmed in comparative studies of phantom and clinical power spectra and parenchymal texture. We present a novel method for simulating the hierarchical organization of breast tissue subcompartments, seen in detailed histological images. The subcompartmentalization introduces microstructure in breast phantoms, resulting in improved realism of phantom images. The qualitative validation of phantoms with simulated microstructure is discussed in this paper; the quantitative validation in ongoing.

Keywords: Software breast phantoms, virtual clinical trials, small-scale tissue simulation, stereology, testing realism.

1   Introduction

Virtual clinical trials (VCTs) have received considerable attention recently; a VCT is an efficient way to perform optimization and preclinical validation of novel breast imaging systems (1, 2). VCTs are based upon sophisticated computer simulations of breast anatomy, image acquisition, image processing and display. The synthetic images generated by VCT can be assessed by model or human observers.

The quality of a VCT depends upon a number of factors including phantom realism; the phantom realism needs to be commensurate with the diagnostic task in question. The University of Pennsylvania (UPenn) breast anatomy model is based upon the simulation of large-scale and meso-scale anatomical structures; a variety of features are modelled, including the overall breast outline, the skin, the matrix of Cooper's ligaments and tissue compartments, and the assignment of adipose and fibroglandular tissue to these compartments.(3) The validity of this design has been confirmed for a number of tasks, and the visual realism of the anatomy model is

H. Fujita, T. Hara, and C. Muramatsu (Eds.): IWDM 2014, LNCS 8539, pp. 348–355, 2014.
© Springer International Publishing Switzerland 2014

supported by a number of comparative studies of phantom and clinical power spectra (4, 5) and parenchymal texture (6-8).

That said, we are constantly striving to improve the breast anatomy model further. In this paper, we present a novel method for simulating the hierarchical organization of breast tissue subcompartments, seen in detailed histological images. The introduction of a hierarchy of subcompartments into our breast anatomy model results in more realistic phantom images.

2   Methods

2.1   Histological Analysis

Our existing method for simulating breast tissue structures was motivated by the observed appearance of tissue compartments in existing histology and computed tomography breast images. In this paper we present a new analysis of histology slices from two breasts specimens; one obtained after breast reduction and another after mastopexy. The patients were aged 33 and 50, respectively. No abnormalities were detected in the two analysed breast specimens. The histologic analysis was performed at the University of Padova, Italy. Ten histology slices were analysed, at least one slice from each breast quadrant.

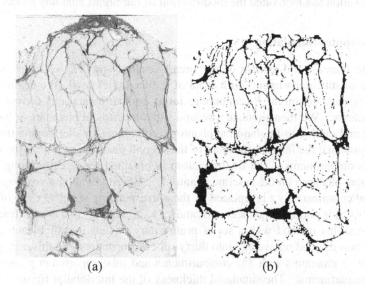

(a)   (b)

Fig. 1. An example of a breast histology image used in the size and shape analysis of adipose tissue compartments: (a) histology section with the Azan-Mallory staining; two analysed compartments are highlighted; (b) a binarized version of the same histology section

Fig. 1(a) shows a detailed microscopic image of the breast obtained using Azan-Mallory staining. The Azan-Mallory staining technique combines the original Mallory connective tissue stain with azocarmine (9); as a result, collagen is stained blue, nuclei and cytoplasm are red, and elastic fibres are pink or unstained. The section in Fig. 1(a) is oriented so that the areolar region is superior. In this example, the adipose tissue compartments are clearly encapsulated by the blue stained Cooper's ligaments. Two individual compartments have been highlighted to illustrate this observation.

Digital images of the stained histologic slices were binarized by thresholding. A binarized image of the matching tissue section is shown in Fig. 1(b). The binarized sections were used to estimate the size and shape of the tissue compartments. Two parameters, mean volume and axial ratio, were calculated using the stereological unfolding method by Saltykov, which assumes an ellipsoidal compartment shape (10). From this, compartment size and shape distributions were calculated.

Examination of Fig. 1 suggests that the thickness of the Cooper's ligaments depends upon the volume of the associated compartments. Thus, we have also estimated the volumetric fraction of the connective tissue and the average thickness of the Cooper's ligaments.

Finally, as seen in Fig. 1(a), the individual adipose compartments appear to be divided into smaller compartments by interlobular fibrous septa. Due to their small thickness, these interlobular fibrous septa may not be clearly visible in clinical breast images; however, they certainly contribute to the small-scale tissue variations seen in clinical images. The combination of the thicker Cooper's ligaments and the thinner interlobular fibrous septa indicate a hierarchical organization of tissue compartments. This observation has motivated the modification of our breast anatomy model.

2.2   Computer Simulation

In order to increase the realism of our breast anatomy model, we have included a simulation of subcompartments with septa of reduced thickness. We begin by simulating a baseline phantom, P, containing large compartments and correspondingly thick ligaments. We then simulate a second subcompartment phantom, S, having the same size and outline as the baseline phantom, containing smaller compartments and thinner ligaments; the internal structure of the second phantom will form the structure of the subcompartments. The final phantom is obtained by superimposing the subcompartment phantom on the baseline phantom. Algorithmically, a voxel $v_p(x,y,z)$ of P at spatial coordinate x,y,z is replaced by the corresponding voxel $v_s(x,y,z)$ of S if and only if $v_s(x,y,z)$ is part of a ligament in S, and $v_p(x,y,z)$ belongs to a compartment in P.

We tested this method with a set of preliminary models in which each compartment in P was divided on average into thirty subcompartments. In this test, we simulated baseline phantoms with 333 compartments and subcompartment phantoms with 10,000 compartments. The simulated thickness of the interlobular fibrous septa was selected to be 200μm in the subcompartment phantoms, 3 times smaller than the 600μm thickness of the primary Cooper's ligaments in the baseline phantoms.

The simulated microstructure was assessed subjectively based upon synthetic mammographic projections of phantoms with or without subcompartments. The synthetic images were generated using the breast anatomy and imaging simulation pipeline, developed at the University of Pennsylvania for the purpose of conducting VCTs of breast imaging systems (1). The pipeline includes modules for the simulation of normal breast anatomy, insertion of lesions, breast positioning and deformation, clinical image acquisition, image reconstruction and post-processing, image display, and image interpretation by model observers. External modules may be included in the pipeline as plugins.

The software breast phantoms with and without subcompartments were subject to simulated mammographic compression using a finite element deformation method (11). Mammographic imaging was then simulated using a ray tracing projection method, assuming a poly-energetic x-ray beam without scatter, and an ideal detector model. The quantum noise was simulated by adding a random Poisson process. The simulated image acquisition geometry corresponds to the Hologic Selenia Dimensions full-field digital mammography system (Hologic Inc., Bedford, MA). The resulting synthetic raw projections are post-processed using a commercial software package (Adara, Real Time Tomography, Villanova, PA).

3 Results and Discussion

3.1 Histological Analysis

Table 1 gives the values of average compartment volume, axial ratios and ligament thickness, as estimated from histology slides, in three different regions of the breast: subcutaneous ("Sub-Q"), posterior, and periglandular. These values have been averaged over 30 analysed adipose compartments. Adipose tissue compartments have a larger volume in the subcutaneous (0.84 ml) and posterior (0.94 ml) regions, as compared to the periglandular region (0.26 ml). Visually, these estimates of compartment volume agree with the observed appearance of breast tissue structures in these regions of clinical images.

The orientation of the breast tissue compartments had relatively little dependence upon region; the axial ratio varied from 2.02 in the subcutaneous region to 2.91 in the posterior region. This range of axial ratios corresponds to an angular difference of just 7 degrees. The variation in angular ratios is considerably larger in the posterior region (0.30; i.e., 10% of the average angular ratio), as compared to the subcutaneous region (0.14; 6%) and periglandular region (0.12; 6%). This suggests that some underlying structure may exist in these areas, which constrains the shape and orientation of the compartments.

Table 2 shows the volume fraction and thickness of the connective tissue, estimated from the binarized images of the stained Cooper's ligaments. The tabulated values have been averaged over 10 analysed tissue slices. The estimated average volume fraction was 12.3%, while the average thickness of Cooper's ligaments was 289 μm. The estimated ligament thickness fits well within the range of thicknesses used in our previous computer simulation of Cooper's ligaments: 200-600 μm. The volume fraction showed 11% variation relative to the mean value, while the ligament thickness showed 5% variation relative to the mean value.

Table 1. Average values of compartment volumes and axial ratios in various breast regions, estimated from breast histological sections

Region	Volume (cm^3)	Axial ratio
Sub-Q	0.84 ± 0.04	2.02 ± 0.14
Posterior	0.94 ± 0.07	2.91 ± 0.30
Periglandular	0.26 ± 0.01	2.04 ± 0.12

Table 2. Average values of the connective tissue volume fraction and thickness, estimated from Cooper's ligaments in breast histological sections

	Volume fraction (%)	Thickness (μm)
Cooper's ligaments	12.3 ± 1.4	289.2 ± 13.0

3.2   Computer Simulation

Fig. 2 shows preliminary results of the simulation of subcompartments in a breast phantom.   Fig. 2(a) show a cross-section of a baseline phantom simulated with

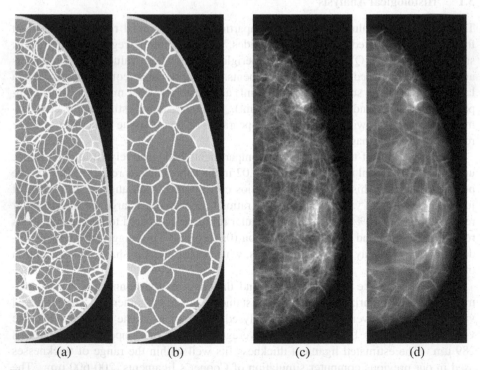

(a)   (b)   (c)   (d)

Fig. 2. Simulation of breast tissue microstructure by subcompartmentalization.   Shown are sections of a software phantom (a) with and (b) without subcompartments, with corresponding synthetic mammographic projections (c) with and (d) without subcompartments.

subcompartments, while Fig. 2(b) shows the same phantom without subcompartments. Figs. 2(c-d) show the corresponding synthetic mammographic projections of these phantoms. In both cases, the phantoms have a total volume of 450 cm^3, with 100 μm voxels. Subjectively, the projection image of the subcompartmentalized phantom shows a higher level of realism. The simulated parenchymal pattern is enriched by the addition of small-scale structures. In addition, the simulated Cooper's ligaments appear less prominent and less geometric, as compared to the projection of the phantom without subcompartments.

A quantitative analysis was performed by comparison of the Laplacian Fractional Entropy (LFE) in clinical and synthetic images. The LFE measure describes the relative content of non-Gaussian statistics in breast images (12). The LFE analysis of the phantoms confirmed that the addition of subcompartments yields a considerable improvement in the LFE measure; the phantom with subcompartments is much closer to clinical images (8). The results of the LFE analysis are shown in Fig. 3. At low spatial frequencies, the phantom without subcompartments exceeds the LFE estimated in clinical mammograms. The peak LFE value of 92% occurs at 0.35 cyc/mm. At spatial frequencies above this peak, the LFE drops to zero at 1.0 cyc/mm. Subcompartmentalization reduces the LFE values, thus matching closely those estimated in mammograms. Based upon our current simulation method, subcompartmentalization increases the simulation time proportional to the square root of the number of compartments. This may be potentially prohibitive for real-time VCT simulations. As a viable alternative, we could pre-compute a number of subcompartment phantoms to be combined randomly with baseline phantoms created in real time.

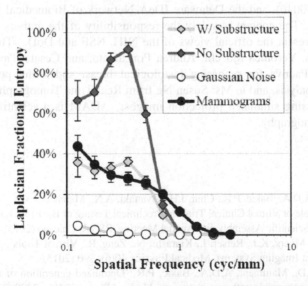

Fig. 3. Laplacian Fractional Entropy (LFE) as a function of spatial frequency, estimated from phantoms generated with and without subcompartments. The phantom LFE values are shown in comparison with those estimated from clinical mammograms and simulated Gaussian noise. Error bars show ±1 standard deviation. (Reproduced with permission from Ref. #8.)

Our future work will include a more detailed analysis of phantoms containing sub-compartments, and a more complete exploration of the various simulation parameters for each of the tissue regions analysed in this work (subcutaneous, deep, and periglandular). In this way, we hope to add spatial dependence to our anatomy simulation method, further improving realism.

4 Conclusions

We have simulated the microstructure of breast tissue by adding subcompartments to our current design of anthropomorphic breast phantoms. This modification was motivated by the hierarchical organization of Cooper's ligaments and interlobular fibrous septa, as shown by Azan-Mallory stained breast histologic slices.

Subjectively, synthetic images of phantoms with subcompartmentalization show an improved level of realism; the simulated parenchymal pattern has been enriched, while the simulated Cooper's ligaments appear less geometric. The observed improvement in the appearance of phantom images is in agreement with a preliminary quantitative validation based upon Laplacian Fractional Entropy analysis.

Acknowledgements. This work was supported in part by the US National Institutes of Health (R01 grant #CA154444), the US Department of Defense Breast Cancer Research Program (HBCU Partnership Training Award #BC083639), the US National Science Foundation (CREST grant #HRD-0630388 and III grant # 0916690), and the US Department of Defense/Department of Army (45395-MA-ISP, #54412-CI-ISP, W911NF-11-2-0046), and the Delaware IDeA Network of Biomedical Research Excellence award. The content is solely the responsibility of the authors and does not necessarily represent the official views of the NIH, NSF and DoD. The authors are thankful to Drs. Veronica Macchi, Andrea Porzionato, and Cesare Tiengo from the University of Padova for preparing histological breast slides and performing the stereological analysis, and to Ms. Susan Ng from Real-Time Tomography (Villanova, PA) for processing simulated projection images. ADAM is a scientific advisor to Real-Time Tomography.

References

1. Maidment, A.D.A., Bakic, P.R., Chui, J.H., Avanaki, A.N., Marchessoux, C., Pokrajac, D.D., et al.: The Role of Virtual Clinical Trials in Preclinical Testing of Breast Imaging Systems. In: 99th RSNA Scientific Assembly and Annual Meeting. RSNA, Chicago (2013)
2. Bakic, P.R., Myers, K.J., Reiser, I., Kiarashi, N., Zeng, R.: Virtual Tools for Validation of X-Ray Breast Imaging Systems. Medical Physics 40(6), 390 (2013)
3. Pokrajac, D.D., Maidment, A.D.A., Bakic, P.R.: Optimized generation of high resolution breast anthropomorphic software phantoms. Medical Physics 39(4), 2290–2302 (2012)
4. Bakic, P.R., Lau, B., Carton, A.-K., Reiser, I., Maidment, A.D.A., Nishikawa, R.M.: An Anthropomorphic Software Breast Phantom for Tomosynthesis Simulation: Power Spectrum Analysis of Phantom Projections. In: Martí, J., Oliver, A., Freixenet, J., Martí, R. (eds.) IWDM 2010. LNCS, vol. 6136, pp. 452–458. Springer, Heidelberg (2010)

5. Lau, A.B., Bakic, P.R., Reiser, I., Carton, A.-K., Maidment, A.D.A., Nishikawa, R.M.: An Anthro-pomorphic Software Breast Phantom for Tomosynthesis Simulation: Power Spectrum Analysis of Phantom Reconstructions. Medical Physics 37, 3473 (2010)

6. Kontos, D., Bakic, P.R., Carton, A.-K., Troxel, A.B., Conant, E.F., Maidment, A.D.A.: Parenchymal Pattern Analysis in Digital Breast Tomosynthesis: Towards Developing Imaging Biomarkers of Breast Cancer Risk. Academic Radiology 16(3), 283–298 (2008)

7. Bakic, P.R., Keller, B., Zheng, Y., Wang, Y., Gee, J.C., Kontos, D., et al.: Testing Realism of Software Breast Phantoms: Texture Analysis of Synthetic Mammograms. In: Nishikawa, R.M., Whiting, B.R., Hoeschen, C. (eds.) SPIE Physics of Medical Imaging, vol. 8668. SPIE, Lake Buena Vista (2013)

8. Abbey, C.K., Bakic, P.R., Pokrajac, D.D., Maidment, A.D.A., Eckstein, M.P., Boone, J.M.: Non-Gaussian Statistical Properties of Virtual Breast Phantoms. In: Mello-Thoms, C.R., Kupinski, M.A. (eds.) SPIE Image Processing, Observer Performance, and Technology Assessment. SPIE, San Diego (2014)

9. Bergman, R.A.: Anatomy Atlases; A digital library of anatomy information, http://www.anatomyatlases.org/ (cited March 8, 2014)

10. Weibel, E.R.: Stereological Methods. Academic Press, London (1979)

11. Lago, M.A., Maidment, A.D.A., Bakic, P.R.: Modelling of mammographic compression of anthropomorphic software breast phantom using FEBio. In: Int'l Symposium on Computer Meth-ods in Biomechanics and Biomedical Engineering. UT 2013, Salt Lake City (2013)

12. Abbey, C.K., Nosrateih, A., Sohl-Dickstein, J., Yang, K., Boone, J.M.: Non-Gaussian statistical properties of breast images. Medical Physics 39, 7121–7130 (2012)

A Virtual Human Breast Phantom Using Surface Meshes and Geometric Internal Structures

Ann-Katherine Carton[1], Anthony Grisey[1], Pablo Milioni de Carvalho[1], Clarisse Dromain[2], and Serge Muller[1]

[1] GE Healthcare, 283 rue de la Minière, 78533 Buc, France
[2] Gustave Roussy, 114 rue Edouard-Vaillant, 94805 Villejuif Cedex, France
ann-katherine.carton@ge.com

Abstract. A highly realistic virtual imaging chain including a model of the human breast could become an important tool for breast imaging system development, optimization and performance assessment. Here we propose a virtual modular breast model with mathematically defined complex anatomical structures that are each represented by a surface mesh. The anatomical structures are designed based on previously published descriptions of internal breast anatomy. Several phantom iterations were performed to tune simulated breast phantom x-ray images visually to real patient images. X-ray image simulation was performed using a polygonal projector. Visual assessment of simulated images of our breast phantoms has shown that our phantom can mimic the range of local features seen in mammograms, contrast-enhanced spectral mammography images and breast CT slices. Further understanding of the fibroglandular tissue structure and its spatial distribution are needed to improve our simulations.

Keywords: Anthropomorphic breast phantom, simulation, breast imaging.

1   Introduction

Today, the diagnostic value of new breast imaging techniques is evaluated through clinical feasibility studies which are complex, require a huge amount of work and can be very expensive. A highly realistic virtual imaging chain including a computational model of the human breast might become an important tool to get an early indication of diagnostic accuracy without actual clinical study. Ultimately, such studies might allow for faster, cheaper and broader clinical trials - all happening in silica. During the last decade, there has been a considerable effort to develop virtual models of breast anatomy. They can be classified according to how the internal breast structures are modeled; either using mathematically defined structures [1,2,3] or based on segmented clinical breast images [4,5]. Today's mathematical breast phantom models are voxelized. The various anatomical structures are defined by relative simple geometric primitives and a 3D fractal noise model is used to simulate the fibroglandular tissue. These models allow simulating an infinite variety of breast morphometries, but their realism is limited due to the simplicity of the geometric primitives. Also, the uniform voxel size makes phantom and image simulations very time-consuming when small

H. Fujita, T. Hara, and C. Muramatsu (Eds.): IWDM 2014, LNCS 8539, pp. 356–363, 2014.
© Springer International Publishing Switzerland 2014

voxels are used. Today's empirical breast phantoms are created by segmenting high-spatial resolution (~0.2 mm voxel size) clinical breast CT images according to breast tissue composition (*i.e.* adipose, fibroglandular, or skin) and then a surface mesh is created for each segmented tissue region boundary. The current phantom database is extended to 100 including a variety of breast morphmetries [5]. The flexibility to adapt mesh resolution according to the complexity of the segmented tissues allows minimizing phantom and image generation time. Simulated x-ray images have shown to be very realistic. Because phantoms are represented using a limited number of tissue region boundaries based on x-ray attenuation properties, and not individual anatomical breast structures, its customizability for specific (multimodality) optimization tasks may be somehow limited.

We propose an alternative breast phantom model whereby complex anatomical structures are mathematically defined and each individual structure has its own surface mesh. Due to its inherent characteristics, our model allows for an infinite variety of breast morphometries and is very highly customizable. We describe the methods used to create the model and we demonstrate the phantom's ability to simulate multimodality imaging data.

2   Phantom Simulation

Our virtual breast model includes the skin with subcutaneous adipose columns, Cooper's ligaments, adipose tissue compartments, ductal network, fibroglandular tissue and blood vessels. These are designed based on literature descriptions on clinical radiological [6,7,8,9] and histology images [10,11,12,13,14] and in-vivo observations [13]. Several iterations were performed to tune simulated breast phantom x-ray images visually to patient images. Internal structures are defined by triangular surface meshes and they are modeled using a variety of geometric mesh primitives, Bézier curves and Voronoi cells. Computerized operations, such as surface subdivision and mesh decimation, are used for geometry deformation, curve to mesh conversion and mesh simplification. Internal structures are constructed with Blender (v 2.63) [15], a free and open source computer graphics software product developed for creation of 3D animation, with Python (v 2.6.5) as internal scripting language and Voro++ [16], a free software library for computing 3D Voronoi tessellations. The main program is written in C++; C++ scripts serve to call Python for Blender scripts, to assess the Voro++ library and to convert the vertex and face coordinates of the mesh objects exported from Blender in a format compatible with our imaging simulation chain.

Two breast outline configurations were modeled (**Fig. 1**); one outline represents a compressed breast in CC view during a mammography exam and one outline represents an uncompressed breast of a woman in prone position during a dedicated breast CT exam. The *skin* is modeled as a single layer with uniform user-configurable thickness (1 to 5 mm range [6]) by scaling a copy of the breast outline. Our model allows to model *subcutaneous adipose columns* by displacing the mesh vertices of the skin inner layer along the local normal (**Fig. 2**).

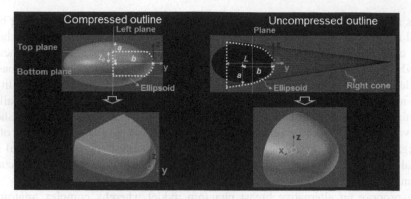

Fig. 1. Illustration of compressed and uncompressed breast outlines. The compressed outline is approximated by an ellipsoid truncated by three planes. The semi-axis lengths of the ellipsoids allow modifying the breast surface area and the shape of the breast edge that is not compressed while z_p determines the compressed breast thickness. The uncompressed outline is modeled as a combination of a truncated right cone with circular base and a section of an ellipsoid. The cone height and the ellipsoidal semi-axis lengths are configurable so as to modify the total length and thickness of the uncompressed breast phantom.

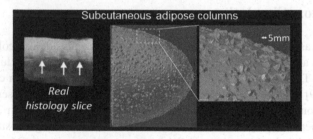

Fig. 2. Subcutaneous adipose columns are modeled by displacing the mesh vertices of the skin inner layer along the local normals using a Blender-specific "Displace modifier". The simulated subcutaneous adipose columns are 2 to 3 mm spaced apart and their depth is on average 1 mm. These values are consistent with reported measurements on histological sections [14].

*Subcutaneous, retromammary and intraglandular **adipose tissues*** are modeled as cells of a 3D Voronoi diagram (**Fig. 3**) similarly as in the breast model of Pokrajac *et al* [2]. Seed points are randomly positioned over the phantom volume using two different uniform distributions; seed points in the intraglandular region are more closely positioned than those in the subcutaneous and retromammary regions. For each seed point, a single Voronoi cell is then computed as a collection of vertices connected by edges [16]. The number of adipose compartments is configurable by the user; typically 150-350 compartments are simulated. The Voronoi cell meshes are subdivided to smooth their edges and to create spaces between them of ~100-200 µm representing the ***Cooper's ligaments***.

Lactiferous ducts are modeled as a concatenation of duct segments forming the branches of a random binary tree model [3]. Each duct segment is modeled starting from a Bézier curve which is converted to a 3D extruded tube. To match anatomical realism, 5 to 9 ducts are simulated [13]. To mimic the radial divergence of real ducts, simulated ducts are positioned along virtual ellipsoids with apices at 1.2 cm from the areola (**Fig. 4 a**). *Fibroglandular tissue* (**Fig. 4 b** and **c**) is modeled around the lactiferous ducts. The fraction of ducts surrounded by fibroglandular tissue is user-defined (range 0 to 1). Fibroglandular tissue segments are also modeled starting from Bézier curves which are then converted to extruded mesh-type tubes. Next, large scale fibroglandular structures are created by displacing the mesh vertices along the local normal using Blender-specific displace modifiers. These modifiers allow for different breast tissue parenchymal patterns as observed in mammograms. To mimic fine fibrous tissue details, a second displace modifier is applied along the principal axis of the duct branch. The fibroglandular tissue distribution within the phantom is configured by controlling 1) the minimum distance between the fibroglandular tissue and the skin surface, 2) the positions of the ducts in the breast quadrants and 3) the ellipsoid semi-axis lengths along which the fibroglandular tissue is positioned. *Blood vessels* are modeled similarly as the lactiferous ducts but they have a smaller diameter.

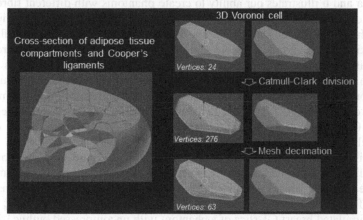

Fig. 3. (Left) Adipose tissue is modeled by modified 3D Voronoi cells. (Right) Illustration of Catmull-Clark mesh subdivision and decimation to smooth the Voronoi cell edges and simplify the meshes without noticeable reduced geometric detail. Catmull-Clark subdivision also creates ~100-200 µm spaces between Voronoi cells representing the Cooper's ligaments.

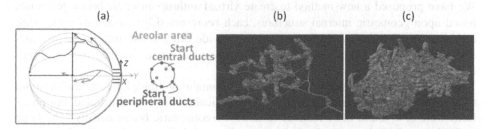

Fig. 4. (a) Illustration of the positioning of simulated ducts along virtual ellipsoids with apices at 1.2 cm from the areola. Illustration of fibroglandular tissue modeled around (b) a single duct and (c) around all ducts.

3   Simulated Breast X-Ray Images

Breast phantom x-ray images were simulated using a polygon projector implemented in CatSim, a virtual imaging platform previously developed and validated at GE Healthcare [17]. Typical system topologies were considered using perfect energy-integrating, quantum-noise limited detectors. Acquisitions were simulated using mono-energetic x-ray beams and assuming only primary x rays.

Fig. 5 shows mammographic realizationsof a 5 cm thick breast phantom with compressed outline. Fig. 5 a, b, c and d illustrate that different clinical realistic mammographic fibroglandular textures can be generated by using different Blender-specific mesh displacement modifiers to create the fibroglandular tissue. Fig. 5 e shows a mammographic projection through a region containing only adipose tissue. Note that the projections of the compartment boundaries, depicting the Cooper's ligaments, are rather straight. Fig. 5 f demonstrates a mammographic depiction of the skin with adipose columns seen as radiolucent spots.

Fig. 6 a and b illustrates our ability to create phantoms with different fibroglandular tissue distributions; the two mammograms were generated from 5-cm thick compressed phantoms whereby the minimum distance between the fibroglandular tissue and the skin surface and the ellipsoid semi-axis lengths along which the fibroglandular tissue is developed were set different while all other phantom parameters were the same. The volumetric breast densities of these phantoms, defined as the volume fraction of fibroglandular tissue, were also calculated. For this calculation the mesh data were first converted to 0.2 mm cubed voxels. Volumetric breast densities are equal to 8% and 10%. These values are fairly realistic based on volumetric breast densities found in clinical images [18].

Fig. 7 illustrates that our phantom design is highly customizable for various imaging modalities; a simulated dual-energy recombined contrast-enhanced mammography image is shown whereby the composition of the fibroglandular tissue was set as a mixture of pure fibroglandular tissue and 0.2 mg iodine/ml (Fig. 7 a). Fig. 7 b illustrates a simulated breast CT slice of a phantom with uncompressed outline.

4   Discussion

We have proposed a new method to create virtual anthropomorphic breast phantoms based upon geometric internal structures, each represented by surface meshes, using computer graphics software. Our phantoms provide full ground truth tissue information and high flexibility in covering wide anatomical variations and they are very highly customizable.

Qualitatively, mammographic sub-regions containing fibroglandular and adipose tissue and skin provide a fairly high level of clinical realism. As illustrated, our phantoms were also found to be realistic in terms of volumetric breast density. The large scale tissues, including the physical breast edge and the borders between the adipose and fibroglandular tissue regions, as well as the borders of the adipose tissue compartments appeared with a more or less regular appearance in simulated mammograms degrading the subjective perception of reality.

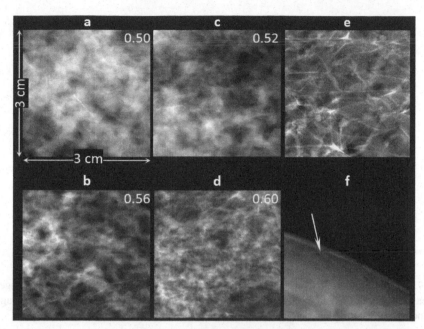

Fig. 5. Regions of interest showing mammographic depiction of (**a, b, c, d**): fibroglandular texture patterns obtained by using different displace modifiers to create the fibroglandular tissue, (**e**): adipose tissue compartments and Cooper's ligaments, (**f**): the skin with adipose columns seen as radiolucent spots (arrow)

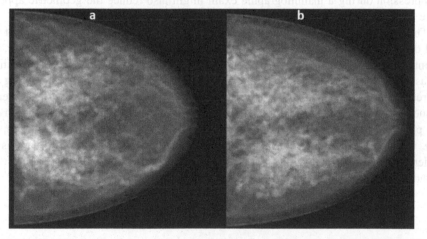

Fig. 6. (**a, b**): Simulated mammograms of two phantoms with different fibroglandular tissue distribution but otherwise created with the same parameters; each phantom contains eight ducts of which 80% are surrounded with fibroglandular tissue that is created with the same Blender mesh modifiers

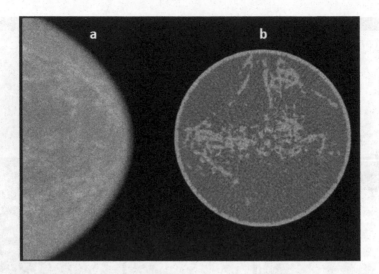

Fig. 7. (a): Illustration of a dual-energy recombined contrast-enhanced mammography image of a breast phantom of which the fibroglandular tissue exhibits a 0.2 mg/ml iodine contrast agent enhancement. (b): Simulated breast CT slice of an uncompressed breast phantom.

Further understanding of the fibroglandular tissue structure and its spatial distribution is needed to improve the realism of our simulations. Application of finite element methods to deform the breast phantom with uncompressed outline to simulate breast compression during a mammographic exam might also reduce the geometric appearance and thus improve realism.

The use of the phantom is illustrated by simulated digital mammograms, breast CT and dual-energy recombined contrast-enhanced mammography images. However, the phantom design is also appropriate for simulating other imaging modalities such as breast MRI and breast ultrasound; these modalities can be simulated by applying the corresponding image acquisition model with appropriate physical properties of each tissue type. Considerable flexibility is provided through a script allowing to convert the phantom format from mesh-based data to voxels-based data. As said before, today, we haven't taken into consideration to simulate the deformation of breast tissue under compression. Inclusion of a model of breast compression will allow for a more broad use including straight multi-modality image comparison.

5   Conclusion

An alternative phantom model to simulate the female breast, based on mathematically defined complex anatomical structures that are each represented by a surface mesh, was demonstrated. Future work will involve full characterization and further optimization of the realism of the internal anatomical structures. The proposed model may provide an important tool to assess the performance of different breast imaging modalities.

References

1. Bliznakova, K., Suryanarayanan, S., Karellas, A.: Evaluation of an improved algorithm for producing realistic 3D breast software phantoms: Application for mammography. Med. Phys. 37, 5604–5617 (2010)
2. Pokrajac, D.D., Maidment, A.D.A., Bakic, P.R.: Optimized generation of high resolution breast anthropomorphic software phantoms. Med. Phys. 39, 2290–2302 (2012)
3. Bakic, P.R., Albert, M., Brzakovic, D., et al.: Mammogram synthesis using a three-dimensional simulation. III. Modeling and Evaluation of the Breast Ductal Network. Med. Phys. 30, 1914–1925 (2003)
4. Li, C.M., Segars, W.P., Tourassi, G.D., et al.: Methodology for generating a 3D computerized breast phantom from empirical data. Med. Phys. 36, 3122–3131 (2009)
5. Segars, W.P., Veress, A.I., Wells, J.R., et al.: Population of 100 realistic, patient-based computerized breast phantoms for multi-modality imaging research. SPIE Paper 9033-9067 (2014)
6. Ulger, H., Erdogan, N., Kumanlioglu, S., et al.: Effect of age, breast size, menopausal and hormonal status on mammographic skin thickness. Skin Res. Technol. 9, 284–289 (2003)
7. Teboul, M., Halliwell, M.: Atlas of ultrasound and ductal echography of the breast: The introduction of anatomic intelligence into breast imaging. Blackwell Science, 398 (1995)
8. Ramsay, D.T., Kent, J.C., Hartmann, R., et al.: Anatomy of the lactating human breast redefined with ultrasound imaging. Journal of Anatomy 206, 525–534 (2005)
9. Huang, S.-Y., Boone, J.M., Yang, K., et al.: The characterization of breast anatomical metrics using dedicated breast CT. Med. Phys. 38, 2180–2191 (2011)
10. Shotgun Histology Active Breast, http://www.youtube.com/watch?v=GXAKSuEU4Ms (accessed: February 3, 2014)
11. Shotgun Histology Inactive Breast, http://www.youtube.com/watch?v=rUD8zHC-fx4 (accessed: February 3, 2014)
12. Page, A.L., Anderson, T.J.: Diagnostic histopathology of the breast, p. 362. W.B. Saunders Company (1987)
13. Love, S.M., Barsky, S.H.: Anatomy of the nipple and breast ducts revisited. Cancer 101, 1947–1957 (2004)
14. Kopans, D., Rusby, J.: Cutaneous Caves and Subcutaneous Adipose Columns in the Breast: Radiologic-Pathologic Correlation. Radiology 249, 779–784 (2008)
15. Blender Foundation, Blender Homepage, http://www.blender.org/ (accessed: September 4, 2013)
16. Rycroft, C.: Voro++ homepage, http://math.lbl.gov/voro++/ (accessed: September 4, 2013)
17. De Man, B., Basu, S., Chandra, N., et al.: CatSim: A new computer assisted tomography simulation environment. Proc. SPIE 6510, 1–8 (2007)
18. Yaffe, M., Boone, J.M., Packard, N., et al.: The myth of the 50-50 breast. Med. Phys. 36, 5437–5443 (2009)

Characterisation of Screen Detected and Simulated Calcification Clusters in Digital Mammograms

Lucy M. Warren[1,2], Louise Dummott[1,2], Matthew G. Wallis[3,4],
Rosalind M. Given-Wilson[5], Julie Cooke[6], David R. Dance[1,2], and Kenneth C. Young[1,2]

[1] National Coordinating Centre for the Physics of Mammography,
Royal Surrey County Hospital NHS Foundation Trust, Guildford, UK
[2] Department of Physics, University of Surrey, Guildford, UK
[3] Cambridge Breast Unit, Cambridge University Hospitals NHS Foundation Trust, Cambridge, UK
[4] NIHR Cambridge Biomedical Research Centre, Cambridge, UK
[5] Department of Radiology, St. George's Healthcare NHS Trust, London, UK
[6] Jarvis Breast Screening and Diagnostic Centre, Guildford

Abstract. Simulated microcalcifciation clusters have been used in studies performed to investigate the effect of different imaging conditions on cancer detection in breast screening. This work compares the characteristics of the simulated clusters to screen-detected calcification clusters. Using a database of 271 screen-detected cancers it was found that 67 (25%) presented radiographically as calcification clusters. The characteristics of 1215 microcalcifications from all 67 clusters and 304 microcalcifications from 30 simulated clusters were quantitatively analysed. The diameter of simulated calcifications were within the range of 99% of real calcifications. The cluster diameters of the simulated clusters were within the range of 70% of the real clusters. Our simulated calcifications had similar characteristics to real calcifications but were representative of smaller clusters which represent 17% of screen-detected cancers. Consequently, a significant change in detection of our simulated clusters due to change in imaging condition has a predictable impact on cancer detection in screening.

Keywords: Calcification, digital mammography, simulation, virtual clinical trials.

1 Introduction

Simulated cancers have been used in virtual clinical trials to determine if there are significant differences in cancer detection in breast screening between different imaging conditions, such as different image processing or different detectors [1-3]. It is particularly useful to use simulated cancers in breast screening applications where prevalence of cancer is low and the use of real images of cancers may introduce a selection bias. In this work we concentrate on the use of simulated calcification clusters. In order to relate the results of these studies to cancer detection in screening it is necessary to know how the simulated clusters compare to screen-detected cancers.

H. Fujita, T. Hara, and C. Muramatsu (Eds.): IWDM 2014, LNCS 8539, pp. 364–371, 2014.

In this work quantitative characteristics such as calcification diameter and cluster diameter were compared for screen-detected calcification clusters and simulated clusters.

2   Method

2.1   Screen-Detected Cancers

In the United Kingdom (UK) the National Health Service Breast Screening Programme (NHSBSP) invites women aged 50-70 (extending to 47-73) years to undergo mammographic screening every 3 years. The examination consists of two views of each breast, a cranial-caudal (CC) view and a medio-lateral oblique view (MLO). In our department we have a large database containing digital mammography images collected from two breast screening sites in the UK. Images from the database of all 267 patients with screen-detected cancers detected between June 2011 and December 2012 were analysed. All of the images were obtained using Hologic Selenia X-ray systems and processed and unprocessed images were available. Along with the digital images, the database also contains the associated biopsy and surgery results from the national breast screening information system (NBSS). For four patients the NBSS and image data were inconsistent and these were excluded from the analysis. The remaining 263 patients contained 271 biopsy confirmed cancers. These will be termed the 'real' cancers. The mammograms were annotated by an experienced radiologist, who outlined the lesion on the mammogram corresponding to the cancer, and provided a description of the radiological appearance by selecting as many as appropriate from the following list: mass, architectural distortion, focal asymmetry or suspicious calcification. Finally, the radiologist categorised the conspicuity of the lesion as 'obvious', 'subtle', 'very subtle' or 'occult'.

The percentage of cancers of each radiological type (non-calcification lesions, suspicious calcifications and both) was calculated. Next the conspicuities of the lesions were analysed. Each patient has two views of each breast acquired during a breast screening examination and so a lesion can assigned one of the four conspicuities above in each view. Therefore, each lesion has two conspicuities, or a conspicuity pair). In order to be marked a lesion had to be visible in at least one view and so the conspicuity pair "occult/occult" was not an option. Therefore there are nine different conspicuity pairs. Finally, using the NBSS data it was possible to determine the proportion of invasive and in-situ cancers for each radiological type of cancer. These two categories were then further divided according to histological grade.

2.2   Simulated Calcification Clusters

The simulated calcification clusters were generated using our published and validated method [4]. In this method images of calcification clusters were extracted from images of sliced mastectomy samples acquired at times five magnification in a digital specimen cabinet. The simulated clusters were created from these extracted images and then inserted into digital mammograms taking account of the physical characteristics of the imaging system. A radiologist has inspected all the images of the simulated lesions and verified that the clusters were realistic in appearance.

The expert radiologist also graded the conspicuity of each simulated calcification cluster within the mammogram. The simulated clusters were only inserted into a single view since the simulated clusters were extracted from 2D images of mastectomy samples and could not be reoriented into the second view. As such there were only three possible conspicuities – obvious (ob), subtle (s) and very subtle (vs).

2.3   Quantification of the Characteristics of Real and Simulated Calcification Clusters

The real and simulated calcification clusters were segmented from the unprocessed mammograms using a region-growing algorithm to form a binary image. This was used to determine the boundaries of each calcification and two parameters were calculated; diameter of individual calcifications and diameter of cluster.

Diameter of a Calcification. The diameter of each calcification was calculated by counting the number of pixels in each calcification. From this the diameter of a disc with the same area was calculated. This diameter was defined as the diameter of the calcification.

Diameter of a Cluster. The diameter of each cluster was calculated by encompassing the calcifications by the convex hull. The area of the polygon was then calculated and the diameter of a disc with the same area was determined. This diameter was defined as the diameter of the cluster.

For each statistic described above the percentage of real calcifications or clusters with characteristics within the range of the characteristics of the simulated clusters was calculated.

3   Results and Discussion

3.1   Screen-Detected Cancers

It was found that 60% of the screen-detected cancers were identified as non-calcification lesions, 29% were suspicious calcifications and 11% had a lesion with both calcification and non-calcification features. The proportion of conspicuity combinations for the calcification lesions is shown in Figure 1. For the calcifications the conspicuity was often similar in the two views. The proportion of conspicuity combinations for the non-calcification lesions is shown in Figure 2.

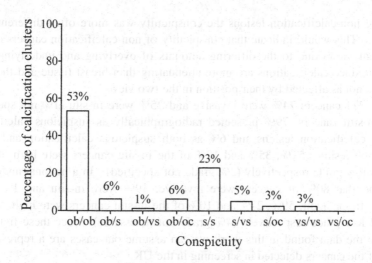

Fig. 1. Percentage of suspicious calcifications with each pair of conspicuities. A cancer can appear in an image as obvious (ob), subtle (s), very subtle (vs) or occult (oc). Each cancer is imaged in two views and so has a pair of conspicuities.

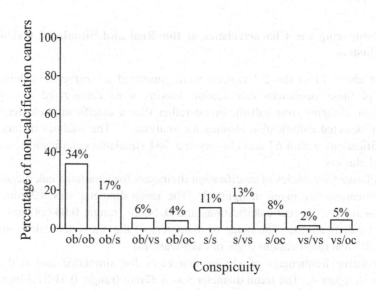

Fig. 2. Percentage of non-calcification lesions with each pair of conspicuities. A cancer can appear in an image as obvious (ob), subtle (s), very subtle (vs) or occult (oc). Each cancer is imaged in two views and so has a pair of conspicuities.

For the non-calcification lesions the conspicuity was more often different in the two views. This would indicate that conspicuity of non-calcification cancers changes in different views due to the differing amounts of overlying and underlying breast tissue, but since calcifications are more attenuating than breast tissue and their conspicuity is not as affected by their position in the two views.

Of the 271 cancers 74% were invasive and 25% were in-situ (1% not specified). Of the in-situ cancers, 79% presented radiographically as suspicious calcification, 15% non-calcification lesions and 6% as both suspicious calcification and a non-calcification lesion. 51%, 35% and 12% of the in-situ cancers were high, intermediate and low grade respectively (2% grade not specified). In a national audit [5], it was found that 80% of cancers were invasive, 19% were in-situ and 1% micro-invasive. In the audit, 59%, 27% and 10% of the in-situ cancers were high, intermediate and low grade respectively (4% grade not assessable). Since these figures are similar to the data found in this work we can assume our cases are a representative sample of the cancers detected in screening in the UK.

3.2   Simulated Calcification Clusters

The radiologist also marked the conspicuities of the simulated clusters. 58% of the simulated clusters were obvious, 32% were subtle and 10% were judged to be very subtle in appearance.

3.3   Comparing the Characteristics of the Real and Simulated Calcification Clusters

As stated above 79 of the 271 cancers were annotated as suspicious calcifications. Twelve of these suspicious calcification lesions were categorized as segmental calcification covering over half the breast rather than a calcification cluster, leaving 67 screen-detected calcification clusters for analysis. The analysis included 1215 real calcifications within 67 real clusters and 304 simulated calcifications within 30 simulated clusters.

The relative frequencies of calcification diameters for simulated calcifications and real calcifications are given in figure 3. The mean diameter was 0.26mm (range: 0.07-1.16mm) for the real calcifications and 0.24mm (range: 0.08-0.83mm) for the simulated calcifications. The range of diameters of the simulated calcifications included 1207 real calcifications (99% of calcifications).

The relative frequencies of cluster diameters for simulated and real clusters are given in figure 4. The mean diameter was 8.37mm (range: 0.91-31.34mm for the real clusters and 3.80 (range: 1.90-9.27mm) for the simulated clusters. The range of diameters of simulated clusters included 47 real clusters (70% of calcification clusters).

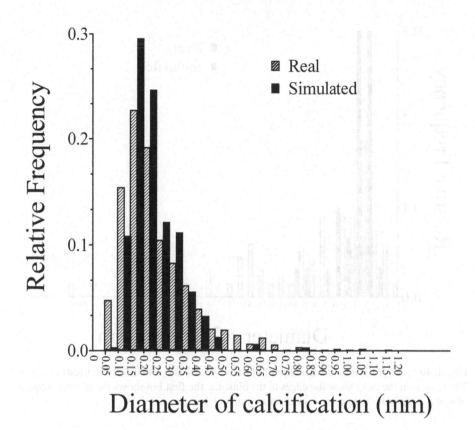

Fig. 3. Relative frequency of diameter of real and simulated calcification clusters. The values on the ticks show the minimum and maximum values of each bin, i.e. the first bin shows the relative frequency of real and simulated calcifications of the diameter range 0-0.05mm.

The limiting characteristic for the simulated clusters was the cluster diameter since this is representative of the smallest number of real clusters. This is not a surprising result and is due to the simulation methodology. The simulated calcification clusters were extracted from digital images of mastectomy samples. These were imaged at times five magnification on a digital specimen cabinet, at which the field of view was 10×10mm. Therefore all simulated clusters had a diameter less than 10mm. However, encouragingly, the simulated clusters were representative of 70% of real calcification clusters, or 60% of suspicious calcifications if areas of segmental calcification are also included. Therefore, since suspicious calcification was 29% of the 271 screen-detected cancers in this study, our simulated calcifications represent 17% of screen-detected cancers.

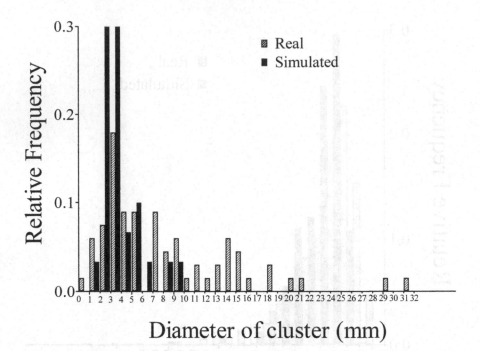

Fig. 4. Relative frequency of diameter of cluster for real and simulated calcification clusters. The values on the ticks show the edges of the bins, i.e. the first bin shows the relative frequency of real and simulated clusters of the diameter range 0-1mm.

4   Conclusion

From our analysis of 271 screen-detected cancers we found that 29% of screen-detected cancers were detected as suspicious calcification only. Our simulated calcifications were representative of 99% of real calcifications in terms of calcification ldiameter. Due to the limited field of view of the images from which the simulated calcification clusters were extracted the simulated calcification clusters were typical of 60% of screen-detected cancers identified as suspicious calcifications. Therefore, the simulated clusters represent 17% of screen-detected cancers. Consequently, a change in detection of our simulated calcification clusters due to change in imaging condition is an important finding with a predictable impact on the detection of cancers in screening.

Acknowledgements. This work is part of the OPTIMAM project and is supported by Cancer Research-UK & EPSRC Cancer Imaging Programme in Surrey, in association with the MRC and Department of Health (England).

The authors are grateful to Dr Mark Halling-Brown and Dr Mishal Patel for their assistance querying the image database and NBSS for the data used in this work.

References

1. Warren, L.M., Mackenzie, A., Cooke, J., Given-Wilson, R.M., Wallis, M.G., Chakraborty, D.P., Dance, D.R., Bosmans, H., Young, K.C.: Effect of image quality on calcification detection in digital mammography. Med. Phys. 39, 3202–3213 (2012)
2. Warren, L.M., Cooke, J., Given-Wilson, R.M., Wallis, M.G., Halling-Brown, M., Mackenzie, A., Chakraborty, D.P., Bosmans, H., Dance, D.R., Young, K.C.: The effect of image processing on detection of cancers in digital mammography. AJR (in press, 2014)
3. Mackenzie, A., Warren, L.M., Dance, D.R., Chakraborty, D.P., Cooke, J., Halling-Brown, M.D., Looney, P.T., Wallis, M.G., Given-Wilson, R.M., Alexander, G.G., Young, K.C.: Using image simulation to test the effect of detector type on breast cancer detection. In: Proc. SPIE, vol. 9037 (in press, 2014)
4. Warren, L.M., Green, F.H., Shrestha, L., Mackenzie, A., Dance, D.R., Young, K.C.: Validation of simulation of calcifications for observer studies in digital mammography. Phys. Med. Biol. 58, N217-N228 (2013)
5. NHS Breast Screening Programme and Association of Breast Surgery, An audit of screen detected breast cancers for the year of screening April 2010 to March 2011, NHS Cancer Screening Programmes (2012)

Development of a Micro-Simulation Model for Breast Cancer to Evaluate the Impacts of Personalized Early Detection Strategies

Rasika Rajapakshe[1], Cynthia Araujo[1], Chelsea Vandenberg[1],
Brent Parker[1], Stephen Smithbower[1], Chris Baliski[1], Susan Ellard[1],
Laurel Kovacic[1], Melanie Reed[1], Scott Tyldesley[2], Gillian Fyles[1],
and Rebecca Mlikotic[1]

[1] BC Cancer Agency, Centre for the Southern Interior, 399 Royal Avenue, Kelowna,
BC Canada
[2] BC Cancer Agency, Vancouver Centre, 600 W 10th Avenue, Vancouver, BC Canada
{RRajapak,Brent.Parker}@bccancer.bc.ca

Abstract. Breast cancer screening with mammography has been shown to reduce breast cancer mortality. However the frequency and the age range for screening eligibility has been controversial. Individual risk based screening regimens have recently been proposed to overcome some of the weaknesses of screening mammography. However, it is not possible to evaluate the full impact of such risk based individualized screening strategies in Canadian context. Therefore a mathematical cancer control model for breast cancer using care paths and cancer control data from the province of BC is being developed to model different early detection strategies. The model will incorporate the incidence, detection, diagnosis, progression, and case fatality of breast cancer in BC as baseline to make projections of the population health and economic impacts of different early detection methods for breast cancer. Once the model is validated, it will be possible to test early detection pathways and strategies, frequencies and durations, as well as any health care costs associated with detection, diagnosis, treatment and on-going care of breast cancer patients.

Keywords: Breast Cancer, Screening, Modeling, Micro-Simulation.

1 Introduction

Breast cancer screening by mammography has been shown to reduce breast cancer mortality and screening stratiges continue to evolve as an understanding of the benefits and risk of screening are understood and new technologies become availible [1-4].

In addition, it is well known that the health benefits and cost utility of screening mammography may be strongly influenced by a woman's risk for breast cancer, which can be estimated based on numerous risk factors such as her age, breast

H. Fujita, T. Hara, and C. Muramatsu (Eds.): IWDM 2014, LNCS 8539, pp. 372–379, 2014.
© Springer International Publishing Switzerland 2014

density, history of breast biopsy and family history of breast cancer [5]. Therefore, there is a growing interest in personalized cancer screening [6,7]. Furthermore, other technologies such as tomosynthesis, ultrasound, and MRI are continuing to be considered for their potential role in screening.

Although randomized clinical trials have long been the gold standard in assessing the benefit of screening strategies, these screening trials are very difficult to implement as they require a large population, significant organizational and implementation resources and long-term follow-up of at least 10 to 15 years. In addition, they are not able to identify the downstream impacts associated with a change in screening policy. For this reason, it would be valuable to be able to propose 'what if' scenarios that could evaluate the impact of a new population based screening strategy based on limited factors such as a new strategy's sensitivity, specificity and cost per screen.

Mathematical models have the potential to help answer these questions for which empirical evidence is scarce or unattainable. One type of model known as microsimulation models operate at the level of the individual behavioral entity, such as a person, family, or group and simulate large representative populations of these low-level entities in order to draw conclusions that apply to higher levels of aggregation such as an entire country. Once a base population is created, these models enable the entry of various known parameters associated with a proposed screening strategy. From this, a simulation can be performed and proposed outcomes, along with margins of confidence can be assessed. This approach enables multiple variations of proposed screening strategies to be investigated within hours or days [8,9].

Recognizing the potential that these mathematical models have, the Cancer Intervention and Surveillance Modeling Network was developed [10]. These models have been able evaluate and provide evidence for various controversial topics in the area of cancer screening which have helped to guide screening policies in the USA. In addition, the Canadian Partnership Against Cancer (CPAC) recently developed and implemented the Cancer Risk Management Model (CRMM) platform to answer important questions in cancer control in a Canadian context [11]. The CRMM currently incorporates the lung and colorectal and cervical cancer however, there are no current, validated breast cancer models available that are based on data and care paths from Canada.

2   Objectives

At the BC Cancer Agency we are working to build a breast cancer microsimulation model based on professional practice guidelines, expert opinion and data from British Columbian Health and Oncology administrative data sources.

This model will enable evaluation of the impact of different screening strategies for breast cancer and will incorporate incidence, detection, diagnosis, progression, case fatality and costing of breast cancer as baseline to make projections of the population health and the economic impacts of different screening regimens. Unlike existing models which are built exclusively on professional opinion or screening data from decades ago, we are incorporating modern data sources from the early 2000s.

Availability of such a model will enable researchers and policy makers to evaluate the effects and effectiveness of different screening strategies on population health and costs to the health care system before implementation. The ultimate goal is to improve the early detection of breast cancer.

3   Methods

The first step in developing the breast cancer micro-simulation model was to generate breast cancer care paths. The care paths were developed using information from expert opinions in the fields of radiology, radiation oncology, surgical oncology, medical oncology and palliative care, as well as concepts from the NCCN Oncology Guidelines, BC Provincial Breast Health Strategy, Cancer Care Ontario, and the Canadian Partnership Against Cancer's Cancer Risk Management Lung Cancer Model & the Screening Mammography Program of British Columbia (SMPBC) and the Medical Services Plan of British Columbia & Ontario's Case Cost Initative. This pathway was further revised and populated with one year of diagnosis and treatment data from the BC Cancer Agency Administrative Data Warehouses.

4   Results

The care pathway begins with early detection of breast cancer by screening mammography or referral by a general practitioner as shown in Figure 1 and abnormalities found proceed to the diagnostic pathway. Patients with false findings return to routine screening. In the case of a positive finding, the clinical staging largely determines the treatment pathway which includes surgery, radiation therapy and systemic therapy as shown in Figures 2-4.

The distribution of patients that flow through various treatment strategies (surgery, radiation, chemo/biological therapy and hormone therapy) is incorporated and stratified by TNM staging and sub-section of this component of the path is depicted in Figure 5 showing rates and corresponding confidence intervals from our preliminary 1 year of data. This figure highlights the transition percentages, along with 95% confidence intervals, associated with each post-mastectomy treatment option for the patients who underwent mastectomy for T stage T1-T2, node negative breast cancer.

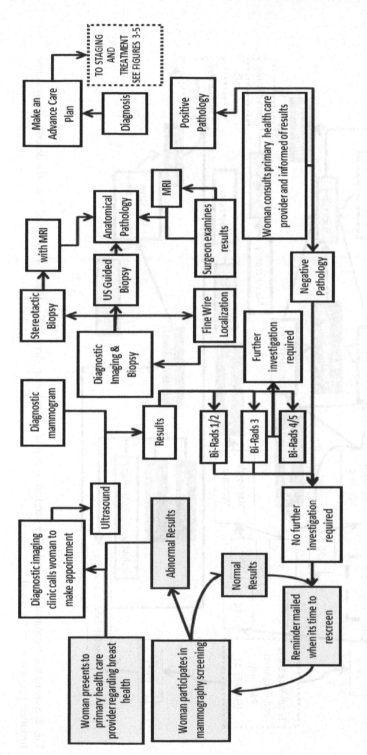

Fig. 1. Breast cancer screening (grey) and diagnosis (white)

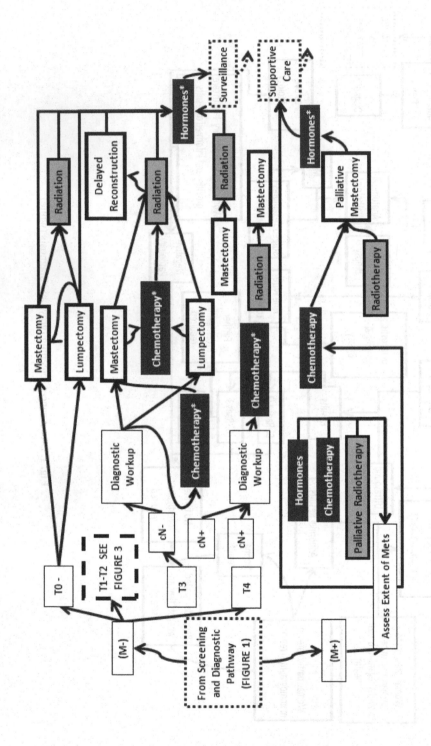

Fig. 2. Staging and treatment paths including surgical, systemic and radiation therapy. See Figure 4 for * and ^ which describe the systemic treatment pathway in greater detail.

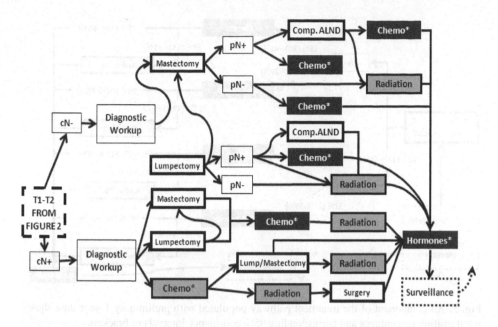

Fig. 3. Treatment paths for T1-T2 cancers. See Figure 4 for * and ^ which describe the systemic treatment pathway in greater detail.

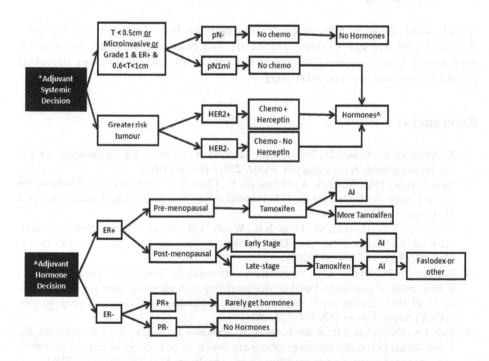

Fig. 4. Systemic therapy treatment path for non-metastic breast cancer patients

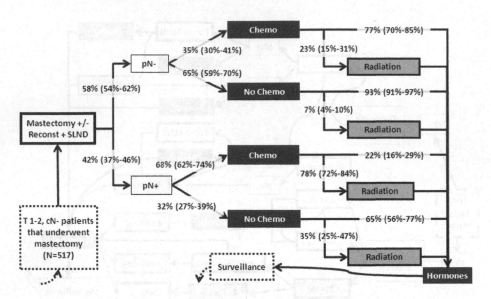

Fig. 5. An component of the treatment pathway populated with preliminary 1-year data showing transition percentages and corresponding 95% confidence intervals in brackets

5   Conclusion

A preliminary model of a breast cancer care path has been developed and has been populated with one year of data. Efforts are underway to expand the initiative by integrating full data (screening through to mortality) for breast cancer cases diagnosed in British Columbia between 2000-2005.

References

1. Kerlikowske, K., Grady, D., Rubin, S.M., Sandrock, C., Ernster, V.L.: Efficacy of screening mammography. A meta-analysis. JAMA 273, 149–154 (1995)
2. Nelson, H.D., Tyne, K., Naik, A., Bougatsos, C., Chan, B.K., Humphrey, L.: Screening for Breast Cancer: An Update for the U.S. Preventive Services Task Force. Annals of Internal Medicine 151, 727–737 (2009)
3. Humphrey, L.L., Helfand, M., Chan, B.K., Woolf, S.H.: Breast cancer screening: A summary of the evidence for the U.S. Preventive Services Task Force. Ann. Intern. Med. 137(5, pt. 1), 347–360 (2002)
4. Hellquist, B.N., Duffy, S.W., Abdsaleh, S., Bjorneld, L., Bordas, P., Tabar, L., et al.: Effectiveness of population-based service screening with mammography for women ages 40 to 49 years: Evaluation of the Swedish Mammography Screening in Young Women (SCRY) cohort. Cancer 117, 714–722 (2011)
5. Tice, J.A., Cummings, S.R., Smith-Bindman, R., Ichikawa, L., Barlow, W.E., Kerlikowske, K.: Using clinical factors and mammographic breast density to estimate breast cancer risk: Development and validation of a new predictive model. Ann. Intern. Med. 148, 337–347 (2008)

6. Gail, M., Rimer, B.: Risk-based recommendations for mammographic screening for women in their forties. J. Clin. Oncol. 16, 3105–3114 (1998)
7. Schousboe, J.T., Kerlikowske, K., Loh, A., Cummings, S.R.: Personalizing mammography by breast density and other risk factors for breast cancer: Analysis of health benefits and cost-effectiveness. Ann. Intern. Med. 155, 10–20 (2011)
8. Mandelblatt, J.S., Cronin, K.A., Berry, D.A., Chang, Y., de Koning, H.J., Lee, S.J., et al.: Modeling the impact of population screening on breast cancer mortality in the United States. Breast 20(suppl. 3), S75–S81 (2011)
9. Feuer, E.J.: Modeling the impact of adjuvant therapy and screening mammography on U.S. breast cancer mortality between 1975 and 2000: Introduction to the problem. J. Natl. Cancer Inst. Monogr. 36, 2–6 (2006)
10. Cancer Intervention and Surveillance Modeling Network. CISNET Publication, http://cisnet.cancer.gov/publications/ (accessed March 8, 2014)
11. Canadian Partnership Against Cancer. Cancer Risk Management Model Website, http://www.cancerview.ca (accessed March 8, 2014)

Modelling Vascularity in Breast Cancer and Surrounding Stroma Using Diffusion MRI and Intravoxel Incoherent Motion

Colleen Bailey[1], Sarah Vinnicombe[2], Eleftheria Panagiotaki[1],
Shelley A. Waugh[2], John H. Hipwell[1], Daniel C. Alexander[1],
Kathryn Kitching[2], Patsy Whelehan[2], Sarah E. Pinder[3],
Andrew Evans[2], and David J. Hawkes[1]

[1] Centre for Medical Image Computing, University College London, Engineering
Front Building, London, UK, WC1E 6BT
colleen.bailey@ucl.ac.uk
[2] Dundee Cancer Centre, Ninewells Hospital and Medical School, Dundee, UK,
DD1 9SY
[3] Breast Research Pathology, Research Oncology, Division of Cancer Studies,
King's College London, Guy's Hospital, London, UK, SE1 9RT

Abstract. Contrast-enhanced magnetic resonance imaging (MRI) has
shown variation in the stroma with distance from the tumor and this
correlates with histological microvessel density. To date, however, conventional diffusion MRI has demonstrated limited sensitivity to these
changes. This study modelled the diffusion signal by intravoxel incoherent motion (IVIM) to obtain parameters related to the vasculature and
tissue diffusion. This revealed a small vascular contribution to the signal
in tumor and peri-tumoral stroma within 8 mm. Monoexponential fitting
performed worse than the IVIM model in tumor and stroma within 8 mm,
but was sufficient in more distal stromal regions where lower microvessel
density is expected. Modelling diffusion MRI by IVIM provided a measure of vascularity that may complement information from DCE-MRI
and yielded additional information about diffusion in the extravascular
tissue.

Keywords: diffusion MRI, vascularity, stroma, modelling, IVIM, breast
cancer.

1 Introduction

As breast cancer treatment options increase, tools to predict tumor invasiveness and recurrence are needed. Changes in peri-tumoral stroma are potential
markers of outcome. For example, signal enhancement from Dynamic Contrast-
Enhanced Magnetic Resonance Imaging (DCE-MRI) correlates with tumor recurrence [1] and survival [2]. There is also spatial variation: signal enhancement
ratio becomes less prominent with distance from the tumor, an effect that correlates with microvessel density [3]. However, DCE-MRI signal at low temporal

H. Fujita, T. Hara, and C. Muramatsu (Eds.): IWDM 2014, LNCS 8539, pp. 380–386, 2014.

resolution depends on many physiological parameters, including the microvessel density, blood flow, vessel permeability and the extracellular space into which contrast agent leaks.

Diffusion MRI is also sensitive to the vasculature. The intravoxel incoherent motion (IVIM) model separates vascular pseudodiffusion from diffusion in the extravascular tissue and has recently been used to model the diffusion signal from breast tumors [4,5], demonstrating a pseudodiffusive contribution to the signal of 6-10% for malignant tissues. This component was less than 2% in non-cancerous fibroglandular tissue (FGT), but the regions analysed were in the contralateral breast or at a distance from the tumor. The peri-tumoral stroma region remains unexamined by IVIM.

McLaughlin et al. examined the diffusion signal in the peri-tumoral stroma following taxane treatment with a monoexponential model and measurements at two b-values [6]. They found a weak correlation between change in tumor volume and change in monoexponential apparent diffusion coefficient (ADC) from pre-treatment values. Furthermore, there was no significant difference between ADC in stroma near (2-5 mm) and far (9-13 mm) from the tumor. This is somewhat puzzling since microvessel density decreases with distance from the tumor [3] and the protein content and density of the extracellular matrix also vary. This may be because ADC lacks specificity to microstructural changes: a decrease in vascular pseudodiffusion can be compensated for by faster diffusion in the extravascular space.

The DCE-MRI signal enhancement variations in the peri-tumoral stroma and the low specificity of monoexponential diffusion measures to vascular effects suggest that a more complex diffusion model may be needed in the stroma. This study modelled diffusion MRI data in breast using IVIM to examine vascular perfusion and tissue diffusion effects in the tumor and the peri-tumoral stroma. Results were compared to a monoexponential ADC method using the Akaike Information Criterion (AIC).

2   Methods

2.1   Patients and Data Acquisition

Three pre-chemotherapy patients presenting with breast cancer were imaged on a 3 T Siemens Trio (Siemens Healthcare, Erlangen) with a 7-channel InVivo breast coil in compliance with Local Research Ethics Committee approval.

Diffusion data were acquired with a 2D fat-saturated Twice-Refocused Spin Echo sequence at 5 b-values (50, 100, 200, 400-450 and 800 s/mm^2), with at least one unweighted image. Sequence parameters were: effective repetition time $TR_{eff} = 65$ ms, echo time TE = 159 ms, 5 averages, in-plane resolution 1.77 x 1.77 mm^2, slice thickness 4 mm, field of view 12.7 x 34.0 cm^2 and 24-34 slices.

DCE-MRI data were acquired with a 3D fat-saturated Spoiled Gradient Recalled sequence: TR = 3.8 ms, TE = 1.38 ms, 1 average, resolution 1.08 x 1.08 x 0.90 mm^3, field of view 35.6 x 38.0 x 14.4 cm^3. Patients received 0.1 mmol/kg body weight Gadoteric acid (Dotarem, Guerbet). Temporal resolution was 49 s, but only the subtraction of the baseline image from the two-minute post-contrast image was used to define the tumor region.

2.2   Registration, Region Selection and Noise Correction

Motion was corrected by non-rigid registration of the unweighted images using NiftyReg (University College London, UK), a free-form registration implemented using cubic B-splines [7]. The transformation was then applied to the corresponding diffusion-weighted images in each direction.

Tumors were selected using a region-growing algorithm (MITK segmentation) on the DCE-MRI subtraction images and verified by a radiologist. These were transformed to the nearest diffusion-weighted slice and regions of interest (ROIs) at varying distances from the tumor (0-4, 4-8, 8-12 and 12-16 mm; see Figure 1) were generated. Each region was adjusted to exclude non-fibroglandular voxels based on a manual breast contour and decrease in signal of less than 30% from the 50 to 800 s/mm^2 images. Signal from voxels in each ROI was averaged to obtain a mean. Non-Gaussian noise was corrected by subtracting a factor dependent on the local noise [8]. All three diffusion-weighted directions were averaged to obtain signal for fitting and all unweighted image values were combined to get a single signal value for b=0 to use for fitting.

2.3   Data Fitting

Data were fitted to two different models: a monoexponential model

$$S = S_0 \exp\left(-b \cdot ADC\right), \tag{1}$$

where S_0 is the signal in the absence of diffusion weighting and ADC is the apparent diffusion coefficient; and the biexponential IVIM model

$$S = S_0 \left[f_p \exp\left(-b \cdot D_p\right) + (1 - f_p) \exp\left(-b \cdot D_t\right)\right], \tag{2}$$

where S_0 is as above, f_p is the fraction of signal decay from pseudodiffusion, D_p is the pseudodiffusion coefficient and D_t is the tissue diffusion coefficient.

Weighted least squares fits were performed using Python and the scipy optimize minimize module with L-BFGS-B minimization. A lower bound of 0 was used for all parameters and upper bound of 5x the unweighted signal for S_0, no bound for ADC or D_t and 1 for f_p. The data have low sensitivity to D_p, so it was fixed at 2 x 10^{-2} mm^2/s similar to previous work [4,5].

The AIC indicates information lost by fitting while accounting for model complexity (lower values indicate less loss) and was calculated by

$$AIC = \chi^2 + 2k, \tag{3}$$

where χ^2 is the reduced chi-squared and k is the number of fit parameters.

Parameter and AIC values were averaged across slices with visible tumor (n = 2, 5 and 1 for patients 1, 2 and 3 respectively) from all patients. Voxel-by-voxel maps of the parameters were also generated.

Statistical errors in the fitted parameters were calculated by adjusting one parameter at a time and re-fitting the remaining parameters until

$$\chi^2 \geq \chi_0^2 \left[1 + \frac{n_p}{N - n_p} F\left(n_p, N - n_p, 0.68\right) \right], \tag{4}$$

where χ^2 is the reduced chi-squared from the fit with one fixed parameter, χ_0^2 is the reduced chi-squared from a fit where all parameters vary, n_p is the number of parameters in the fit, N is the number of data points and F is the F distribution function, calculated here for a 68% confidence interval.

3 Results

Figure 1 shows sample DCE and diffusion-weighted (b=200 s/mm^2) images with the tumor outlined in cyan and the surrounding fibroglandular regions (0-4 mm, 4-8 mm, 8-12 mm and 12-16 mm) in blue and purple. The mean SNR of the unweighted images was 69 and in the surrounding regions (increasing distance): 40, 42, 38 and 27. In the second patient, regions beyond 0 mm had low SNR and could not be analysed.

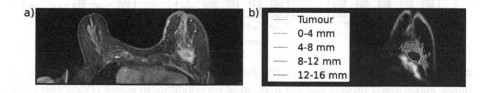

Fig. 1. (a) The post-contrast DCE and (b) diffusion-weighted (b=200 s/mm^2) images with the tumor (*cyan*) and surrounding ROIs of fibroglandular stroma outlined

Figure 2a shows the fits of the models to the diffusion data for one slice of a tumor. Residuals are shown in 2b. Monoexponential fits are in solid blue (lines for the 68% confidence interval of the ADC parameter calculated by Eq. 4 are dotted) and biexponential fits are in red.

Figure 3 summarizes the parameters (mean +/- SD across the slices from all patients) from the monoexponential and biexponential fits as a function of distance from the tumor, as well as the AIC for each fit. Figure 4 shows maps of the fit parameters through one slice of the tumor volume. The 68% confidence intervals for the fit parameters in the tumor, given by Eq. 4, were 4% for S_0 and 15% for ADC for the monoexponential fit and 6% for S_0, 25% for D_t, 86% for the lower error of f_p and 107% for the upper error of f_p for the biexponential fit. Because the values of f_p are relatively small, this translates to a parameter range of 0.02 - 0.21.

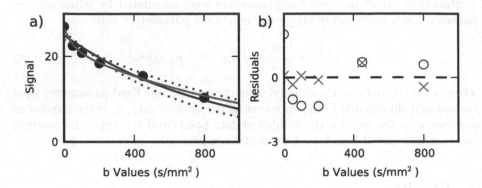

Fig. 2. Results of data fitting. (a) Signal as b value increases. Monoexponential fits to the data are in *solid blue* and biexponential fits are in *red*. The dotted line shows the fit using the ADC parameter error for the 68% confidence interval. (b) Residuals.

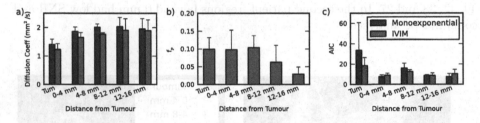

Fig. 3. Monoexponential (*blue*) and IVIM (*red*) fit parameters (a) ADC and D_t in tumor and stromal regions and (b) fraction of pseudodiffusive signal (IVIM only). (c) AIC. Bar graphs mean +/- SD for all patients, all tumor-containing slices.

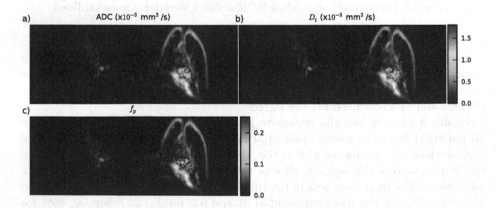

Fig. 4. Maps of fit parameters. (a) ADC from the monoexponential fit, (b) D_t from IVIM and (c) f_p from IVIM.

4   Discussion

For peri-tumoral stroma within 8 mm of the tumor, IVIM provided a better fit to the diffusion data, shown by the lower and comparable AICs in this region, as well as the residuals (blue points in Figure 2b), which were consistently below zero for b-values of 100-200 s/mm^2 and then rose above zero. Residuals for the IVIM fit were more evenly distributed. IVIM did not add significant information in more distal stroma, however.

The values of the diffusion coeffecient $D_t = (1.4 +/- 0.2)$ x 10^{-3} mm^2/s and the pseudodiffusion fraction $f_p = 0.10 +/- 0.03$ in the tumors themselves agreed with previous IVIM results: $D_t = (1.3 +/- 0.3)$ x 10^{-3} mm^2/s and $f_p = 0.06 +/-$ 0.03 in [4] and $D_t = (1.2 +/- 0.4)$ x 10^{-3} mm^2/s and $f_p = 0.10 +/- 0.05$ in [5]. It should be noted that Bokacheva et al. excluded tumor edges, which tend to be more vascular, from their analysis, which may account for their slightly lower average. The parameter maps (Figure 4) demonstrated some heterogeneity of the parameters within the tumor. In addition, there may be differences in the patient populations.

In the stroma, D_t was near that for free water and demonstrated an increasing trend further from the tumor, which could be due to less dense extracellular matrix or less cross-linking in this region. The monoexponential ADC showed little variation with distance from the tumor, in agreement with [6]. The pseudodiffusion fraction, f_p, decreased with distance from the tumor (Figure 3b), consistent with lower microvessel density [3] and previous DCE data [2]. These IVIM parameters suggest that the smaller contribution of vascular perfusion to the signal further from the tumor is compensated for by freer diffusion in the extravascular space, resulting in a similar calculated ADC value throughout the stroma when a two-point ADC method is used. Future work will attempt to validate the IVIM findings using histological measures of microvessel density.

The IVIM model assumes that the extravascular tissue can be represented by a single diffusion decay contribution. In the peri-tumoral stroma, there are very few cells relative to the tumor itself and low b-values are insensitive to cellular restriction, so this assumption is reasonable in this region. However, more complex models may be needed to describe the tumor, such as those incorporating restricted and hindered water diffusion by cells [9]. IVIM also assumes that water does not move between the vasculature and the tissue during measurement, which may affect parameter accuracy for leaky tumor vasculature.

This is the first study examining the diffusion signal in peri-tumoral stroma for non-monoexponential behavior. Although this preliminary work examined only a small number of patients, the results showed that a significant vascular contribution to the signal exists in the stroma close to the tumor. These differences could not be detected by a conventional monoexponential ADC model. In light of the correlations observed previously between DCE-MRI stromal enhancement and tumor recurrence, models of MR diffusion signal that account for vascular contributions deserve further study.

Acknowledgements. This work is supported by funding from EPSRC grant "MIMIC": EP/K020439/1 and EU FP7 Virtual Physiological Human grant: "VPH-PRISM" (FP7-ICT-2011-9, 601040).

References

1. Kim, M.Y., Cho, N., Koo, H.R., Yun, B.L., Bae, M.S., Chie, E.K., Moon, W.K.: Predicting local recurrence following breast-conserving treatment: Parenchymal signal enhancement ratio (SER) around the tumor on preoperative MRI. Acta Radiol. 54, 731–738 (2013)
2. Hattangadi, J., Park, C., Rembert, J., Klifa, C., Hwang, J., Gibbs, J., Hylton, N.M.: Breast stromal enhancement on MRI is associated with response to neoadjuvant chemotherapy. Am. J. Roentgenol. 190, 1630–1636 (2008)
3. Nabavizadeh, N., Klifa, C., Newitt, D., Lu, Y., Chen, Y.-Y., Hsu, H., Fisher, C., Tokayasu, T., Olshen, A.B., Spellman, P., Gray, J.W., Hylton, N., Park, C.C.: Topographic enhancement mapping of the cancer-associated breast stroma using breast MRI. Integr. Biol. 3, 490–496 (2011)
4. Bokacheva, L., Kaplan, J.B., Giri, D.D., Patil, S., Gnanasigamani, M., Nyman, C.G., Deasy, J.O., Morris, E.A., Thakur, S.B.: Intravoxel incoherent motion diffusion-weighted MRI at 3.0 T differentiates malignant breast lesions from benign lesions and breast parenchyma. J. Magn. Reson. Imaging. Early View (2013)
5. Sigmund, E.E., Cho, G.Y., Kim, S., Finn, M., Moccaldi, M., Jensen, J.H., Sodickson, D.K., Goldberg, J.D., Formenti, S., Moy, L.: Intravoxel incoherent motion imaging of tumor microenvironment in locally advanced breast cancer. Magn. Reson. Med. 65, 1437–1447 (2011)
6. Mclaughlin, R.L., Newitt, D.C., Wilmes, L.J., Jones, E.F., Wisner, D.J., Kornak, J., Proctor, E., Joe, B.N., Hylton, N.M.: High Resolution In Vivo Characterization of Apparent Difusion Coefficient at the Tumor-Stromal Boundary of Breast Carcinomas: A Pilot Study to Assess Treatment Response Using Proximity-Dependent Diffusion-Weighted Imaging. J. Magn. Reson. Imaging. Early View (2013)
7. Modat, M., Ridgway, G.R., Taylor, Z.A., Lehmann, M., Barnes, J., Fox, N.C., Hawkes, D.J., Ourselin, S.: Fast free-form deformation using graphics processing units. Comput. Methods Programs Biomed. 98, 278–284 (2010)
8. Henkelman, R.M.: Measurement of signal intensities in the presence of noise in MR images. Med. Phys. 12, 232–233 (1985)
9. Panagiotaki, E., Schneider, T., Siow, B., Hall, M.G., Lythgoe, M.F., Alexander, D.C.: Comparment models of the diffusion MR signal in brain white matter: A taxonomy and comparison. NeuroImage 59, 2241–2254 (2012)

Monte Carlo Modeling of the DQE of a-Se X-Ray Detectors for Breast Imaging

Yuan Fang[1,2,*], Andreu Badal[1], Karim S. Karim[2], and Aldo Badano[1]

[1] Division of Imaging and Applied Mathematics, Office of Science and Engineering Laboratories, Center for Devices and Radiological Health, U.S. Food and Drug Administration. Silver Spring, MD
[2] Department of Electrical and Computer Engineering, University of Waterloo, Waterloo, ON, Canada

Abstract. We study the resolution characteristics of a-Se semiconductor x-ray detectors using ARTEMIS, a detailed Monte Carlo transport code that simulates the three-dimensional spatial and temporal transport of electron-hole pairs under an external electric field. The model takes into account generation and re-absorption of characteristic x rays, spreading due to Compton scattering and high-energy secondary electron transport, and drift and diffusion of electron-hole pairs under applied bias. The point responses for a 200 μm thick mammography detector for RQA radiation qualities are simulated using parallel processing. Line spread functions and modulation transfer functions show a dependence on incident x-ray energy and spatial frequency.

Keywords: detective quantum efficiency, ARTEMIS, Monte Carlo simulation, amorphous Selenium.

1 Introduction

Semiconductor based x-ray detectors convert x-ray photons directly into charge signal without a scintillator material, and can be used to improve spatial resolution compared to indirect based detectors. In particular, detectability of microcalcifications and small lesions in mammography has driven the development of high spatial resolution imagers with small pixel pitch. Amorphous selenium (a-Se) flat-panel x-ray imagers offer high resolution[1,2] and are currently used clinically for mammography applications and actively researched for other novel breast imaging modalities.

In this work, we study the resolution characteristics of an a-Se direct x-ray detector for a range of RQA radiation qualities using Monte Carlo methods with detailed simulations of charge carrier transport under the influence of applied electric field.

---

* yuan.fang@fda.hhs.gov

H. Fujita, T. Hara, and C. Muramatsu (Eds.): IWDM 2014, LNCS 8539, pp. 387–393, 2014.

2   Method

2.1   Monte Carlo Simulations

This work utilizes an open source Monte Carlo transport code, ARTEMIS[3,4,5] (pArticle transport, Recombination, and Trapping in sEMiconductor Imaging Simulations) specifically developed for detailed simulation of electron-hole-pair transport in direct x-ray detectors. The simulation of the signal formation process in ARTEMIS is based on PENELOPE[6] for the simulation of photon and secondary electron transport coupled with a detailed transport code for the spatiotemporal simulation of electron-hole pairs, and the general-purpose simulation package for PENELOPE[7], which contains a modular main program and several tally options and source models that facilitate the simulation of medical physics applications. This version of ARTEMIS includes a parallel processing option, based on message passing interface (MPI) and allows for speed-ups in simulations proportional to the number of processor cores available. This improvement is achieved by utilizing different computers and processing cores by sending messages over the network to combine the simulation results in each MPI thread.

For mammography applications, we model an a-Se detector with a thickness of 200 μm. The line spread function (LSF) is calculated from the point response across detector pixels, and the modulation transfer function (MTF) is obtained by taking the Fourier transform of the LSF. The detective quantum efficiency (DQE) at zero frequency is calculated with the expression[8]:

$$DQE(0) = \eta As, \tag{1}$$

where η is the interaction efficiency, and As is the Swank factor. The detective quantum efficiency (DQE) as a function of spatial frequency, is given by[9]:

$$DQE(\nu) = \frac{MTF^2(\nu)}{NNPS(\nu)}, \tag{2}$$

where $MTF(\nu)$ is the modulation transfer function and $NNPS(\nu)$ is the normalized noise power spectrum.

2.2   Clinical Spectra

We used RQA beam qualities generated with methods described by Boone *et al.*[10], with the parameters listed in Table 1. All beam qualities are taken from the table of radiation qualities for the determination of MTF and DQE and corresponding parameters in IEC document 62220-1-2 (2007) and 61267 (2005)[11,12]. The radiation qualities are shown in Figure 1.

3   Preliminary Results

Figure 2 and 3 show the simulated LSF and MTF. A million histories of incident photons are simulated in each case, with the source incident perpendicular to a

Table 1. Radiation Quality (IEC 61267:2005) for the determination of DQE

Radiation Quality	Tube voltage (kV)	HVL (mm Al)	Filter (mm Al)
RQA3	50	4.0	10.0
RQA5	70	7.1	21.0
RQA7	90	9.1	30.0
RQA9	120	11.5	40.0

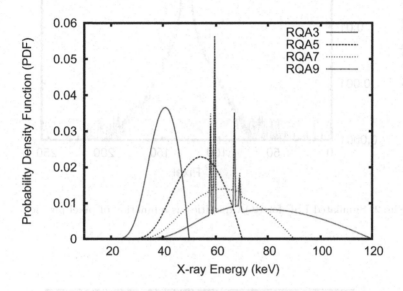

Fig. 1. RQA beam qualities used for Monte Carlo simulations

200 μm thick a-Se detector biased at 10 V/μm. A pixel size of 5 μm is used with 256 pixels in both x and y directions.

The simulated DQE results are shown in Figure 4. The simulated DQE was calculated by adding the frequency response of the signal and noise transfer and taking into account the aperture of the sensor pixel, as shown in Equation 2. The ARTEMIS code has been updated with the MPI parallel processing option, and Table 2 and Figure 5 shows a comparison of the MPI processing times for single core and multi-core processors for 1000 incident photons. The total time is calculated from summing the initialization and simulation times. With the MPI option, doubling the number of processors from one to two show a similar linear increase in the number of simulated histories per second. However this improvement is not linear for the one hundred threads case, mainly due to the amount of time required to save a large amount of data, and relatively low number of histories per core.

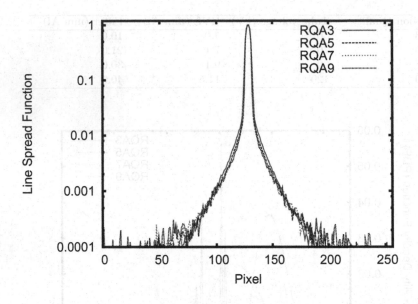

Fig. 2. Simulated LSF for RQA qualities as a function of pixel position

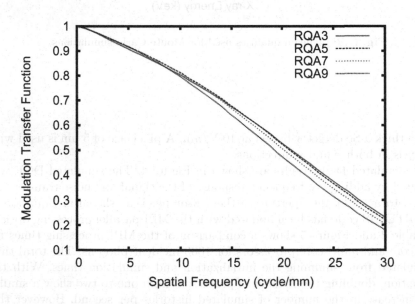

Fig. 3. Simulated MTF for RQA qualities as a function of spatial frequency

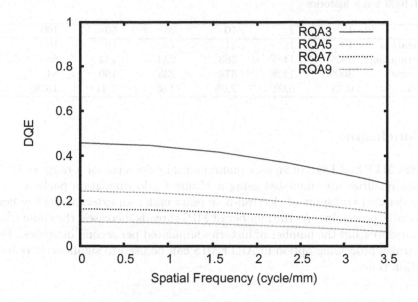

Fig. 4. Simulated DQE for RQA qualities as a function of spatial frequency

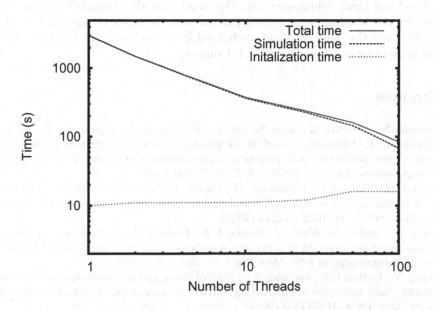

Fig. 5. Simulation time as a function of number of MPI threads

Table 2. Simulation time in seconds as a function of number of MPI threads for a total of 1000 x-ray histories

	1	2	10	25	50	100
Initialization	10	11	11	12	16	16
Simulation time	2999	1487	363	223	144	68
Total time	3009	1498	374	235	160	84
Hist/sec	0.34	0.69	2.95	4.88	7.41	15.30

4 Conclusion

The LSF, MTF and DQE of an a-Se mammography detector for a range of RQA radiation qualities are simulated using a Monte Carlo simulation package that include detailed transport of electron-hole pairs under an external electric field with parallel processing. As the number of MPI threads increases, the simulation speed improves and the number of histories simulated per second increases. The MPI parallel processing option in ARTEMIS can be used to signficantly reduce simulation time.

Acknowledgments. The author (Y.F.) acknowledge funding by an appointment to the Research Participation Program at the Center for Device and Radiological Health administered by the Oak Ridge Institute for Science and Education through an interagency agreement between the U.S. Department of Energy and U.S. Food and Drug Administration. This work was also financially supported in part by the Natural Sciences and Engineering Research Council of Canada (NSERC), and the Mitsui Canada Scholarship (Grand prize of the Canadian National and Ontario Japanese Speech Contest).

References

1. Irisawa, K., Yamane, K., Imai, S., Ogawa, M., Shouji, T., Agano, T., Hosoi, Y., Hayakawa, T.: Direct-conversion 50 μm pixel-pitch detector for digitial mammography using amorphous selenium as a photoconductive switching layer for signal charge readout. In: Proc. SPIE, vol. 7258, 72581I (2009)
2. Zentai, G., Partain, L., Richmond, M., Ogusu, K., Yamada, S.: 50 μm pixel size a-Se mammography imager with high DQE and increased temperature resistance. In: Proc. SPIE, vol. 7622, 762215 (2010)
3. Fang, Y., Badal, A., Allec, N., Karim, K.S., Badano, A.: Spatiotemporal Monte Carlo transport methods in x-ray semiconductor detectors: Application to pulse-height spectroscopy in a-Se. Med. Phys. 39, 308–320 (2012)
4. Fang, Y., Karim, K.S., Badano, A.: Effect of burst and recombination models for Monte Carlo transport of interacting carriers in a-Se x-ray detectors on Swank noise. Med. Phys. 41, 011904 (2014)
5. Sharma, D., Fang, Y., Zafar, F., Karim, K.S.: Badano, Recombination models for spatio-temporal Monte Carlo transport of interacting carriers in semiconductors. Appl. Phys. Lett. 98, 242111 (2011)

6. Salvat, F., Fernandez-Varea, J.M., Sempau, J.: PENELOPE-2006: A code system for Monte Carlo Simulation of Electron and Photon Transport. Issy-les-Moulineaux. OECD/NEA Data Bank, France (2006)
7. Sempau, J., Badal, A., Brualla, L.: A PENELOPE-based system for the automated Monte Carlo simulation of clinacs and voxelized geometries—application to far-from-axis fields. Med. Phys. 38, 5887–5895 (2011)
8. Swank, R.K.: Absorption and noise in x-ray phosphors. J. Appl. Phys. 44, 4199 (1973)
9. Cunningham, I.A.: Applied Linear-Systems Theory. In: Beutel, J., Van Metter, R.L. (eds.) The Handbook of Medical Imaging. Physics and Psychophysics, vol. 1, p. 122. SPIE Press (2008)
10. Boone, J.M., Fewell, T.R., Jennings, R.J.: Molybdenum, rhodium, and tungsten anode spectral models using interpolating polynomials with application to mammography. Med. Phys. 24, 1863–1874 (1997)
11. Medical electrical equipment – Characteristics of digital X-ray imaging devices – Part 1: Determination of the detective quantum efficiency. IEC62220-1 (2007)
12. Medical diagnostic X-ray equipment - Radiation conditions for use in the determination of characteristics. IEC61267 (2005)

kVp Tool for Digital Mammography Using Commercial Metallic Foils

Héctor A. Galván and Yolanda Villaseñor

Instituto Nacional de Cancerología, Av. San Fernando 22, Sección XVI, 10400, México
hgalvane@gmail.com

Abstract. An alternative method to evaluate the kVp on digital mammography units was developed using commercial metallic foils of different elements and an aluminum step wedge contained in a mammography test phantom developed at National University of México (UNAM) as a low cost tool. Relative response of metallic foils *(Cu+5Al+8Al) / (Mo+Rh+Ag) vs kVp*, for a numerical analysis and in experimental method of three FFDM systems, shows a linear behavior and permits to calculate kVp with precision of ±0.4 kV. First results are shown and further work is still in process.

Keywords: Digital mammography, quality control, kVp.

1 Introduction

One of the quality control tests for the mammography system is the evaluation of the kilovoltage (kV). Although the invasive methods to evaluate this parameter are more accurate these are not so practical to do, instead the non-invasive methods are preferred. There are several commercial systems to measure the kV, like those that use radiographic film or those that use digital detectors which can be expensive. Anther method using metallic foils have been developed[2].

The HG breast phantom[1], developed at the National University of México (UNAM) as low cost tool to evaluate the performance of analog mammographic systems (film/screen), has several metallic foils to evaluate kV when a three system equation is applied to the optical density (OD) values produced by these foils on the film. This phantom was a master's thesis work and is being used at the National Cancer Institute of México (INCan) to further evaluate its utility.

This phantom is composed of an acrylic block with dimensions of 10 cm long, 10 cm width and 4.3 cm height, with a cavity of 0.3 cm height where several components are placed; the acrylic density used is $1.17\pm0.01 \text{g/cm}^3$ (figure 1). Within the cavity there are 6 different diameters of nylon fibers to simulate glandular fibers, 5 different widths of polyethylene foils to simulate tumor masses, 5 different diameters of compressed talc to simulate microcalcifications, a nonhomogeneous zone to simulate breast structure, an aluminum step wedge to evaluate the film processor and 6 different metallic foils to evaluate the kV. The costs of the elements that composed the HG phantom is close to the $150 USD.

H. Fujita, T. Hara, and C. Muramatsu (Eds.): IWDM 2014, LNCS 8539, pp. 394–398, 2014.
© Springer International Publishing Switzerland 2014

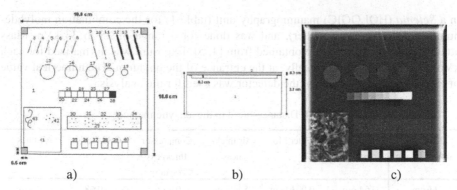

Fig. 1. a) Front view diagram of HG phantom, b) lateral view. C) Radiographic image of HG phantom.

The aluminum step wedge produces a known attenuation pattern on the film, and when fix kVp and mAs are used, OD variations of the film due to the film processor can be tested. In order to use this phantom element, an initial calibration of the film and film processor must be done.

The metallic foils of this phantom use the effect of k-edge discontinuity to evaluate the peak kilo-voltage (kVp). When an X-ray spectrum passes through a metalic material, the attenuation it experiences will depend on the material's properties. If the material has a k-edge value within the spectrum's energy interval, it is possible to observe a drastic change on its attenuation due to the k-edge. Thus, using metalic materials with k-edge values within the clinical mammography energy range (22-33 keV) is effective to evaluate the kV. To perform such evaluation using the HG phantom, the OD produced by three different metalic materials is measured and three equations are applied. This method also require an initial calibration

In this work we report a new and easy method to evaluate the kVp in FFDM systems using the step wedge and the aluminum foils of the HG phantom.

2 Materials and Methods

The step wedge is made of commercial aluminum, with 9 steps of 0.111, 0.222, 0.333, 0.444, 0.555, 0.666, 0.888 and 1.110 mm thickness, and a step of 1.110 aluminum plus 1.0 mm lead. All steps have an area of 0.5 x 0.5 cm². The measured aluminum density is 2.9±0.1 g/cm³. The metallic foils and its thickness are: copper (Cu) of 25 μm, molybdenum (Mo) of 25 μm, rhodium (Rh) of 25 μm, silver (Ag) of 25 μm, cadmium (Cd) of 100 μm, and tin (Sn) of 25 μm. All metallic foils have an area of 0.5 x 0.5 cm², and purity above 99.9%. The thicknesses of the foils were determined by the commercial availability of the manufacturer.

2.1 Analytical Method

To understand the behavior of the metallic foils an analysis of the spectrum's attenuation was performed. The spectrums curves were obtained from [3] and the scatter radiation was not considered. The analysis reproduces the geometry parameters found in a *Selenia* (HOLOGIC) mammography unit (table 1) for the combination molybde-num/molybdenum (target/filter), and was done for a range of 25 to 33 kVp. Mass attenuation coefficients were obtained from [4, 5]. Exposure was normalized for each kVp to the value found clinically, at the entrance of the phantom. The numerical value of exposure at the entrance of the detector was used for the analysis.

Table 1. Distances used in the analytic method

Distance source image	Distance source base	Filter Mo	Air thick-ness	Compressor thickness (lexan)	Grid factor	Air thick-ness
66 cm	64 cm	0.0030 cm	59.8 cm	0.2 cm	0.68	cm^2

2.2   Experimental Method

The The radiographic images from the HG phantom were obtained using a *Selenia* (HOLOGIC) mammography unit at the National Cancer Institute (INCan) and a *Senographe DS* (GE) mammography unit at the UNAM Physics Institute. For the *Selenia* units the mode *semi* was used, where the kVp is manually selected and the mAs is set by the unit; for the *Senographe DS* unit the *MANUAL* mode was used, where the kVp and mAs were fixed. The nominal values of the kVp used were 25 to 33 in steps of 1. Images were acquired in *for processing* mode and FIJI software was used to measure the mean pixel value (MPV) and the regions of interest used had dimensions 3mm x 3mm.

3   Results

Values of the step wedge and the metallic foils from the analytical method are shown in figures 2a y 2b, which are normalized to the base value. Figure 2c shows the value for six selected elements.

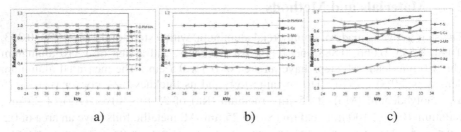

a)   b)   c)

Fig. 2. a) Response of the step wedge normalized to base value. b) Response of the 6 metallic foils normalized to base value. c) Response of 6 selected elements.

The numerical value of the step wedge and the copper foil shows an increase of the signal as the kVp increases; on the other hand the signal of the molybdenum, rhodium and silver foils shows a decrease in the signal as the kVp increases. The tin and cadmium foils show no dependency with kVp. Then, a relationship using this results was proposed as:

$$(Cu+5Al+8Al) / (Mo+Rh+Ag) \qquad (1)$$

This result is plotted as a function of kVp, and is shown in figure 3.

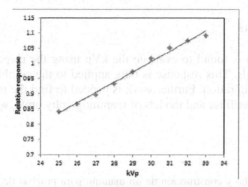

Fig. 3. The numerical value of (Cu+5Al+8Al)/(Mo+Rh+Ag) as a function of kVp for the analytical method

The result of figure 3 is adjusted to a linear fit whit a correlation coefficient of r^2=0.992, a slope of m=0.0337 and interception of b=-0.0061. Performing a similar analysis to experimental data from the three mammography units, using the MPV produced by the same elements and kVp values, leads to the results shown on figure 4. Table 2 lists the corresponding values of slope and interception for the three systems. Using this analysis, kVp can be computed with a precision of ± 0.4.

Table 2. Values of the lineal fit for the relative response as a function of kVp for the 3 mammography units

System	Slope	Interception	r^2
Selenia 1	0.0443	-0.2286	0.998
Selenia 2	0.0439	-0.2203	0.998
Senographe DS	0.0306	0.1072	0.996

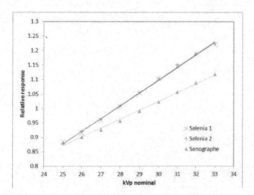

Fig. 4. Numerical value of (Cu+5Al+8Al)/(Mo+Rh+Ag) as a function of nominal kVp for the 3 mammography units

The three systems and the analytical method have a linear response, although the values of slope and interception are different. The origins of these differences could be due to differences in X-ray spectrum produced by each model of X-ray tube.

4   Conclusions

A linear relationship is found to evaluate the kVp using the response produced by a series of metallic foils. This response is only applied to the combination Mo/Mo and requires an initial calibration. Further work is needed to find the response to different combinations of target/filter and models of mammography units, which is in progress.

References

1. Galván, H.A.: Diseño y construcción de un maniquí para pruebas de control de calidad en equipos de mamografía convencional, Master's thesis,UNAM (2006)
2. Napolitano, M.E., Trueblood, J.H., Hertel, N.E., David, G.: Mammographic x-ray unit voltage test tool based on k-edge absorption effect. Medical Physics 29(9), 2169–2176 (2002)
3. Boone, J.M., Fewell, T.R., Jennings, R.J.: Molybdenum, rhodium, and tungsten anode spectral models using interpotating polynomials with application to mammography. Medical Physics 24(12), 1863–1874 (1997)
4. National Institute of Standards and Technology,
   http://www.nist.gov/pml/data/xraycoef/
5. Jeffrey, A.: Fessler web page,
   http://web.eecs.umich.edu/~fessler/irt/irt/ct/
   xray-mass-atten/compound/lexan

Possibility of Exposure Dose Reduction in Contrast Enhanced Spectral Mammography Using Dual Energy Subtraction Technique : A Phantom Study

Noriko Nishikawa, Kaori Yanagisawa, Kuniji Naoi, Yutaka Ohnuma,
and Yoshihisa Muramatsu

Department of Radiology, National Cancer Center Hospital East 6-5-1,
Kashiwanoha, Kashiwa-City, Chiba 277-8577 Japan
nonishik@east.ncc.go.jp

Abstract. Contrast Enhanced Spectral Mammography using energy subtraction technique (CESM) with iodinated contrast media is promising technology to improve the contrast of the image and detectability of tumor. One of the issues to be solved on this technique is giving additional radiation exposure to the patient compared with conventional mammography. We investigated phantom study to optimize scan protocol and parameter setting for reducing radiation dose without image degradation. We acquired the images with two different imaging conditions, fully-automated mode and manual mode, and evaluated image quality by image noise, contrast and exposure dose. On image quality evaluation in manual mode, the normalized noise power spectrum (NNPS) at low-energy image was increased and image quality became worse, but the quality of recombined image was not significantly different comparing to fully-automated mode. The contrast at low-energy image in manual mode was slightly deteriorated, but at recombined image was not much different comparing to auto mode. On the other hand, average glandular dose (AGD) was able to be reduced to 1.41 mGy from 1.96 mGy by setting manual mode. These results suggest it may possible to reduce the exposure dose by using manual mode instead of fully-automated mode when CESM has performed in clinical service.

1   Introduction

Mammography is one of the most popular and widely used methods to detect breast cancer in clinical service. But it is sometimes difficult to identify a tumor lesion due to the low contrast image against the normal breast tissue. Contrast Enhanced Spectral Mammography (CESM) using dual energy subtraction technique is a new application system and recently available as the product for clinical service.

CESM is a unique application in digital mammography system. About 2 min before data acquisition, iodinated contrast media was injected intravenously. Then, a pair of low- and high-energy X-ray was exposed to the patient sequentially as the one series of data acquisition. Data acquisition was performed completely same as standard mammography with both left and right breast in totally 4 views. It has been completed within 5 min from the beginning to the end of acquisition. Low energy of

H. Fujita, T. Hara, and C. Muramatsu (Eds.): IWDM 2014, LNCS 8539, pp. 399–406, 2014.

X-ray has set below K-edge absorption of iodine and higher energy has upper K-edge and it has obtained the contrast enhanced image, so called recombined image, by subtracting and processing low- and high-energy image data. This technique is used for detection of angiogenesis by tracking contrast media up-take and wash-out in tissues same as CT scan because of the use of same iodinated contrast media. Low-energy image is made of the exposure of X-ray at 26-32 kVp, and is used in interpretation as with conventional mammography. High-energy image is 45-49 kVp, and is used only for recombined image calculated with low-energy image. As the result, image can be obtained by the user is two : 1) low-energy image, 2) recombined image enhanced iodinated contrast media by processing[1-4].

In the clinical experience at our hospital, it was useful for dense breast and cases that can not be visualized a tumor in conventional mammography. However, this technique has a drawback to increase radiation exposure as compared with conventional mammography. We found there are 2 main reasons of increasing radiation exposure. The first reason is coming from high-energy X-ray exposure. Another reason is CESM mode can not use Automatic Exposure Control system (AEC) at low-energy exposure and the dose is determined by only the breast thickness. High-energy exposure is an essential for CESM and the ratio of radiation dose from high-energy exposure is relatively small. On the other hand, the conditions at the individual breast such as different breast density is varied even if the breast thickness is the same. And it has observed the exposure parameter is not optimized and the dose becomes excessive in many cases. So, there is some possibility to reduce the dose by optimizing exposure parameter at low-energy considering with not only breast thickness but also breast density and other parameters.

The objectives of this study is to find optimal exposure parameter in CESM mode considering to both exposure dose and image quality using the phantom.

2   Materials and Methods

The study were performed with Senographe Essential made by GE Healthcare (Chalfont St. Giles, UK). It is full-field digital mammography system consisted of in-direct conversion flat panel detector with CsI absorber that has 1914 x 2294 pixels and pixel size of 100 micro-mm. The X-ray tube is available to deliver low (26-32 kVp) and high (45-49 kVp) energy X-ray by changing the voltage, materials of tube target and pre-filter. System is available to perform not only conventional mammography but also CESM with the specific software and hardware for data acquisition and image processing.

Image data were acquired 3 times and calculated the average of these as the final result. ACR Mammographic Accreditation Phantom (Gammex 156) were used with the thickness of 45 mm. Focal spot size was 0.3 mm.

The system is available to perform both conventional mammography mode and CESM mode. Both mode are available to perform manual mode. AEC is available when it is performed with fully-automated mode and exposure parameter is determined by pre-exposure. There are 3 selectable exposure mode in the system, namely "contrast", "standard" and "dose". We use "standard" at this time as we normally use this mode in clinical service.

First, we performed the study and took the image of 156 phantom with fully-automated "standard" mode to identify exposure parameter in standard procedure. And then, we recorded target material, pre-filter, tube voltage, beam current and duration of exposure (mAs), entrance skin exposure (ESE) and average glandular dose (AGD). AGD was calculated the following formula proposed by Wu et al[5-7].

$$D_g = D_g N \times X_a \tag{1}$$

where D_g denotes AGD (mGy); X_a denotes the breast entrance skin exposure in air needed to produce a proper density image; $D_g N$ denotes the average glandular dose resulting from a breast entrance skin exposure in air 1 R (2.58×10^{-4} Ckg^{-1}).

Next, we performed the study and took the image of 156 phantom with fully-automated "CESM" mode and recorded the same parameter in both low and high energy exposure.

Then, we performed the study and took the image of 156 phantom with CESM mode with manual mode at low energy exposure. Parameter at high energy exposure had set to a configurable parameter value closest to value derived in fully-automated CESM mode.

We analyzed NNPS of low-energy image and re-combined image about fully-automated mode and manual mode. NNPS was calculated by setting the ROI in uniform area of 156 phantom and by performing digital Fourier transformation obtained from the power spectrum variation of digital values[8]. The analysis method was setting and measuring ROI at 128 x 128 pixels, and used two-dimensional fast Fourier transform by "Image J" of a free analysis software.

About contrast evaluation, a simulated mass with a diameter of 15mm was made from a filter paper impregnated with iodinated contrast media (300mgI/ml) that was diluted 40 times with water. The dilution ratio is the result of adjusting so that the value at which the digital value is not saturated. We put a simulated mass on 156 phantom and measured digital values within the ROI at the portion of background and a simulated mass. We defined the difference of these average values as the contrast.

$$Contrast = |D_{signal} - D_{B.G.}| \tag{2}$$

where D_{signal} denotes average digital values within the ROI of a simulated mass on phantom; $D_{B.G.}$ denotes average digital values within the ROI of uniform area on phantom. $D_{B.G.}$ was overlap part of the wax block and PMMA block at 156 phantom moreover nothing of the fibers, calcifications and masses.

3 Results

Exposure parameter and dose with fully-automated mode were following (Table.1).

Table 1. Exposure parameter and dose with fully-automated mode

		target material	pre-filter	tube voltage	beam current and duration of exposure	ESE	AGD
standard		Rh	Rh	29 kV	40.4 mAs	3.90 mGy	1.05 mGy
CESM	low-energy	Rh	Rh	29 kV	61.7 mAs	5.53 mGy	1.47 mGy
	high-energy	Rh	Cu	45 kV	161.8 mAs	0.47 mGy	0.49 mGy

AGD of CESM is represented by the total AGD, namely the sum of AGD of high-energy image and low-energy image. This also applies to the ESE. Therefore, total ESE and total AGD were the followings,

total ESE = 5.53 mGy (low) + 0.47 mGy (high) = 6.00mGy

total AGD = 1.47 mGy (low) + 0.49 mGy (high) = 1.96mGy

Exposure parameter with CESM mode with manual mode was following (Table.2).

Table 2. Exposure parameter with manual mode. Parameter at low energy exposure had set to condition at fully-automated "standard" mode. Parameter at high energy exposure had set to a configurable parameter value closest to value derived in fully-automated CESM mode.

		target material	pre-filter	tube voltage	beam current and duration of exposure
CESM	low-energy	Rh	Rh	29 kV	40.0 mAs
manual	high-energy	Rh	Cu	45 kV	160.0 mAs

Result of total ESE and total AGD at manual mode were the followings,

total ESE = 3.58 mGy (low) + 0.47 mGy (high) = 4.05mGy

total AGD = 0.94 mGy (low) + 0.47 mGy (high) = 1.41mGy

In the comparison of NNPS, manual mode was larger than the fully-automated mode at low-energy image (Fig 1-2). Although NNPS value of manual mode was slightly higher, they are not widely different from each other (Fig.3-4).

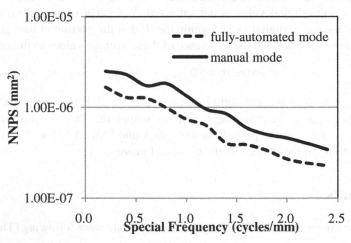

Fig. 1. NNPS about horizontal of CESM with fully-automated mode and manual mode at low energy image

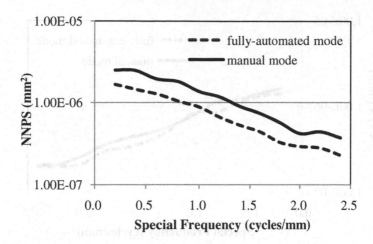

Fig. 2. NNPS about vertical of CESM with fully-automated mode and manual mode at low energy image

In the comparison of contrast obtained between fully-automated mode and manual mode, when there were differences of areal 60 in the digital value, it was at the same at recombined image (Fig. 1) and

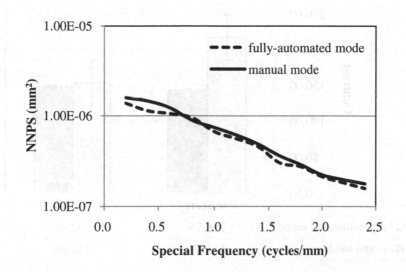

Fig. 3. NNPS about horizontal of CESM with fully-automated mode and manual mode at re-combined image

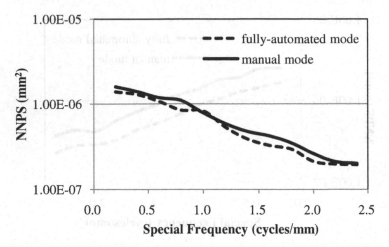

Fig. 4. NNPS about vertical of CESM with fully-automated mode and manual mode at re-combined image

In the comparison of contrast, although between fully-automated mode and manual mode were slight differences, there were only difference of about 60 in the digital value. It was almost the same at re-combined image (Fig.5).

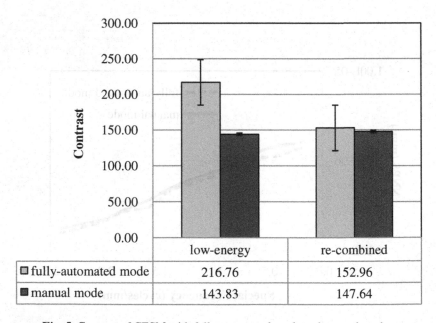

	low-energy	re-combined
▢ fully-automated mode	216.76	152.96
▪ manual mode	143.83	147.64

Fig. 5. Contrast of CESM with fully-automated mode and manual mode

4   Consideration

The comparison of low-energy image between fully automated mode and manual mode, the value of NNPS in fully-automated mode is better than manual mode. This comes from lower X-ray beam current at manual mode, namely manual mode was exposed about 20 mAs lower than fully-automated mode. However, there is no significant difference on NNPS value between fully-automated mode and manual mode in re-combined image. Re-combined image is calculated with specific software and image processing. The detailed algorithm and method has not opened yet and it seemed there were some correction and/or processing, such as filtering, smoothing etc. that control re-combined image with certain noise level. In this study, there is almost same value of NNPS even if we acquire the data with reducing the exposure dose. In image contrast, there are some difference between fully-automated mode and manual mode on low-energy image but no significant difference on re-combined image.

It is important to consider how to perform the interpretation in actual clinical site. Interpretation of CESM at our department is the followings,

1. Read the low-energy image with conventional manner
2. Confirm the presence or absence of abnormal legion using re-combined image
3. 1) and 2) are performed iteratively

Considering to this image reading process, the contrast of re-combined image is more important than that of low-energy image especially the case of dense breast and cases that can not be visualized abnormal legions in conventional mammography. Regarding to exposure dose, AGD was able to reduce 28 % from 1.96 mGy at fully-automated mode to 1.41 mGy at manual mode in CESM mode. In comparison of total radiation dose, CESM with fully-automated mode was 1.86 times higher than conventional mammography when it has performed with fully-automated mode but it becomes 1.34 times with manual mode. Based on mentioned above, we think there seems to be the worth to perform manual mode imaging condition at CESM.

5   Conclusion

CESM has very good tumor visualization capability among to the various application of digital mammography and it is promising technique in clinical diagnosis especially for dense breast patient. Further investigation for low-dose imaging is important and must be a positive impact for the diagnosis of breast cancer.

References

[1] Dromain, C., et al.: Contrast-enhanced digital mammography. European Journal of Radiology 69, 34–42 (2009)
[2] Dromain, C., et al.: Evaluation of Tumor Angiogenesis of Breast Carcinoma Using Contrast-Enhanced Digital Mammography. AJR 187, W528–W537 (2006)

[3] Jong, R.A., et al.: Contrast-enhanced digital mammography: Initial clinical experience. Radiology 228, 842–850 (2003)

[4] Lewin, J.M., et al.: Dual-energy contrast enhanced digital subtraction mammography: Feasibility. Radiology 229, 261–268 (2003)

[5] Ishiguri, K. (ed.): Mammography Technology. Iryo kagakusya (2009)

[6] Wu, X., et al.: Spectral Dependence of Glandular Tissue Dose in Screen-Film Mammography. Radiology 179, 143–148 (1991)

[7] Sobel, W.T., Wu, X.: Parametrization of mammography normalized average glandular dose table. Med. Phys. 24(4), 547–554 (1997)

[8] Ichikawa, K., Ishida, T. (eds.): Image quality measurement of digital radiography. Ohmsha (2010)

A Protocol for Quality Control Testing for Contrast-Enhanced Dual Energy Mammography Systems

Jennifer Oduko[1], Peter Homolka[2], Vivienne Jones[3], and David Whitwam[3]

[1] National Coordinating Centre for the Physics of Mammography, Guildford, UK
jenny.oduko@nhs.net
[2] Centre for Medical Physics and Biomedical Engineering, Medical University of Vienna,
Vienna, Austria
peter.homolka@meduniwien.ac.at
[3] Medical Physics Department, Northampton General Hospital, Northampton, UK
{vivienne.jones,david.whitwam}@ngh.nhs.uk

Abstract. Physics and radiographer QC procedures are urgently needed as the first few contrast-enhanced dual energy systems have been installed in the U.K. Preliminary work on one commercially available system has enabled us to propose new tests, relevant to the properties of dual energy imaging systems. Results are presented for measurements with the chosen phantom, which contains disks with a range of iodine content from 0.25 to 2 mg/cm^2. Breasts of different thicknesses and different glandularity were simulated by adding slabs of CIRS material, of a range of compositions, on top of the phantom. The system tested had a response which was proportional to the iodine content of disks in the phantom, had good reproducibility, and did not change significantly when simulated breast thickness and composition were varied.

Keywords: mammography, contrast-enhanced, dual energy.

1 Introduction

The first few contrast-enhanced dual energy systems have been installed in the U.K. The performance of the low-energy component of the system can be tested in the usual way, following the U.K. and European protocols [1-2]. However, physicists also need to test the high-energy X-ray output and half-value layer (HVL), and the special imaging characteristics relating to iodine contrast medium in the image, in order to complete the acceptance and commissioning tests. As imaging of patients commences, initially as part of clinical trials, radiographers also need a protocol for routine quality control (QC) tests, to ensure the reproducible behavior of the system on a day-to-day basis. The tests and results presented here have been developed by working on one system (GE SenoBright). When other systems become commercially available the proposed protocol may be revised or extended so as to be generally applicable.

H. Fujita, T. Hara, and C. Muramatsu (Eds.): IWDM 2014, LNCS 8539, pp. 407–414, 2014.

2   Equipment and Methods

2.1   Equipment

After some initial work with diluted solutions of Iopamidol, a new phantom was made available for this work. It contains six rows of five disks, 5 mm in diameter, embedded in 20 mm thick polymethyl methacrylate (PMMA). In each row the disks have the same Iopamidol content, giving a range of values from 0.25 to 2 mg/cm^2 of iodine. A row with no Iopamidol and an empty row are also present. The phantom is described in detail in [3], and a dual-energy image is shown in Figure 1. Breasts of different thickness and different glandularity were simulated by adding slabs of CIRS material on top of the phantom. The following were used: 0%, 50% and 100% glandular material, and randomly patterned CIRS BR3D, which is a 50:50 mixture of 0 and 100% glandular material. A low-energy image of the phantom with this material is also shown in Figure 1. In addition, layers of PMMA were used, as these are commonly available, although not exactly tissue-equivalent.

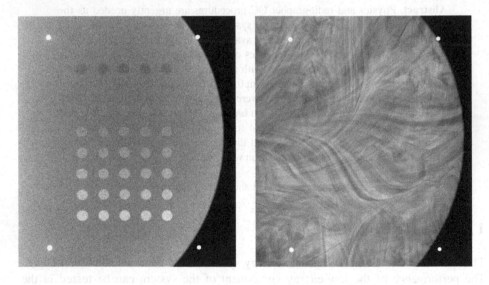

Fig. 1. "Recombined" image (left) and low-energy image (right) of the iodine phantom with added CIRS BR3D tissue-equivalent material

2.2   Measurement of Output and HVL

Measurement of the high-energy component of the exposure presented some initial challenges, because 40-49kV is outside the normal mammographic range, and because the high energy exposure is always preceded by a low-energy exposure. Measurements were made with a mammography ion chamber, after verifying that the results agreed with those obtained using an ion chamber designed for general radiographic use, which had been calibrated over this kV range. Using the "pulse exposure" mode allowed the high-energy component to be measured without any contribution from the low-energy component.

2.3   Mean Glandular Dose

The mean glandular dose D was calculated using the equation

$$D = K g c s \tag{1}$$

where K is the incident air kerma calculated at the top of the breast with the compression paddle in place, and g,c, and s are published conversion factors [4, 5].

2.4   Reproducibility, Signal Variation with Iodine Content and Noise

The phantom alone was imaged five times under automatic exposure control (AEC) and the reproducibility of the iodine signal difference (the difference between mean pixel values in the iodine disk and the adjacent background) was determined. Measurements were made with ImageJ on the "combined" image, displayed by the system after suitably combining the low and high energy images. This processed image is the appropriate one for measuring the iodine signal as it is the one used clinically.

The phantom was then imaged four times in manual exposure mode, using the same kV, target and filter for both high and low energy exposures as under AEC control, but with the mAs for each component selected to be 0.5, 0.75, 1.5 and then 2 times the AEC-selected values. The signal difference, noise and signal difference to noise ratio (SDNR) were determined.

2.5   Simulating Breasts of Different Thickness and Glandularity

The phantom was imaged under AEC control, with 2-5 cm of CIRS BR3D material added on top, and subsequently with 2-5 cm of the different uniform CIRS materials in turn. The glandularity of the phantom and CIRS material combined varied between 16% and 99.5% in the central region (excluding 5 mm adipose "skin" layers, in accordance with the Dance model). Finally 2-5 cm of PMMA was used, with spacers to adjust the paddle height to the appropriate equivalent breast thicknesses.

3   Results

3.1   Output and HVL

The results for the low and high energy exposures are shown in Table 1.

Table 1. Output and HVL

kV target filter	Output (µGy/mAs at 1m)	HVL (mm Al)	kV target filter	Output (µGy/mAs at 1m)	HVL (mm Al)
25 Mo Rh	21.50	0.373	40 Mo Cu	0.485	2.68
28 Mo Rh	32.33	0.412	43 Mo Cu	0.781	2.99
31 Mo Rh	44.34	0.442	46 Mo Cu	1.158	3.27
34 Mo Rh	57.54	0.463	49 Mo Cu	1.617	3.52
28 Rh Rh	29.48	0.415	40 Rh Cu	0.538	2.65
31 Rh Rh	40.46	0.458	43 Rh Cu	0.860	2.97
34 Rh Rh	52.64	0.495	46 Rh Cu	1.271	3.25
37 Rh Rh	66.02	0.524	49 Rh Cu	1.770	3.50

3.2   Mean Glandular Dose

Typical high-energy doses are shown in Table 2. These are for the iodine phantom with 10-50 mm 0% glandular CIRS material added. The calculated MGDs differ from those determined by the system, which are based on a different breast model.

Table 2. Exposure factors, calculated MGD and organ dose displayed by the system, for the high energy exposure (phantom with added 0% glandular material)

Phantom thickness (mm)	kV target filter	mAs	HVL (mm Al)	Glandularity of central portion (%)	Calculated MGD (mGy)	Organ dose (mGy)
20	46 Mo Cu	72.3	3.3	97	0.21	0.26
30	46 Mo Cu	72.3	3.3	49	0.21	0.26
40	45 Mo Cu	112	3.2	32	0.28	0.35
50	45 Rh Cu	165	3.2	24	0.43	0.48
60	47 Rh Cu	185	3.4	19	0.60	0.71
70	49 Rh Cu	185	3.5	16	0.72	0.91

3.3   Reproducibility, Signal Variation with Iodine Content and Noise

Reproducibility was satisfactory, with mean signal difference for 2 mg/cm^2 of iodine details 73.8 ± 1.5 (2 SEM); the maximum deviation from the mean was 3.6%. The signal difference was linear with iodine concentration in the disks, as shown in Figure 2. When incident air kerma K was varied, the signal difference remained constant, noise decreased as $K^{-0.37}$, and SDNR increased as $K^{0.37}$, as shown in Figure 3.

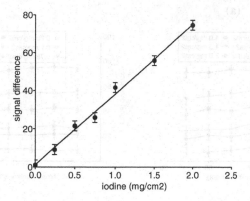

Fig. 2. Signal difference as a function of iodine concentration in the disks. Error bars are 2 SEM.

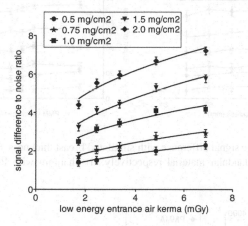

Fig. 3. SDNR variation with incident air kerma. Error bars are 2 SEM.

3.4   Simulating Breasts of Different Thickness and Glandularity

The iodine signal difference varied little over the wide range of thicknesses and materials of different glandularity used. Three representative graphs, shown in Figure 4 (a) to (c), were obtained when using different CIRS materials of glandularity 0%, 50% and 100%. PMMA showed a different variation of signal with breast thickness, but the signal difference variation was broadly similar, as shown in Figure 4(d).

The response of PMMA differs from that of the tissue-equivalent materials, as shown by the variation of iodine signal (mean pixel value) with thickness in Figure 5. All the tissue-equivalent materials show a linear increase in signal, but for PMMA the signal remains constant.

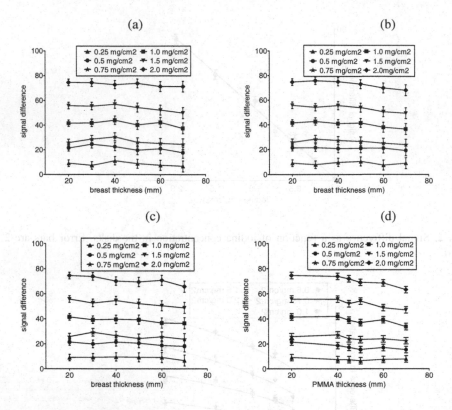

Fig. 4. Variation of iodine signal difference with simulated breast thickness. (a), (b), (c) phantom with 0%, 50%, 100% glandular material respectively, d) phantom with PMMA and spacers. Error bars are 2 SEM.

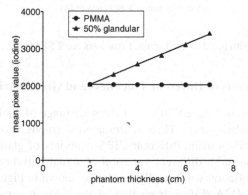

Fig. 5. Variation of mean pixel value for an iodine insert with thickness, for CIRS 50% glandular material and PMMA

4   Discussion

The results of the tests carried out indicate properties of the system tested that are desirable for clinical imaging, i.e. the signal difference has good reproducibility, does not change with incident air kerma, and is proportional to the iodine content of the phantom details. There is little change in the results when materials of different glandularity are used. This suggests that iodine contrast would be equally visible in breasts of different densities, in the uniform background of the combined image.

As other contrast-enhanced dual energy imaging systems become available, the tests may need to be developed further to ensure applicability to all systems. Eventually, performance standards could be set.

There seems to be no phantom with a range of iodine content commercially available at the present time. The phantom used in this study enabled a range of performance tests to be carried out. Such a phantom, or as a minimum one with two or three different iodine area concentrations, could suffice for commissioning and routine physics testing. PMMA, while not tissue-equivalent, was found to give signal difference results that were broadly similar to those obtained with different CIRS materials. It could be used for routine testing if type-testing included PMMA results for reference.

If a suitable phantom were available, radiographer QC could comprise a subset of the tests described here. There should be a daily constancy check of exposure parameters under AEC control, with a measurement of the iodine signal difference. Weekly or monthly tests should include measurements with added thicknesses of PMMA, which is similar to tests in the current QC protocols for 2-D imaging and tomosynthesis.

5   Conclusion

The suggested tests are practicable and form the basis of physics and radiographer testing protocols. A suitable phantom is needed to carry them out, and one with iodine-containing inserts embedded in PMMA was found to be practical and convenient to use.

The results of the physics tests carried out on the GE SenoBright system showed performance characteristics that would be desirable for clinical use.

References

1. Kulama, E., Burch, A., Castellano, I., Lawinski, C.P., Marshall, N., Young, K.C.: Commissioning and Routine Testing of Full Field Digital Mammography Systems (NHSBSP Equipment Report 0604). NHS Cancer Screening Programmes, Sheffield (2009)
2. Van Engen, R., Young, K.C., Bosmans, H., Thijssen, M.: The European Protocol for the Quality Control of the Physical and Technical Aspects of Mammography Screening. In: European Guidelines for Quality Assurance in Breast Cancer Screening and Diagnosis, 4th edn. European Commission, Luxembourg (2006)

3. Leithner, R., Knogler, T., Homolka, P.: Development and Production of a Prototype Iodine Contrast Phantom for CEDEM. Phys. Med. Biol. 58, N25–N35 (2013)
4. Dance, D.R., Skinner, C.L., Young, K.C., Beckett, J.R., Kotre, C.J.: Additional Factors for the Estimation of Mean Glandular Breast Dose using the UK Mammography Dosimetry Protocol. Phys. Med. Biol. 45, 3225–3240 (2000)
5. Dance, D.R., Young, K.C.: Estimation of Mean Glandular Dose for Contrast Enhanced Digital Mammography: Factors for use with the UK, European and IAEA Breast Dosimetry Protocols. Phys. Med. Biol. 59(9), 2127–2137

Trends in Mammogram Image Quality, Dose and Screen-Detected Cancer Rates in an Organized Screening Mammography Program

Brent Parker[1,2], Rasika Rajapakshe[1,2], Ashley Yip[1], Teresa Wight[2], Nancy Aldoff[2], Janette Sam[2], and Christine Wilson[2]

[1] BC Cancer Agency, Centre for the Southern Interior, Kelowna, BC Canada
[2] Screening Mammography Program of BC, Vancouver, BC Canada

Abstract.

BACKGROUND: The Screening Mammography Program of British Columbia (SMPBC), Canada is a population based program that regularly performs quality assurance testing and outcomes analysis.

METHODS: A study was conducted to analyze the trends in the SMPBC quality assurance data from 1994 onwards to investigate any correlation between improvements in image quality (IQ), changes in radiation dose delivered per screen and detection of breast cancers.

RESULTS: Both IQ and cancer detection rates of invasive tumours ≤5 mm increased over 1994-2011 which came at the cost of a 127% increase in radiation dose delivered to the breast between 1994-2005 (IQ increased 21%, tumours ≤5 mm increased 107%). In subsequent years, as digital units started to replace film units the programs' average IQ and CDRs remained unchanged, while the integration of digital units reduced the dose delivered at a populational level.

CONCLUSION: Improvements in IQ coincided with increased detection of small tumours.

Keywords: Quality Assurance, Screening Mammography, Cancer Detection Rates.

1 Introduction

Mammography has been a principal method of screening for breast cancer over the past several decades since randomized control trials suggested its benefit [1, 2]. Furthermore, epidemiological modeling and meta-analysis studies have confirmed that mammographic screening is associated with a reduction in breast cancer mortality [3]. These studies demonstrate a benefit of screening mammography on breast cancer mortality; however, since these trials, image quality has significantly improved. The extent at which image quality has improved in recent decades is important when evaluating the effectiveness of mammography for the purposes of screening as trials that use less sensitive and specific imaging techniques may underestimate the impact of screening [4-7].

H. Fujita, T. Hara, and C. Muramatsu (Eds.): IWDM 2014, LNCS 8539, pp. 415–422, 2014.
© Springer International Publishing Switzerland 2014

Both technological advances in film screen mammography (FSM) (1990s) as well as the advent of digital mammography (2000s) have led to noticeable improvements in image quality. Studies from the U.S. FDA National Mammography Quality Standard's Act and Screening Mammography Program of British Columbia (SMPBC), a population based screening mammography program, have shown that improvements in mammographic technologies improved image quality (IQ) over the 1990s and early 2000s [8, 9]. These observations have been made from regular IQ quality assurance testing.

Associated with the technological advances with FSM in the 1990s and early 2000s, these quality assurance studies also show that the increases in image quality for film mammography came at the expense of roughly doubling the mean glandular dose (MGD), which is an estimate of the radiation delivered to the average women per mammogram. This dose increase can be attributed to the development of Min R 2000 film and new x-ray tube target materials which necessitated radiation dose increases for an improved image quality. Ideally, mammographic images should give optimal image quality with minimal radiation exposure for the patient because it has been shown that radiation exposure has the potential to induce cancer [10].

Although this observed increase in dose and IQ has been described before, to our knowledge there is a limited understanding regarding if these increases in IQ influenced the detection of cancers in a screening setting.

Because increases in IQ for FSM also required increased radiation exposure it is relevant to understand if this increased radiation exposure risk also came with a benefit of an increased detection of cancers. Furthermore, as full field digital mammography (FFDM) units replaced FSM units, it is relevant to understand how dose and cancer detection rates change at a populational level.

This study reports the trends of SMPBC quality assurance data from 1994 onwards and investigates potential relationship between improvements in film based mammographic image quality and cancer detection rates that occurred over 1995-2005. In addition, the study quantifies how the integration of digital screening units into the program is changing the program's IQ, MGD and screening cancer detection rate (CDR).

2   Methods

The SMPBC was established in 1988 and was the first population based mammography screening program in Canada. Women who are residents of British Columbia and aged 40 years and older are eligible to participate in screening mammography at no charge. The SMPBC began transitioning from FSM to FFDM in 2007 and currently 52% of the screening centers employ FFDM. In order to ensure a safe and effective screening service, the program performs regular quality tests on all of their units at each of their centers. IQ and MGD calculations were extracted for each unit's annual quality assurance report. The average IQ was measured by a Mammography Accreditation (ACR) Phantom for each year. The phantom is a lucite block used to simulate the x-ray attenuation of a compressed 4.2 cm human breast composed of 50% adipose tissue and 50% glandular tissue, containing details (masses, fibers and specks) ranging from visible to invisible on a mammographic image. An increase in image quality is defined as an increase in specks, masses and fibers being visible on the phantom image. The minimum performance criterion to pass accreditation is visibility on a mammographic test image of four of the largest fibers, three of the largest speck groups and three of the largest masses.

Furthermore, the MGD, defined as the mean (average) dose to the glandular tissue was calculated for each year between 1994-2013. The MGD is considered to be a reasonable measure for comparing relative risk from different mammography procedures and the acceptable limit for the dose for the phantom is 3 mGy [11-13].

In order to evaluate the differences between FSM and FFDM in ACR and MGD scores, a one-way between groups Analysis of Variance (for MGD) and Student's T Test (for ACR) for the years were calculated where both FSM and FFDM quality assurance tests were available (years 2008- 2013). Both the average MGD and IQ score along with 95% confidence intervals were plotted in Figures 1 and 2 for each year between 1994-2013.

The SMPBC publishes annual reports that describe participation and screening outcomes. From these reports, basic demographic and program performance data was extracted for each year from 1994-2013. In these reports, cancer detection rates are stratified by both the size of the tumour and by age. From this data, the annual age-standardized screen detected cancer rates for women between the ages of 40-79 between the years 1994-2011 were calculated for each range of tumour size reported ($\leq$ 5mm, 6-10mm, 11-15mm, 16-20mm, > 20mm). Age-standardized cancer detection rates (CDRs) were reported in rates per 10,000 screens. The calculation of this data enabled longitudinal comparison of CDRs against the provincial average IQ score.

In order to determine the extent of IQ, MGD and CDRs trends, a linear regression model based on mean values of IQ and MGD and the age standardized CDR were developed. Residuals were plotted to assess for model fit, and an analysis of variance testing was used to assess if trends significantly greater than 0.

All statistical analyses were performed in SPSS and statistical significance was set at $p < 0.05$.

3   Results

Program Performance

The screening program grew from 123,881 screens per year with 19 sites in 1994 to 281,715 screens per year with 38 fixed and 3 mobile sites in 2012. Cancer detection rates fluctuated between 3.4-4.8 per 1000 screens and the programs' sensitivity and specificity ranged from 84-88% and 39-94% respectively. These results suggest that as the program expanded to provide improved coverage to the population of BC, it was able to maintain a quality program with minimal year-to-year variability.

Image Quality, Dose and CDR Years 1994-2005

Both IQ and MGD increased from 1994-2005 (Figures 1-2). During this period, IQ increased 21% (average 1994 ACR=10.2 to average 2004 ACR=12.3) and MGD increased by 127% (average 1994 MGD= 0.98 mGy to average 2004 MGD= 2.22 mGy). As described in Figure 3, there was also a significant increase in the detection of invasive tumours ≤5 mm over this time period. The age standardized CDR for tumors ≤ 5mm increased from 1.49 per 10,000 screens to 3.09 per 10,000 screens (a 107% relative increase). This increasing trend was not observed for tumours greater > 5mm (11% increase in CDR for tumours 6-10mm, 8% increase in CDR for tumours 11-15mm, 3% decrease in CDR for tumours 16-20mm, and 11% increase for tumours > 20mm).

Image Quality, Dose and CDR Years 2006-Current
As depicted in Figure 1 and 2, in the years following 2005, IQ and MGD leveled off in the SFM units. As FFDM started to become integrated into the program (data available for years 2007-2013), MGD was reported to be significantly lower in FFDM units compared to SFM units (Average Film MGD = 1.88mGy, Average Digital, measured 45&8 method, MGD= 1.63mGy, Average Digital RMI method=1.49mGy, p=<.001)

IQ scores were quite variable for FFDM units at the beginning, however, as the number of units within the program increased, and as quality assurance testing became more developed and standardized, the variability in scores decreased, which can be visually seen by observing the confidence intervals in Figure 2. Although when comparing the aggregated IQ scores between the film and digital units for the years with digital IQ data available (2007-2013), there was no statistically significant difference in IQ between screening modalities (Film N=208, mean =12.4, Digital N=80, mean=12.3, p=.552).

Following 2005, CDRs of invasive tumours ≤5 mm varied significantly from 2.07 to 3.23 cases per 10,000 screens. The most recent CDR data available is 2011 data, which suggest a CDR of 2.93 per 10,000 screens (97% increase from the 1994 CDR) and therefore most recent five year average CDR is 2.88 per 10,000 screens (93% increase from 1994 the CDR). No significant trends were observed for tumours >5mm with the exception of the CDR for tumours >20mm, which increased incrementally from 6.0 per 10,000 screens in 2005 to 8.5 per 10,000 screens in 2011.

Correlation between IQ and MGD and IQ and CDRs
For the years 1994-2005, based on linear modeling there was a significant correlation between ACR scores and dose (y=0.42x-3.13, R^2= 0.92, p<.001) and a modest correlation between ACR scores and CDR ≤ 5mm (y=0.58x-3.99, R^2= 0.58 p<.001). However, when the correlation for average ACR scores (both digital and film unit scores included in average calculation) and CDR ≤ 5mm was extended to 2011, the resulting model suggested a lesser but still significant increasing relationship (y=.41x-2.13, R^2=.33, p=.016).

4   Discussion

In the late 1990s and early 2000s the increased detection of small cancers within the SMPBC coincided with increases of image quality. To our knowledge this is the first study that suggests that improvements in image quality in the context of screening mammography may be associated with increased detection of small cancers at a populational level; an improvement that came without a reduction in the program's sensitivity or specificity. In absolute terms, the increased CDR is modest (an increased CDR of 1.6/10,000 screens, or an additional 41 cancers detected in 2005 in this size category when compared to 1994 ≤ 5mm CDRs). Although the data compiled from 2006 to 2011 suggests some variability, if an increased detection in these small tumours is to be sustained in upcoming years, without a significant change in the overall screen detected cancer rate, it is possible that this could have an effect in shifting the T stage distribution of screened detected cancers towards a lower stage. In theory this could improve prognosis as reoccurrence, metastatic potential and prognosis of a breast cancer is thought to be significantly dependant on tumour size [14, 15]. However, a detailed and quantified estimation of this potential impact is beyond the scope of this study.

With regards to the changes in dose over the course of the period of study, although the MGD more than doubled between 1994-2005, this reported average MGD of 2.22 mGy is significantly less than the dose delivered in the early era of screening mammography in the United States when the MGD was estimated to be an average of 14 mGy in 1974 [11]. The integration of digital units into the program has led to a decreased average dose being delivered to the screening population as a whole. Although the risk of radiation-induced breast cancers from breast screening is thought to be minimal, such reductions implemented at a populational level may have relevant implications.

There are a number of limiting factors that may influence this study results. It should be noted that the ACR score is a semi-qualitative score which is subject to a degree of intra- and inter- observer variability. However, it is likely that the potential variability would be minimized in our calculation of the average ACR score due to the large number of units measured each year. Finally, and perhaps most significantly, it is noteworthy to suggest that although there was an increased rate of detecting small cancers that correlated with increases in image quality, other factors, could be influencing the observed change in CDRs of these small tumours. For example, it is possible that there was an improvement in the performance of the program's radiologists between the years 1994-2005 which led to the increased detection of these small tumours.

5   Conclusion

These results describe a correlation between increase in image quality and the detection of small tumours in a population based organized screening mammography program. This increased image quality originally came at the cost of an increased dose, but the MGD is now trending downward as digital units replace the film-screen mammography. These results suggest that improvements in image quality may influence the detection of small invasive cancers at a population based level.

6   Figures

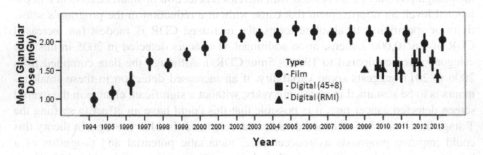

Fig. 1. Changes in Mean Glandular Dose (MGD) of the SMPBC with 95% confidence intervals. The mean MGD peaks in 2005 at 2.22mGy (average based on the 49 available SFM unit MGD measurements). As of 2013, the integration of FFDM units has reduced the programs mean MGD to 1.69 mGy (average based on the 19 available SFM and 30 FFDM unit MGD measurements).

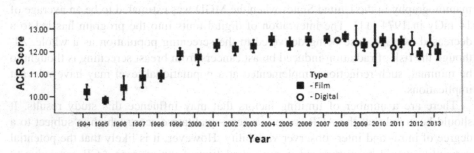

Fig. 2. Changes in cumulative ACR IQ of the SMPBC with 95% confidence intervals. An increase in image quality indicates more specks, masses and fibers visible on the phantom image.

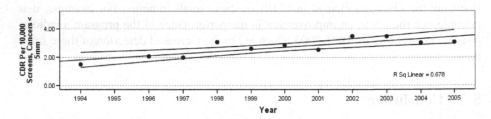

Fig. 3. Age adjusted CDRs of invasive cancers ≤ 5mm per 10,000 screens between the years 1994-2005. A linear trendline and 95% confidence interval of trendline is included. These CDRs encompass SMPBC screen detected cancer in women ages 40-79. The increasing trend seen above between years 1994-2005 was specific to invasive carcinomas ≤ 5mm and not observed in cancers > 5mm.

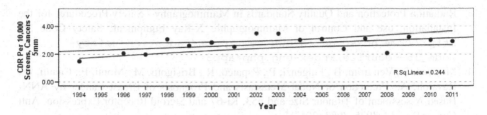

Fig. 4. Age adjusted CDRs of invasive cancers ≤ 5mm per 10,000 screens with trendline and confidence intervals extended to 2011

References

1. Shapiro, S., Venet, W., Strax, P., Venet, L., Roeser, R.: Selection, Follow-Up, and Analysis in the Health Insurance Plan Study: A Randomized Trial with Breast Cancer Screening. Natl. Cancer Inst. Monogr. 67, 65–74 (1985)
2. Tabar, L., Gad, A., Holmberg, L., Ljungquist, U., Fagerberg, C., Baldetorp, L., Gröntoft, O., Lundström, B.: Reduction in Mortality from Breast Cancer After Mass Screening with Mammography: Randomised Trial from the Breast Cancer Screening Working Group of the Swedish National Board of Health and Welfare. The Lancet 325, 829–832 (1985)
3. Cronin, K.A., Feuer, E.J., Clarke, L.D., Plevritis, S.K.: Impact of Adjuvant Therapy and Mammography on US Mortality from 1975 to 2000: Comparison of Mortality Results from the CISNET Breast Cancer Base Case Analysis. JNCI Monographs, 112–121 (2006)
4. Boyd, N.F., Byng, J.W., Jong, R.A., Fishell, E.K., Little, L.E., Miller, A.B., Lockwood, G.A., Tritchler, D.L.: Quantitative Classification of Mammographic Densities and Breast Cancer Risk: Results from the Canadian National Breast Screening Study. J. Natl Cancer Inst. 87, 670–675 (1995)
5. Kopans, D.B., Feig, S.A.: The Canadian National Breast Screening Study: A Critical Review. Am. J. Roentgenol. 161, 755–760 (1993)
6. Caro, J.J., O'Brien, J.A., Hartz, S.C.: Canadian National Breast Screening Study. CMAJ. 148(6), 876–877; author reply 880–883 (1993)
7. Basinski, A.S.: The Canadian National Breast Screening Study: Opportunity for a Rethink. CMAJ. 147, 1431–1434 (1992)
8. Rajapakshe, R.: Prospective Analysis of Quality Control Data from the Screening Mammography Program of British Columbia (SMPBC), 500 (2007)
9. Trends in Mammography Dose and Image Quality 1974-2005,
   `http://www.fda.gov/RadiationEmittingProducts/MammographyQual`
   `ityStandardsActandProgram/FacilityScorecard/ucm113352.htm`
10. Henderson, T.O., Amsterdam, A., Bhatia, S., Hudson, M.M., Meadows, A.T., Neglia, J.P., Diller, L.R., Constine, L.S.: Systematic Review: Surveillance for Breast Cancer in Women Treated with Chest Radiation for Childhood, Adolescent, Or Young Adult Cancer. Ann. Intern. Med. 152, 444,455, W144–W154 (2010)
11. Conway, B.J., Suleiman, O.H., Rueter, F.G., Antonsen, R.G., Slayton, R.J.: National Survey of Mammographic Facilities in 1985, 1988, and 1992. Radiology 191, 323–330 (1994)
12. Mammography Quality Standards Act Regulations,
    `http://www.fda.gov/radiationemittingproducts/mammographyqual`
    `itystandardsactandprogram/regulations/ucm110906.htm`

13. Radiation Protection and Quality Standards in Mammography - Safety Procedures for the Installation, use and Control of Mammographic X-Ray Equipment: Safety Code 36, http://www.hc-sc.gc.ca/ewh-semt/pubs/radiation/safety-code_36-securite/index-eng.php#app3

14. Mojarad, S., Venturini, B., Fulgenzi, P., Papaleo, R., Brisigotti, M., Monti, F., Canuti, D., Ravaioli, A.: Prediction of Nodal Metastasis and Prognosis of Breast Cancer by ANN-Based Assessment of Tumour Size and p53, Ki-67 and Steroid Receptor Expression. Anti Cancer Res. 33, 3925–3933 (2013)

15. Soerjomataram, I., Louwman, M.W., Ribot, J.G., Roukema, J.A., Coebergh, J.W.: An Over view of Prognostic Factors for Long-Term Survivors of Breast Cancer. Breast Cancer Res. Treat. 107, 309–330 (2008)

Power Spectrum Analysis of an Anthropomorphic Breast Phantom Compared to Patient Data in 2D Digital Mammography and Breast Tomosynthesis

Lesley Cockmartin[1,*], Predrag R. Bakic[2], Hilde Bosmans[1], Andrew D.A. Maidment[2], Hunter Gall[3], Moustafa Zerhouni[3], and Nicholas W. Marshall[1]

[1] KU Leuven, Department of Imaging and Pathology, Division of Medical Physics and Quality Assessment, Herestraat 49, 3000 Leuven, Belgium
[2] University of Pennsylvania, Department of Radiology, 1 Silverstein Building HUP, 3400 Spruce Street, Philadelphia, PA 19104-4206
[3] Computerized Imaging Reference Systems (CIRS), Inc., 2428 Almeda Ave, Suite 316 Norfolk, Virginia 23513 USA
{Lesley.Cockmartin,Hilde.Bosmans,Nicholas.Marshall}@uzleuven.be,
{Predrag.Bakic,Andrew.Maidment}@uphs.upenn.edu,
{hgall,zerhounim}@cirsinc.com

Abstract. Digital breast tomosynthesis (DBT) images of a novel anthropomorphic breast phantom (UPenn phantom) acquired on two breast tomosynthesis systems were analyzed in terms of their power spectra (PS). The β and κ power law coefficients were estimated from 2D planar, tomosynthesis projection images and reconstructed planes. These data were compared to the PS characteristics as retrieved from a group of patient data. Power spectra of the UPenn phantom images were very similar to the patient data, with power law parameters in the range of values found in patients. Power law exponents were 2.99 and 3.45 for 2D, 2.87 and 2.75 for DBT projections and, 1.92 and 3.10 for DBT reconstructions for the Siemens and Hologic system respectively. The agreement was better than with other (non-anthropomorphic) 3D structured phantoms, making this phantom a good candidate test object for DBT performance testing.

Keywords: digital breast tomosynthesis, digital mammography, phantom, breast structure, power spectrum analysis.

1 Introduction

Digital breast tomosynthesis (DBT) acquires a series of projections of the breast from which a stack of slices is reconstructed. DBT should improve the detection and characterization of breast lesions based on two main features: (1) lesions show up in one or a few planes, providing depth information; (2) the tissue superposition from breast structures at a distance from the plane of interest is reduced, improving the detectability and

---

[*] Corresponding author.

H. Fujita, T. Hara, and C. Muramatsu (Eds.): IWDM 2014, LNCS 8539, pp. 423–429, 2014.
© Springer International Publishing Switzerland 2014

delineation of the lesions. In order to compare existing breast imaging modalities to DBT, these aspects have to be taken into consideration. Proper performance testing should define a task and an associated figure of merit. In the case of comparative studies between 2D mammography and DBT, the detection of a 3D lesion in a structured background would be a good candidate performance test.

Most existing anthropomorphic test objects, developed for projection mammography, have structures in a relatively thin 3D slab. There is therefore a need for another type of phantom, preferably a 3D anthropomorphic test object. This study focuses on a newly designed breast phantom (UPenn phantom, CIRS Inc., VA, USA), which is based on a previously developed anthropomorphic software phantom [1, 2]. The UPenn phantom had been developed for the use in preclinical and clinical assessment of image quality in 2D and 3D breast imaging systems. Whereas the anatomy of the breast has been mimicked as closely as possible, it remained to be determined how this structured phantom would compare to real patient data. In this paper, planar 2D and DBT images of this phantom, acquired on two different DBT systems, were evaluated in terms of power spectrum analysis. We calculated power spectra and power law coefficients of the newly designed phantom, acquired at different dose levels in 2D and DBT mode. Then we compared the resulting power spectra to previously published power spectra of a group of patients and additionally also to the power spectra of three other phantoms developed for DBT [3]. Finally, mean glandular doses (MGD) of the phantom were compared to patient doses.

2   Methods and Materials

2.1   Anthropomorphic Phantom

The design of the physical UPenn phantom (CIRS Inc., VA, USA) was based on the previously developed anthropomorphic software UPenn phantom which contains realistically arranged anatomical structures, including skin, adipose tissue compartments, Cooper's ligaments and regions of dense fibro-glandular tissue [1, 2]. By simulating a realistic arrangement of breast tissue structures, the phantom provides an anatomically correct complex tissue background, designed for consistent validation of various breast imaging modalities. The phantom consists of precisely distributed breast equivalent materials that mimic the realistic arrangement of tissue structures, thus demonstrating in projection images how underlying targets can be masked by overlapping normal tissue structures. The complete phantom simulates a 450 ml breast with compressed thickness of 5 cm and volumetric breast density of 17% (excluding the skin). The accompanying software phantom provides detailed ground truth of the anatomy simulation, allowing for direct quantitative assessment of measurements.

2.2   Phantom Acquisitions and Patient Dataset

Patient datasets together with their power spectrum and power law parameter calculations were previously described in literature [3]. Patients had been imaged on a Siemens Inspiration (Siemens, Erlangen, Germany) and a Hologic Selenia Dimensions system (Hologic, MA, USA) using the routine DBT settings. In total 50 lesion-free patient cases with 80 mammograms and 80 DBT image series were selected for the Siemens dataset and 26 patient cases including 48 mammograms and 48 DBT series for the Hologic system. Given that our hospital mainly performs DBT for further investigation of BIRADS 3, 4, or 5 cases, the majority of the lesion-free breasts contained dense fibroglandular structures.

The Siemens system acquires 25 projections covering an angle of 50 degrees and uses a W anode and Rh filter of 50 μm thick for both 2D and DBT acquisitions. The Hologic system is equipped with a W anode and Rh or Ag filter for 2D image acquisitions while for DBT Al filtration with a thickness of 700μm is used. The unit acquires 15 projections over a 15 degree angular range. Both systems are using a version of filtered back projection for the reconstruction of DBT projection images and neither system uses an anti-scatter grid in DBT mode.

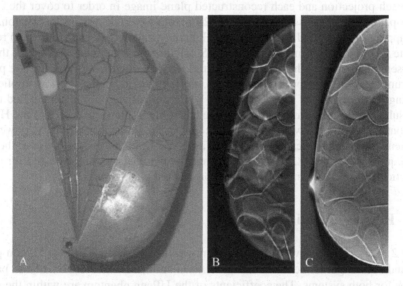

Fig. 1. Photograph of the UPenn phantom (A) and reconstructed DBT planes (B, C) acquired on the Hologic and Siemens system respectively

Table 1. Image exposure settings acquired under AEC control for the UPenn phantom, together with linearized mean PVs of the region used for the power spectrum analysis in 2D and DBT projection images. For DBT, the given tube load is the total tube load for the complete DBT acquisition.

System	Modality	Anode/filter	Tube voltage (kV)	Tube load (mAs)	$PV_{linearized}$ (~μGy)
Siemens	2D	W/Rh	29	69	70
	DBT	W/Rh	29	158	12
Hologic	2D	W/Rh	29	108	100
	DBT	W/Al	31	55	17

The UPenn phantom was imaged on a Siemens Inspiration and a Hologic Selenia Dimensions tomosynthesis system in 2D and DBT mode under automatic exposure control (AEC) (Figure 1). Automatically selected exposure settings for both modalities are tabulated in Table 1. Afterwards, a dose series was acquired by decreasing and increasing the automatically selected tube load (mAs) by 25% and 50% for both modalities.

2.3   Power Spectrum Analysis

Prior to the PS calculation, projection images were linearized using the detector response curve. Since pixel values in the reconstructed planes are largely independent of the exposure used to acquire DBT images, linearization was not possible for reconstructed images. A squared region adapted to the size of the phantom, was extracted from each projection and each reconstructed plane image in order to cover the center of the phantom. Records of size 128 × 128 pixels were taken from this region, half overlapping in both x and y directions. A Hanning window was applied to each record and the records were then input to a 2D PS calculation. The radial average of the 2D PS ensemble, including the 0° and 90° spatial frequency axes, was used for the power spectrum analysis. For projection images, normalization of the PS was applied by dividing by the square of the mean signal, while normalization was not applied to the PS results for the reconstructed planes. The changing in-plane pixel size of the Hologic reconstructed images was taken into account in the PS analysis. Finally, power law exponents and magnitudes, β and κ, were assessed from power law fits over the spatial frequency range of 0.2–0.7 mm^{-1}. Power law parameters were averaged for all 15 projection images and similarly for all reconstructed planes.

3   Results and Discussion

Table 2 gives an overview of the β and κ power law coefficients of the UPenn phantom and the range of these coefficients (mean, min, max and stdev) of the patient images for both systems. The coefficients of the UPenn phantom are within the range of those of the patients, confirming that the phantom structure consists of a similar texture as in patients. Additionally, figure 2 illustrates the PS curves of the phantom images, acquired at different dose levels and plotted against the average patient PS curve. Figure 2a shows the comparison for 2D mammographic images of the Hologic system and figure 2b for the central ~0° DBT projection images of Siemens. These graphs show that the change in dose did not influence the slope and the magnitude of the PS curve (β and κ) in the low frequency region with coefficients of variation (COV) ranging from 1% to 6% in 2D and DBT projections. This indicates that there is no influence of quantum noise within the power law region and that the PS in this region is dominated by the phantom structure. At higher frequencies, however, the quantum x-ray noise dominates and the PS curves are decreasing with increasing dose as the PS data are normalized for the signal at the detector. Figure 2 also shows the close agreement between phantom and patient PS curves, confirming the earlier agreement in power law coefficients.

Table 2. Power law exponents (β) and magnitudes (κ) for 2D, DBT projections and DBT reconstructed planes of the UPenn phantom, together with the data obtained from patient images

		2D		DBT projections		DBT reconstructed planes	
		β	κ (mm²)	β	κ (mm²)	β	κ (mm²)
Siemens							
Phantom		2.99	3.21E-05	2.87	1.54E-05	1.92	1.57E+02
Patients	Mean	3.37	1.55E-05	2.92	9.02E-06	2.31	3.49E+01
	Min	2.63	5.44E-06	2.09	5.65E-06	1.39	6.39E+00
	Max	3.94	3.47E-05	3.45	1.60E-05	3.07	2.71E+02
	Stdev	0.29	5.97E-06	0.34	1.90E-06	0.38	4.77E+01
Hologic							
Phantom		3.45	2.22E-05	2.75	1.16E-05	3.10	2.23E+01
Patients	Mean	3.57	1.60E-05	2.94	4.92E-06	3.61	3.12E+01
	Min	2.81	3.28E-06	2.36	1.81E-06	2.49	1.40E+00
	Max	4.06	3.29E-05	3.71	9.55E-06	4.59	1.81E+02
	Stdev	0.26	5.91E-06	0.25	1.99E-06	0.47	3.19E+01

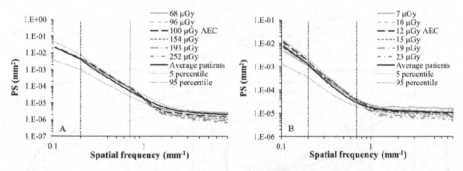

Fig. 2. Power spectrum curves of the UPenn phantom acquired at different dose levels and plotted together with the average, 5th and 95th percentile of the patient PS data for 2D mammograms of the Hologic system (A) and central DBT projection images of the Siemens system (B). The dashed vertical lines define the frequency region of the power law fit.

Next, the UPenn phantom was compared against three other structured phantoms, developed for DBT, namely the BR3D phantom (CIRS Ltd., VA, USA), the Voxmam phantom (Leeds Test Objects, UK) and the spheres in water phantom. A detailed description of these phantoms can be found in Cockmartin et al. [3]. The PS curve of the UPenn phantom falls within the patient PS range for both systems and both 2D and DBT images and therefore performs better than the other three structured phantoms. The PS curve of the spheres in water phantom falls within the patient range only for 2D and DBT projections of the Siemens system. The power spectrum magnitude of the Voxmam phantom structure appears to be overall high. The BR3D CIRS phantom follows the patient curves closely in terms of power spectrum magnitude but previously reported β coefficients are generally slightly lower than the ones observed in patients [3]. Thus, the PS of the newly designed UPenn phantom has the best match to the PS of the patient data and, therefore, validates its anthropomorphic character.

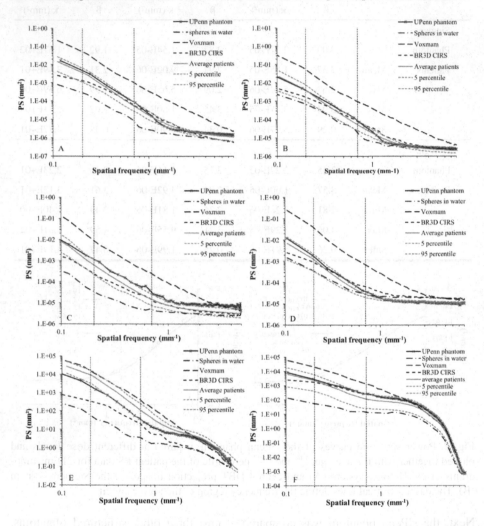

Fig. 3. Power spectrum curves of the UPenn phantom compared to three other structured phantoms and patients for the Hologic system (left) and the Siemens system (right) for 2D images (A) and (B), central DBT projections (C) and (D), and central reconstructed planes (E) and (F).

Finally, the mean glandular dose (MGD) was calculated for the UPenn phantom exposures under AEC for 2D and DBT, and the values were plotted against previously assessed patient doses [3]. For Hologic, the MGD is 1.21 mGy and 1.38 mGy while for Siemens, it is 0.74 mGy and 1.70 mGy for 2D and DBT respectively. The phantom doses are within the patient dose range and below the achievable dose level set up for 2D mammography. However, 2D and DBT phantom doses fall within the lower segment of the patient dose range for Siemens. For Hologic, only a small difference in dose for 2D and DBT phantom exposures is found.

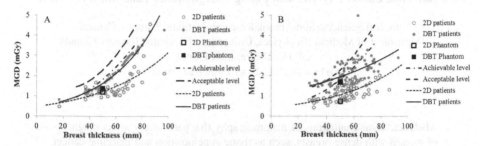

Fig. 4. Mean glandular doses for 2D and DBT phantom and patient images for Hologic (A) and Siemens (B)

A limitation of this study is that only a limited amount of patient data are included in our patient dataset. The launch of a general phantom validation procedure should start from a database that is representative for a general screening population. Finally, given the large technical differences between DBT systems, a general conclusion is only possible after tests on other DBT systems are completed.

4   Conclusions

In conclusion, this study tested the anthropomorphic structure of the newly designed UPenn phantom against patient breast structure for 2D and DBT imaging in terms of power spectra and power law coefficients. The phantom structure was found to be a good candidate for DBT performance testing with dose properties similar to patient doses. In future, simulated lesions or lesion-like objects will be inserted in the phantom, allowing clinically relevant detection tasks.

References

1. Pokrajac, D.D., Maidment, A.D.A., Bakic, P.R.: Optimized generation of high resolution breast anthropomorphic software phantoms. Med. Phys. 39(4), 2290–2302 (2012)
2. Brunner, C.C., Acciavatti, R.J., Bakic, P.R., Maidment, A.D.A., Williams, M.B., Kaczmarek, R., Chakrabarti, K.: Evaluation of various mammography phantoms for image quality assessment in digital breast tomosynthesis. In: Maidment, A.D.A., Bakic, P.R., Gavenonis, S. (eds.) IWDM 2012. LNCS, vol. 7361, pp. 284–291. Springer, Heidelberg (2012)
3. Cockmartin, L., Bosmans, H., Marshall, N.W.: Comparative power law analysis of structured breast phantom and patient images in digital mammography and breast tomosynthesis. Med. Phys. 40(8), 0189201–01892017 (2013)

Contrast-Enhanced Digital Mammography Image Quality Evaluation in the Clinic

Melissa L. Hill[1,2,*], Aili K. Bloomquist[1], Sam Z. Shen[1], James G. Mainprize[1], Ann-Katherine Carton[3], Sylvie Saab-Puong[3], Serge Muller[3], and Martin J. Yaffe[1,2]

[1] Physical Sciences, Sunnybrook Research Institute, Toronto, Canada
[2] Department of Medical Biophysics, University of Toronto, Toronto, Canada
[3] GE Healthcare, Buc, France
melissa.hill.sri@gmail.com

Abstract. Some limitations of mammography that particularly affect diagnosis of women with dense breasts, such as tissue superposition and marginal cancer image contrast, can be overcome with the use of contrast-enhanced digital mammography (CEDM). CEDM uses iodinated contrast agents to increase attenuation in areas exhibiting hyper-vascularization, potentially due to tumour angiogenesis, and image subtraction to cancel normal tissue signal. Here, we propose a method for objective task-based image quality evaluation of CEDM that can be routinely carried out in the clinic. A phantom was designed with features that allow for practical measurements of MTF, NPS, and iodine contrast that were used to estimate a CEDM detectability index for a given imaging task. We present results from several months of weekly testing of a commercial dual-energy CEDM system. From these data, we demonstrate measurement sensitivity to variations from standard acquisition conditions, suggesting the potential to identify system failure modes using this approach.

Keywords: CEDM dual-energy mammography iodine detectability phantom.

1   Introduction

Contrast-enhanced digital mammography (CEDM) is a technique that uses intravenous administration of a contrast agent to identify breast cancer on the basis of iodine signal enhancement from tumour angiogenesis [1–3]. CEDM potentially offers tissue functional information and image subtraction largely eliminates the tissue superposition that can limit mammography performance. Commercial systems for CEDM were introduced relatively recently and are generally being used in a diagnostic setting. It is important to monitor these systems to ensure consistent, high performance.

Because CEDM systems are extensions of digital mammography (DM), many of the image quality elements are likely to be in common with those of DM, and are monitored through quality control procedures already in place. These include tests of x-ray beam quality, radiation dose, beam collimation, detector sensitivity, and system

---

* Corresponding author.

H. Fujita, T. Hara, and C. Muramatsu (Eds.): IWDM 2014, LNCS 8539, pp. 430–437, 2014.

resolution [4, 5]. However, compared to mammography where the detection task primarily consists of the identification of calcifications and suspicious soft tissue masses, in CEDM iodine enhancement detectability is of main importance. Iodine detection can place different demands on the imaging system, and requires some adjustment to the conventional mammographic technique. For example, greater x-ray beam energies and specialized image processing are used [2, 3].

Model observers have been proposed as an efficient and objective means to predict human performance for mammography tasks of interest [6]. In this work we propose CEDM task-based performance evaluation that can be efficiently implemented in the clinic for routine quality assurance testing using a single phantom image.

2   Methods

2.1   Detectability Index

One model observer that accounts for the contrast sensitivity of the human eye is the nonprewhitening observer with eye filter (NPWE) [7]. The NPWE detectability index, d'_{NPWE}, was calculated for dual-energy (DE) CEDM (no internal noise) as:

$$d'^2_{\mathrm{NPWE}} = \frac{\left[\iint MTF^2(f_x, f_y) W^2_{\mathrm{task}}(f_x, f_y) E^2(f_x, f_y) df_x df_y \right]^2}{\iint NPS^2(f_x, f_y) MTF^2(f_x, f_y) W^2_{\mathrm{task}}(f_x, f_y) E^4(f_x, f_y) df_x df_y}, \tag{1}$$

where MTF is the system modulation transfer function, NPS is the noise power spectrum, W_{task} is the product of a task function and the object-to-background contrast, C_{task}, and E is an eye filter. The task function is written as the Fourier transform of the difference between two hypotheses, in this case between signal present (hyp_1) and signal absent (hyp_2) to describe a detection task [8]:

$$W_{\mathrm{task}}(f_x, f_y) = C_{\mathrm{task}} |\mathcal{F}\{hyp_1 - hyp_2\}|. \tag{2}$$

The applied eye filter has the form [7]:

$$E(f) = f^n \exp(-cf^2), \tag{3}$$

where f denotes the radial spatial frequency, and n and c are scalar factors that can vary with the viewing conditions and task. Values of $n = 1.3$ and $c = 3$, were used here that are consistent with common viewing conditions (50 cm distance) and have been shown to give reasonable agreement with human observers [7, 9].

In DE CEDM, a low-energy (LE) mammogram is acquired at x-ray energies below the K-edge of iodine and a high-energy (HE) image is acquired at energies predominantly above the K-edge. Richard and Siewerdsen demonstrated that when LE and HE image MTFs differ, the effective resolution in a DE image decomposed by weighted log-subtraction will be dependent on the object composition and weighting factor [10]. This situation can arise for a CsI-based detector under CEDM imaging conditions [11], where the effective DE image MTF can be described as [10]:

$$MTF_{DE}(f_x, f_y, w_B) = MTF_{LE}(f_x, f_y) \left| \frac{H_{HE}(f_x, f_y) - w_B k_{rel}}{1 - w_B k_{rel}} \right|, \tag{4}$$

where H_{HE} is the ratio of the MTFs for the HE and LE imaging, MTF_{HE}/MTF_{LE}, and k_{rel} is the ratio of the LE-to-HE signal(task)-to-background differences.

2.2   Phantom Design

A 22×20 cm^2, 4 cm thick poly(methyl methacrylate) (PMMA) phantom body was machined to mimic clinical imaging conditions to allow for system testing under automatic exposure control (AEC) operation. A 12.5 μm thick, 5×5 cm^2 tin MTF tool was placed on the PMMA to represent a 10 mg/cm^2 iodine detection task (higher than clinically expected, but practical for manufacture) against a uniform background.

Two contrast-detail regions with 1 cm thick iodinated-epoxy resin discs were embedded for contrast measurement [12]. Disc diameters of 3, 5 and 10 mm represent clinically relevant lesion sizes with iodine areal densities of 0.2, 0.6 and 1.0 mg/cm^2 [1]. One insert was embedded under uniform PMMA, and the other under a textured insert. The textured structure was fabricated by casting epoxy (no iodine) in a mold designed from a clinical mammogram region. These inserts were placed at the phantom periphery, leaving a uniform 6×6 cm^2 central region for NPS measurement. The proposed CEDM phantom is shown in Fig. 1, and is used at our institution for weekly physics testing of a commercial system (Senobright® and Senographe® Essential, GE Healthcare, Chalfont St. Giles, UK).

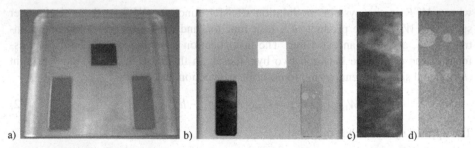

Fig. 1. CEDM phantom; (a) photograph; (b) HE image (Mo/Cu, 45 kV); (c) HE image texture insert; and (d) DE decomposed image of (c) and the LE image (not shown), revealing discs with 1.0, 0.6 and 0.2 mg/cm^2 iodine areal densities from top to bottom, at diameters of 10, 5, and 3 mm from left to right

2.3   Measurement Repeatability

Reference detectability values were established by imaging the phantom 10 times at 2 min intervals using an AEC-selected technique, moving the phantom slightly between exposures. The LE AEC technique used a Mo anode and Rh filter, 28 kV and 67 mAs, while a Mo anode, Cu filter and 45 kV, 110 mAs were used for the HE images. All DE image decomposition was performed using an algorithm integrated in the commercial imaging system [13].

The system MTF, NPS and contrast from the largest disc at each iodine areal density were measured from DE decomposed images and used to calculate d'_{NPWE} for disc detection. The task function was defined analytically as the 2D Fourier Transform of a disc. The system MTF was measured using the oversampled edge technique, sampling all four edges on the Sn MTF tool [14]. The 2D MTF was estimated using the MTF measurements in the x- and y-directions and calculating the 2D MTF radially. This is an approximation to the true 2D MTF, which likely has non-rotationally symmetric components, for example, due to rectangular detector elements and an anti-scatter grid. The 2D NPS was measured using a uniform phantom region, 512 pixels on a side [8]. The signal difference (termed 'contrast', C_{task}, in this work) between the average image intensity in a circular region within the largest iodinated disc, and the average of 6 regions surrounding the disc in the adjacent phantom background was measured to scale the task function.

2.4   Sensitivity

The tube potential (kV) and current and exposure time (mAs) for LE and HE images were each varied from the AEC-selected parameters to test detectability index sensitivity to the imaging technique in the combinations listed in Table 1.

Table 1. Technique factors used for CEDM disc detectablity sensitivity tests

Test #	LE image		HE image		Test #	LE image		HE image	
	kV	mAs	kV	mAs		kV	mAs	kV	mAs
1	26		45		7		32		110
2	30		45		8		63		56
3	28	63	43	110	9	28	32	45	56
4	28	63	47	110	10	28	90	45	110
5	25		42		11		63		160
6	31		49		12		90		160

3   Results

Fig. 2 shows the average of parameters used to calculate the reference d'_{NPWE}. The DE system MTF, the contrast between a 1 cm diameter disc and background, and the NPS normalized by the mean ROI intensity squared (NNPS) are shown in plots (a) through (c), respectively.

In Fig. 3(a) the NNPS, and C_{task} in 3(b), for cases 3 and 5 from Table 1, with lowered tube potentials than those selected by the AEC, are compared to the average from the 10 reference repeated AEC-acquired images. The images in Fig. 3(c) to (e) illustrate the disc appearance for each case and the corresponding change in the values of d'_{NPWE}. Example DE decomposed disc images are displayed at 100 ADU window width and a constant level relative to the image background signal.

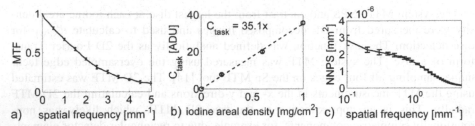

a)   spatial frequency [mm⁻¹]   b) iodine areal density [mg/cm²] c)   spatial frequency [mm⁻¹]

Fig. 2. Experimental decomposed DE image average of: (a) MTF; (b) disc contrast (C_{task}) vs iodine areal density; and (c) NNPS, for 10 AEC image acquisitions (LE: Mo/Rh, 28 kV, 67 mAs; HE: Mo/Cu, 45 kV, 110 mAs). Selected points are shown with error bars in (a)-(c) represent the standard deviation.

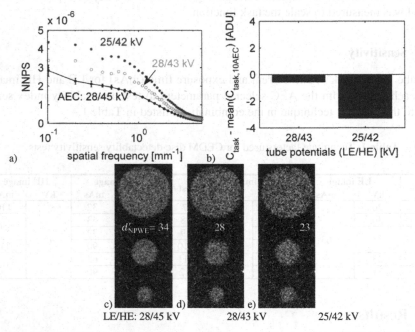

Fig. 3. (a) NNPS of DE decomposed images with LE and HE image kV of 25/42 kV (∗), 28/43 kV (○), and reference AEC kV (28/45, ●), respectively. (b) Difference between contrast in DE images with varied kV and the $C_{task,10AEC}$ acquired at the reference settings.. DE images and d'_{NPWE} for 1cm, 1 mg/cm² iodine disc detection acquired using (c) AEC, 28/45 kV; (d) 28/43 kV; and (e) 25/42 kV.

A reference d'_{NPWE} value, d'_{ref}, was established using the AEC-selected imaging technique, and making 10 repeated phantom images in a single session on a commercial CEDM system. In Fig. 4, the differences between individual d'_{NPWE} values estimated from DE decomposed images of 1) 10 successive reference acquisitions, and 2) 12 instances of weekly phantom imaging over a 3 month period, and d'_{ref} are shown for 1 cm, 1 mg/cm² iodine disc detection. Cases with non-AEC techniques (Table 1) are displayed on the same plot when the differences were more than 3 standard deviations from d'_{ref}.

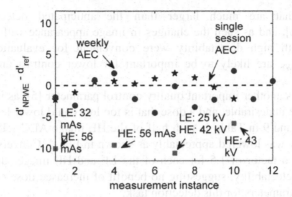

Fig. 4. Difference between individual and average reference d'_{NPWE} (single session, d'_{ref}) for 1 cm diameter, 1 mg/cm^2 iodine discs in DE decomposed images acquired using the AEC (LE: Mo/Rh, 28 kV, 67 mAs; HE: Mo/Cu, 45 kV, 110 mAs), in one session (★), at weekly intervals (●), and acquired with the given technique factor (■) varied from the AEC as in Table 1

4   Discussion

A single DE decomposed phantom image was used to estimate disc detectability in CEDM for routine quality control testing. This work is based on the underlying assumption that the NPWE observer can be predictive of human observer performance. While this has been shown to be a reasonable approximation in conventional mammography[15] and DE chest radiography [9], it remains to be tested in CEDM. Nonetheless, relative values of d'_{NPWE} are expected to be useful to monitor CEDM imaging performance, and changes from a reference detectability value were studied.

The standard deviation in d'_{ref} was about 1.4, and represents the expected variation of detectability for a single imaging session for this system. However, some drift in the system parameters from day-to-day is anticipated, and can be tolerable, such as from variations in the number of image acquisitions made prior to system testing, affecting lag and ghosting, and temperatures of the detector and anode at the time of imaging. Indeed, these day-to-day variations, as monitored over a 3 month period, were observed to result in a greater spread in the differences between d'_{ref}, and the individual measurements than imaging on a single day, as shown in Fig. 4. The d'_{NPWE} weekly estimates fell within a range of ± three standard deviations of d'_{ref}. As such, we set this range as a threshold, beyond which changes in detectability may indicate a degradation of system performance.

Although it is expected to be a relatively rare failure mode [5], kV accuracy is important in CEDM to ensure good iodine contrast. Two cases, at lines 3 and 5 in Table 1, where the HE image kV was too low, resulted in relatively large decreases in disc detectability as indicated in Fig. 4. The reasons for this drop in detectability are explored in Fig. 3(a) and (b), where it is revealed that a combination of increased NNPS and decreased contrast contribute to the lower detectability. Increased noise is visible in the phantom images by a comparison of Fig. 3(c) to (d) or to (e), and a marginally lower contrast is noticeable in Fig. 3(d) vs (c). Note that the discs displayed here have detectabilities that are much larger than the anticipated detection threshold ($d'_{NPWE}{\sim}1.9$) [16], and as such the changes in image appearance with kV are subtle. While discs with high detectability were convenient for evaluation here, small changes in d'_{NPWE} are likely to be important for lower contrast and smaller disc detection.

Tube output is another important quality control parameter [5], as increased radiation dose may be undesirable, and a dose that is too low could lower lesion detectability. For cases 8 and 9 in Table 1, with half of the HE image AEC-selected exposure, disc detectability was lowered appreciably as shown in Fig. 4. Conversely, increasing the exposure by a factor of 1.5 for each of the LE and HE images did not result in improved disc detectability, suggesting no benefit of increased dose compared to the AEC-selected parameters for this detection task.

It is interesting to note that in the tests of kV accuracy and tube output, detectability changes were largest when the HE technique was varied. When the LE image acquisition parameters were varied alone, the detectability did not change appreciably. For example, when the exposure was cut in half for the HE image (lines 8 and 9 of Table 1) the detectability decreased substantially, but not when the exposure was similarly decreased for the LE image alone (line 7 of Table 1). Thus, our results indicate that d'_{NPWE} for the given task is more sensitive to technique changes for the HE image than for the LE image. This suggests that monitoring these technique factor elements for DE CEDM system performance may be more important than for conventional mammography systems, which use acquisition techniques similar to LE images.

5   Conclusions

An efficient and robust method to estimate DE CEDM system performance from a single image was demonstrated. The parameters required to estimate d'_{NPWE} could be directly measured from a DE decomposed image of the CEDM phantom. Estimates of d'_{NPWE} from DE decomposed images concurrently test system image quality factors, the DE algorithm, and can likely be used to predict human diagnostic performance. We have shown that d'_{NPWE} is sensitive to CEDM image acquisition technique variations, which could be used to identify deleterious changes in system performance.

Future work will involve establishing thresholds for the detectability index by calibrating the index values to those identified in a human reader study. Also, as more clinical experience is gained with this modality, relevant diagnostic morphologies and tasks can be identified and added to the testing protocol for a more comprehensive CEDM performance evaluation.

Acknowledgements. This project is funded by the Ontario Institute for Cancer Research. The authors wish to acknowledge Jacqueline Craig, David Green, and Gordon Mawdsley for their contributions to the design and manufacture of the phantom.

References

1. Jong, R.A., Yaffe, M.J., Skarpathiotakis, M., Shumak, R.S., Danjoux, N.M., Gunesekara, A.: Contrast-enhanced digital mammography: Initial clinical experience. Radiology 228, 842–850 (2003)
2. Dromain, C., Balleyguier, C., Muller, S., Mathieu, M.-C., Rochard, F., Opolon, P., Sigal, R.: Evaluation of tumor angiogenesis of breast carcinoma using contrast-enhanced digital mammography. Am. J. Roentgenol. 187, W528–W537 (2006)
3. Lewin, J.M., Isaacs, P.K., Vance, V., Larke, F.J.: Dual-energy contrast-enhanced digital subtraction mammography: Feasibility. Radiology 229, 261–268 (2003)
4. Van Engen, R., Young, K.C., Bosmans, H.: The European protocol for the quality control of the physical and technical aspects of mammography screening. Part B: Digital mammography, pp. 1–114. European Comission, National Expert and Training Centre for Breast Cancer Screening, Nijmegen (2005)
5. Bloomquist, A.K., Yaffe, M.J., Pisano, E.D., Hendrick, R.E., Mawdsley, G.E., Bright, S., Shen, S.Z., Mahesh, M., Nickoloff, E.L., Fleischman, R.C., Williams, M.B., Maidment, A.D.A., Beideck, D.J., Och, J., Seibert, J.A., Fajardo, L.L., Boone, J.M., Kanal, K.: Quality control for digital mammography in the ACRIN DMIST trial: Part I. Med. Phys. 33, 719–736 (2006)
6. Monnin, P., Marshall, N.W., Bosmans, H., Bochud, F.O., Verdun, F.R.: Image quality assessment in digital mammography: Part II. NPWE as a validated alternative for contrast detail analysis. Phys. Med. Biol. 56, 4221–4238 (2011)
7. Burgess, A.E.: Statistically defined backgrounds: Performance of a modified nonprewhitening observer model. J. Opt. Soc. Am. A 11, 1237–1242 (1994)
8. Sharp, P., Metz, C.E., Wagner, R.F., Myers, K.J., Burgess, A.E.: ICRU Report No. 54 Medical imaging: The assessment of image quality. Bethesda, MD (1996)
9. Richard, S., Siewerdsen, J.H.: Comparison of model and human observer performance for detection and discrimination tasks using dual-energy x-ray images. Med. Phys. 35, 5043–5053 (2008)
10. Richard, S., Siewerdsen, J.H.: Cascaded systems analysis of noise reduction algorithms in dual-energy imaging. Med. Phys. 35, 586–601 (2008)
11. Rowlands, J.A., Ji, W.G., Zhao, W.: Effect of depth dependent modulation transfer function and K-fluorescence reabsorption on the detective quantum efficiency of indirect conversion flat panel x-ray imaging systems using CsI. In: Proc. SPIE, vol. 4320, pp. 257–267 (2001)
12. Hill, M.L., Mainprize, J.G., Mawdsley, G.E., Yaffe, M.J.: A solid iodinated phantom material for use in tomographic x-ray imaging. Med. Phys. 36, 4409–4420 (2009)
13. Puong, S., Bouchevreau, X., Patoureaux, F., Iordache, R., Muller, S.: Dual-energy contrast enhanced digital mammography using a new approach for breast tissue canceling. In: Proc. SPIE, vol. 6510, p. 65102H (2007)
14. Fujita, H., Tsai, D.Y., Itoh, T., Doi, K., Morishita, J., Ueda, K., Ohtsuka, A.: A simple method for determining the modulation transfer function in digital radiography. IEEE Trans. Med. Im. 11, 34–39 (1992)
15. Burgess, A.E., Jacobson, F.L., Judy, P.F.: Human observer detection experiments with mammograms and power-law noise. Med. Phys. 28, 419–437 (2001)
16. Beutel, J., Kundel, H.L., Metter, V.: Handbook of Medical Imaging. Physics and Psychophysics, vol. 1. SPIE Press (2000)

BREAST: A Novel Strategy to Improve the Detection of Breast Cancer

Patrick C. Brennan[1], Phuong Dung Trieu[1], Kriscia Tapia[1], John Ryan[2],
Claudia Mello-Thoms[1], and Warwick Lee[1,3]

[1] Faculty of Health Sciences, The University of Sydney, Australia
{patrick.brennan,phuong.trieu,kriscia.tapia,
claudia.mello-thoms}@sydney.edu.au
[2] Ziltron, Ireland
john.ryan@ziltron.com
[3] BreastScreen New South Wales, Cancer Institute, Australia
Warwick.LEE_ext@cancerinstitute.org.au

Abstract. Early diagnosis of breast cancer is highly dependent on quality breast imaging and precise image interpretation. The BREAST programme is an innovative strategy for reader performance self-evaluation in breast cancer detection. Using an online system, detailed feedback on reader/image interpretation is given instantly. Our strategy is currently focused on mammograms but has the potential to be available for a wide range of medical imaging modalities. BREAST also serves a solution to researchers requiring large observer numbers by facilitating the involvement of experts wherever they are located. In summary, BREAST improves the efficacy of mammographic cancer detection through a system of reader performance monitoring and enables research studies with a large amount of robust data.

Keywords: early diagnosis, mammograms, reading performance, reporting assessment.

1 Introduction

Breast cancer is one of the most common types of cancer diagnosed in women. The rate of females developing breast cancer in Australia is one in nine [1] and the risk of mortality is one in thirty seven [2]. Mammography is a fundamental screening method in breast cancer detection, and in Australia breast x-rays are performed on over 800,000 women each year. Nevertheless, approximately a third of cancers are not detected by radiologists when reading screening mammograms, although not all missed abnormalities were invisible on the images [3,4,5,6,7,8,9]. The success of screening programs depends on the accurate image interpretation of radiologists, implying that if reader efficacy is monitored and individual-specific errors highlighted, underperformance can be identified and addressed.

H. Fujita, T. Hara, and C. Muramatsu (Eds.): IWDM 2014, LNCS 8539, pp. 438–443, 2014.
© Springer International Publishing Switzerland 2014

Aiming to improve radiologist performance in breast cancer detection, a novel web-based solution known as Breast Screen Reader Assessment Strategy (BREAST) has been developed by the collaboration of experts in medical imaging at the University of Sydney, BreastScreen New South Wales and an information technology partner (Ziltron). BREAST has been implemented in Australia since 2011 with the financial support of the Australian Department of Health and Aging. The scheme has recently secured additional funding from the National Breast Cancer Foundation for further infrastructure development.

BREAST contains a comprehensive database of mammographic images and reading decisions of radiologists that are widely accessible to researchers interested in identifying reasons for errors in mammogram reporting and in creating innovative solutions to reduce error rates. In order to acquire the data, our strategy uses an evaluation tool from Ziltron (Ireland) which enables over 300 BreastScreen readers in Australia and New Zealand to access test sets at their workstations and provide instant feedback. Performance metrics such as specificity, sensitivity, location sensitivity, receiver operating characteristics (ROC) area under the curve (AUC) and Jacknife alternate free response operating characteristic (JAFROC) figure of merit (FOM) are presented promptly after readers have completed a single test set. Also our system enables participants to review their performance as their correct and incorrect decisions are scored on each image. Although participant identity information is not provided to authors, data distributions of reader performance levels are available for investigation.

As well as having clinical benefit, the system supports substantially the research activities of our group. With a large number of radiologists examining high quality image data bases, topics such as the impact of disease prevalence, characteristics of missed cancers, the importance of breast density on detection, the efficacy of novel computer-aided diagnostic programs and the relevance of reader test set methodologies compared to clinical audit are being investigated [10,11,12,13].

2   Methodology

2.1   Test Sets

Since being established in 2011, the BREAST has three high quality, clinically-relevant image test sets known as Hobart, Sydney and Darwin. Each set consists of 60 cases in two view (craniocaudal and mediolateral oblique) bilateral mammograms and each case is classified as normal or malignant. All images were acquired by digital technology and de-identified after being collected from BreastScreen New South Wales Digital Breast Image Library.

Cases were selected in order to be challenging to participants and thus offer both self-assessment as well as training value. Malignant cases were biopsy proven whilst negative cases were assessed by the consensus reading of at least two senior radiologists following the negative screen reports of two clinical radiologists.

2.2   Participants

Participants are Australia BreastScreen readers, who might be radiologists or other accredited medical practitioners. BREAST has recently been introduced as a quality assurance and training tool to New Zealand's BreastScreen Aotearoa. The demographic background of screen readers were collected via an on-line questionnaire including details on mammographic reading practice and the training interpretation courses that might have been undertaken.

2.3   Procedure

The BREAST program has been implemented as a quality assurance and training tool throughout BreastScreen Australia. Along with access details to Ziltron's online system, an external hard drive containing images in the test set was distributed to BreastScreen in each state to enable screen readers to investigate the images using the full resolution available through local Picture Archiving and Communication System (PACS) systems.

For each image in the test set, readers are asked to record whether the case is normal or abnormal and for each abnormal finding that would warrant further mammographic assessment, lesion localization is required (Fig. 1). The radiologists need to classify according to the Australian version of the Breast Imaging Reporting and Data (BIRADS) system's 5 point confidence rating system: 1-normal, 2-benign, 3-indeterminate, 4-probally malignant and 5-definitely malignant. Ratings of 3, 4 and 5 indicate a need for further assessment and constitute a positive result. Ratings of 1 and 2 indicate that no further assessment is required and a negative result. The participants are not informed of the overall number of cancers that are present in the test set.

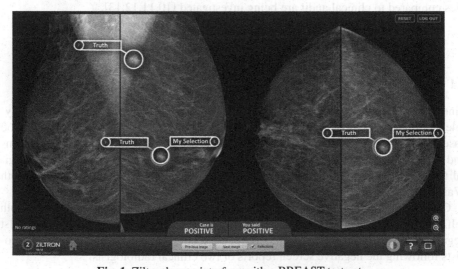

Fig. 1. Ziltron's user interface with a BREAST test-set

3   Results

After 3 years, the BREAST programme is broadly available and well accepted in all states across Australia and has been introduced to New Zealand in late 2013. From 2011 to 2013, over 300 readings have been performed by 180 screen readers, accounting for approximately 78% of BreastScreen readers. Australian Capital Territory is currently leading in program engagement where 100% of breast radiologists have completed at least one BREAST test set. South Australia and Tasmania have 89% and 83% participation respectively. Two thirds of radiologists in New South Wales have undertaken the test sets and in Victoria, 55% of readers have participated. As Queensland has recently implemented the program, the participation rate currently is lower than the national average, standing at 25%.

From the data generated, it is possible to produce useful regional and national performance distributions so that each reader's performance can be judged against these distribution values. Each reader receives a report with details on correct recall cases, the percentage of correct negative cases, percentage of correct lesions, ROC AUC and JAFROC FOM scores. The Clinical Director of each BreastScreen Service also receives a quarterly report of participants within their service. The report provides the information relating to the performance across all participating screen readers and the level of variation across BreastScreen Australia along with potential reference levels of good performance (25th, 50th, 75th percentiles) (Fig. 2). Individuals with poor performance can be encouraged to undertake another dedicated training set which is targeted at mammographic features responsible for individual-specific errors.

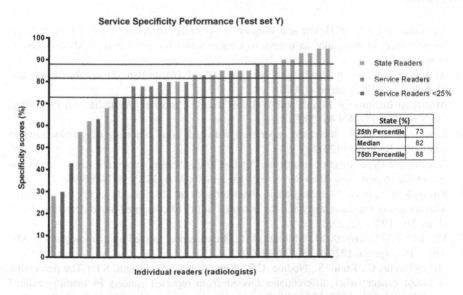

Fig. 2. Example of the data reported for participants and BreastScreen Services

According to the radiologists, BREAST has been playing an essential role in improving the readers' experience in breast cancer detection. In a recent survey, 96% of participants indicated that BREAST test sets have been important to their on-going professional development, and a further 86% of readers highlighted the value of this learning activity as an effective strategy for training them.

4   Conclusion

Over the last three years, the introduction of BREAST in Australia has been recognized as an important strategy by scientists, clinicians and BreastScreen managers. With the highly encouraging level of reader engagement, it is anticipated that our novel approach will assist the optimization of mammographic readings and increase the radiologists' ability to detect breast cancer. The data has served our research community well with a series of publications in the leading radiologic journals. We welcome collaborations to expand the use of the BREAST program.

Acknowledgements. BREAST project has been funded by Royal Australian and New Zealand College of Radiologists and the Department of Health and Ageing since 2011. Funds have recently been acquired for the next four years from the National Breast Cancer Foundation following an application in 2012 with support from our local and international collaborators.

References

1. Australian Institute of Health and Welfare & Australasian Association of Cancer Registries: Cancer in Australia: an overview. Cancer series no. 60, Cat no CAN 56. AIHW, Canberra (2010)
2. Australian Institute of Health and Welfare: ACIM (Australian Cancer Incidence and Mortality). AIHW, Canberra (2010)
3. Australian Institute of Health and Welfare. Breast Cancer in Australia: An Overview, Canberra. Cat no CAN 46 (2009)
4. Brennan, P.C., et al.: Increased experience with soft copy reporting may reduce expert specificity. Radiology (2011)
5. Government Department of Health and Ageing: BreastScreen Australia Evaluation: Evaluation Final Report. Australian Screening Monograph (2009) ISBN: 1-74186-968-4
6. Birdwell, R.L., et al.: Mammographic characteristics of 115 missed cancers later detected with screening mammography and the potential utility of computed-aided detection. Radiology 219, 192–202 (2011)
7. Martin, J.E., Moskowitz, M., Milbrath, J.R.: Breast cancer missed by mammography. AJR Am. J. Roentgenol. 132(5), 737–739 (1979)
8. Mello-Thoms, C., Dunn, S., Nodine, C.F., Kundel, H.L., Weinstein, S.P.: The perception of breast cancer: what differentiates missed from reported cancers in mammography? Acad. Radiol. 9(9), 1004–1012 (2002)
9. Patnick, J.: Annual review 2005: One vision – NHS Breast screening programme, Sheffield, England, Fulwood House (2005)

10. Rawashdeh, M.A., Bourne, R.M., Ryan, E.A., Lee, W.B., Pietrzyk, M.W., Reed, W.M., Borecky, N., Brennan, P.C.: Quantitative measures confirm the inverse relationship between lesion spiculation and detection of breast masses. Academic Radiol. (2013) (in press)
11. Soh, B.P., Lee, W.B., McEntee, M.F., Kench, P.L., Reed, W.M., Heard, R., Chakraborty, D.P., Brennan, P.C.: Test set data can reasonably describe actual clinical reporting in screening mammography. Radiology (2013) (in press)
12. Mousa, D.A., Brennan, P.C., Ryan, E., Lee, W.B., Pietrzyk, M.W., Reed, W.M., Alakhras, M.M., Li, Y., Mello-Thoms, C.R.: Effect of mammographic breast density on radiologists' visual search pattern. In: SPIE Proceedings (in press, 2014)
13. Soh, B.P., Lee, W.B., Mello-Thoms, C.R., Tapia, K., Ryan, R.T., Hung, W.T., Thompson, G.J., Heard, R., Brennan, P.C.: Does sensitivity measured from screening test-sets predict clinical performance?. In: SPIE Proceedings (in press, 2014)

A Regional Web-Based Automated Quality Control Platform

Stephen Smithbower, Rasika Rajapakshe, Janette Sam, Nancy Aldoff,
and Teresa Wight

BC Cancer Agency, British Columbia, Canada
{ssmithbower,rrajapak,jsam,naldoff2,twight}@bccancer.bc.ca
http://www.bccancer.bc.ca

Abstract. Quality control is a key factor in ensuring a high standard
of care in the field of mammography. We have found that abrupt ir-
regularities in image quality from mammography units can arise as the
result of factors ranging from vendor software upgrades, having software
parameters modified during unit maintenance, or even having detectors
replaced. We have developed both a simple weekly quality control test
performed on processed images that can quickly capture these changes in
image quality, as well as a centralized software platform that automates
our test across several mammography centers. Technologists acquire a
phantom exposure and upload it to our regional PACS network. The
images are then automatically downloaded, analysed, and the results
stored by the mammoQC software. These results are instantly available
to technologists via a web dashboard, where reports can be generated automatically. Our platform currently services over 25 locations in British
Columbia.

Keywords: mammography, quality control, qa, quality assurance,
mammo, web, online, dashboard, automated, image, processing.

1 Introduction

With the advent of digital mammography there have been many efforts to develop quality assurance tests, programs, and policies in order to ensure and
maintain the performance of the equipment in digital mammography systems
- one of the most demanding imaging modalities with the most stringent requirements. Great effort has been made to develop and recommend a uniform
set of quality assurance programs with tests designed to be the same across
multiple technologies, technical designs, and manufacturers. With the great improvements made in the technologies and technical designs utilized by modern
digital mammography systems, in addition to the advantages conferred by being digital, we propose a *"minimalist"* approach for a simple and easy "quality
monitoring" test that can be performed with ease by a technologist, in order
to monitor changes in quality for the acquisition components of a digital mammography system. Due to the complexity of the various components that can

H. Fujita, T. Hara, and C. Muramatsu (Eds.): IWDM 2014, LNCS 8539, pp. 444–451, 2014.
© Springer International Publishing Switzerland 2014

be changed within a digital system, information regarding such changes made, for example, by service personnel or by other colleagues, may not necessarily be communicated properly to the operators or quality assurance staff of an institution. Even if such information were communicated properly, it can sometimes be difficult to judge whether or not a full-blown assessment of the changes is necessary.

2 Design

2.1 Signal Difference to Noise Ratio

Signal difference to noise ratio (SDNR), also sometimes referred to as contrast to noise ratio, is considered to be the most critical image quality metric in acquisition if only a single IQ metric is to be monitored [1]. It is defined as:

$$SDNR = \frac{|Object\ Signal - Background\ Signal|}{\sigma(Background)} \tag{1}$$

For an imaging system with output linear to x-ray exposure the SDNR value will remain constant both before and after proper conversion to logarithmic space, which is the data space within which image processing algorithms typically operate.

SDNR is often measured with a relatively large object providing a sizable surface area within the image, and a background with similar surface area, so as to allow for an adequate assessment of the required signals and standard deviation for the SDNR calculation. The choice of thickness for the SDNR object should reflect the minimum subject contrast relevant to the imaging modality. Currently a 25mm in diameter circular disk made of PMMA with a thickness of 1mm has been proposed. The 1mm of PMMA represents roughly 5% of the subject contrast in a typical x-ray spectrum used for imaging 53mm of breast. Shown in Figure 1 is a photograph of the D-shaped phantom with the circular disk under compression and ready for exposure.

2.2 SDNR Tracking

Depending on the resolution vs. noise trade off strategy, the image processing algorithm applied to digital mammograms may change. This will impact the SDNR value calculated from the processed image, relative to the raw, unprocessed image; this can lead the SDNR value to lose its connection to the underlying physics of the image (keeping in mind that the image processing algorithm is often a black box). To ensure the quality of a black box is then to at least measure any change in its output. Our proposal is to calculate the SDNR value using the processed images, so as to include the effect of any applied image processing. This is a different approach than that which is employed by most other similar test proposals.

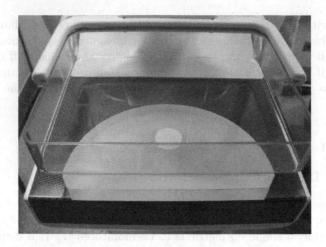

Fig. 1. Photograph of the D-shaped phantom (double-stacked) and a circular disk with a thickness of 1mm

We believe any measurable change to image quality should be reflected in both the SDNR values and the background signal level. The extent of this impact, such as the result of a reduction in resolution or increase in electronic noise, has not yet been fully quantified. However, by monitoring changes in both SDNR and background signal values, we should be able to determine any trends that may indicate whether or not an issue has arisen that has a meaningful impact on the images being produced. From practical experience, the quality assurance staff in our screening program were once made aware of an image processing software update that had not been communicated to them solely due to changes in monitored SDNR values.

2.3 Image Acquisition

Images of the D-shaped phantom with the circular disk should be acquired under the same exposure method used for typical imaging of 53mm of breast. For instance, if an automatic exposure control (AEC) mode is used for image acquisition, the same AEC mode should be used to acquire a diagnostic image of the 45mm thick D-shaped phantom. In such a case, the x-ray technique factors selected by the AEC should be tracked together with the SDNR values. These are critical pieces of information, and any significant change in their settings should warrant further attention. For example, in most cases the kVp and target/filter combination should remain the same for repeated phantom image acquisitions, and any change in the mAs value determined by the AEC represents a change in dose. In the event that the mAs values under the AEC remain unchanged, but the background signal level drops significantly, there is a likely indication of a reduction in the detector gain.

3   mQC Software

3.1   Image Processing

In order to take full advantage of the nature of a digital system, calculating SDNR values and tracking both SDNR and x-ray techniques should be fully automated. To do this, we have developed an algorithm that analyzes the D-shaped phantom image, detects the circular disk, selects an appropriate background ROI, and finally calculates the an SDNR value without any user intervention required. This algorithm has been developed in to a DICOM server that can be configured as a designated DICOM destination for the acquisition workstation, and has been named "mQC". This software can be installed on any Windows-based computer that has a network connection to the acquisition workstation. The attending technologist is only required to send the acquired phantom images to the mQC server, and the rest is taken care of automatically.

mQC automatically calculates SDNR values, and extracts all relevant x-ray technique factors available in the DICOM header of the phantom image. This information, along with acquisition date and time, is inserted in to a database organized by location, and the stations within each location (so that individual station results may be readily retrieved). As such, a single instance of mQC can track phantom images from multiple independent stations.

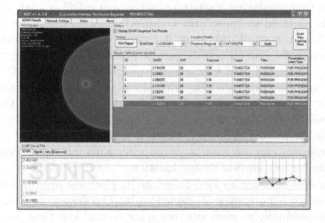

Fig. 2. Screen capture of the mQC software. The processed D-shaped phantom image is displayed in the upper left corner of the screen, along with the automatically detected ROIs used for the SDNR calculation. Each row in the table on the right represents the test results for individual phantom images, including x-ray factors as well as the calculated SDNR values. The chart at the bottom of the screen shows trends for the track data.

Figure 2 displays a screen capture of the mQC Server software. Currently mQC uses the mean value of the first 5 images to establish a baseline SDNR value (indicated in blue on the trend graph in figure 2). Subsequent SDNR values are then compared against this baseline, and plotted on the trend graph. Two yellow lines on the graph represent the $\pm$ 10% difference from baseline and act as warning margins. Two additional red lines represent the $\pm$ 15% margins and indicate actionable limits. The baseline may be adjusted by the station operator. In addition to SDNR values, both kVp and mAs values may also be plotted. A detailed report on the station using windowed data (phantom image results acquired within a specified time frame) can be generated for printing.

3.2 Web Application

A version of mQC that operates on a "cloud" infrastructure has also been developed for institutions that consist of many digital mammography units located at remote sites, such as the Screening Mammography Program of British Columbia, Canada. It utilizes an existing DICOM network infrastructure that enables the phantom images to be transferred from the aforementioned remote sites, to a central server. In the BC Screening Mammography Program many of the remote screening sites are operated by regional health authorities. Digital mammograms can be transferred through each authority via internal networks, and transferred province-wide through a provincial network (the "transfer grid"). In a setup such as this, rather than deploying a separate instance of mQC at each site, technologists are only required to "push" the acquired phantom images to the transfer grid directly from the acquisition unit. A custom watchdog application periodically polls the transfer grid for new diagnostic phantom images using the DICOM C-FIND query command, and forwards the images to a central mQC server instance. The results are processed like normal and stored in a database. The final SDNR results, x-ray technique factors, and a preview image of the phantom and the selected ROIs are then pushed to a secondary external database. This database feeds the mQC Dashboard, which is a web interface that our technologists and physicists can use from any computer with internet access to review QC test results for any station at any location.

The advantages of using a cloud-based mQC platform are obvious for institutions with many remote sites of operation. mQC software no longer needs to be deployed individually to each site, negating several logistical issues (such as obtaining a workstation to install mQC on, networking issues when connecting with acquisition workstations, user accounts, remote tech support, etc). Future software upgrades for bug fixes and feature enhancements can be applied immediately, with all connected sites receiving the benefit of the upgrade simultaneously, as opposed to slowly rolling out the update to individual sites. Collection and review of multiple sites is also made significantly easier and more efficient, as the reviewing agency has immediate access to the most recent test results via the web interface. Results no longer need to be collated at each respected site and forwarded to the reviewing agency at regular intervals.

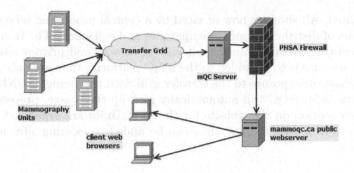

Fig. 3. mQC architectural diagram. Phantom images are pushed to the transfer grid and pulled down and processed by the mQC server. The results are then pushed out through the PHSA firewall to a public webserver which hosts the mQC dashboard, allowing the results to be reviewed online immediately.

3.3   DICOM Attribute Collection

Due to a number of incidents involving both detector changes and software upgrades in various units utilizing the platform, the detector description, id, calibration date, and current software version are tracked in addition to x-ray technique factors. We have found that a change in software or detector is behind the majority of test result discontinuities and it is helpful to be able to diagnose this immediately via the mQC dashboard.

Currently only a preview of the processed image is stored in the database, however in the future we may extend mQC to also store a copy of the raw pixel data that the test was performed on, in order to allow us to retroactively perform analyses. A large collection of such images is already being manually curated in order to perform regression testing when software patches are being developed.

4   Results

4.1   Deployment Procedure

In its original implementation, the mQC software was developed as a single stand-alone application that was installed on individual workstations at multiple mammography centres. However issues with administrative permissions on the workstations, firewall policies, and interference with retrieving the locally-collected test results made it clear that this approach would require a fair bit of labour to scale. The greatest difficulty came with attempting to upgrade the installed software, as the lack of a remote upgrade capability often required one of the researchers to travel to each site and perform the upgrade manually.

In response, the current centralized system was developed. While more complicated (now consisting of the PHSA Transfer Grid, Grid Watchdog, mQC Processing Server, and web dashboard) almost all of the aforementioned issues have been alleviated. All sites are now serviced by a central processing server, negating the issues of distributing software upgrades and collection. The transfer grid was a pre-existing network solution, alleviating firewall and privacy issues.

When a new site is to be added to the mQC platform, they are only required to push a phantom exposure to the transfer grid with the string "SDNR" in the patient name field. mQC will automatically pick up the image, process it, and create a new section on the website for the unit. Units are organized by their site location automatically. New units can be added to existing sites using the same process.

4.2   Issues

The most immediate issue with the current design relates to using the location and station identifiers stored in the DICOM header of each test image for categorization of results. Often, after maintenance is performed on a unit, one or both of these attributes has been modified. Because categorization of results utilizes a string comparison, this will result in misplacing the new results from the unit (usually by creating a new unit entry). Manual amalgamation of results is then required.

4.3   Performance

mQC has been servicing public digital mammography screening sites across the province of British Columbia for over 2 years. There are currently 27 sites and 34 units which have collected had 1594 test results analyzed. Some sites have multiple units, and these sites in particular have voiced a noticeable improvement in workflow (though we have not performed a rigorous study of this).

During its tenure mQC has identified several QA issues. In each of these cases either a detector change or a unit software upgrade was responsible. On more than one occasion routine unit maintenance by the vendor included a software upgrade which altered the processed image output, but QA staff were not made aware of the adjustments until after mQC detected the change and prompted an investigation.

5   Future Development

mQC provides an efficient platform for collecting, organizing, storing, and reviewing QA test data. We hope to extend the platform using a software plugin architecture, so that arbitrary tests may utilized the platform ad-hoc.

For example, the uniformity test is performed as a routine quality control check to ensure relatively even output of radiation across the field of view of the detector. We plan to implement automated versions of this test as specified by various vendors in order to determine which method is most effective in an automated system, alongside the existing SDNR implementation.

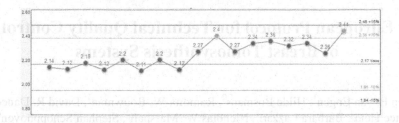

Fig. 4. A graph of consecutive results generated by the mQC dashboard for technologists. The jump in SDNR values starting in the center was due to a detector change in the unit, which was caught by mQC.

6   Conclusions

The "Double D" phantom with a circular disk, and its companion mQC software, is intended to serve as a simple and easy test suite to monitor changes in digital mammography systems that impact image quality. It is not intended as a comprehensive tool that will check or benchmark all aspects of digital image quality. Rather, it simply monitors several critical factors to ensure consistency in the operation of the digital system. Various reviews and calls to action can be automatically triggered when test results surpass the user-defined warning/error margins. Our platform provides an immediate feedback mechanism for major changes in image quality, whilst requiring a minimum of operator effort. The mQC software provides data analysis, data tracking and database management, charting, and automatic report generation, and we hope to extend the platform to include further QA tests.

Reference

1. Yaffe, M.J.: Digital Mammography. In: Beutel, J., Kundel, H.L., Van Metter, R.L. (eds.) Handbook of Medical Imaging. SPIE Press, Bellingham (2000)

A European Protocol for Technical Quality Control of Breast Tomosynthesis Systems

Ruben E. van Engen[1], Hilde Bosmans[2], Ramona W. Bouwman[1], David R. Dance[3],
Patrice Heid[4], Barbara Lazzari[5], Nicholas W. Marshall[2], Stephan Schopphoven[6],
Celia Strudley[3], Martin Thijssen[7], and Kenneth C. Young[3]

[1] National Expert and Training Centre for Breast Cancer Screening (LRCB), Nijmegen,
The Netherlands
[2] Department of Radiology, University Hospitals Leuven, Belgium
[3] National Coordinating Centre for the Physics of Mammography (NCCPM), Royal Surrey
County Hospital, Guildford, UK
[4] Arcades, Marseille, France
[5] General Hospital Pistoia, Italy
[6] Mammografie Screening Referenzzentrum Südwest, Marburg, Germany
[7] Rijnstate Ziekenhuis, Arnhem, The Netherlands
r.vanengen@lrcb.nl

Abstract. Quality control (QC) procedures for digital breast tomosynthesis (DBT) systems are a crucial part of the acceptance of a new modality. In contrast to the situation in the US, the European approach is to provide a device independent protocol with limiting values that should be applied to all systems. A European QC protocol that deals with this challenge is being developed and is currently work-in-progress. In this paper four specific QC tests for DBT, which have reached an (almost) final stage, are presented: reproducibility, system projection MTF, z-resolution and missed tissue at the top and bottom of the reconstructed volume. The proposed tests have been evaluated on several DBT systems. The encouraging results show that these tests will form an appropriate and necessary part of QC procedures for DBT.

Keywords: Quality control, tomosynthesis.

1   Introduction

Digital breast tomosynthesis (DBT) systems are currently available on the market and their use is being considered for breast cancer screening. Therefore guidance on quality control (QC) measurements for DBT systems is required. In contrast to the situation in the US, the European approach is to provide a device independent protocol with limiting values that should be applied to all systems. In Europe QC using this approach on full field digital mammography (FFDM) systems is performed according to the fourth edition of the European Guidelines for breast cancer screening and diagnosis [1] and its supplement [2]. These documents are the starting point in the development of a QC protocol for breast tomosynthesis systems [3]. The protocol remains

H. Fujita, T. Hara, and C. Muramatsu (Eds.): IWDM 2014, LNCS 8539, pp. 452–459, 2014.
© Springer International Publishing Switzerland 2014

work-in-progress. However dosimetry for DBT systems has already been established [4] and the design and implementation of some other tests have are close to being finalized. In this paper four newly developed QC tests are presented.

2   Methods

2.1   Reproducibility

DBT systems need to be sufficiently stable to provide high quality images and therefore the testing of reproducibility is a key aspect of QC procedures. The following reproducibility measurement is proposed: a 45 mm thick homogeneous polymethyl methacrylate (PMMA) phantom covering the whole image receptor is positioned on the bucky and 5 tomosynthesis images are acquired in the clinically used automatic exposure control (AEC) mode. The exposure factors and the angle of the projections are recorded from the DICOM header. From each exposure, the mean pixel value (MPV) and the standard deviation (SD), is recorded in the reference region of interest (ROI) of the first projection image. This reference ROI is defined as a square of 5x5 mm 6 cm from chest wall side and centered laterally in the image. From these ROIs the average pixel value and standard deviation (SD) are measured and the signal-to-noise ratio (SNR) calculated by dividing the pixel value by the SD. Projection images are low dose, therefore a higher precision might be obtained by summing the pixel values in the reference ROI for all projections and calculating SD over all projections as the square root of the summed variances to obtain the SNR over all projection images. For both methods the variance in SNR for the acquired DBT images is calculated.

2.2   System Projection MTF

In some DBT systems the X-ray tube moves during the exposure of a projection image. This implies that the image is blurred in the direction of movement. This QC test quantifies this blur by measuring the MTF in projection images.

For the determination of the amount of blurring it is important to use clinically relevant exposure factors. Therefore the exposure factors for a 45 mm thick homogeneous block of PMMA in fully automatic mode are used to measure system projection MTF. An aluminium attenuator of 2 mm thickness is positioned near the X-ray tube and the MTF test object is placed at the bucky at a slight angle to the columns and rows of the detector. An exposure in manual mode is made mimicking the exposure of the PMMA block. The MTF is calculated, as described in the 4th edition of the European Guidelines [1] for the zero degree projection image. The system projection MTFs for two DBT systems have been measured: one with step-and-shoot approach and one with continuous movement of the X-ray tube.

2.3   z-Resolution

The z-resolution is related to the ability to remove overlying structures and the amount of artefact and noise due to out-of-focus structures in the image. The z-resolution of reconstructed images is determined by the angular range at which the projection images are made. This implies that the z-resolution of images for the currently available DBT systems will differ. For the z-resolution measurement it is proposed to image a 60 mm thick PMMA phantom containing a 1.0 mm diameter aluminium sphere in the middle of the phantom in the clinically used AEC mode. On the resulting reconstructed tomosynthesis image the Slice Sensitivity Profile (SSP) along the z-direction is measured and the Full Width Half Maximum (FWHM) is determined [3]. This FWHM is taken as a measure of z-resolution. Results are given below for two types of DBT systems: one with a small angular range and one with a large angular range.

2.4   Missed Tissue at the Top and Bottom of the Reconstructed Tomosynthesis Image

It is important that the reconstructed tomosynthesis image extends from the bucky surface to the compression paddle to avoid missing any breast tissue. To assess potential missed tissue several small pins are taped underneath the compression paddle and on the bucky. One pin is positioned near each corner of the expected reconstructed image using the indications on the bucky and compression paddle and one pin is positioned at the centre of the image on the bucky and underneath the compression paddle. By positioning pins at several places, missed tissue is evaluated for the whole top and bottom of the reconstructed image. A homogeneous PMMA phantom (45 mm thick) is positioned on the bucky. The phantom is subsequently imaged in fully automatic mode. In the resulting reconstructed tomosynthesis image, it is determined whether the pins are in focus in any of the focal planes.

3   Results

3.1   Reproducibility

Typical reproducibility data from a single tomosynthesis acquisition are shown in table 1. The first exposure listed is the pre-exposure in zero degree position; the second exposure corresponds to projection image 1 and so on. Either projection image 1, or all projections, are used for the calculations. It is noted from the DICOM header that the angles of the projection images range from -25 to + 20 degrees. The angle is not symmetrical with respect to the zero degree position, which was expected for this system. Note also the trend in pixel value in the reference ROI on the projection images due to the variation of the angle of incidence of the X-rays.

Table 1. Data from the DICOM header and average pixel value in the reference ROI of the projection images of one of the reproducibility measurement images

Exposure	Angle (°)	mAs	Average Pixelvalue ROI	Exposure	Angle (°)	mAs	Average Pixelvalue ROI
1	0.00	5.00	229.5	14	-3.00	5.38	193.0
2	-25.02	5.38	151.5	15	-1.07	5.38	193.4
3	-24.06	5.38	157.6	16	0.84	5.38	193.6
4	-22.12	5.38	163.0	17	2.70	5.38	193.4
5	-20.20	5.38	168.3	18	4.63	5.38	192.5
6	-18.28	5.38	173.0	19	6.54	5.38	191.4
7	-16.39	5.38	177.3	20	8.48	5.38	189.8
8	-14.48	5.38	180.6	21	10.40	5.38	188.1
9	-12.56	5.38	183.9	22	12.29	5.38	185.4
10	-10.64	5.38	186.7	23	14.23	5.38	183.0
11	-8.70	5.38	188.8	24	16.16	5.38	180.0
12	-6.82	5.38	190.6	25	18.08	5.38	176.8
13	-4.89	5.38	192.3	26	19.98	5.38	173.1

In Table 2 the results for the reproducibility measurement are given using projection image 1 and using the summed projection images. The variation of SNR between the images five tomosynthesis acquisitions is lower for the summed projections (0.4%) than for measurements made using only the first projection image (3.7%).

Table 2. Reproducibility measurements using projection image 1 and using the combined projection images. Exposure factors: W/Rh 28 kV, 5.38 mAs per projection.

DBT image	$SNR_{projection\ 1}$	$SNR_{summed\ projections}$
1	42.0	145.0
2	40.7	144.7
3	41.5	145.3
4	41.9	145.2
5	42.3	145.1
Average	41.7	145.1
Variation (%)	3.7	0.4

3.2   System Projection MTF

In figure 1 the results of the system projection MTF are shown. For the system using a step-and-shoot approach, it is observed that the MTFs in the x- and y-directions are almost equal. For the system using a continuous tube movement the MTF in direction of the tube movement (y-direction) is lower than in x-direction. This result is similar to that found previously by Marshall et al [5].

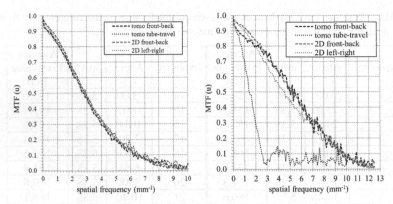

Fig. 1. MTF in x- and y-direction for a DBT system using a step-and-shoot approach (left) and a DBT system using a continuous tube movement (right)

3.3   Z-Resolution

In figure 2 the results of the z-resolution measurement are given for two different brands of DBT system. The FWHM for system 1 (small angular range) is 11.2 mm, for system 2 (large angular range) the FWHM is 5.5 mm.

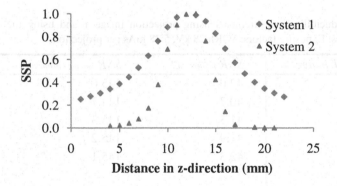

Fig. 2. Slice sensitivity profiles for two different types of DBT systems, system 1: FWHM = 11.2 mm, system 2: FWHM = 5.5 mm

3.4   Missed Tissue at the Top and Bottom of the Reconstructed Tomosynthesis Image

Figure 3 shows that the images of the object (small pin) in the top and bottom focal planes of the reconstructed tomosynthesis image are in focus. In this example the reconstructed tomosynthesis image therefore extends from bucky to the compression paddle and all tissue in z-direction is included in the reconstructed image.

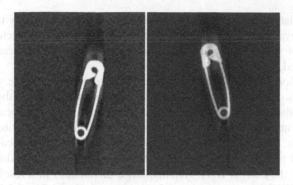

Fig. 3. View of an object (a small pin) taped on the bucky (left) and directly underneath the compression paddle (right) in respectively the top and bottom focal plane

4 Discussion

It is proposed to perform reproducibility measurements in projection images, due to the fact that advanced image reconstruction methods may influence the pixel values and SD in the reconstructed focal planes to such an extent that potential problems of reproducibility might not be detected. Reproducibility measured in the first projection image showed large variations in SNR due to the low detector air kerma per projection. Summing all projection images increases the accuracy of the measurement. It is suggested that the same limiting values as used in FFDM are applied: the variation in tube-time product for 5 subsequent images should be smaller than 5% and the variation in SNR in the reference ROI should be less than 10%. It can be seen that the system for which this measurement was performed did not have a symmetrical distribution of the projection images around the zero degree position, which was as expected according to the specifications. The effect of this asymmetrical distribution of projection images on the quality of the reconstructed image is not known. At this moment most, but not all, DBT systems give access to unprocessed projection images. For the evaluation of reproducibility it is essential that access to this type of image is obtained for all brands of system.

It is clear from the system projection MTF measurement that resolution in the tube movement direction will decrease for DBT systems with continuous tube movement. This result is in line with the study by Marshall and Bosmans [5]. It is likely that this will influence visibility of objects, however further study is required to investigate this more thoroughly. The MTF in both x- and y direction could be checked regularly to detect potential changes in the resolution of projection images over time. For this purpose the accuracy of the measurement technique proposed should be sufficient. However, due to the fact that projection images are low dose, it might be considered to use a 1 mm thick attenuator to increase the number of X-ray quanta reaching the image receptor which would reduce the noise on the measurement. The amount of blurring due to the movement of the X-ray tube depends on the distance from the point of interest in the imaged volume to the rotational axis of the tube and the distance from the detector. Therefore at acceptance or in type tests system projection

MTF could be also measured a number of positions above the bucky table (e.g. at 40 and 70 mm) to evaluate blurring at different heights in the reconstructed volume. For the evaluation of system projection MTF access is given to unprocessed projection images is required.

The z-resolution of DBT systems is related to the angular range over which the projections are acquired. The z-resolution influences the ability of the system to remove/minimize the influence of noise due to overlying tissue in a focal plane and the loss of signal of an object due to the distribution of the signal over one or more adjacent focal planes. This will influence the visibility of objects clinically, but further study is required to estimate the impact on tumor detection. Due to differences in the angular range of the current DBT systems, large differences in z-resolution are seen. The measured FWHM for system 1 and 2 are respectively 11.2 and 5.5 mm, differing by a factor of 2. Therefore we propose to quantify z-resolution in a QC test, even if the clinically required z-resolution in not (yet) known. Measured FWHM values could be used as a reference for subsequent QC tests. However, a disadvantage of this measure is the dependence of the FWHM on the attenuation and size of the imaged object. Therefore the object used for the measurement should always be specified when FWHM values are given. For the measurements in this paper the FWHM of an aluminium sphere with diameter of 1 mm has been chosen. This choice of material and size is a result of availability of materials and experience with measurements on several brands of DBT systems [6]. The z-resolution might also differ over the reconstructed volume of a DBT system, due e.g. to the smaller number of projection images which are used in the reconstruction of the top lateral edges of the image. Therefore the z-resolution measurement could be performed at different positions in the reconstructed volume in acceptance tests or typetests. It is also important to note that the measured z-resolution is larger than the spacing between focal planes in the reconstructed image (typically 1 mm).

In FFDM missed tissue is evaluated by measuring the distance between bucky edge and the edge of the image at chest wall side. This small part of the breast will not be imaged. In DBT, an additional measurement to evaluate missed tissue at the top and bottom of the reconstructed image seems reasonable. The proposed test checks whether all breast tissue is visualized in the z-direction. In the results obtained it is observed that all pins are in focus on both top and bottom focal plane of the image. This means that for the system under evaluation, the reconstructed image in z-direction just extends from the bucky to the compression paddle.

At this moment limiting values are difficult to set. For some measurements common sense is sufficient to set limits (e.g. no missing tissue between the bucky and compression paddle), for other tests results from clinical trials are required (e.g. what z-resolution is required for DBT systems, or which decrease of the MTF in the direction of tube movement could be allowed). Due to this lack of limiting values quality control at this moment assures stability of a system and does not have the ability to set major pass/fail criteria. This is a topic for further study.

Beside this a test to quantify the image quality of the reconstructed image remains a work-in-progress. Existing methods of measurement and accompanying (non anthropomorphic) phantoms cannot be used in DBT, because they do not take into account the effect of removing overlying breast tissue.

5   Conclusions

Results are encouraging and show that the tests presented will form an appropriate and necessary part of QC procedures. For some of the proposed tests access to unprocessed projection images is required, at this moment however this type of images cannot be obtained on all brands of system. Therefore access to such is requested in our draft QC protocol for DBT systems [3].

Quality control procedures for DBT systems are still in development and the development of a test to quantify the reconstructed image quality and the setting of limiting values are challenges. A suitable image quality test is necessary for a QC protocol which aims at giving quantitative pass/fail criteria for DBT systems. The QC tests outlined here can assure system stability, but cannot separate good from suboptimal systems. Our future work is therefore focused on the development of an overall image quality test and the setting of limiting values.

References

1. Van Engen, R.E., Young, K.C., Bosmans, H., Thijssen, M.: European protocol for the quality control of the physical and technical aspects of mammography screening. Chapter 2b: Digital mammography. In: Perry, N., Broeders, M., de Wolf, C., Törnberg, S., Holland, R., von Karsa, L. (eds.) European Guidelines for Quality Assurance in Breast Cancer Screening and Diagnosis, 4th edn., pp. 105–165. European Commission, Office for Official Publications of the European Communities, Luxembourg (2006)
2. Van Engen, R.E., Bosmans, H., Dance, D.R., Heid, P., Lazzari, B., Marshall, N., Schopphoven, S., Thijssen, M., Young, K.C.: Digital mammography update. European protocol for the quality control of the physical and technical aspects of mammography Screening S1, Part 1: Acceptance and constancy testing. In: Perry, N., Broeders, M., de Wolf, C., Törnberg, S., Holland, R., von Karsa, L. (eds.) European Guidelines for Quality Assurance in Breast Cancer Screening and Diagnosis, 4th edn., pp. 1–54. Office for Official Publications of the European Communities, Luxembourg (2013)
3. Van Engen, R.E., Bosmans, H., Bouwman, R., Dance, D.R., Heid, P., Lazzari, B., Marshall, N.W., Schopphoven, S., Strudley, C., Thijssen, M.A.O., Young, K.C.: Protocol for the quality control of the physical and technical aspects of digital breast tomosynthesis systems, draft version 0.15, EUREF (2014), can be downloaded from http://www.euref.org
4. Dance, D.R., Young, K.C., van Engen, R.E.: Estimation of mean glandular dose for breast tomosynthesis: Factors for use with the UK, European and IAEA breast dosimetry protocols. Phys. Med. Biol. 56, 453–471 (2011)
5. Marshall, N.W., Bosmans, H.: Measurements of system sharpness for two digital breast tomosynthesis systems. Phys. Med. Biol. 57(22), 7629–7650 (2012)
6. Bouwman, R., Visser, R., Young, K., Dance, D., Lazzari, B., van der Burght, R., Heid, P., van Engen, R.: Daily quality control for breast tomosynthesis. In: Hsieh, J., Samei, E. (eds.) Medical Imaging 2010: The Physics of Medical Imaging (2010)

Conventional Mammographic Image Generation Method with Increased Calcification Sensitivity Based on Dual-Energy

Xi Chen and Xuanqin Mou[*]

Institute of Image Processing & Pattern Recognition,
Xi'an Jiaotong University, Xi'an, Shaanxi, China
{xi_chen,xqmou}@mail.xjtu.edu.cn

Abstract. The visualization of calcifications could be obscured in mammograms because of overlapping of tissue structures. Dual-energy digital mammography (DEDM) can generate tissue-subtracted image for improving the detectability of breast calcifications, but the mass information is missing. This paper proposes a conventional mammographic image generation method with increased calcification sensitivity based on DEDM. Firstly, a conventional mammographic image is generated with low-energy and high-energy images based on multi-scale decomposition and reconstruction. Secondly, the tissue-subtracted "calcification image" is generated using a nonlinear inverse mapping function with calcification pixels marked. Finally, the density values of the marked calcification pixels in the reconstructed mammographic image are increased for better visualization. Preliminary results show that the proposed DEDM method can generate both calcification and conventional mammogram-like images and the calcification sensitivity is increased. The CNR of calcifications of 50% glandular ratio has been increased from 2.75 to 9.32.

Keywords: digital mammography, dual-energy, multi-scale, calcification sensitivity.

1 Introduction

Mammography is the gold standard for breast cancer screening. Calcifications are one of the earliest and main indicators of breast cancer. However, the visualization of calcifications could be obscured in mammograms because of overlapping of tissue structures. Dual-energy digital mammography (DEDM) is a promising technique to improve the detectability of calcifications since it can be used to suppress the contrast between adipose and glandular tissues of the breast. In DEDM, a pair of digital mammographic images, with low-energy (LE) and high-energy (HE), are acquired and a tissue-subtracted "calcification image" is generated using appropriate mathematical manipulation [1, 2]. However, the masses, if present, are missing in tissue-subtracted calcification image. The patient may need an extra conventional mammography which is unacceptable.

---

[*] Corresponding author.

H. Fujita, T. Hara, and C. Muramatsu (Eds.): IWDM 2014, LNCS 8539, pp. 460–467, 2014.

The purpose of this work is to develop a new technique based on DEDM. In this investigation, LE and HE images are combined to generate conventional mammographic image using multi-scale image decomposition and reconstruction method. At the same time, the tissue-subtracted calcification image is generated by the scatter corrected LE and HE images.

The calcifications are more apparent in the "calcification image". However, the radiologists don't get used to reading this image because there is no tissue structure for reference [3]. So the calcifications are detected in the calcification image, and the calcification information is overlaid onto the generated conventional gray scale mammogram for radiologist reviewing. This technique is presented as a practical way to use the increased calcification sensitivity of DEDM. We present the performance of this technique by breast phantom studies implemented on a commercial full-field digital mammography system.

2   Method

In DEDM, if HE and LE spectra are known, two unknowns (glandular ratio g and calcification thickness t_c of the breast) can be solved pixel by pixel. If the spectrum is known, mammogram of any kV can be retrieved. In practice, it is hard to get the exact distribution of spectra, so we use inverse-map technique [4] to calculate t_c and g and multi-scale technique [5] to reconstruct conventional mammographic image.

2.1   Conventional Mammographic Image Generation

Conventional mammographic image generation has four steps based on multi-scale decomposition and reconstruction frame.

Data Preprocessing. A breast phantoms with 50% glandular ratio was exposed at fixed mAs and multi kVs, from the kV of LE to kV of HE with 2kV interval. The average gray value of each image was measured and the ratio coefficients between these gray values were calculated. And then, if we would like to generate a conventional mammographic image of a certain kV, we should first do LE and HE images multiplied by the corresponding coefficients.

Multi-scale Decomposition. After the preprocessing procedure, LE and HE images are decomposed from coarseness to detail as the scale of filter decreased. As illustrated in Fig.1, F_0 is the input image data (LE or HE image), G_k ($k = 0, 1, 2,.., N - 1$) is the 3×3 Gaussian filter kernel, and * is the convolution operator. In each step, the previous high-pass residual image D_{k-1} is smoothed by the filter kernel G_k [6]. N is the decomposition level and we adopted $N=5$ in this experiment.

Component Reconstruction. For LE and HE images, we have $F^L_1, F^L_2, ..., F^L_5, D^L_4$ and $F^H_1, F^H_2, ..., F^H_5, D^H_4$. Let F^R_k ($k = 1, 2,.., 5$) and D^R_4 be the corresponding reconstructed components. For low frequency components ($k = 1, 2$):

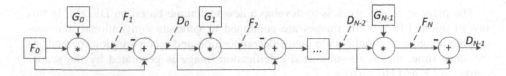

Fig. 1. Decomposition Architecture

$$F^R_k = 0.5F^L_k + 0.5F^H_k, \quad k = 1, 2. \tag{1}$$

For high frequency components, F^R_k ($k = 3, 4, 5$) and D^R_4 were reconstructed using a fusion strategy based on similarity measure [7]. M ($M= F_{3, 4, 5}$ or D_4) level was adopted as an example to illustrate the reconstruction process. $F_M(x, y)$ is the component value of the pixel (x, y), the local energy $E_M(x, y)$ of 3×3 neighborhood centered on the pixel is:

$$E_M(x, y) = \sum_{i=-1}^{1} \sum_{j=-1}^{1} F_M^2(x+i, y+j) \tag{2}$$

We define the correlation coefficient $C_M(x, y)$ between LE and HE images in the M level neighborhood as:

$$C_M(x, y) = \frac{2\sum_{i=-1}^{1}\sum_{j=-1}^{1} F^L_M(x+i, y+j)F^H_M(x+i, y+j)}{E^L_M(x, y) + E^H_M(x, y)} \tag{3}$$

λ is defined as the similarity threshold and is 0.75 in this investigation. If $C_M(x, y) > \lambda$, the weights are:

$$W^L_M(x, y) = \begin{cases} 0.5\left(1 - \dfrac{1 - C_M(x, y)}{1 - \lambda}\right) & E^L_M(x, y) < E^H_M(x, y) \\[2mm] 0.5\left(1 + \dfrac{1 - C_M(x, y)}{1 - \lambda}\right) & E^L_M(x, y) \geq E^H_M(x, y) \end{cases}$$

$$W^H_M(x, y) = 1 - W^L_M(x, y) \tag{4}$$

The reconstructed component F^R_M is:

$$F^R_M(x, y) = W^L_M(x, y)F^L_M(x, y) + W^H_M(x, y)F^H_M(x, y) \tag{5}$$

If $C_M(x, y) \leq \lambda$, the reconstructed component F^R_M is:

$$F^R_M(x, y) = \max\left\{F^L_M(x, y), F^H_M(x, y)\right\} \tag{6}$$

Conventional Mammographic Image Generation. The conventional mammographic image can be generated by the reconstructed components. The high frequency components were suppressed in order to reduce the quantum noise. The generation formulation is:

$$F^R{}_0 = \sum_{k=1}^{4} F^R{}_k + 0.4F^R{}_5 + 0.1D^R{}_4 \tag{7}$$

2.2   Optimized Calcification Image Generation

A nonlinear inverse mapping technique was used to generate DE calcification images from separately acquired LE and HE images. An inverse mapping function could adequately model the calcification thickness (t_c) as a function of the LE and HE log-signal (f_l, f_h):

$$t_c = \frac{a_0 + a_1 f_l + a_2 f_h + a_3 f_l^2 + a_4 f_l f_h + a_5 f_h^2 + a_6 f_l^3 + a_7 f_l^2 f_h + a_8 f_l f_h^2 + a_9 f_h^3}{b_0 + b_1 f_l + b_2 f_h + b_3 f_l^2 + b_4 f_l f_h + b_5 f_h^2} \tag{8}$$

where $f_j = \ln(I_{rj}/I_j)$ $(j=l,h)$. This equation is applied pixel-by-pixel to the image. I_{rj} is the reference signal. I_j is the transmitted fluence of the phantom. An algorithmic scatter correction method [8] was applied to in order to get an optimized DE calcification image. So there is no scatter fraction in I_j. The coefficients of the inverse-map function, a_k $(k=0,\ldots,9)$ and b_k $(k=0,\ldots,5)$, were determined by a least-squares fit of the calibration data [4].

2.3   Calcification Sensitivity Enhancement

Noise reduction techniques have been investigated to counteract the noise increase in DE calcification signal. In this study, a median filter (kernel = 3) was applied to the DE calcification image, and then a histogram of the smoothed image was made. The pixels, which had density values at highest 0.2% of the image, as determined in the histogram analysis were flagged. This essentially created a binary image, with 0.2% of the pixels labeled 1. Since the conventional mammographic image and calcification image were both generated by LE and HE images, they are exactly registered. In the conventional mammographic image, the pixels, whose corresponding pixels in the calcification image were labeled 1, were determined as calcification pixels. The density values of the marked calcification pixels in the generated conventional mammographic image were increased by 10%.

3   Results

The full-field digital mammography systems used in this study was GE Senographe Essential system. 28 kV/50 mAs and 48 kV /12.5 mAs were used for DEDM with Rh target and Rh filter. A breast phantom and a calcification phantom were used as the imaged object. The breast model was a density step phantom that simulated different ratios of glandular and adipose tissues. The calcification phantom was a rectangular block of 50% glandular ratio with embedded calcification clusters. The imaged object was constructed by placing the calcification phantom on the breast phantom. For example, we would like to generate a mammographic image of 34kV. Fig.2 presents the LE, HE, reconstructed (34kV) and actual conventional mammographic images. Tables 1 and 2 lists the contrast and image noise in different glandular ratios of Fig.2. The reconstructed image is close to the actual image.

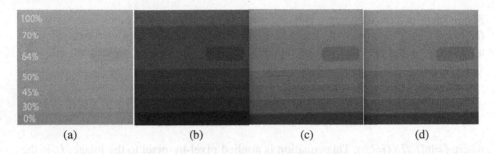

Fig. 2. Images of phantoms. (a) 28kV; (b) 48kV; (c) 34kV (reconstructed); (d) 34kV (real).

Table 1. Contrast (%) between different glandular ratios

Image	0%/30%	30%/45%	45%/50%	50%/70%	70%/100%
LE	24.9	10.8	5.2	19.2	30.1
HE	14.8	5.7	3.1	10.4	15.5
Reconstructed	23.0	9.5	4.2	16.1	25.9
Real	21.8	9.0	4.5	16.2	25.2

Table 2. Image noise (%) of ROIs in different glandular ratios

Image	Glandular ratio (%)					
	0	30	45	50	70	100
LE	1.03	1.00	1.32	1.12	1.27	1.52
HE	0.86	0.86	1.01	0.91	0.94	0.95
Reconstructed	0.72	0.66	1.01	0.71	0.78	0.82
Real	0.72	0.86	1.09	0.92	0.99	1.05

Fig.3 shows a section of images of calcification and breast phantoms. The image section corresponds to glandular ratios of 30%, 45% and 50% with calcification sizes of 230–280 μm. Fig.3(a) shows the reconstructed image of 34kVp, the image brightness and contrast were adjusted for display .Fig.3(b) shows the calcification image calculated based on Eq.(8) with scatter correction. Since DEDM is an imaging tech-

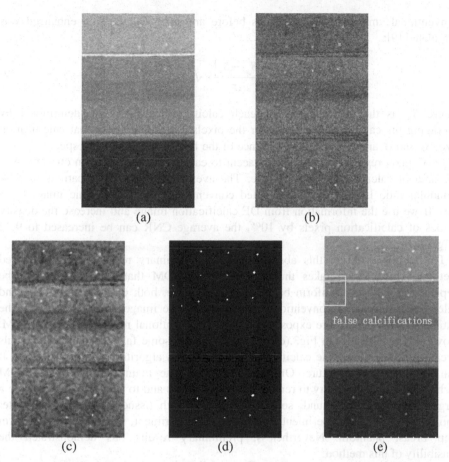

Fig. 3. A 250 × 145 pixel section of images showing calcifications with size of 230–280μm over 30% (bottom), 45% and 50% (top) glandular ratio tissue-equivalent material. (a) Reconstructed mammographic (34kV) image with adjustment of the image brightness and contrast (b) DE calcification image; (c) DE calcification image after median filter (kernel=3); (d) Binary DE calcification image; (e) Reconstructed mammographic (34kV) image with calcification enhancement and with adjustment of the image brightness and contrast.

nique whose resultant calcification signal is sensitive to image noise in LE and HE images, the DE calcification image was smoothed with median filter (kernal=3) as shown in Fig.3(c). After noise reduction the clacification image is converted to binary image by suitable threshold (Fig.3(d)). In the reconstructed conventional mammographic image, the density values of pixels, whose corresponding pixels in Fig.3(d) were labeled 1, were increased by 10% (Fig.3(e)). And then, the calcification sensitivity was increased.

A simple visual evaluation of the calcifications was performed. Firstly, the ensemble average of 5 LE images was used to determine the pixel locations of the calcifications in the image. And then, the CNR of each calcification in the generated conventional mammographic images before and after calcification enhanced was calculated [9]:

$$CNR = \frac{\left| S_{\mu c} - S_B \right|}{\sigma} \times \sqrt{A} \qquad (9)$$

where $S_{\mu c}$ is the mean signal for each calcification which was determined by averaging the calcification signal over the pixels corresponding to that calcification size. S_B and σ are the mean and variance of the background signal respectively of a 31×31 pixel region in the image adjacent to each of the calcification clusters. A is the area of calcification in the image. The average CNR of calcifications of 50% glandular ratio is 2.75 in the generated conventional mammographic image(Fig.3 (a)). If we use the information from DE calcification image and increase the density values of calcification pixels by 10%, the average CNR can be increased to 9.32 (Fig.3 (e)).

The results listed in this abstract are the preliminary results of the proposed method. This method takes the advantage of DEDM that calcifications can be depicted in a largely uniform background. Therefore, both calcification image and calcification enhanced conventional mammogram-like image can be generated; the patient will not need more exposure to get the conventional mammogram in DEDM. However, as indicated in Fig3.(d) and (e), there are some false calcification signals because we used a simple calcification determination algoritnm while we believe it can be improved in future. On the other hand, the main advantage of DEDM techinique lies in its ability to remove tissue structures and to show calcifications in a largely uniform background, so breast phantom with tissue structures is a better choise for validation experiment. In the present experiment, we just used a uniform step breast phantom. Nevertheless, preliminary results has demonstrated the feasibility of this method.

4   Conclusions

A conventional mammographic image generation method from DEDM is proposed based on a multi-scale decomposition and reconstruction framework. The calcification pixels were detected in DE calcification image, and the density values of the corresponding pixels in the reconstructed conventional mammogram-like image were increased. Preliminary results demonstrated that the proposed DEDM method can generate both calcification and conventional mammogram-like images, and calcification sensitivity was increased. In the future, we will validate the proposed method by tissue structured phantoms and improve calcification detection algorithm.

Acknowledgement. This work was supported in part by the National Natural Science Foundation of China (Grant No. 61172163).

References

1. Lemacks, M.R., Kappadath, S.C., Shaw, C.C., Liu, X., Whitman, G.: A Dual-energy Subtraction Technique for Microcalcification Imaging in Digital Mammography-A Signal-to-noise Analysis. Med. Phys. 29, 1739–1751 (2002)
2. Kappadath, S.C., Shaw, C.C.: Quantitative Evaluation of Dual-energy Digital Mammography for Calcification Imaging. Phys. Med. Biol. 49, 2563–2576 (2004)
3. Boone, J.M.: Color Mammography: Image Generation and Receiver Operating Characteristic Evaluation. Investigative Radiology 26, 521–527 (1991)
4. Kappadath, S.C., Shaw, C.C.: Dual-energy Digital mammography: Calibration and Inverse-mapping Techniques to Estimate Calcification Thickness and Glandular-tissue Ratio. Med. Phys. 30, 1110–1117 (2003)
5. Wang, Y.-P., Wu, Q., Castleman, K., Xiong, Z.: Chromosome Image Enhancement Using Multiscale Differential Operators. IEEE Trans. Med. Imaging 22, 685–693 (2003)
6. Zhang, M., Mou, X.: A Novel Contrast Equalization Method for Chest Radiograph. In: Proc. SPIE, vol. 6144, p. 61446R (2006)
7. Burt, P.T., Lolczynski, P.J.: Enhanced Image Capture through Fusion. In: Proc. 4th Int. Conf. on Computer Vision, pp. 173–182. IEEE (1993)
8. Chen, X., Nishikawa, R.M., Chan, S., Lau, B.A., Zhang, L., Mou, X.: Algorithmic Scatter Correction in Dual-energy Digital Mammography. Med. Phys. 40, 111919 (2013)
9. Luo, T., Mou, X., Tang, S.: An Applicability Research on JND Model. In: Proc. SPIE, vol. 6146, p. 614610 (2006)

Development of Mammography System Using CdTe Photon Counting Detector for Exposure Dose Reduction
- Study of Effectiveness of the Spectrum by Simulation -

Naoko Niwa, Misaki Yamazaki, Sho Maruyama, and Yoshie Kodera

Department of Radiological Sciences, Graduate School of Medicine,
Nagoya University, Nagoya, Japan
niwa.naoko@e.mbox.nagoya-u.ac.jp

Abstract. We have proposed a new mammography system using a cadmium telluride photon counting detector to reduce exposure dose. In conjunction with this, we propose a new high x-ray energy spectrum with tungsten/barium (W/Ba) as a target/filter. In this study, the usefulness of the W/Ba spectrum, in terms of image quality and dose distribution is evaluated through Monte Carlo simulation. The contrast-to-noise ratio and dose distribution are measured using polymethyl methacrylate phantoms of 2, 4, and 7 cm thickness. In each case, the result obtained using the W/Ba spectrum is better than that from conventional mammographic spectra. The results of this study indicate that, by using a higher energy x-ray than in conventional mammography, it is possible to obtain significant exposure dose reduction without loss of image quality.

Keywords: photon counting, mammography, dose reduction, Monte Carlo simulation.

1 Introduction

Recently digital mammography with photon counting technology has applied to silicon detector [1]. To reduce exposure dose, we have proposed a new mammography system using a cadmium telluride (CdTe) photon counting detector. Because CdTe has high absorption efficiency over a wide energy range and electrical noise is not mixed in the proposed photon counting technique, we can utilize energy spectra that differ from the energy band used in conventional mammography, allowing for a significant exposure dose reduction without loss of image quality.

The purpose of this study is to investigate the effectiveness of high x-ray energy spectrum. Using Monte Carlo simulation, we evaluated the image quality and exposure dose.

H. Fujita, T. Hara, and C. Muramatsu (Eds.): IWDM 2014, LNCS 8539, pp. 468–474, 2014.
© Springer International Publishing Switzerland 2014

2   Materials and Method

2.1   Monte Carlo Simulation Geometry

All simulations were performed using the Electron Gamma Shower ver.5 (EGS5) Monte Carlo code. Fig.1.(a) shows the simulation geometry used; the source-to-image-distance was 66 cm and the exposure area was 12×16 cm^2. Polymethyl methacrylate (PMMA) phantoms of differing thickness (2, 4, and 7 cm) were compressed by a 0.25 cm compression plate (also composed of PMMA) and placed directly onto 0.1 cm-thick detector of pixel size 0.1×0.1 mm^2. All scattered radiations were rejected, and neither electrical nor system noise were taken into account.

Table 1 lists the simulation conditions for each PMMA phantom thickness. In order to clearly compare our new system with a conventional mammography system, each condition of spectrum and detector was different.

To test the new system, the detector was simulated as a type of photon counting detector. It was composed of CdTe and can set several bins. By setting the threshold to 25 keV in the lowest bin, it is possible to discard the photons of 25 keV or less with the electrical noise. Fig.1.(b) shows the spectral distribution of high energy x-rays used in the simulation, which were produced by an x-ray unit KXO-50G/DRX-2924HD (TOSHIBA, Tochigi, Japan) with the tube voltage set to 40 kV and an imaging plate (BaFX2+: Eu, X= Cl, Br, I) (FUJIFILM, Tokyo, Japan) added as a Ba filter.

The standard mammography detector used for comparison was of a selenium-based flat panel detector. It measured the amount of absorbed energy in each pixel. The spectra used were based on published data [2] for a Molybdenum anode filtered with Molybdenum (30 μm) and Rhodium (25 μm) with the tube voltages set to 26, 28, and 32 kV. These spectra are also represented by Fig.1.(b).

Table 1. Simulation conditions

PMMA thickness	Target / filter	Tube voltage	Detector	Pixel value
20mm	Mo/Mo	26kV	a-Se 1mm	Absorbed energy
	W/Ba	40kV	CdTe 1mm	Number of count
40mm	Mo/Mo	28kV	a-Se 1mm	Absorbed energy
	W/Ba	40kV	CdTe 1mm	Number of count
70mm	Mo/Rh	32kV	a-Se 1mm	Absorbed energy
	W/Ba	40kV	CdTe 1mm	Number of count

To match the display characteristics of an analog system using the x-ray film, the pixel values were obtained by using a logarithmic transform.

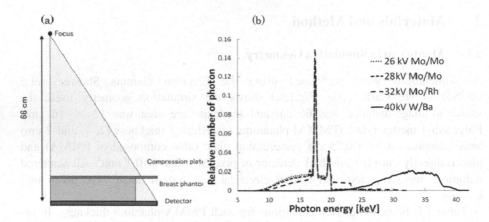

Fig. 1. (a). Simulation geometry (b). X-ray spectra used in the simulation

2.2   Calculations of Absorbed Dose Distribution and CNR

To compare the performances under the high energy W/Ba spectrum with those under the conventional spectra, we scored the absorbed dose distribution of the PMMA phantom, and calculated the contrast-to-noise ratio (CNR) in simulation images produced by an acrylic step phantom. Fig. 2 shows a schematic image of the acrylic step phantom on top of the PMMA phantom, and the actual image obtained by simulation. The region of interest in the simulation image was arranged at each step, and we calculated the CNR using:

$$\mathrm{CNR} = \frac{m_{\mathrm{BG}} - m_{\mathrm{SIGNAL}}}{\sqrt{\dfrac{\sigma_{\mathrm{BG}}^2 + \sigma_{\mathrm{SIGNAL}}^2}{2}}} \tag{1}$$

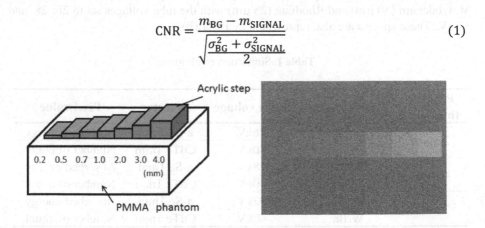

Fig. 2. Acrylic step phantom and simulation image

where m_{BG} is the mean pixel value of background area, m_{SIGNAL} is the mean pixel value in each step region, σ_{BG} is the standard deviation of the background area, and σ_{SIGANL} is the standard deviation of each step region. In order to ensure that the conditions more closely approximated those found in the real mammographic imaging, about 3×10^5 transmission photons per unit area (mm^2) was used for each PMMA thickness; these conditions were confirmed through x-ray spectrometer measurements using Mo/Mo and Mo/Rh target/filters.

3   Results

3.1   Dose Distribution

Figs. 3, 4, and 5 show the absorbed dose distributions inside each phantom when absorbing identical doses. The absorbed doses at depth were normalized by the value of the surface dose under conventional conditions, in which the entrance surface dose (ESD) was high and the absorbed dose decreased with distance from the phantom surface. Under high energy W/Ba conditions, the ESD decreased by more than 60% as compared with conventional conditions, while the absorbed dose decreased slowly with distance from the phantom surface.

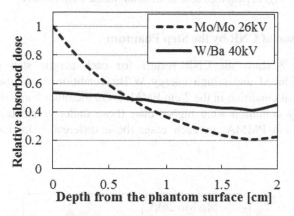

Fig. 3. Absorbed dose distribution inside 2 cm PMMA

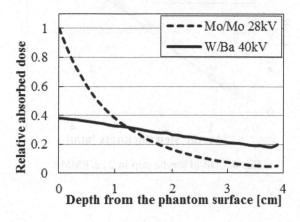

Fig. 4. Absorbed dose distribution inside 4 cm PMMA

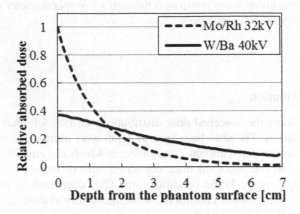

Fig. 5. Absorbed dose distribution inside 7 cm PMMA

3.2   Comparison of CNR by the Step Phantom

Figs. 6, 7, and 8 show the CNR results for each acrylic step phantom. The CNR values produced under high energy W/Ba condition were lower than those under conventional condition in the 2 cm PMMA. On the other hand, the CNR values with high energy condition were higher than those under conventional conditions in 4 cm and 7 cm PMMA. In each case, these differences increased with step thickness.

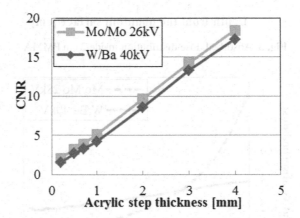

Fig. 6. CNR of acrylic step in 2 cm PMMA

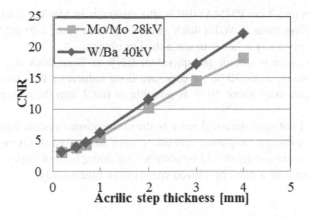

Fig. 7. CNR of step phantom with 4 cm PMMA

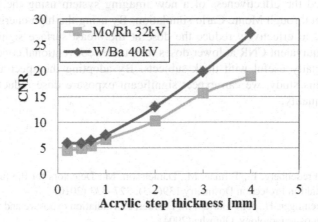

Fig. 8. CNR of step phantom with 7 cm PMMA

4   Discussion

Though this simulation, the CNRs in the W/Ba condition were mostly better than those in the conventional conditions. The contrasts under conventional spectrum are superior to those under high energy spectra for a low contrast object. With respect to the noise values, the signal-to-noise ratio (SNR) under high energy condition is high compared with those under conventional condition. This is the reason why the incident photons to detector are small by using conventional spectra because the photons are attenuated largely inside PMMA phantom. In calculating the CNR of a low contrast object, the influence of the noise value is highly dependent on the number of photons incident on the detector [3]. Correspondingly, the CNRs under high energy W/Ba spectra were higher than those by conventional spectrum in the 4 cm and 7 cm PMMA. However, the result of simulation in the 2cm PMMA was not similar to the ones in the 4 cm and 7 cm PMMA; that is, the contrasts in Mo/Mo 26kV are extraordinarily higher than those in W/Ba 40kV. Based on these results, to get the effectiveness of high energy x-ray is better to use a thicker object.

In Fig. 7, in order to obtain an equivalent CNR at 2mm-thick step in the 4 cm PMMA, it is able to about 30 % for exposure dose reduction. It is seen from Fig. 8 that a dose reduction of about 50 % is possible at the 2 mm-thick step of the 7 cm PMMA.

This study did not take electrical noise in the conventional system into account, nor did it employ an energy weighting process to take advantage of energy discrimination; improved future results should be obtained by doing both of these. It will also be necessary to determine a more optimized spectrum in future study.

5   Conclusion

We investigated the effectiveness of a new imaging system using the high energy W/Ba spectrum through Monte Carlo simulation. By using the high energy spectrum, it was possible to effectively reduce the dose at the breast surface significantly, by obtaining an equivalent CNR at lower doses than under conventional conditions. This effect is especially useful with thick subjects. By adopting the spectral conditions examined in this study, we can expect significant exposure dose reduction without loss of image quality.

References

1. Åslund, M., Fredenberg, E., Telman, M., Danielsson, M.: Detectors for the future of X-ray imaging. Radiation Protection Dosimetry 139(1-3), 327–333 (2010)
2. Säbel, M., Aichinger, H., Joite-Barfuß, S., Dierker, J.: Radiation exposure and image quality in X-ray diagnostic radiology. Ohmsha (2004)
3. Evans, D.S., Workman, A., Payne, M.: A comparison of the imaging properties of CCD-based devices used for small field digital mammography. Phys. Med. Bio. 47, 117–135 (2002)

Development of Mammography System Using CdTe Photon-Counting Detector for Exposure Dose Reduction
- Evaluation of Image Quality in the Prototype System -

Misaki Yamazaki, Niwa Naoko, Sho Maruyama, and Yoshie Kodera

Department of Radiological Sciences, Graduate School of Medicine,
Nagoya University,
Nagoya, Japan
yamazaki.misaki@d.mbox.nagoya-u.ac.jp

Abstract. We discuss a new mammography system using a cadmium telluride (CdTe) photon-counting detector for exposure dose reduction. We created a prototype system that uses a CdTe detector and an automatic moving stage. For a variety of conditions, we measured the image properties and evaluated the image quality produced by reconstructing scanning images from several thousand frame data elements obtained by shift-and-add method, from which it was demonstrated that the basic detector performance in terms of output linearity with respect to X-ray intensity was good. The spatial resolution under various conditions and the linearity of the relationship between the thickness of the acrylic step and reconstructed scanning images were also measured. Finally, we evaluated the image quality obtained by scanning a breast phantom. Our results show that the developed prototype system can improve image quality by optimizing the balance between the shifting-and-adding operation and the output of the X-ray tube.

Keywords: photon counting, digital mammography, dose reduction.

1 Introduction

In the field of X-ray imaging, it is important to attain both high quality of images and low exposure dose. In this paper, we discuss the development of a new mammography system that uses a cadmium telluride (CdTe) photon-counting detector in order to reduce exposure dose without loss of image quality. Because CdTe has a high absorption efficiency over a wide energy range and electrical noise is not mixed in the proposed photon-counting technique, we can utilize a new energy spectrum that differs from the energy band used in conventional mammography.

In this study, we created a prototype system consisting of a CdTe detector and an automatic movement stage, and we measured and evaluated the image properties and image quality produced by this system.

H. Fujita, T. Hara, and C. Muramatsu (Eds.): IWDM 2014, LNCS 8539, pp. 475–481, 2014.

2   Materials and Methods

2.1   Prototype System Using CdTe Photon-Counting Detector

Figure 1 shows a schematic of a prototype scanning system based on a CdTe photon-counting detector. The automatic moving stage is so positioned that the subject is moved between the CdTe detector and the X-ray tube; we operated the moving stage by remote control from a computer located outside of the X-ray laboratory. The photon-counting detector, which uses a 1 mm-thick CdTe detector, can perform data collection at 300 frames per second (fps) with a pixel size of 0.2×0.2 mm^2 and a matrix size of 50×1573 pixels per frame. Figure 2 shows a photograph of experimental system. Table 1 lists the specifications of the CdTe detector.

We reconstructed images from several thousand frame data elements that were obtained by scanning using the shift-and-add method. The correct amount of shift to be used in the shift-and-add operation was calculated on the basis of the magnification of the image and the speed of the moving stage.

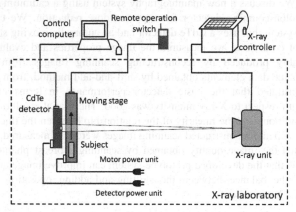

Fig. 1. Schematic of experimental system

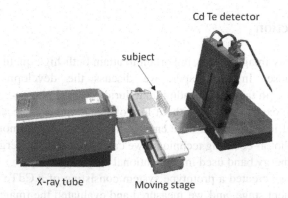

Fig. 2. Photograph of prototype scanning system

Table 1. Specifications of the CdTe detector

Specification	Realized Value
Active area	8×144 mm^2
Modules	18
Size of module	8×8 mm^2
Array configuration	40×40
Pixel size	200×200 μm^2
Pixel depth	16 bits
Matrix size	50×1573
Frame rate	300 fps (×4 Bin)
Material	CdTe 1mm thick

2.2   Detector Performance

To evaluate the linearity of the relationship between detector output and X-ray intensity, we employed a digital X-ray unit, KXO-50G/DRX-2924HD (TOSHIBA, Tochigi, Japan), with the tube voltage set at 40 kV. Using an imaging plate (BaFX^{2+}: Eu, X = Cl, Br, I) (FUJIFILM, Tokyo, Japan) installed as a Ba filter, the output of the detector was measured while changing the X-ray intensity from 0.032 to about 8.8 μC/kg at 1.6×10^4 counts/s (cps) /pixel. By obtaining calibration data prior to data collection, the sensitivities of each module and of each pixel in the detector were corrected.

2.3   Evaluation of Image Properties

To measure the input-to-output linearity of the detector, we used the digital X-ray unit described above to image 10 acrylic steps with 1 mm intervals. The tube voltage and current were set at 50 kV and 4 mA, respectively, and a 0.5 pixel shift was used to implement the shifting-and-adding operation.

To measure spatial resolution, we utilized a micro focus X-ray tube, L7901 (Hamamatsu Photonics, Hamamatsu, Japan). A resolution chart with eleven slit patterns (0.5, 1.0, 1.5, 2.0, 2.5, 3.0, 4.0, 5.0, 6.0, 8.0, and 10.0 lp/mm) and a tungsten edge were used to obtain, respectively, digital and presampled modulation transfer functions (MTFs).The tube voltage and current were set at 40 kV and 0.25 mA, respectively, the data acquisition time was 12 seconds, and several amounts of shift were used. Because the pixel size was 200 μm, the images were produced at a magnification of two in accordance with the planned use of the prototype for mammography.

In experiments to evaluate the overall performance of the prototype as a mammography system, we obtained breast phantom RMI-156 images through scanning. In this case, the digital X-ray unit KXO-50G/DRX-2924HD was used with the tube voltage and current set at 50 kV and 4 mA, respectively, at a source-image distance (SID) of 60 cm and a shift of 0.25 pixel. In addition, to compare the prototype system with the conventional mammography system, Mermaid (KONIKAMINOLTA, Tokyo, Japan) was used with the same surface dose conditions. In order to reduce the surface dose of conventional mammography system to that of the prototype system, the beam quality used as an input for the conventional mammography system was RQA-M2, which was installed a 2-mm thick aluminum filter. Therefore, the beam quality of the conventional mammography system became hard.

3   Results

Figure 3 shows the relationship between dose and detector output. The graph exhibits a high degree of linearity at a count rate of 1.6×10^4 cps/pixel and within the energy band used. In addition, there was a high degree of linearity between acrylic step thickness and the pixel values of the reconstructed scanning images, as shown in Fig. 4.

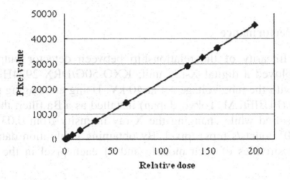

Fig. 3. Relationship between dose and detector output

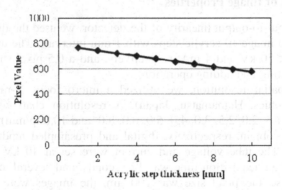

Fig. 4. Linearity of the relationship between thickness of the acrylic step and pixel value of panorama image

Figure 5 shows a reconstituted image of the resolution chart and its density profile. From this image, we found that a chart of up to about 6.0 cycles/mm could be reconstructed clearly. Figure 6 shows the outputs of several digital MTFs calculated from square wave response functions (SWRFs) by using a resolution chart, and the presampled MTF calculated using the edge method with a shift of 0.25 pixel is shown in Fig.7.

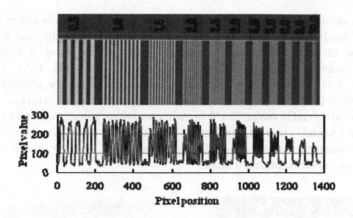

Fig. 5. Reconstructed image of resolution chart (top) and its profile (bottom)

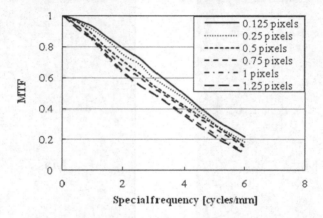

Fig. 6. Digital MTF results at several amounts of shift

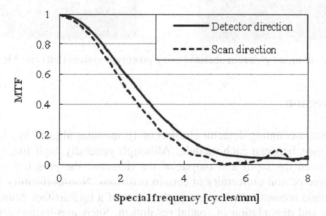

Fig. 7. Presampled MTF results (shift of 0.25 pixel)

Figure 8 shows the breast phantom images. The exposure dose used to produce this image was much less than that used in conventional mammography, and the surface dose of the breast phantom was measured during a scan using a Radcal 9015 ionization chamber dosimeter (Radcal Corporation, Monrovia, CA). Owing to the lack of X-ray tube capacity available for this experiment, the phantom surface dose was only 0.117 mGy. In conventional mammography, an average glandular dose (AGD) of 1.6 mGy under 28 kV Mo/Mo conditions will correspond to a surface dose of about 8.0 mGy in a 4 cm polymethyl methacrylate (PMMA) phantom. Despite the much lower surface dose produced in our experiment, however, it was possible to see a mass on the breast phantom image.

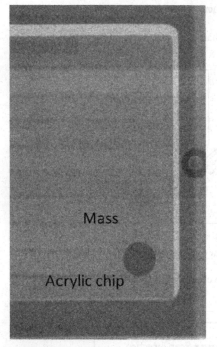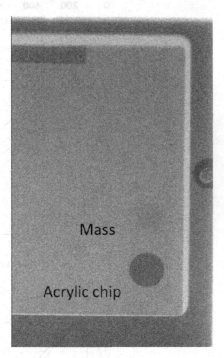

Fig. 8. Images of breast phantom obtained using prototype system (left) and Mermaid (right)

4   Discussion

The CdTe photon-counting detector consists of 18 modules aligned in a linear manner with several gaps between each module. Although generally high linearity could be obtained between the input and output of the detector, the presence of these gaps caused a degree of non-uniformity at certain positions. Non-uniformity also occurred in the panoramic reconstructed image in the form of a line artifact caused by factors such as noise and degradation of spatial resolution. Such non-uniformities generally occur owing to the lack of input for a detector, which almost disappears with the increase in the number of incident photons.

In the proposed imaging system, the pixel size is larger (0.2×0.2 mm^2) than that obtained using conventional mammography. However, by magnifying acquired images by a factor of two, the high frequency part of a chart clearly becomes 6.0 cycles/mm. Our results show the change in MTF values in terms of the amount of shifting performed in the shift-and-add operation; that is, image quality improves as scanning speed and amount of shift decrease, although doing so increases the exposure dose as the scanning time increases. The values of digital MTF were higher than those of presampled MTF; however, we could not determine the reason for this. The spatial resolution in the detector direction was higher than in the scan direction; this result is similar to that of previous work [1].

Because of the lack of X-ray tube capacity available for this experiment, we were not able to compare the images obtained by our prototype system with that produced in conventional mammography under identical practical conditions. Although we would need to use an X-ray tube with larger output to obtain clinically useful images, we were able to see a mass on the breast phantom image even under the low exposure dose conditions in these experiments.

5   Conclusion

In this study, we developed a prototype mammography system using a CdTe detector to enable exposure dose reduction. In this system it is possible to improve image quality by optimizing the balance of shifting-and-adding with the output of the X-ray tube; correspondingly, in future work we will assess optimizing conditions and improvements based on the relationship between the amount of shift and the output of the X-ray tube as well and we will also determine an optimal X-ray spectrum.

Reference

1. Magnus, Å., Björn, C., Mats, L., Mats, D.: Physical characterization of a scanning photon counting digital mammography system based on Si-strip detectors. Med. Phys. 34, 1918–1925 (2007)

Investigation of Dependence on the Object Orientation in Visibility-Contrast Imaging with the X-Ray Talbot-Lau Interferometer

Takayuki Shibata[1], Shohei Okubo[1], Daiki Iwai[1], Junko Kiyohara[2],
Sumiya Nagatsuka[2], and Yoshie Kodera[1]

[1] Department of Radiological Sciences,
Nagoya University Graduate School of Medicine, Nagoya, Japan
[2] Konica Minolta, Inc. Tokyo, Japan
takayuki.shibata@g.mbox.nagoya-u.ac.jp

Abstract. Visibility-contrast image obtained by the X-ray grating interferometer reflects reduction of coherence due to the object's structures. In the case of the one-dimensional grating, visibility-contrast image is affected by relative angle between the structures of the object and the grating. In this study, we have investigated the features of the visibility-contrast signal at the edge of the object. We imaged the acrylic cylinder with the Talbot-Lau interferometer (Konica Minolta, Inc.) by rotating from -90 degrees to +90 degrees with respect to the grating's periodic direction, and measured its edge signal. The signal became its maximum at -90 degrees and +90 degrees, and became zero at 0 degree. This result showed a good agreement with the angle dependency of the x-ray refraction at the edge of the cylindrical structure.

Keywords: Talbot-Lau interferometer, phase contrast, soft tissue.

1   Introduction

Talbot-Lau interferometer, which consists of a conventional x-ray tube, an x-ray detector, and three gratings arranged between them, is a new x-ray imaging s ystem using phase-contrast method for excellent visualization of soft tissue. So, lit is expected to be applied to an imaging method for soft tissue in the medical field, such as mammograms. Using the Talbot-Lau interferometer, three types of images, i.e., the absorption image, the differential phase contrast image and the visibility-contrast image can be obtained. The absorption image is equivalent to the conventional x-ray image. The differential phase contrast image shows the gradient of the refractive index of the object along the periodic direction of the grating. The visibility-contrast image reflects reduction of coherence due to the object's structures. Its well-known feature is the contrast due to the x-ray small-angle scattering.

H. Fujita, T. Hara, and C. Muramatsu (Eds.): IWDM 2014, LNCS 8539, pp. 482–487, 2014.
© Springer International Publishing Switzerland 2014

2   Purpose

The purpose of this study is to investigate the features of the visibility-contrast image. As mentioned above, the visibility-contrast image is sensitive to the object with tiny structures which generate x-ray small angle scattering. The visibility contrast also shows the distinct signal at the edge of the object. In the case of the one-dimensional grating, the signal value in visibility-contrast image is affected by relative angles formed by object's structure and grating. In this study, we investigated the influence of the object orientation to the grating by experiment and evaluate the signal quantitatively in visibility-contrast image.

3   Materials and Methods

3.1   Talbot-Lau Interferometer

Talbot-Lau interferometer is combined Talbot effect and Lau effect.
- Talbot effect
  Talbot effect is a phenomenon in which coherent light transmitted through the diffraction grating (G1 gating) forms an image of same pattern as the grating (self image) on a fixed distance downstream of the grating.
- Lau effect
  Talbot effect requires a coherent light source such as synchrotron radiation facility or micro-focus x-ray tube. However, we can utilize Talbot effect using an incoherent x-ray source by Lau effect. The G0 grating with x-ray source works as line source which emits partial coherent x rays. The pitch of the G0 grating is designed to make the self images generated by each line source overlapped.
- Fringe scan method
  If we try directly to detect the phase sift, the spatial resolution of the detector is not sufficient. The fringe scan method introduces the moiré pattern by using G2 grating with the same period as the G1 grating. Then, it is required to obtain several images for detecting the phase sift of moiré pattern changed by sliding the G0 grating. In this experiment, the amount of sliding of the grating has a one-fourth of the period of G0 grating, and it is imaged four times to reconstruct one image (4 steps method).

3.2   Imaging Methods

We imaged acrylic cylinder (8 mm in diameter) using Talbot-Lau interferometer (Konica Minolta, Inc.) on the following imaging conditions while rotating by 15 degrees from -90 degrees to +90 degrees with respect to the grating's periodic direction.
- Imaging conditions
  X-ray tube voltage: 40kV
  X-ray tube current: 100mA
  Current time product: 250mAs × 4 steps (1000mAs)

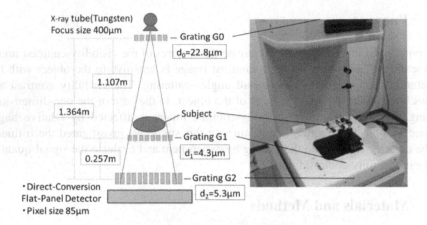

Fig. 1. Talbot-Lau Interferometer

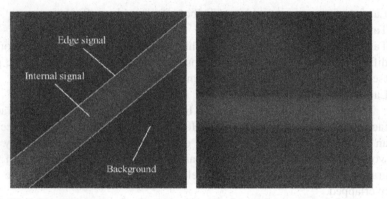

Fig. 2. Visibility-contrast image of acrylic cylinder with 45 degrees left and 0 degree right

3.3   Measurement

At first, we were converted raw data to text data using ImageJ (ver. 1.46r). Here, in visibility-contrast image, signal value shows 1.0 if there is no subject (background).

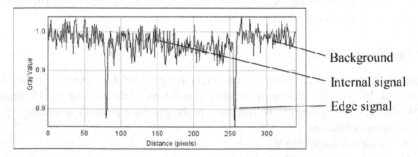

Fig. 3. Signal profile of acrylic cylinder in visibility-contrast image

However, signal value becomes lower than 1.0 if there is a subject. Therefore, we picked up minimum value in each row and column and calculated their average using spread sheets. The averaged minimum value in each row and column was compared, and the smallest signal at the edge of the acrylic cylinder was determined. In addition, we measured internal signal value which is the averaged signal value in acrylic cylinder, and we carried out these calculations on all angles.

4 Results

In visibility-contrast image, the object orientation affected to the edge signal of acrylic cylinder, and the edge signal value became the maximum when the angle of acrylic cylinder with respect to the periodic direction of grating is -90 and +90 degrees. And the edge signal decreased as it approached to 0 degree, and the edge signal became zero when the 0 degree.

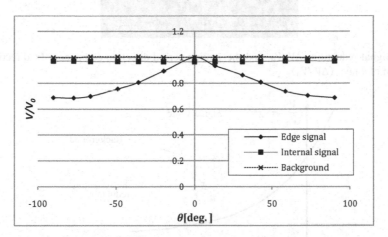

Fig. 4. Measured signal (edge signal, internal signal and background)

5 Introduction of the Estimation

According to the value of the edge signal of the visibility-contrast image, only the edge signal increased or decreased by a change in the angle, and there was no effect on the internal signal. We thought that the signal value of visibility-contrast image had a relation to the x-ray refraction. In the case of the one-dimensional grating, Talbot-Lau interferometer detects the parameters along the periodic direction of the grating.

5.1 Methods of Estimation

As mentioned above, we thought that the signal value of visibility-contrast image reflected only the component of grating period direction in the refraction of x ray. So, we calculated the angle dependence of the x-ray refraction along the grating periodic direction. If the maximum value of the signal reduction due to edge of acrylic cylinder is $\Delta V/V_0$, the edge signal $(\Delta V/V_0)_x$ which is proportional to the grating period direction the component of the refraction of x ray(the grating's periodic direction is x direction) can be formulated as Equations (1) and (2).

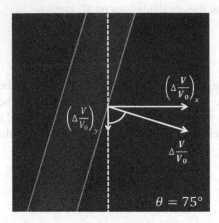

Fig. 5. Signal reduction; $\Delta V/V_0$, and the grating period direction component (x direction) of refraction of x ray; $(\Delta V/V_0)_x$

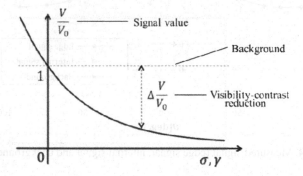

Fig. 6. Signal value (V/V_0) of visibility-contrast image is lower than background $(=1.0)$

$$\left(\Delta \frac{V}{V_0}\right)_x = \left|\Delta \frac{V}{V_0}\sin\theta\right| \tag{1}$$

$$\left(\Delta \frac{V}{V_0}\right)_y = \left|\Delta \frac{V}{V_0}\cos\theta\right| \tag{2}$$

$$\frac{V}{V_0} = \left(\frac{V}{V_0}\right)_{BG} - \left(\Delta \frac{V}{V_0}\right)_x = \left(\frac{V}{V_0}\right)_{BG} - \left|\Delta \frac{V}{V_0}\sin\theta\right| \tag{3}$$

V/V_0: Visibility-contrast value
$\Delta V/V_0$: Visibility-contrast reduction
$(V/V_0)_{BG}$: Background value, $(V/V_0)_{BG} = 1$

Then, the signal value of another angle φ from the signal value of the object angle θ can be estimated as Equation (4).

$$\left(\frac{V}{V_0}\right)_{\text{Estimated Value}} = \left(\frac{V}{V_0}\right)_{\text{BG}} - \left|\left(\left(\frac{V}{V_0}\right)_{\text{BG}} - \frac{\left(\Delta\frac{V}{V_0}\right)_x}{\sin\theta}\right)\sin\varphi\right| \qquad (4)$$

5.2   Relationship

We compared the measured value obtained by the experiment and the estimated value obtained by calculation. As a result, the difference between the measured value and the estimated value was 2.7% at most and 1.1% on average. They were consistent with high accuracy.

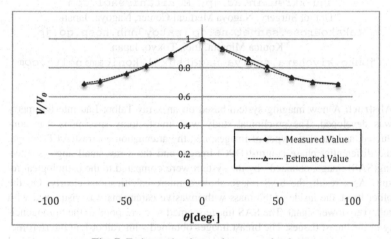

Fig. 7. Estimated value and measured value

6   Conclusion

Visibility-contrast signal at the edge of the object obtained by X-ray Talbot-Lau interferometer has a strong correlation with the refraction along the periodic direction of the one-dimensional grating. We were able to estimate the effect of the object orientation to the edge signal.

References

1. Yashiro, W., et al.: On the origin of visibility contrast in x-ray Talbot interferometry. Optics Express 18(16), 16890 (2010)
2. Yashiro, W., et al.: Distribution of unresolvable anisotropic microstructures revealed in visibility-contrast images using x-ray Talbot interferometry. Physical Review B 84, 094106 (2011)
3. Jensen, T.H., et al.: Directional x-ray dark-field imaging. Phys. Med. Biol. 55, 3317 (2010)

Development of New Imaging System Based on Grating Interferometry : Preclinical Study in Breast Imaging

Tokiko Endo[1,2], Shu Ichihara[3], Suzuko Moritani[3], Mikinao Ooiwa[2], Misaki Shiraiwa[2], Takako Morita[4], Yasuyuki Sato[4], Junko Kiyohara[5], and Sumiya Nagatsuka[5]

[1] Dpt. of Breast Surgery, Higashi Nagoya National Hospital, Nagoya, Japan
endot@toumei.hosp.go.jp
[2] Dpt. of Advanced Diagnosis, Nagoya Medical Center, Nagoya, Japan
kk6m-ooiw@asahi-net.or.jp, misaki-s@db3.so-net.ne.jp
[3] Dpt. of Pathology, Nagoya Medical Center, Nagoya, Japan
shu-kkr@umin.ac.jp, MoritaniS@aol.com
[4] Dpt. of Surgery, Nagoya Medical Center, Nagoya, Japan
takako@rose.sannet.ne.jp, satoy@nnh.hosp.go.jp
[5] Konica Minolta, Inc., Tokyo, Japan
{junko.kiyohara,sumiya.nagatsuka}@konicaminolta.com

Abstract. A new imaging system based on an x-ray Talbot-Lau interferometry was developed. The preclinical study with mastectomy specimens was conducted, and the three types of images, i.e., the attenuation contrast(ATT) image, the differential phase contrast(DPC) image, and the x-ray small angle scattering(SAS) image, obtained by the system were compared to the pathological result. As a result, the SAS image showed micro-calcifications clearly. On the other hand, the inside of the mass with invasive carcinoma was visualized with relatively lower signal. The SAS image seemed to correspond to the homogeneity of the breast tissues. The breast images obtained with Talbot-Lau interferometry showed the different aspects which cannot be depicted with the conventional x-ray image. Comparative reading of the three images would enable us to get additional information of breast tissues.

Keywords: x-ray, phase contrast.

1 Introduction

X-ray imaging have been widely used in medical field since its discovery in 1895. The x-ray is one of the electromagnetic waves. When x-rays pass through an object, their phases as well as amplitudes are altered. Conventional x-ray imaging is based on the change in the amplitude by the interaction with objects. Therefore inside of the human body can be visualized by the attenuation of the amplitude depending on organs or tissues. The soft tissues like articular cartilage, however, cannot be visualized with the conventional x-ray imaging, because the attenuation by them are weak and their attenuation characteristics are rarely different from their surroundings. On the other hand, x-ray phase contrast imaging has higher sensitivity to image soft tissues than the attenuation based imaging and its clinical application is expected.

H. Fujita, T. Hara, and C. Muramatsu (Eds.): IWDM 2014, LNCS 8539, pp. 488–493, 2014.
© Springer International Publishing Switzerland 2014

X-ray phase contrast imaging has been actively studied since 1990s. However, most of the methods were limited to academic study. This is because it needed the special x-ray source, such as a synchrotron facility or a micro-focus x-ray tube. Recently, an x-ray grating interferometer which works with a conventional x-ray tube has been developed. This is the modification of the x-ray grating interferometry based on the Talbot effect with one more grating aligned just behind the x-ray source[1,2]. This is called an x-ray Talbot-Lau interferometer. As it can utilize a medical x-ray tube, the imaging system based on a Talbot-Lau interferometry could be applied to clinical imaging.

In the case of breast imaging, preclinical studies with mastectomy specimens have been already reported by some groups[3,4]. We also found that the intraductal components which would contain micro-calcifications appeared more clearly in the images obtained by the Talbot-Lau interferometry[5]. In order to investigate the further features of the breast images obtained with grating interferometry, we imaged partial mastectomy specimens after formalin fixation and then compared to the pathological results.

2   Methods

2.1   Imaging System

An X-ray Talbot-Lau interferometer consists of a conventional x-ray tube, an x-ray detector, and three gratings arranged between them. The left side of Fig.1 shows the arrangements of these devices. When the phase grating(G1) is exposed in coherent x-rays, its self-image is generated downstream. This is Talbot effect. If an object is in

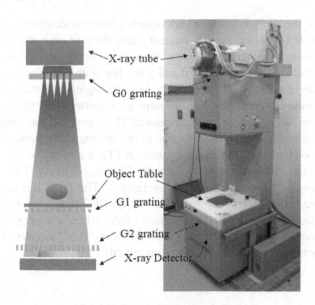

Fig. 1. Talbot-Lau interferometer

the x-ray path, this self-image is deformed. The direct detection of this deformation, however, is difficult, because the pitch of the G1 grating is too small to be detected with a medical x-ray detector. Then, the absorption grating(G2) which has the same pitch as that of the G1 self-image is installed to generate the moiré image between them. The source grating installed just after the x-ray tube (G0) transforms incoherent x-rays by the x-ray tube to partial coherent x-rays as multiple line sources. The pitch of the G0 grating is designed to make x-rays emitted by each line sources overlap each other on the G2 grating.

The right hand of Fig.1 shows imaging system we developed. The system was designed at 28keV. The x-ray tube with a tungsten anode was operated at 40kV. A nominal size of the x-ray focus was 0.4mm.The x-ray detector was a flat panel detector with pixel size of 85μm. The distance between G0 and G2 grating was 1.36m. The sample position was in front of the G1 grating. Magnification factor at the object table was 1.23. The G2 grating used in this study was fabricated with LIGA process and the Au electroplating [6]. The pitch of the G2 grating was 5.3μm.

2.2   Characteristics of the Images Obtained with Talbot-Lau Interferometry

Imaging with grating interferometry is performed with one of the gratings scanned along the periodic direction of the grating. During the scan, the amount of the x-rays reaching to each pixel in the detector changes according to the relative positions of the gratings and it can be approximated by equation(1).

$$I(x, y) = a_0(x, y) + a_1(x, y)\cos\left(2\pi\frac{\chi}{d} + \phi_x(x, y)\right)$$ (1)

where I(x, y) is the x-ray intensity which detected with the detector pixel at the position(x, y). The a0(x, y) is the average intensity, and the a1(x, y) is the amplitude of the moiré fringe created by three gratings, and the $\phi_x(x, y)$ is the phase shift of the interference pattern due to the object. The d and χ are the pitch of the scanned grating and the relative shift of the grating, respectively. In our imaging system, four images were obtained while the G0 grating scanned in steps of a quarter of its pitch, 5.7μm. Then, three parameters, a0, a1/a0, ϕ_x were calculated[7]. In general, the imaging with and without object compensate the imperfection of the gratings. The parameters a0, a1/a0, and ϕ_x correspond to the attenuation contrast(ATT), the x-ray small angle scattering(SAS), and the differential phase contrast(DPC), respectively. The ATT image is almost the same as the conventional x-ray images. The DPC image visualizes the refraction angle between different materials. As the DPC image has higher sensitivity to the soft tissues in human body, the surface of the articular cartilage was observed with this system[8]. The SAS image reflects the x-ray small angle scattering by microscopic structures comparable to the grating pitch[9].

2.3   Breast Tissues

In order to investigate how these three images depict breast tissues, formalin fixed mastectomy specimens were imaged with this system. A specimen was slightly compressed with plastic plates of 5mm thickness. We also imaged a piece of the specimen whose thickness was about 3.5mm. In this case, in order to eliminate artifact due to the air, the specimen was bathed in ethanol. Then, imaging results were compared to the pathological results. The protocol of this study was approved by the institutional review board of Nagoya Medical Center, Japan.

3   Results

According to the pathological result, the specimen included the tumor which consisted of the invasive ductal carcinoma and the ductal carcinoma in situ(DCIS) around it. The invasive carcinoma partially showed the scirrhous component. Fig.2(a) shows the sliced specimens which positioned at the center of the lesion, and the results of the pathological examination are overplotted. The regions circled with red and yellow lines correspond to the area where the invasive ductal carcinoma and the DCIS were observed, respectively. Fig.2(b) is the pathological image of T11.

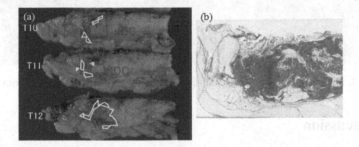

Fig. 2. Pathological result of the imaging specimen

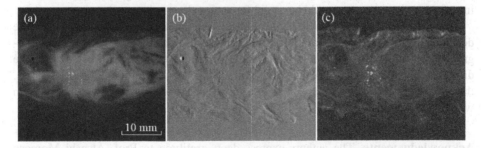

Fig. 3. Images of the sliced specimen with Talbot-Lau interferometry

The imaging result of T11 are shown in Fig3. Fig.3(a), (b) and (c) are the ATT image, the DPC image, and the SAS image, respectively. All three images depicted the calcifications clearly. In the SAS image, the calcifications as well as their surroundings showed higher scattering signal. This result indicated that the region around the calcifications consisted of full of microscopic structures. On the other hand, the part of the mass was shown as low scattering signal, i.e., dark area in Fig3.(c). In the DPC image, the area was shown relatively flat. These results indicated that the invasive carcinoma observed in T11 was composed of relatively homogeneous structure.

Fig.4 shows the imaging result of the partial mastectomy specimen, which was imaged before sliced as Fig.2(a). Thickness of the specimen was 19mm. Fig.4(a),(b), and (c) shows the ATT image, the DPC image, and the SAS image, respectively. The invasive ductal carcinoma and DCIS were observed on the lower left of each images. The SAS image showed the same features as that of the sliced specimen, i.e., the clear depiction of the calcifications and the lower signals inside the mass. The calcifications which were vague in the ATT image were distinctly observed in the SAS image. This result indicated that the SAS image would visualize the homogeneity of the breast tissues which could not be obtained with the conventional mammography.

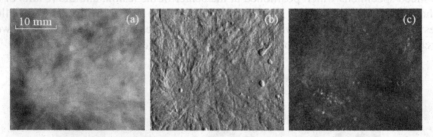

Fig. 4. Images of the partial mastectomy specimen with Talbot-Lau interferometry

4   Discussion

The breast images obtained with Talbot-Lau interferometry showed the different aspects which cannot be depicted with the conventional x-ray image. Comparative reading of these three images would be useful for image diagnosis.

In order to realize the clinical applications, some challenging subjects remain. The dose level of the imaging is more than ten times as high as the conventional mammography in this study. And, the imaging area is limited to the $50\times50mm^2$ due to the difficulty in the fabrication of the G2 grating. In order to overcome these problems, the upgrade of the gratings as well as the further optimization of the imaging system would be required.

Acknowledgements. The authors express deep gratitude to Prof. Atsushi Momose with Institute of Multidisciplinary Research for Advanced Materials, Tohoku University, for his various technological instructions in this study. This study was supported by SENTAN, JST.

References

1. Momose, A., Kawamoto, S., Koyama, I., Hamaishi, Y., Takai, K., Suzuki, Y.: Demonstration of X-ray Talbot Interferometry. Jpn J. Appl. Phys. 42, L866-L868 (2003)
2. Pfeiffer, F., Weitkamp, T., Bunk, O., David, C.: Phase retrieval and differential phase-contrast imaging with low-brilliance X-ray sources. Nat. Phys. 2, 258–261 (2006)
3. Stampanoni, M., Wang, Z., Thuring, T., David, C., Roessl, E., Trippel, M., Kubik-Huch, R.A., Singer, G., Hohl, M.K., Hauser, N.: The First Analysis and Clinical Evaluation of Native Breast Tissue Using Differential Phase-Contrast Mammography. Invest. Radiol. 46, 801–806 (2011)
4. Anton, G., Bayer, F., Beckmann, M.W., Durst, J., Fasching, P.A., Haas, W., Hartmann, A., Michel, T., Pelzer, G., Radicke, M., Rauh, C., Rieger, J., Ritter, A., Schulz-Wendtland, R., Uder, M., Wachter, D.L., Weber, T., Wenkel, E., Wucherer, L.: Grating-based darkfield imaging of human breast tissue. Z. Med. Phys. 23, 228–235 (2013)
5. Endo, T., Ooiwa, M., Shiraiwa, M., Morita, T., Ichihara, S., Moritani, S., Hasegawa, M., Satoh, Y., Hayashi, T., Katou, A., Kiyohara, J., Nagatsuka, S., Momose, A.: Development of a New Breast Imaging Method Based on X-ray Talbot-Lau Interferometry. In: RSNA 2011 SSC15 (2011)
6. Noda, D., Tanaka, M., Shimada, K., Hattori, T.: Fabrication of Diffraction Grating with High Aspect Ratio Using X-ray Lithography Technique for X-ray Phase Imaging. Jpn J. Appl. Phys. 46, 849–851 (2007)
7. Pfeiffer, F., Bech, M., Bunk, O., Kraft, P., Eikenberry, E.F., Bronnimann, C., Grunzweig, C., David, C.: Hard X-ray dark-field imaging using a grating interferometer. Nat. Mater. 7, 134–137 (2008)
8. Tanaka, J., Nagashima, M., Kido, K., Hoshino, Y., Kiyohara, J., Makifuchi, C., Nishino, S., Nagatsuka, S., Momose, A.: Cadaveric and in vivo human joint imaging based on differential phase contrast by X-ray Talbot-Lau interferometry. Z. Med. Phys. 23, 222–227 (2013)
9. Yashiro, W., Terui, Y., Kawabata, K., Momose, A.: On the origin of visibility contrast in x-ray Talbot interferometry. Opt. Express 18, 16890–16901 (2010)

Basic Study on the Development of a High-Resolution Breast CT

Atsushi Teramoto[1], Tomoyuki Ohno[2], Fumio Hashimoto[1], Chika Murata[1],
Keiko Takahashi[1], Ruriha Yoshikawa[3], Shoichi Suzuki[1], and Hiroshi Fujita[4]

[1] Graduate School of Health Sciences, Fujita Health University, Aichi, Japan
teramoto@fujita-hu.ac.jp
[2] Fujita Health University Hospital, Aichi, Japan
[3] Gifu University Hospital, Gifu, Japan
[4] Graduate School of Medicine, Gifu University, Gifu, Japan

Abstract. X-ray breast computed tomography (breast CT) was developed by some research groups to overcome the limitations of mammography. Breast CT is expected to be an effective diagnostic tool because it can generate three-dimensional images of a breast. However, the spatial resolution of the existing system is not satisfactory for identifying microcalcifications within the breast. The purpose of this study was to develop a prototype of high-resolution breast CT system, and to evaluate the imaging properties of the developed system. Our experimental system consists of a microfocus X-ray tube and a flat panel detector with a C-arm frame, a bed, and their controllers. Images were reconstructed by using cone-beam X-ray projections and the Feldkamp-Davis-Kress algorithm. We used phantoms to experimentally evaluate three imaging properties and exposure dose. Consequently, the modulation transfer function value was 0.1 at the frequency of 6.0 LP/mm, which is higher than that of clinical CT and breast CT. Breast phantom microcalcifications were observed clearly. Furthermore, entrance surface dose in the experimental system was similar to that of mammography. These results indicate that our experimental system overcomes the limitations of both the mammogram and existing breast CT systems.

Keywords: Breast, computed tomography, microfocus X-ray.

1   Introduction

Breast cancer is the most prevailing cancer among women in the world; more than 10% of women are likely to develop invasive breast cancer during their lifetime. Mammography is widely used for the detection of breast cancer. However, overlapping breast tissue creates false shadow in many cases. Furthermore, mammography examination causes pain because of the application of pressure. X-ray breast computed tomography (breast CT) was developed to overcome these mammography limitations [1,2]. Breast CT can acquire a 3-dimensional image without incurring any pain by pressure. Breast CT systems have been installed in some research institutes and are currently under clinical evaluation. However, the spatial resolution of the existing

H. Fujita, T. Hara, and C. Muramatsu (Eds.): IWDM 2014, LNCS 8539, pp. 494–500, 2014.

breast CT systems is lower than that of magnified mammogram; it is not sufficient for identifying microcalcifications within the breast [2]. In this study, we developed an experimental high-resolution breast CT system that aims to improve the spatial resolution. The specific goal of this study was to obtain the sub-50 µm spatial resolution for clear observations of microcalcification. Furthermore, by using the developed system we evaluated its imaging properties and the exposure dose.

2   Materials and Methods

2.1   High-Resolution Breast CT System

Figure 1 shows the scan part of our prototype system. It consists of a microfocus X-ray tube (L7901, Hamamatsu Photonics, focus size: 5 µm, maximum tube voltage: 100 kV, maximum tube current: 0.1 mA) and a flat panel detector (C7942CA, Hamamatsu Photonics, indirect conversion type, pixel pitch: 50 µm, matrix size: 2366 × 2368, bit depth: 12 bits) with C-arm frame, and computer for control. A woman lies face down on a table with one breast suspended through an opening. X-ray tube and flat panel detector rotate around the breast to collect the projection data. The proposed system obtains high-resolution image data by using geometric magnification. It can be adjusted by changing the position of rotational center. The maximum magnification is 2.5; the spatial resolution reaches 20 µm.

The projection images are reconstructed into a 3-dimensional (3D) image by using the Feldkamp-Davis-Kress (FDK) algorithm [3]. We employed ramp filter as the reconstruction function, and matrix size of the 3D image was 2048x2048x2048. Image reconstruction is performed by original software that was developed and optimized by using Intel C++, and calculation is conducted using personal computer (CPU: Intel Xeon 3.06 GHz, 12 cores, Memory: 32 GB).

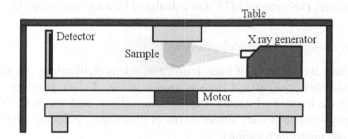

Fig. 1. The structure of the proposed system

2.2   Performance Evaluation

To evaluate the basic imaging characteristics of our system, the following evaluations were conducted. Phantoms, shown in Fig. 2 and Fig. 3, were employed for these evaluations.

(1) Uniformity of CT values

Image uniformity was evaluated by using the uniformity phantom [Fig. 2(a)]. The mean CT values of 5 regions of interest (ROIs) were calculated by using the axial image of the phantom. Then, the standard deviation of mean CT values at 5 locations was determined [4].

(2) Noise level

Noise level was evaluated by using the uniformity evaluation phantom and the noise evaluation phantom [Figs. 2(a) and 2(b)] [4]. Noise level was calculated as follows:

$$\text{Noise level} = \frac{\sigma_{AV} \cdot CS \cdot 100}{\mu_w} \ [\%]. \tag{1}$$

$$CS = \frac{\mu_w - \mu_{air}}{CT_w - CT_{air}} \ [cm^{-1} / CT \ value]. \tag{2}$$

CS: Linearity index of CT value.
σ_{AV}: Standard deviation of mean CT values of water in axial image
μ_w: Absorption coefficient of water ($=0.195 \ cm^{-1}$).
μ_{air}: Absorption coefficient of air ($=0$).
CT_w: Mean CT value of water in axial image inside the uniformity phantom.
CT_{air}: Mean CT value of air part in axial image.

(3) Modulation transfer function

The modulation transfer function (MTF) of our breast CT was evaluated by using the MTF evaluation phantom, as shown in Fig. 2(c). The MTF phantom was scanned under the minimal resolution of 5 µm; cross-sectional image of Cu sheet was obtained. Pre-sampled MTF was calculated by using this image [5-7].

(4) Visibility of mass and microcalcifications

To evaluate the visibility of mass lesion and microcalcifications, we scanned the breast phantom (model013, CIRS) as shown in Fig. 3. This phantom was developed for the training of needle biopsy examinations, and was made from a gel with a physical consistency similar to the human tissue, including simulated mass lesions and microcalcifications.

(5) Entrance surface dose

Entrance surface dose of breast was evaluated by using thermoluminescent dosimeter (MSO-S, Kyokko). It was measured by using total filtration of 3.5 mm Al, tube voltage of 80 kV, tube current of 0.1 mA, and scanning time of 90 seconds.

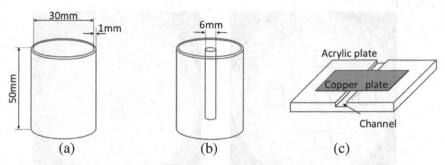

(a)   (b)   (c)

Fig. 2. Phantoms for the performance evaluation of the proposed system. (a) The uniformity evaluation phantom: a water-filled cylindrical vessel. (b) The noise evaluation phantom: an air-filled cylindrical acrylic vessel in (a). (c) The MTF evaluation phantom: a 10 μm thick copper overlaid on an acrylic plate.

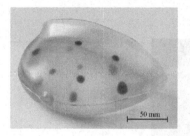

Fig. 3. Breast phantom (model013, CIRS)

3 Results

3.1 Uniformity and Noise

Slice images of uniformity evaluation phantom and noise evaluation phantom are shown in Fig. 4. Uniformity and noise level of our system were 2.35 and 14.95%, respectively. The noise level of the proposed system was about 10-fold higher than that of a typical clinical CT system.

3.2 MTF

The slice image and the MTF evaluation results are shown in Fig. 5. The MTF value of the proposed system became 0.1 at the spatial frequency of 6.0 cycles/mm. As for the clinical CT system, the MTF value became 0.1 at the spatial frequency of around 1.0 cycles/mm. The MTF value of the existing breast CT system was 0.1 at the spatial frequency of 0.7 – 1.5 cycles/mm. Therefore, the spatial resolution of our experimental system was better than that of either a conventional clinical CT or an existing breast CT.

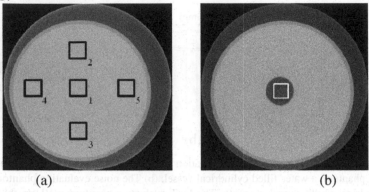

(a)   (b)

Fig. 4. Slice images of uniformity evaluation phantom (a) and noise evaluation phantom (b). Square boxes on these images indicate the regions used for the evaluation.

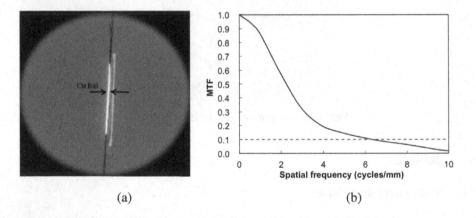

(a)   (b)

Fig. 5. Slice image of the MTF phantom (a) and the MTFs of the proposed system and a clinical CT system (b)

3.3   Evaluation Using Breast Phantom

Figures 6(a) and 6(b) show a cross-sectional image and a 3D-rendered image of the breast phantom, respectively. The 3D structure of the mass region and microcalcifications were clearly identified in the obtained images. By comparing these images with the mammogram results [Fig. 6(c)], we found that the proposed system generated a 3D image structure of the breast with the resolution equivalent to that of the mammogram.

3.4   Exposure Dose

The entrance surface dose of the proposed system was 14.11 mGy. A typical entrance surface dose in mammography is 10-20 mGy per breast [8]; the exposure dose of our system was similar to that of mammography.

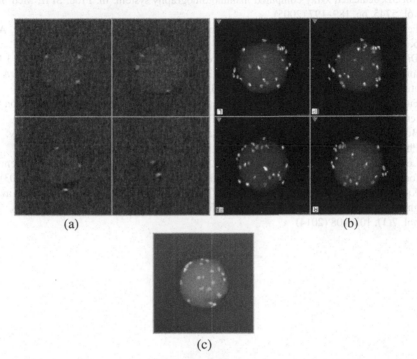

(a)   (b)

(c)

Fig. 6. Images obtained by using the proposed system (a) Axial CT images obtained by using the proposed system. (b) 3D rendered images. Brown regions and yellow dots represent mass lesions and microcalcifications, respectively. (c) Mammographic magnification image (Mammomat Novation, Siemens).

4   Conclusions

We have developed a prototype of high-resolution breast CT system with a microfocus X-ray tube. In addition, we evaluated the imaging properties and the exposure dose of the proposed system. Furthermore, we evaluated the image quality by using breast phantom that included microcalcifications. The MTF of the proposed system was better than that of either a clinical CT or an existing breast CT, and microcalcifications in the breast phantom were observed clearly. These results indicate that our breast CT system overcomes the limitations of both the mammogram and the existing breast CT systems.

References

1. Boone, J.M., Nelson, T.R., Lindfors, K.K., et al.: Dedicated breast CT: Radiation dose and image quality evaluation. Radiology 221, 657–677 (2001)
2. Tornari, M.P., McKinley, R.L., Bryzmialkiewicz, C.N., et al.: Design and development of a full 3D dedicated x-ray computed mammotomography system. In: Proc. SPIE Med. Imag., vol. 5745, pp. 189–197 (2005)
3. Feldkamp, L.A., Davis, L.C., Kress, J.: Practical cone-beam algorithm. J. Opt. Soc. Am. A 6, 612–619 (1984)
4. Diagnostic Radiology Committee Task Force on CT Scanner Phantoms. Report No. 1 Phantoms for Performance Evaluation and Quality Assurance of CT Scanners. American Association of Physicist in Medicine, Chicago, Illinois (1977)
5. Fujita, H., Tsai, D.Y., Itoh, T., et al.: A simple method for determining the modulation transfer functions in digital radiography. IEEE Trans. Med. Imag. 11(1), 34–39 (1992)
6. Boone, J.M.: Determination of the presampled MTF in computed tomography. Med. Phys. 28(3), 356–360 (2001)
7. Lee, S.C., Kim, H.K., Chun, I.K., et al.: A flat-panel detector based micro-CT system: Performance evaluation for small-animal imaging. Phys. Med. Biol. 48, 4173–4185 (2003)
8. Kawaguchi, A., Matsunaga, Y., Otsuka, T., Suzuki, S.: Patient investigation of average glandular dose and incident air Kerma for digital mammography. Radiol. Phys. Technol. 7(1), 102–108 (2014)

Analysis of Dependence of Detector Position on Detected Scatter Distribution in Dedicated Breast SPECT

Steve D. Mann[1,2], Jainil P. Shah[2,3], and Martin P. Tornai[1,2,3]

[1] Medical Physics Graduate Program, Duke University Medical Center, Durham, NC 27705
[2] Department of Biomedical Engineering, Duke University, Durham, NC 27705
[3] Multi Modality Imaging Lab, Duke University Medical Center, Durham, NC 27710
{steve.mann,jainil.shah,martin.tornai}@duke.edu

Abstract. In SPECT, scattered photons contribute to the detected signal, reducing contrast and quantification accuracy. Several methods exist to correct scatter, including the dual-energy window technique, but have not been fully evaluated on non-traditional SPECT trajectories. Using MCNP5, a Monte Carlo study was performed to analyze how incident scatter is affected by detector position for breast SPECT. An ideal detector was positioned at various azimuthal and polar angles relative to a pendant breast geometry. Detected scatter from the breast, heart, liver, torso, and lesion was linearly fit; the slope was used to characterize the distribution. Typical photopeak and scatter energy window ratios were calculated. Results indicate detected scatter depends upon detector position and its vantage of major uptake organs; however, the effect is minimal for non-direct views, with a ratio of 0.37. A single coefficient for dual-energy window scatter correction should suffice for breast imaging trajectories ignoring direct views of the heart/liver.

Keywords: Breast imaging, SPECT, scatter, Monte Carlo, dual-energy window.

1   Introduction

During SPECT acquisitions, scattered photons originating within the body can contribute significantly to the total detected signal. Due to various detector effects, including incomplete charge collection in solid-state detectors, scatter within the detector, and the Poisson nature of photoelectron generation within scintillator detectors, energy resolution is limited, resulting in the need of a relatively large photopeak energy window for counting detected primary events [1-2]. Even with intrinsic, high-Z semiconductor detectors, the need for multiplexing signals in imaging detectors reduces the finer energy resolution possible with those devices. However, the addition of low-angle (high energy) scattered photons hitting the detector contaminates the photopeak window data, resulting in reduced image contrast and quantification accuracy. Several scatter correction methods have been investigated in literature, ranging from simple subtraction methods to Monte Carlo or de-convolution approaches [3-8].

One of the most straightforward and robust scatter correction techniques to implement is the dual-energy window (DEW) method [3]. This approach makes an assumption that,

H. Fujita, T. Hara, and C. Muramatsu (Eds.): IWDM 2014, LNCS 8539, pp. 501–507, 2014.

for a given acquisition geometry and relatively symmetric object shape, the amount of scatter within the photopeak energy window is proportional to the scatter detected in a (lower-energy) scatter energy window. Through a series of calibration experiments, a coefficient (k-factor) can be determined that allows for a scaled subtraction of the scatter in the photopeak window:

$$True = Photopeak - k \cdot Scatter \tag{1}$$

This technique is easily implemented and gives a fast method for scatter correction, provided the k-factor was calibrated for a similar geometry to the object being imaged. However, for non-traditional trajectories that deviate from a simple circular orbit, such as those used in dedicated breast SPECT for improved imaging of the chest wall, the underlying scatter distribution may change due to asymmetry of the breast and additional detected events originating from the torso, heart, and liver [9-10]. The goal of this simulation study is to determine how incident scatter is affected by detector position, especially with non-traditional trajectories that allow better volume imaging, and its effect on the application of the DEW method for scatter correction. This type of study can only be accomplished using Monte Carlo simulation due to the very precise nature and fine energy sampling it affords.

2   Materials and Methods

A dedicated breast SPECT-CT system has been developed that offers the ability to acquire both low-dose, high-resolution 3D anatomical images with the CT subsystem and unique 3D functional images using Tc-99m Sestamibi (140 keV) and the SPECT subsystem [10-13]. The SPECT subsystem is capable of novel detector positioning, including tilting of the gamma camera, to allow projections into the chest wall with nearly-complete sampling trajectories.

The SPECT subsystem, including gamma camera, was modeled using Monte Carlo N-Particle (MCNP5), including the prone-patient bed and detector. The detector has 2.5 mm pixellation and a 2.54 cm long hexagonal lead collimator with 1.2 mm holes (flat to flat) and 0.2 mm Pb septa. The detector was modeled as an ideal detector, with 100% sensitivity and perfect energy resolution, to determine the distribution of true incident scatter, regardless of detector-specific effects. Organs relevant to breast SPECT, including the breast (754mL), heart (251mL), liver (1272mL), torso (6400mL), and a large simulated lesion (33mL), were included in the simulation. The torso was modeled as an elliptical cylinder, while the breast was modeled as the excluded region of the intersection of an ellipsoid and the torso. The heart and liver were both modeled as simple cylinders, while the lesion was a simple sphere near the center of the breast. The simulation was designed from the perspective of the detector, with the patient and bed rotating about a fixed origin to simulate the non-traditional trajectories capable with the physical SPECT subsystem. This point of view was necessary to optimize the simulation due to the number of lattice elements necessary to construct the collimator. No directional bias was implemented, allowing for a full range of angular scatter for each simulated photon. Figure 1 shows example trajectories and slices through the simulation geometry.

For each simulation, the detector was placed at 8 uniformly spaced azimuthal positions (0-315°) and various polar tilts (0-45° in 15° increments) to determine the effects of detector position on detected scatter. Each region (breast, liver, heart, torso, lesion) was simulated as an independent source with 8e8 histories per region to minimize noise. The results from each source were analyzed in total by retrospectively normalizing the detected events to realistic uptake concentration ratios (1x for breast and torso, 12x for liver and heart each, 6x for lesion) and source volumes. Each detected spectrum was linearly fit in the 113-139keV range, and the resultant slope was used to characterize changes in scatter distribution. For each region, the percent contribution of counts within this range was computed to determine the significance of detected scatter from each source. Additionally, two practical energy windows (113-133keV scatter and >134keV photopeak) typically used in our lab for DEW correction were analyzed by taking the ratio of total counts within each window (k-factor) to determine if the integral area changed significantly with detector position. A significant change in k-factor with detector position may result in significant changes in quantification accuracy and image noise within reconstructed images.

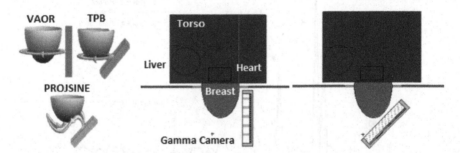

Fig. 1. (LEFT) Examples of various SPECT acquisitions trajectories used for dedicated breast SPECT. Trajectories utilizing detector tilts allow for projections into the chest wall, which is difficult or impossible to image with traditional orbits. (MIDDLE and RIGHT) Images of simulation setup, including gamma camera, breast, torso, liver, and heart, along with the gamma camera shown to two different tilt angles.

3   Results

Reconstructed images acquired with the physical system and phantoms (Figure 2) illustrate the potential contamination of cardiac and hepatic uptake in breast images. The projection data with and without direct views of the heart and liver were reconstructed with the same OSEM reconstruction algorithm.

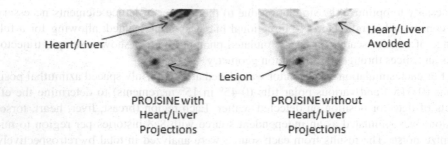

Fig. 2. Reconstructed slices of a breast phantom with torso and lesion obtained with the physical SPECT-CT system. The images represent results from two similar non-traditional trajectories: (LEFT) with direct projection views of heart/liver and (RIGHT) without direct views. Projections including the heart and liver increases both detected photopeak and scattered events originating from these high-uptake organs.

Two examples of different resultant scatter regions, including linear fits, are shown in Fig. 3. The spectra illustrate the difference in magnitude and distribution of detected scatter with gamma camera position.

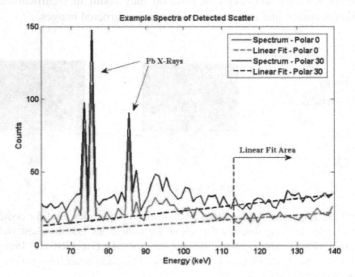

Fig. 3. Plots of the scatter regions of two simulations including all source organs with no lesion. The 113-139keV range was used in the linear fit to characterize detected scatter. The Pb x-ray are due to scatter in the modeled collimator.

The resultant slope from each detector position for the scaled-sum of each source region is shown in Figure 4 for both the lesion and no-lesion cases, along with the total detected scattered events, in the 113-139keV region used in the linear fit.

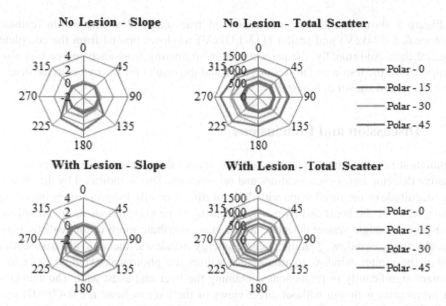

Fig. 4. Azimuthal polar plots of the slope and total scatter detected for simulations with and without a lesion for detector angles of 0-45 degrees. Labels at azimuthal positions on top left plot indicate potential source organs in projection view, depending on polar tilt, which also causes observed asymmetry of total scatter plots.

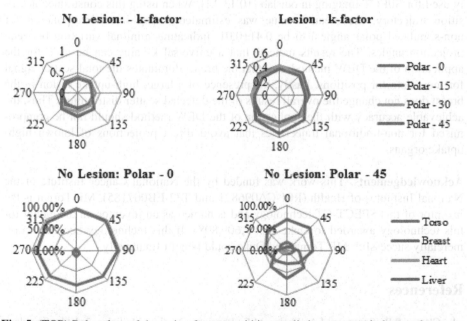

Fig. 5. (TOP) Polar plots of the ratio of scatter within a realistic scatter and photopeak energy window as a function of detector position for simulations with and without a lesion. (BOTTOM) Polar plots of percentage scatter from each source for simulations without lesion. All results are scaled to reflect realistic uptake ratios for each source.

Figure 5 shows the results of the ratio of true scattered events within realistic photopeak (>134keV) and scatter (113-133keV) windows binned from the complete spectral data. Additionally, the percent scatter originating from each source was also computed for the lesion and no-lesion cases, and the results for the two extreme detector tilts are also shown in Figure 5.

4   Discussion and Conclusions

Simulation results indicate that the detected scatter distribution is dependent on the relative detector and source locations and orientations. This is indicated by the changing magnitude of the fitted slope with detector tilt, especially for projections including direct views of the heart and liver. An increasing slope corresponds to an overall increase in low-angle scatter detected, which may contribute more to the realistic photopeak energy window. Within realistic energy windows, the ratio of true-scatter within the scatter window to true-scatter within the photopeak window (k-factor) changes significantly in projections containing the liver and chest wall. The averages for projections with and without direct views of the liver or heart are 0.47 ± 0.04 and 0.37 ± 0.02, respectively. The observed change in k-factor illustrates the need to avoid direct projections of the liver and heart when attempting to more completely image the breast and associated chest wall. We have developed a variation of the presented PROJSINE trajectory (Fig. 1) that avoids direct views of the heart and liver, previously used for SPECT imaging in our lab [10,13-14]. When using this constrained acquisition trajectory, the mean k-value was estimated (using linear-interpolation for non-simulated polar angles) to be 0.41 ± 0.01, indicating minimal variation between projection angles. The results indicate that a universal k-value can be used for the application of the DEW method, and that the breast dominates the total scatter signal for most detector positions. Lastly, the presence of a large, high-uptake lesion in the breast does not change the overall results of the detected scatter distribution. Thus, the achievable accuracy with the application of the DEW method should not be compromised for non-traditional trajectories that avoid direct projections of known high-uptake organs.

Acknowledgements. This work was funded by the National Cancer Institute of the National Institutes of Health (R01-CA096821 and T32-EB007185). MP Tornai is the inventor of this SPECT-CT technology and is named as an inventor on the patent for this technology awarded to Duke (no. 7,609,808). If this technology becomes commercially successful, MP Tornai and Duke could benefit financially.

References

1. Cherry, S.R., Sorenson, J.A., Phelps, M.E.: Physics in Nuclear Medicine, 3rd edn. Saunders, Philadelphia (2003)
2. Knoll, G.F.: Radiation Detection and Measurement. John Wiley & Sons, Inc., Haboken (2000)

3. Jaszczak, R., Greer, K., et al.: Improved SPECT quantification using compensation for scattered photons. J Nucl. Med. 25(8), 893–900 (1984)
4. Harris, C., Greer, K., et al.: Tc-99m attenuation coefficients in water-filled phantoms determined with gamma cameras. Med. Phys. 11(5), 681–685 (1983)
5. King, M., Hademenos, G., Glick, S.: A dual-photopeak window method for scatter correction. J. Nucl. Med. 33(4), 605–612 (1992)
6. Ljungberg, M., Msaki, P., Strand, S.-E.: Comparison of dual-window and convolution scatter correction techniques using the Monte Carlo method. Phys. Med. Bio. 35(8), 1099–1110 (1989)
7. Hutton, B., Buvat, I., Beekman, F.: Review and current status of SPECT scatter correction. Phys. Med. Bio. 56(14), R85–R112 (2011)
8. Buvat, M., Rodriguez-Villafuerte, M., et al.: Comparative assessment of nine scatter correction methods based on spectral analysis using Monte Carlo simulations. J. Nucl. Med. 36(8), 1476–1488 (1995)
9. Perez, K., Cutler, S., et al.: Characterizing the contribution of cardiac and hepatic uptake in dedicated breast SPECT using tilted trajectories. Phys. Med. Biol. 55(16), 4721–4734 (2010)
10. Perez, K., Cutler, S., et al.: Towards quantification of dedicated breast SPECT using non-traditional acquisition trajectories. IEEE Trans. Nucl. Sci. 58(5), 2219–2225 (2011)
11. Brzymialkiewicz, C., Tornai, M., et al.: Evaluation of fully 3-D emission mammotomography with a compact cadmium zinc telluride detector. IEEE Trans. Med. Imag. 24(7), 868–877 (2005)
12. Crotty, D.: Development of an integrated SPECT-CmT dedicated breast imaging system incorporating novel data acquisition and patient bed designs. Ph.D. dissertation, Dept. Biomed. Eng., Duke University, Durham (2010)
13. Perez, K.: Investigating image quality and quantification of functional breast images with a dedicated breast SPECT-CT system. Ph.D. dissertation, Med. Phys. Grad. Prog., Duke University, Durham (2011)
14. Mann, S.D., Perez, K.L., McCracken, E.K.E., et al.: Initial In Vivo Quantification of Tc-99m Sestamibi Uptake as a Function of Tissue Type in Healthy Breasts Using Dedicated Breast SPECT-CT. Journal of Oncology 2012 Article ID 146943, 7 pages (2012), doi:10.1155/2012/146943

Evaluation of Physical and Psychological Burden of Subjects in Mammography

Yongbum Lee and Mieko Uchiyama

Graduate School of Health Sciences, Niigata University, Niigata, Japan
{lee,uchiyama}@clg.niigata-u.ac.jp

Abstract. The realities of physical and psychological burden associated with mammography are not fully understood. We have measured the muscle activity and the sympathetic nervous activity of subjects during mammography to estimate the burden. The experimental results suggested that positioning during mammography affects the muscle activity and the sympathetic nervous activity of the body. We carried out another preliminary experiment for decreasing the examinee's burden using humorous video. In the experiment, two groups ("humor group" and "neutral group") underwent mammography. The humor group was shown a humorous video during mammography. As a result, numerical rating scale scores of humor group on pain and experience time were higher than that of neutral group (no significant difference). In conclusion, the physical and psychological burden of mammography examinees could be evaluated by measuring the muscle activity and the sympathetic nervous activity. Humorous video may be effective at increasing pain tolerance of subjects during mammography.

Keywords: muscle activity sympathetic nervous activity numerical rating scale humorous video.

1 Introduction

Mammography is performed by pressing and stretching the breast using a thin radiolucent compression plate. During mammography, the examinee experiences a physical burden due to the positioning required, such as twisting the neck and raising the arm in addition to the breast compression. As a result, examinees are forced to endure pain caused by breast compression and immobilization. Additionally, in order to obtain the most suitable image for diagnosis, the radiological technologist may directly touch the breast and press it further to spread it if necessary. Breasts are closely related to sexuality for women. Such procedures weigh heavily on examinees in some cases, causing psychological burden in addition to the physical burden. The burden should be measured quantitatively.

As for the physical and psychological burden experienced by the examinees at the time of mammography positioning, we have previously demonstrated the relationship between muscle activity and physical burden [1]. We have also investigated the relationship between sympathetic nervous activity and psychological burden [2]. In this

H. Fujita, T. Hara, and C. Muramatsu (Eds.): IWDM 2014, LNCS 8539, pp. 508–513, 2014.

paper, firstly, some data extracted from the previous papers are indicated in Sections 2 and 3. Next, we describe a preliminary study for decreasing the examinee's burden using humorous video in Section 4. Concluding remarks and discussion on future work are in Section 5.

2   Measurement of Muscle Activity [1]

We measured the muscle activity of subjects during positioning for mammography screening using surface electromyography to clarify the physical burden and pain involved in the positioning. The subjects consisted of 15 women (age: 44.4 ± 6.6 years old, height: 160 ± 6.7 cm, weight: 55.1 ± 3.9 kg, body mass index: 21.4 ± 2.2 %). Measurements were taken in the mediolateral oblique (MLO) position. The target muscles were the sternocleidomastoid, biceps, trapezius and gastrocnemius muscles. A portable multi-purpose bio-amplifier was used for measurements. A numerical rating scale (NRS), which is a tool for self-assessment of subjective pain, was also used for pain measurement.

As a result, analysis of variance showed the difference in the amount of muscle activities to be significant between the relaxation phase before mammography positioning and the stress phase during mammography positioning in all the target muscles (Fig. 1 and Fig. 2). The sites where muscle activity increased were consistent with the sites of pain measured by the NRS (Table 1). These results suggest that positioning during mammography affects the muscle activity of the body and increased muscle activity could be related to the pain. Measurement of muscle activity during mammography is expected to be used effectively, such as in the pain reduction program for the subjects undergoing mammography.

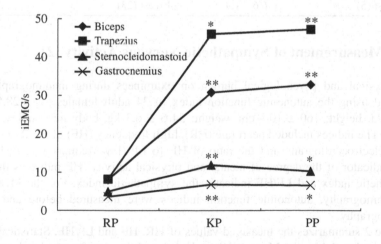

Fig. 1. Muscle activities during right breast positioning. All data are expressed as means. ** P < 0.01 and * P < 0.05 vs. RP values for the same groups.

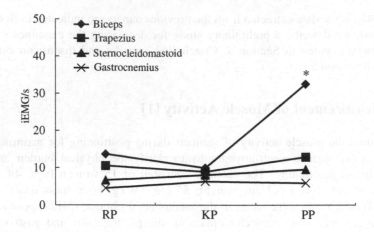

Fig. 2. Muscle activities during left breast positioning. All data are expressed as means. ** P < 0.01 and * P < 0.05 vs. RP values for the same groups.

Table 1. NRS scores at keep phase and pressure phase. The numerical value in parentheses indicates the number of trials. Values are presented as means ± standard deviation.

Keep phase (KP)		Pressure phase (PP)	
For all data (30)	3.7 ± 3.4	For all data (30)	6.7 ± 2.7
shoulder (4)	5.5 ± 1.7	cervix (1)	8.0 ± 0.0
armpit (8)	4.0 ± 3.3	waist (2)	4.8 ± 1.8
breastbone and rib (3)	5.0 ± 5.0	breastbone and rib (3)	3.7 ± 3.2
breast (5)	6.6 ± 1.9	breast (23)	7.5 ± 2.0

3   Measurement of Sympathetic Nervous Activity [2]

The physical and psychological burden on examinees during mammography was analyzed using the autonomic function index in 34 adult females (age: 28.5 ± 9.2 years old, height: 160 ± 10.1 cm, weight: 54.6 ± 6.3 kg, body mass index: 20.2 ± 6.3 %). The indices included heart rate (HR), high frequency (HF) of the R–R interval on an electrocardiogram, and the ratio of HF to LF (low frequency) (LF/HF). HR is an indicator of the degree of mental and physical activity, HF indicates the para-sympathetic index and LF/HF indicates the sympathetic index. For the MLO view in mammography, autonomic function indices were measured before and during mammography.

Table 2 summarizes the measured values of HR, HF and LF/HF. Statistical analysis was performed by the Mann-Whitney U test and the significance level was set at 5 %. The autonomic function indices were compared before and during mammography and all showed no significant differences. The average value before imaging and the reference value at rest were compared. The results showed that HR increased 1.3-fold, HF increased 0.4-fold, and LF/HF increased 3.2-fold over reference values. The values of HR, HF and LF/HF before imaging were all found to be significantly different from the reference values at rest. The chronological values of HR during mammography were consistently more than 80 beats/min up to 120 seconds, showing a tendency to decrease slightly at the end of the mammography imaging (Fig. 3). In addition, chronological changes during mammography showed that HF increased and LF/HF decreased from 120 seconds after the start of imaging (Fig. 4). From these observations, it is evident that the state before mammography is not the same as the resting state and that the sympathetic index is dominant before imaging. They also suggest that some aspects of the psychological burden experienced during mammography are not due to the pain of breast compression alone.

Table 2. Measured values of HR, HF and LF/HF during mammography. Reference values at rest are also indicated [3],[4]. Values are presented as means ± standard deviation. (HR: heart rate, HF: high frequency (0.16 - 0.42 Hz) component, LF/HF: ratio of high frequency to low frequency (0.04 - 0.15 Hz) components).

	Entire mammography	Before imaging	During imaging	Reference values at rest
HR (beats/min)	81.1 ± 13.0	80.4 ± 12.7	81.8 ± 11.8	60.0 [3]
HF (msec^2)	407.3 ± 520.1	429.6 ± 601.7	391.4 ± 444.9	975.0 [4]
LF/HF (msec^2/msec^2)	6.2 ± 4.2	6.5 ± 4.9	5.5 ± 3.9	2.0 [4]

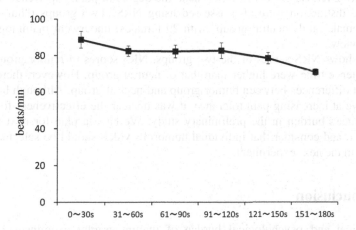

Fig. 3. Chronological changes in HR during mammography. (Standard deviation values are shown in the vertical direction around the mean. 0~30s indicates 0~30 seconds, 31~60s indicates 31~60 seconds, 61~90s indicates 61~90 seconds, 91~120s indicates 91~120 seconds, 121~150s indicates 121~150 seconds, 151~180s indicates 151~180 seconds.)

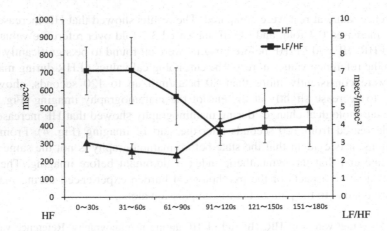

Fig. 4. Chronological changes of HF and LF/HF during mammography

4   Effects of a Humorous Video on Reduction of Examinee's Burden during Mammography

In recent years, there have been claims that humor and laughter possess unique characteristics to help cope with pain [5]. We thought that humorous video might decrease examinee's burden during mammography. Therefore, mammography examinees were shown a humorous video, as a preliminary experiment for decreasing examinee's burden. Humorous video consists of funny-happening scenes which have recorded from television. In the experiment, the degree of pain, experience time, comicality and distraction were also assessed using NRS. Two groups ("humor group" with 15 females and "neutral group" with 29 females) underwent mammography for the MLO view.

Fig. 5 shows NRS scores of the two groups. NRS scores of humor group on pain and experience time were higher than that of neutral group. However, there were no significant differences between humor group and neutral group. Although humor may be effective at increasing pain tolerance, it was unclear the effectiveness for decreasing examinee's burden in the preliminary study. We have a plan for next additional experiment, and consider that individual humorous video should be selected for each examinee in the next experiment.

5   Conclusion

The physical and psychological burden of mammography examinees have been evaluated by measuring the muscle activity and the sympathetic nervous activity. Although humor may be effective at increasing pain tolerance, it was unclear the effectiveness for decreasing mammography examinee's burden in the preliminary study.

The experiment results will be a help of very unique design when further patient-friendly mammographic device is required. The number of subjects was limited in the

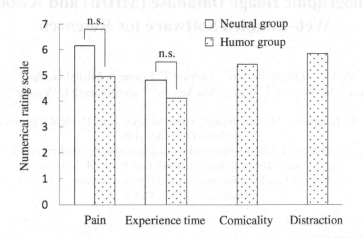

Fig. 5. Mean values of NRS scores of neutral and humor groups

experiments. We have to conduct additional experiments in more subjects. The sense of humor may be different between countries or individuals. The subject should select humorous video in accordance with her sense of humor. Variation of humorous video would be important and required in future work. The effect of humorous video on reduction of mammography examinee's burden need to be discussed with any changes in the physiological measures but this could be for future work.

Acknowledgements. This work was supported by JSPS KAKENHI Grant Number 23593285.

References

1. Uchiyama, M., Lee, Y., Sadakata, M., Sayama, M., Tsai, D.Y.: Measurement of Muscle Activities for Evaluating Physical Burden and Pain during Mammography. Tohoku J. Exp. Med. 228, 53–58 (2012)
2. Uchiyama, M., Lee, Y., Sadakata, M., Tsai, D.Y., Sayama, M.: Effects of Mammography Positioning on the Autonomic Nervous Function. Health 5, 1335–1341 (2013)
3. Mason, J.W., Ramseth, D.J., Chanter, D.O., Moon, T.E., Goodman, D.B., Mendzelevski, B.: Electrocardiographic Reference Ranges Derived from 79, 743 Ambulatory Subjects. J. Electrocardiol. 40, 228–234 (2007)
4. Task Force of the European Society of Cardiology and the North American Society of Pacing and Electrophysiology: Heart Rate Variability: Standards of Measurements, Physiologic Interpretation and Clinical Use. Circulation 93, 1043–1065 (1996)
5. Weisenberq, M., Tepper, I., Schwarzwald, J.: Humor as a Cognitive Technique for Increasing Pain Tolerance. Pain 63, 207–212 (1995)

Mammographic Image Database (MIDB) and Associated Web-Enabled Software for Research

Mark D. Halling-Brown[1,*], Pádraig T. Looney[2], Mishal N. Patel[3],
Lucy M. Warren[2,3], Alistair Mackenzie[2,3], and Kenneth C. Young[2,3]

[1] Scientific Computing, Medical Physics, Royal Surrey County Hospital, Egerton Road,
Guildford, GU2 7XX, UK
[2] National Coordinating Centre for the Physics of Mammography, Medical Physics, Royal
Surrey County Hospital, Egerton Road, Guildford, GU2 7XX, UK
[3] Department of Physics, Faculty of Engineering and Physical Sciences, University of Surrey,
Guildford, GU2 7XH, UK

1 Summary

Current efforts relating to the uptake, evaluation and research into digital medical imaging require the large-scale collection of images (both unprocessed and processed) and data. This demand has led us to design and implement a flexible mammographic image repository, which prospectively collects images and data from multiple screening sites throughout the UK. The MIDB has been designed and created to provide a centralised, fully annotated dataset for research purposes. One of the most important features is the inclusion of unprocessed images. In addition to the images and data, systems have been created to allow expert radiologists to annotate the images with interesting clinical features and provide descriptors of these features. MedXViewer (Medical eXtensible Viewer) is an application we have designed to allow workstation-independent, PACS-less viewing and interaction with anonymised medical images (e.g. for observer studies). With these integrated tools, the MIDB has become a valuable resource for running remote observer studies and providing data and statistics for imaging based-research projects. Previously, studies were run by laborious transfers of images to PACS at remote sites and paper-based data manually curated into databases. Apart from the inconvenience, these approaches also suffer from a lack of accurate location information from the paper-based forms.

2 Introduction

There is a need for comprehensive collections of medical images to be made available for research. Among many requirements are the need for unprocessed images, fully annotated cases and fully representative sets from a variety of disciplines and modalities. Collections of images are required to undertake research and development in Computer Aided Detection (CAD), image perception studies, training and quality assurance. The collection of large set of medical images with full annotation for

---

* Corresponding author.

H. Fujita, T. Hara, and C. Muramatsu (Eds.): IWDM 2014, LNCS 8539, pp. 514–519, 2014.

research purposes is challenging. When the gathering of unprocessed images is required, the difficulties increase massively. The need for accurately curated, comprehensive research sets will only increase as the number of new techniques and modalities increases.

Alongside the need for medical images is the need for more rigorous, consistent and timesaving approaches to managing and undertaking image perception studies. Many studies have previously been run with laborious transfers of images to PACS at remote sites and paper-based data manually curated into databases. Apart from the inconvenience, these approaches suffered from a lack of accurate location information from the paper-based data. One of the most notable items that is lacking from many image perception studies is precise cancer location information. In addition, there are many collaborative image-viewing undertakings, which currently require image transfers between PACS and suffer from a lack of ability to centrally annotate cases with descriptions and regions of interests (ROIs). There are many situations where it would be beneficial to be able to have cases reviewed by experts located at remote sites throughout the country, or indeed the world.

The MIDB systems have been designed to be deployed at multiple remote sites. At these sites, it automatically identifies the relevant cases to collect (e.g. screen detected breast cancers) and then obtains the processed and unprocessed images from the local PACS and associated data from relevant local cancer databases. The images and data are then automatically anonymised and transferred to the central storage. In addition to the data, software (MedXViewer) has been created to allow expert radiologists to annotate the images with interesting clinical features and provide descriptors of these features. In order to avoid subsequent manual transfers of images to multiple remote PACS, the images are streamed from the central location.

The MIDB has been created to provide a centralised, fully annotated dataset for research purposes to meet many of the needs outlined above. One of the most important features is the inclusion of unprocessed images. The MIDB has become a valuable resource with integrated tools for running remote observer studies and providing data and statistics for imaging-based research projects. Initially the database was developed as part of a large research project in digital mammography (OPTIMAM). Hence the initial focus has been digital mammography; as a result, much of the work described will focus on this field and all the current images and data are mammographic.

3   Methods

3.1   Image Database and Collection

A semi-automated process for identifying which cases to collect has been developed. Since we are primarily interested in cancer cases we interrogate local databases of patient/case data to identify these among a much larger set of cases. A full description of the processes is described in more detail elsewhere[1].The processes and systems required to allow semi-automated image collection across multiple heterogeneous sites are extremely complex. The database is made up of several relational databases and a file system for storage of the images. In a very simplified manner, the data models can be split into the image database (ImageDB), observer and training study database (StudyDB) and the associated data schemas (AssocDB). The imageDB maintains the DICOM data, the ground-truth and associated data. Comprehensive loading systems have been created which process the new images and insert the appropriate data into the databases. The observer study database holds details of multiple active observer studies, the observers themselves and the marks and progress made in each study (See Fig 1).

Calculated and derived data can be obtained from the images at the time of collection and include various image feature extractions that are useful for classification, CAD and radiomics applications. Additional annotation, such as features identified by Computer Aided Detection (CAD) systems can be inserted into the database at a later date.

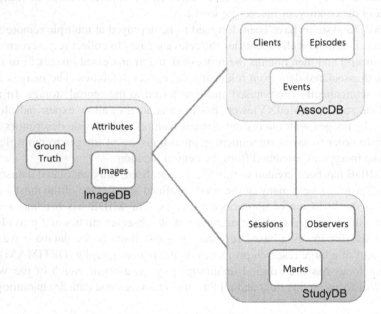

Fig. 1. Overview of main data models involved in OMI-DB. The three main schemas indicated are the Image Database (ImageDB), observer and training study database (StudyDB) and the associated databases (AssocDB).

3.2   Service Layers

In order to allow the tools created to communicate with the OMI-DB, service layer systems were created which manage the messages and transfer between the data and presentation layers. These take the form of web services and are maintained on the same systems as the OMI-DB

3.3   MedXViewer

Various tools enabling interaction with the varying parts of MIDB have been created. Notably, this includes an extensible web-enabled software package designed to facilitate remote studies, collaborative view sessions and training (MedXViewer). Image perception studies and the acquisition of data for research purposes requires the viewing and marking of images, the answering of questions throughout the marking process and the drawing of regions of interests (ROIs) on the images. MedXViewer was initially designed for image perception studies in digital mammography and digital breast tomosynthesis (DBT) but the software can be extended for use in other modalities. One of the key objectives in its development was to allow radiologists to review images and participate in observer studies at multiple remote sites.

MedXViewer was developed in Java and uses the DICOM library Dcm4Che allowing 16-bit images to be created and lookup tables applied. Hence, images can be displayed, as they would appear on a commercial PACS system when MedXViewer is used with clinical quality displays.

The choice of Java as the programming language enables MedXViewer to be used cross-platform on Mac, Linux and Windows environments with no requirement for administrative access or installation. MedXViewer automatically detects the monitor setup and location and places the medical images on the predetermined location. MedXViewer can integrate with the MIDB, allowing images and software to be downloaded from a central store and results to be uploaded to a centralised database. Alternatively the software can be run offline with images and results stored locally. A user is allocated a username and password and their progress and performance can be tracked. The results from MedXViewer can be output in any standard file format (CSV, Excel etc.).

4   Results

The MIDB has been implemented along with the automated collection procedures, anonymisation, associated data gathering, calculated data and expert determined annotations. Currently the full collection system is deployed at three sites and other partial collection processes are in place at two other sites. The database statistics are summarized in Table 1.

When loading the images into the repository, all relevant DICOM tags are extracted to allow a searchable index to be produced. Additionally, CAD predictions are determined and inserted into the database. Expert-determined ground truths are then obtained from our panel of readers (utilising the MedXViewer software) that indicate the relevant ROI and other attributes, such as lesion type and conspicuity. Further annotations are obtained from associated data sources, such as the NBSS. The quantity of additional annotations obtained is large, and includes information on screening history, previous occurrences of cancer, biopsy results and surgical procedures.

Table 1. Database statistics for the MIDB (Correct as of 28/02/2014)

Num of Images	34,014
Num of Studies	4,301
Num of Cases	2,623
Num of Benign Cases	87
Num of Normal Cases	680
Num of Malignant Cases	1,856
Num of Expert Annotated Cases	1,453
Num yet to be Annotated	403

Fig 2 shows the collection of data plotted over time. This is useful to show the projected collection rate and allow us to expect to reach 3,400 cases by the end of April 2014 at the current rate.

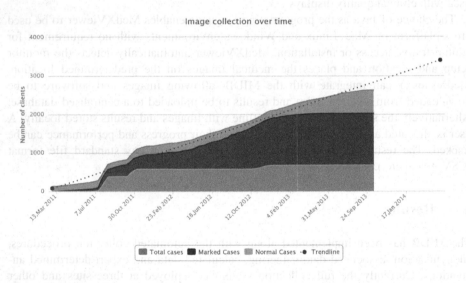

Fig. 2. Image collection over time for the MIDB. Cancer cases often do not become available until several months have passed from the imaging event, hence the lack of recent cases.

Associated tools (including MedXViewer) have been produced which allow interaction with the database in a PACS-less, workstation independent manner. The images from OMI-DB and the associated tools – MedXViewer – have been used in three image perception studies and more are ongoing or planned. The studies investigated the effect of factors such as detector type[2], reader interruption and image processing[3] on cancer detection in digital mammography imaging.

5   Conclusions

A Mammographic Image Database has been created that provides access to a huge number of fully-annotated cases with associated data and unprocessed images. These annotations are obtained from existing cancer databases and from expert opinions. MIDB has already facilitated a number of research projects. The logistics, technology, systems and procedures required bringing together these images and data are extremely difficult to manage and not easily reproduced. We have designed the system to be flexible enough to feasibly allow any site to be added to our collection system. This is facilitated by the provision of multiple differing collection workflows including direct onsite PACS connections. To date we have successfully collected 34,104 2D images from 2,623 clients, run three observer from the MIDB [2,3] and facilitated several studies, including CAD investigations.

In many fields, the retention of unprocessed images is not commonplace. A distinct feature of MIDB is the provision of the unprocessed data that allows certain areas of research to take place, which would otherwise be difficult. An excellent example can be found in Interval Cancer review sessions for mammography. These can be stored, to evaluate whether an abnormality could have been detected on the previous screening films. The provision of unprocessed data from previous screening would allow the comprehensive evaluation of the full raft of factors affecting the reading of images. The effect of image processing can be investigated to find if different processing methods would have facilitated the location of the abnormality.

MedXViewer has been developed which interacts with the MIDB and associated study databases for remote image viewing and interaction. Combined, these provide the ability to run remote paper-less observer studies, provide a training infrastructure or coordinating remote collaborative viewing sessions (e.g. cancer reviews, interesting cases).

Acknowledgements. This work is part of the OPTIMAM project and is supported by CR-UK & EPSRC Cancer Imaging Programme in Surrey, in association with the MRC and Department of Health (England).

References

1. Patel, M.N., Looney, P.T., Young, K.C., Halling-Brown, M.D.: Automated collection of medical images for research from heterogeneous systems: Trials and tribulations. In: Proc. SPIE 9039 Medical Imaging (2014)
2. Mackenzie, A., et al.: Using image simulation to test the effect of detector type on breast cancer detection. In: Proc. SPIE 9037 Medical Imaging (2014)
3. Warren, L.M., Cooke, J., Given-Wilson, R., Wallis, M., Halling-Brown, M.: Effect of image processing on detection of non-calcification cancers in 2D digital mammography imaging. In: Proc SPIE Medical Imaging (2013)

Optimizing High Resolution Reconstruction in Digital Breast Tomosynthesis Using Filtered Back Projection

Shiras Abdurahman, Frank Dennerlein, Anna Jerebko, Andreas Fieselmann, and Thomas Mertelmeier

Siemens AG, Healthcare Sector, Allee am Röthelheimpark 2, 91052 Erlangen, Germany
{shiras.abdurahman.ext,frank.dennerlein,anna.jerebko, andreas.fieselmann,thomas.mertelmeier}@siemens.com

Abstract. In Digital Breast Tomosynthesis, a 3D representation of the breast is reconstructed from low-dose projection images acquired over a limited angular range. Each such image contains high level of noise which is often counteracted by a projection binning to yield the CNR desired in clinical applications. However, this approach reduces spatial resolution and makes imaging of high frequency structures such as micro-calcifications challenging. In this paper, we describe a Filtered Back Projection (FBP) reconstruction method optimized to yield improved CNR without sacrificing spatial resolution. The results from our quantitative evaluation and clinical reading by experienced radiologists indicate that the proposed methods can significantly improve contrast and sharpness of micro-calcifications and reduce noise compared to a baseline FBP method with standard filter settings.

Keywords: Digital Breast Tomosynthesis, Filtered Back Projection, Super-resolution, Artifact Reduction.

1 Introduction

In digital mammography, malignancy predictors such as spiculated masses can be obscured by overlapping tissues especially in dense breasts. Digital Breast Tomosynthesis (DBT) can overcome this limitation by reconstructing a 3D representation of the breast from projection images acquired over a limited angular range. Since the total radiation dose of a DBT exam is split over a number of projection views, the acquired images typically contain higher level of image noise than the standard FFDM images. To improve CNR in these images and in the DBT volume, projection binning is often used. However, this approach reduces 3D spatial resolution and might blur micro-calcifications. In this paper, an optimized, high-resolution DBT method* is presented that yields reconstructions with desired, high CNR without compromising on visibility of micro-calcifications.

---

* The concepts and information presented in this paper are based on research and are not commercially available.

H. Fujita, T. Hara, and C. Muramatsu (Eds.): IWDM 2014, LNCS 8539, pp. 520–527, 2014.
© Springer International Publishing Switzerland 2014

2 Method

DBT imaging involves acquisition of 25 projection images with the standard DBT mode of a MAMMOMAT Inspiration system[1] (Siemens AG, Erlangen, Germany). In this standard mode, the final volume is reconstructed into slices with 1 mm separation, each having an in-plane sampling of 0.085 mm × 0.085 mm which is identical to that of a projection image. The steps of our proposed reconstruction method are depicted in Fig. 1 and described in more details in the following sections.

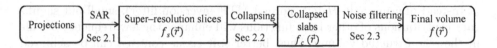

Fig. 1. Block diagram describing the major steps in optimized high resolution reconstruction. $\vec{r} = (x, y, z)^T$ defines location in 3D.

2.1 Super-Resolution Reconstruction with Statistical Artifact Reduction (SAR)

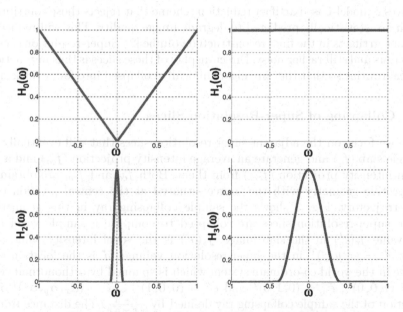

Fig. 2. Basis functions for MTF inversion filter

---

[1] Breast Tomosynthesis with Siemens MAMMOMAT Inspiration is an investigational practice and is limited by U.S. law to investigational use. It is not commercially available in the U.S. and its future availability cannot be ensured.

Filtering step of FBP in Breast Tomosynthesis often consists of MTF inversion filter, spectral filter and slice thickness filter [1]. MTF inversion filter reduces the blurring in the final reconstructed volume and spectral filter compensates the high frequency noise introduced by the MTF inversion filter [1]. Slice thickness filter is a low pass filter in z-direction which will give constant z-resolution and reduce out-of-plane blurring [1]. In our reconstructions, we used a modified MTF filter kernel which is generated by the linear combination of several basis functions (see Fig. 2) as in Eq. 1.

$$H(\omega) = H_0(\omega) + \beta_1 H_1(\omega) + \beta_2 H_2(\omega) + \beta_3 H_3(\omega) \tag{1}$$

Instead of using only $H_0(\omega)$ (normal MTF inversion filter), small but significant contributions of other basis functions will enhance the low frequency details in the reconstructed volume. Thus, better soft tissue contrast can be achieved without blurring the volume. The weights β_1, β_2 and β_3 are empirically determined by experienced readers.

We used unbinned projections for filtering to maximize the spatial resolution. Slice thickness filter is not used to avoid the blurring of micro-calcifications in the projections with high angle of incidence.

The filtered projections are back projected to produce an initial reconstruction on a super-resolution grid. Here, super-resolution means that DBT slices are separated by only < 0.3 mm such that they can nicely capture and represent even tiny diagnostic structures such as micro-calcifications. The back projection step involves a model-based artifact reduction scheme that rejects those contributions which are statistically predicted to degrade image quality. This will reduce out-of-plane artifacts in the final reconstructed volume [2]. Super-resolution slices are numerous and still rather noisy. Direct display of these slices is thus impractical in clinical routine so that they are algorithmically collapsed into fewer thick slabs.

2.2   Collapsing of Super-Resolution Slices

Here, we focus on the adjacent super-resolution slices that will eventually form a single slab (f_c) and generate an average intensity projection (f_{ca}) and a maximum intensity projection (f_{cm}) from them. Both f_{ca} and f_{cm} are obtained in perspective geometry with the source situated at the central position of the scan trajectory. Fig. 3 shows the sample collapsing ray in this geometry in which super-resolution slices are collapsed to compute a sample voxel intensity value $f_c(\vec{r})$ in the slab image. $f_s(\vec{r})$ is the voxel intensity value at 3D point $\vec{r} = (x, y, z)^T$ in the super-resolution volume. $\vec{a}$ is the location of the source in the world co-ordinate system which is spanned by orthonormal vectors $\vec{e_x} = (1, 0, 0)^T$, $\vec{e_y} = (0, 1, 0)^T$ and $\vec{e_z} = (0, 0, 1)^T$. $\vec{\alpha} = (\alpha_x, \alpha_y, \alpha_z)^T$ is the direction of the sample collapsing ray defined by $\frac{\vec{r} - \vec{a}}{\|\vec{r} - \vec{a}\|}$. The distance from the source along the ray is denoted by δ. Δ is the collapsing range which determines the number of adjacent super-resolution slices and θ is the angle between projected ray and normal to the slices. The voxel intensity value at $\vec{r}$ in f_{cm} and f_{ca} are given by the Eq. 2 and Eq. 3 respectively

$$f_{cm}(\vec{r}, \vec{a}, \Delta) = \max_{\delta} \left\{ f_s \left(\vec{r} + \delta \frac{\vec{r} - \vec{a}}{\|\vec{r} - \vec{a}\|} \right) \middle| \delta \in \left[-\frac{\Delta}{2\cos\theta}, \frac{\Delta}{2\cos\theta} \right] \right\} \qquad (2)$$

$$f_{ca}(\vec{r}, \vec{a}, \Delta) = \frac{1}{\Delta} \int_{-\frac{\Delta}{2\cos\theta}}^{\frac{\Delta}{2\cos\theta}} f\left(\vec{r} + \delta \frac{\vec{r} - \vec{a}}{\|\vec{r} - \vec{a}\|} \right) d\delta \qquad (3)$$

$\cos\theta$ is given by α_z.

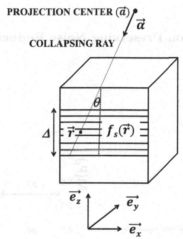

Fig. 3. Perspective geometry for collapsing of super-resolution slices

f_{ca} yields image with reduced noise while f_{cm} will preserve high attenuation structures present in the super-resolution slices. A thick slab is then obtained by combining f_{cm} and f_{ca} contributions, according to the following decision rule that is based on the distribution of the values that lie along the collapsing ray: If the maximum of these values exceeds their mean by more than a threshold t, we can assume the presence of a micro-calcification and therefore decide for the f_{cm} contribution. For all other areas, the f_{ca} value will be used in favor for high CNR. Instead of applying a purely binary decision rule which may cause artificial, high intensity outliers at random locations, we use a weighted combination f_{cm} and f_{ca} for slab generation according to the Eq. 4.

$$f_c(\vec{r}) = k\, f_{cm}(\vec{r}, \vec{a}, \Delta) + (1 - k)\, f_{ca}(\vec{r}, \vec{a}, \Delta) \qquad (4)$$

The weight k is calculated according to Fig. 4. The value t and w were manually optimized on clinical data sets to yield better visibility of micro-calcifications.

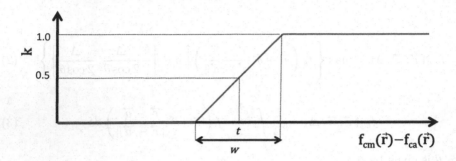

Fig. 4. The weight coefficient k for linear combination of $f_{cm}(\vec{r})$ and $f_{ca}(\vec{r})$

2.3 Micro-calcification Preserving Noise Reduction

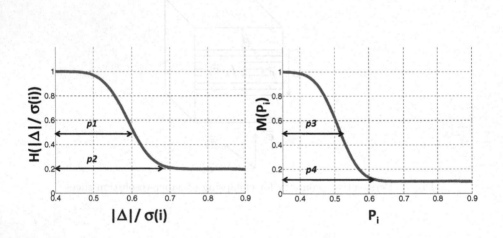

Fig. 5. Smoothing prior functions

In the final step, an iterative, edge and micro-calcification preserving noise filtering scheme is applied on each thick slab to further improve CNR. Eq. 5 and Eq. 6 describe iterative filtering in image domain in which local gradient in the slab image is minimized by number of iterations along with the constraints to preserve local edges and micro-calcifications.

$$f_c(i)^{k+1} = f_c(i)^k - \gamma \, \nabla R(f_c(i)^k) \tag{5}$$

$$\nabla R(f_c(i)^k) = \sum_{j \in N} d_j \Delta_{ji} H\left(\frac{|\Delta_{ji}|}{\sigma(i)}\right) M(P_i) \text{ with } \Delta_{ji} = f_c(j)^k - f_c(i)^k \tag{6}$$

$f_c(i)^k$ is the voxel intensity value at discrete location i in k^{th} iteration. γ is the relaxation factor and $\frac{|\Delta_{ji}|}{\sigma(i)}$ defines the local Contrast to Noise Ratio (CNR) around voxel location i with N adjacent neighborhood voxels. d_j is the filter coefficients.

H is the smoothing prior function as depicted in the Fig. 5 (left). Smoothing strength decreases nonlinearly and thus homogeneous regions are smoothed heavily compared to the the regions with high CNR. Iterative smoothing with only H may deteriorate the CNR of micro-calcifications in tomosynthesis images. $M(P_i)$ function penalizes the smoothing strength in the regions where micro-calcifications are present (see Fig. 5 (right)). In order to compute the pixel-wise likelihood of micro-calcifications (P_i) in the image, homogeneous background image is created by morphological open operation with a predefined structuring element s. Subtracting homogeneous image from original image and subsequent clipping of negative values yields image with probable micro-calcifications (P_i) as it is expressed in Eq. 7.

$$P = f - f \circ s \tag{7}$$

$M(P_i)$ is used to control the noise reduction. Smoothing is therefore strongest in homogeneous areas (contrasts lower than $p1$, see Fig.5 (left)) and practically nonexistent around micro-calcifications and other structures of interest (contrasts greater than $p1$).

The parameters of the noise reduction filter were manually optimized on clinical data sets to yield better visibility of micro-calcifications while maintaining minimal noise level.

3   Results

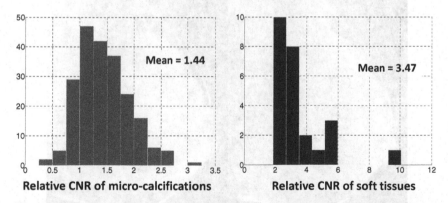

Fig. 6. Histogram of relative CNR for, left: Micro-calcifications; right: Masses

We used FBP with slice thickness filter in which thick slices of 1 mm separation are reconstructed as a baseline reconstruction method. To analyze the improvement of CNR in the new reconstruction method, we segmented 214 faint micro-calcifications in baseline reconstructions of 59 patient images and 25 soft tissue structures in focus from 25 reconstructed volumes. The relative CNR of each micro-calcification and soft tissue structure is computed as the ratio of CNR in images reconstructed with optimized high resolution reconstruction to their CNR in baseline reconstruction. Fig. 6 shows the histogram of the relative CNR of all micro-calcifications and soft tissue structures.

CNR is improved for 83% of the calcifications with an average improvement of 44%(p < 0.001). Fig. 8 presents representative micro-calcifications, clearly showing the improvement of contrast of calcifications (e.g right image, pointed by red arrow) and morphology of calcifications (e.g. left image). CNR is improved for all segmented soft tissue structures with an average improvement of 247% (p < 0.001). Fig. 7 shows the soft tissue contrast in two reconstructions. The new reconstruction method has also been evaluated in a clinical study by experienced readers [3]. Three radiologists evaluated 54 image pairs and compared optimized high resolution reconstruction with baseline FBP. The clinical study study validated our quantitative evaluations and confirmed the statistically significant improvement of new reconstruction method especially in visibility of micro-calcifications and soft tissue structures [3].

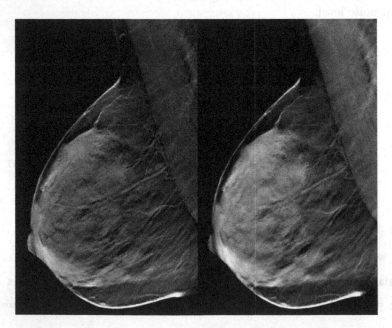

Fig. 7. Soft tissue structures obtained with, left: Baseline reconstruction; right: Optimized high resolution reconstruction. Images courtesy of Leuven University Hospital, Belgium.

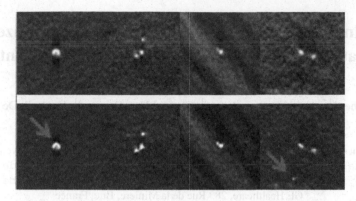

Fig. 8. Micro-calcifications obtained with, top: Baseline reconstruction; bottom: Optimized high resolution reconstruction. Images courtesy of Leuven University Hospital, Belgium.

4   Conclusion

Our results have shown that optimized high resolution reconstructed volumes preserve micro-calcification at high spatial resolution while maintaining noise level acceptable for clinical interpretations. Contrast and sharpness of micro-calcifications have been increased with reduced blurring and thus morphology of calcification clusters are preserved. Our results also show that the new reconstruction method improved CNR of soft tissue regions while preserving the details of spiculated masses such as architectural distortions. The results are validated by a reading study conducted by experienced radiologists.

References

1. Mertelmeier, T., Orman, J., Haerer, W., Dudam, M.K.: Optimizing filtered backprojection reconstruction for a breast tomosynthesis prototype device. In: Proc. SPIE 6142, 61420F-61420F-12 (2006)
2. Abdurahman, S., Jerebko, A., Mertelmeier, T., Lasser, T., Navab, N.: Out-of-Plane Artifact Reduction in Tomosynthesis Based on Regression Modeling and Outlier Detection. In: Maidment, A.D.A., Bakic, P.R., Gavenonis, S. (eds.) IWDM 2012. LNCS, vol. 7361, pp. 729–736. Springer, Heidelberg (2012)
3. Uchiyama, N., Machida, M., Tani, H., Kikuchi, M., Arai, Y., Otsuka, K., Fieselmann, A., Jerebko, A., Mertelmeier, T.: Clinical Efficacy of Novel Image Processing Techniques in the Framework of Filtered Back Projection (FBP) with Digital Breast Tomosynthesis (DBT). To be appeared in Breast Imaging. LNCS. Springer, Heidelberg (2014)

The Investigation of Different Factors to Optimize the Simulation of 3D Mass Models in Breast Tomosynthesis

Eman Shaheen[1,*], Frédéric Bemelmans[1], Chantal Van Ongeval[1], Frederik De Keyzer[1], Nausikaä Geeraert[1,2,3], and Hilde Bosmans[1]

[1] Department of Radiology, University Hospitals Leuven, Herestraat 49, 3000 Leuven, Belgium
{eman.shaheen,frederic.bemelmans,chantal.vanongeval,frederik.dek
eyzer,nausikaa.geeraert,hilde.bosmans}@uzleuven.be
[2] GE Healthcare, 283 Rue de la Miniere, Buc, France
[3] Institut Mines-Télécom, Telecom ParisTech, CNRS LTCI, 46 Rue Barrault, Paris, France
nausikaa.geeraert@student.kuleuven.be

Abstract. The development of 3D mass models of different shapes, margins and degrees of malignancy may allow more profound and clinically relevant testing and optimization of the performance of the newly introduced 3D modalities such as breast tomosynthesis and breast-CT. Three dimensional mass models had been developed earlier and were validated for the realism of their appearance after simulation into 2D and tomosynthesis patient images. Based on the feedback of the readers and the results of the simulations of the earlier study we initiated the present study in which we investigated the effect of insertion position and background glandular tissue estimation on the appearance of these masses. A subset of these masses was re-simulated in another position and using a different background estimator. These simulated masses were subsequently evaluated by an experienced radiologist on a 5-point scale realism score. The results showed that the insertion position of simulated masses is a significant factor in the appearance of realism of these masses and careful choices should be made.

Keywords: Digital mammography, breast tomosynthesis, 3D mass models, simulation.

1 Introduction

Mammography is the standard method for breast cancer screening. However, due to the projection of the 3D breast volume into a 2D image, lesions may stay hidden, with repercussions on detectability. Diagnostic radiology is embracing 3D modalities such as digital breast tomosynthesis (DBT) and breast computer tomography (breast-CT) that can overcome the issue of overlapping tissues. Simulation approaches are currently used to test and optimize the clinical performance of new modalities. They can be the basis for virtual clinical trials or for observer studies of patient images with

---

* Corresponding author.

H. Fujita, T. Hara, and C. Muramatsu (Eds.): IWDM 2014, LNCS 8539, pp. 528–535, 2014.

simulated lesions. Due to the 3D nature of these new modalities, the development of virtual 3D abnormalities including masses and microcalcification clusters is required.

A method was presented to simulate 3D mass models with a variety of margins and shapes. These masses have been validated for the realism of their appearance when inserted into 2D and DBT patient images [1]. This earlier validation study had revealed a more realistic performance of the masses when simulated in 2D than in DBT. In this study, we investigated parameters adjusted during the insertion procedure that affect the appearance of the masses in DBT without changing the 3D mass models in order to further improve the simulations.

2   Materials and Methods

2.1   Database of Mass Models

The previously presented method [1] for developing 3D mass models started from a collection of 25 contrast enhanced breast MRI lesions that were manually segmented and were further processed to represent high resolution isotropic 3D mass models. These models are categorized as "non-spiculated" masses and were then used as nuclei on which spicules were grown following an iterative branching algorithm [2]. We generated 30 "spiculated" masses. The realism of the appearance of the 55 models was assessed in two separate studies after insertion in 2D digital mammography and breast tomosynthesis patient images by means of a validated simulation framework [3, 4].

2.2   The Choice of the Investigated Factors

The fact that the simulation of masses in DBT versus 2D mammography is more challenging can be explained. First, DBT shows more details of the margins of the masses compared to 2D mammography. Second, the simulation of masses in acquired patient images is difficult as the simulation procedure cannot replace the original tissue by a mass: in our approach, a mass is simulated using an expected density difference with the present background structure.

Following the feedback of the radiologists who participated in the validation studies, the main causes for scoring a lesion to be unrealistic included: (1) the higher density of some masses compared to the surrounding background tissues; (2) some masses looked artificially superimposed and this was especially the case with some irregular or spiculated masses that did not integrate well with the background tissue. Therefore, we studied two main parameters: (1) the effect of another estimate of the glandularity (the percentage of dense glandular tissue) at the insertion position (Volpara) [5]; (2) the influence of insertion position presuming that this is determining for how the lesion can integrate with the background.

2.3   Simulation Framework

The simulation framework was previously validated [3] and used to simulate microcalcification clusters [4]. In this approach, templates of lesions were created that maximally account for the polychromatic spectrum, for the tissue into which an object is simulated and for detector characteristics. Mass models were ray traced, and the contrast of the output templates was adjusted for the x-ray spectrum that has been used in the patient image into which the mass has to be simulated. The masses were assumed to be 100% glandular tissue and the background was assumed to be a composition of adipose and glandular tissues with attenuation coefficients as found by Hammerstein et al. [6]. The glandularity of the background at the insertion position had been estimated based on the mean pixel value in the ROI of insertion in the raw 2D patient image using a method derived from Kaufhold et al. [7]. The projections of the masses were further modified to include the unsharpness due to focal spot motion blur and scatter. These adjusted templates were then multiplied with raw patient images. All hybrid raw projection images were then reconstructed using the Siemens software (TomoEngine, Siemens, Erlangen, Germany) that is based on the filtered back-projection algorithm (FBP). The reconstructed voxel size was 0.085x0.085x1 mm^3. All 2D raw images were processed using the system's image processing algorithm (Opview2, Siemens, Erlangen, Germany).

2.4   Observer Study

In the earlier validation study [1], 55 3D mass models were developed. Of these, the best five and the worst fifteen in terms of realistic appearance were selected. Ten were non-spiculated masses and the other ten were spiculated ones. Each mass out of the 20, with the original settings, was re-simulated for two new settings: (1) within the same patient at the same insertion position with the glandularity of the background estimated using Volpara that gave slightly lower values compared to the originally used in-house method in the earlier validation study (settings 1); (2) at an another insertion location possibly allowing the lesion to integrate better with the background tissue (settings 2).

Two studies were conducted, one for 2D and the other for DBT, with a total of 80 masses per modality. Twenty were real masses and the remaining 60 were simulated masses: (1) the chosen 20 masses were taken from the earlier study [1], (2) 20 re-simulated masses based on the first proposed settings, (2) the 20 re-simulated based on the second proposed settings. These 80 masses were randomly distributed and read by an experienced radiologist who had participated in the earlier validation study. The radiologist was asked to score the realism of the mass on a 5-point scale and to score the BIRADS [8] of the lesion.

The scores of the 2 proposed settings were compared to the original settings in a paired analysis using the Wilcoxon signed rank test for both 2D and DBT. The scores of the group of masses that had the highest realism score from the three simulated groups were then compared to the scores of the real masses by means of the Mann-Whitney analysis for 2D and DBT. The BIRADS scores were also evaluated for the different settings using the Wilcoxon signed rank test per modality. Then the BIRADS scores of DBT were compared to the corresponding 2D scores per group of masses. P > 0.05 indicates statistically significant difference.

3   Results

Table 1 shows the mean and standard deviation of the realism scores in 2D and DBT for every mass category: the 20 masses with original settings, the 20 masses re-simulated following settings 1, the 20 masses re-simulated following settings 2 and the 20 real masses. The masses re-simulated with settings 2 had the highest scores in both modalities and this group will be used for further analysis.

Table 1. The mean and standard deviation of the realism scores in 2D and DBT for every mass category: the 20 masses with original settings, the 20 masses re-simulated following settings 1, the 20 masses re-simulated following settings 2 and the 20 real masses

Mass Category	2D realism scores		DBT realism scores	
	Mean	Standard deviation	Mean	Standard deviation
Original settings	4.2	±0.85	3.1	±0.89
Settings 1	4.3	±0.71	3.7	±0.91
Settings 2	4.6	±0.80	4.0	±0.67
Real masses	4.6	±0.74	4.3	±1.04

3.1   Results of the 2D Study

Figures 1 and 2 show an example of a non-spiculated and a spiculated mass respectively simulated into 2D images for the different settings: (a) as originally simulated in the earlier study; (b) the mass re-simulated in the original position but using Volpara as estimator (settings 1); (c) the mass re-simulated at an optimized position (settings 2). Table 2 shows the results of comparing the realism scores, in the 2D study, between the different settings. It is clear that no statistically significant difference was found between the original simulation settings compared to settings 1 and 2. For the comparison of the highest scored settings (settings 2) to the real masses, no statistically significant difference was found.

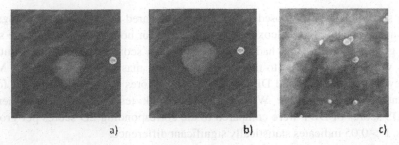

Fig. 1. An example of a non-spiculated mass simulated into 2D patient images with the three different settings. a) The originally simulated mass from the earlier study (realism score = 2). b) The mass re-simulated in the original position using Volpara as estimator (settings 1, realism score = 2). c) The mass re-simulated at an improved position (settings 2, realism score = 5).

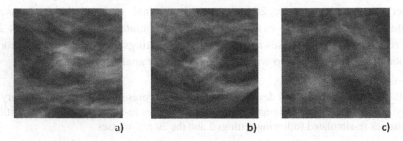

Fig. 2. An example of a spiculated mass simulated into 2D patient images with the three different settings. a) The originally simulated mass from the earlier study (realism score = 4). b) The mass re-simulated in the original position using Volpara as estimator (settings 1, realism score = 5). c) The mass re-simulated at an improved position (settings 2, realism score = 5).

Table 2. The results of the realism scores of the 2D study for the different simulation settings using Wilcoxon ranked test and Mann-Whitney tests reporting the p-values. n.s. indicates that the test revealed none significance but accurate p-value calculation was not possible.

	Wilcoxon p-value	Mann-Whitney p-value
Original vs Settings 1	n.s.	-
Original vs Settings 2	0.201	-
Real vs Settings 2	-	0.787

3.2   Results of the DBT Study

Table 3 shows the results of comparing the realism scores, in the DBT study, between the different settings. It is clear that both new settings (1 and 2) were statistically significantly better than the original simulation settings. When the simulated masses of the highest scored settings (settings 2) were compared to the real masses, no statistically significant difference was found while in the earlier study with the original settings, a statistical significant difference was found between real and simulated masses.

Figures 3 and 4 show an example of a non-spiculated and a spiculated mass respectively simulated into DBT images for the different settings: (a) as originally simulated in the earlier study; (b) the mass re-simulated in the original position but using Volpara as estimator (settings 1); (c) the mass re-simulated at an optimized position (settings 2).

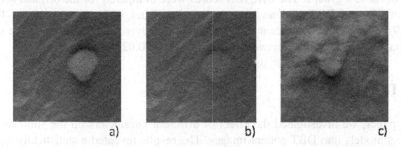

Fig. 3. An example of the non-spiculated mass simulated (as in figure 1) into DBT patient images with the three different settings, the in-focus reconstructed plane is shown. a) The originally simulated mass from the earlier study (realism score = 3). b) The mass re-simulated in the original position using Volpara as estimator (settings 1, realism score = 4). c) The mass re-simulated at an improved position (settings 2, realism score = 5).

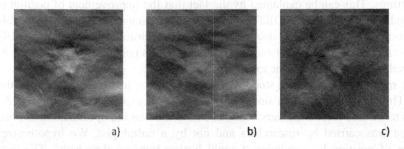

Fig. 4. An example of the spiculated mass simulated (as in figure 2) into DBT patient images with the three different settings, the in-focus reconstructed plane is shown. a) The originally simulated mass from the earlier study (realism score = 3). b) The mass re-simulated in the original position using Volpara as estimator (settings 1, realism score = 4). c) The mass re-simulated at an improved position (settings 2, realism score = 4).

Table 3. The results of the realism scores of the DBT study for the different simulation settings using Wilcoxon ranked test and Mann-Whitney tests reporting the p-values. The asterix (*) indicates statistically significant difference.

	Wilcoxon p-value	Mann-Whitney p-value
Original vs Settings 1	0.024*	-
Original vs Settings 2	0.005*	-
Real vs Settings 2	-	0.085

3.3   Results of the BIRADS Scores

The p-value of the Wilcoxon test applied to the simulated masses with the original settings compared to the masses re-simulated with settings 2 was 0.043 for 2D and 0.001 for DBT indicating statistically significant differences between the BIRADS scores of these 2 groups. The BIRADS scores were compared for the original settings between 2D and DBT and no statistically significant difference had been found (p=0.49). Statistically significant difference was however found comparing the simulated masses with settings 2 between 2D and DBT (p=0.027).

4   Discussion

In this paper, we investigated the effect of different parameters on the simulation of 3D mass models into DBT patient images. The results revealed a statistically significant improvement in the DBT realism scores for the second settings (optimization of position) when compared to the original settings while the realism scores in 2D were unchanged. This indicated that careful choices of insertion positions highly influence the realism of appearance of lesions especially when inserted into a 3D modality such as DBT. The results also revealed a significant change in the BIRADS scores between 2D and DBT for the improved positioning (settings 2) that didn't appear for the original settings. This can be explained by the fact that the improvement of positioning in this study was optimized in DBT regardless the appearance in 2D. Although this optimization didn't affect the realism scores in 2D it occasionally changed the BIRADS scores of some masses to be 1 (normal) because it was not appearing as a mass but as a normal tissue as shown in the example of figure 5.

The main limitation of this study was that only one reader has so far scored the images. This reader was chosen since she was the most experienced with DBT. A next step is to include more observers. Another limitation was the optimization of positioning that was carried by researchers and not by a radiologist. We hypothesize that choices of position by a radiologist could further improve the results. The fact that also non-radiologists are able to position the mass lesions is promising in the frame of the development of extensive studies. The scientist in charge needed on average three

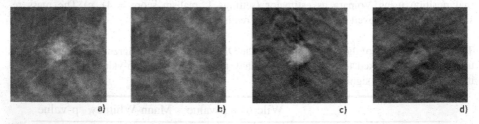

a)   b)   c)   d)

Fig. 5. An example of a simulated spiculated mass in different settings. a) original settings in 2D, BIRADS score = 4. b) improved positioning (settings 2) in 2D, BIRADS score = 1. c) original settings in DBT, BIRADS score = 5. b) improved positioning (settings 2) in DBT, BIRADS score = 3.

iterations before deciding that a new position provided a good new candidate lesion position. All positions in the present study got a final check by either a radiologist or an experienced physicist to reduce the risk of artificially superimposed lesions. Some real lesions can have strange appearances and were sometimes considered unrealistic. As an example, some lesions appeared isolated within the breast region. We have learnt that it was not appropriated to reproduce such rare situations.

5   Conclusion

The simulation of 3D mass models is important to allow the investigation and optimization of the clinical performance of DBT especially when compared to 2D digital mammography. In an earlier study, we developed 55 mass models and validated the realism of their appearance in 2D and DBT. In this study, we attempted to improve their appearance by exploring the limiting factors found in the earlier study such as the estimation of the background composition and a better insertion position. The results showed that the optimization of positioning improved significantly the realism scores in DBT while in 2D the realism scores were unchanged. The BIRADS scores also revealed the influence of this optimization in 2D where some masses were less visible than before. The choices of insertion positions to simulate masses play an important role in the appearance of realism of these masses and should be carried out carefully.

References

1. Shaheen, E., De Keyzer, F., Bosmans, H., et al.: The simulation of 3D mass models in 2D digital mammography and breast tomosynthesis. Submitted to Med. Phys. (December 2013)
2. De Sisternes, L., Zysk, A.M., et al.: Development of a Computational Three-Dimensional Breast Lesion Phantom Model. In: Proc. SPIE, vol. 7622, pp. 7622051–7622058 (2010)
3. Shaheen, E., Zanca, F., et al.: Simulation of 3D objects into breast tomosynthesis images. Radiat. Prot. Dosim. 139, 108–112 (2010)
4. Shaheen, E., et al.: The simulation of 3D microcalcification clusters in 2D digital mammography and breast tomosynthesis. Med. Phys. 38(12), 6659–6671 (2011)
5. Highnam, R., Brady, S.M., Yaffe, M.J., Karssemeijer, N., Harvey, J.: Robust breast composition measurement-volpara. In: Martí, J., Oliver, A., Freixenet, J., Martí, R. (eds.) IWDM 2010. LNCS, vol. 6136, pp. 342–349. Springer, Heidelberg (2010)
6. Hammerstein, G.R., Miller, D.W., White, D.R., et al.: Absorbed radiation dose in Mammography. Radiology 130, 485–491 (1979)
7. Kaufhold, J., et al.: A calibration approach to glandular tissue composition estimation in digital mammography. Med. Phys. 29(8), 1867–1880 (2002)
8. American College of Radiology. Breast Imaging Reporting and Data System (BI-RADS), 4th edn. American College of Radiology, Reston (2003)

Clinical Evaluation of Dual Mode Tomosynthesis

Tokiko Endo[1], Mikinao Ooiwa[1], Takako Morita[1], Namiko Suda[1],
Kazuaki Yoshikawa[2], Misaki Shiraiwa[3], Yukie Hayashi[4], Takao Horiba[5],
Yasuyuki Sato[1], Shu Ichihara[1], Tomonari Sendai[6],
Tetsuro Kusunoki[6], and Takahisa Arai[6]

[1] National Hospital Organization Nagoya Medical Center, Aichi, Japan
[2] National Hospital Organization Hamada Medical Center, Shimane, Japan
[3] Kagawa Prefectural Central Hospital, Kagawa, Japan
[4] Hayashi Clinic, Aichi, Japan
[5] Tokai Central Hospital, Gifu, Japan
[6] FUJIFILM Corporation, Kanagawa, Japan

Abstract. Clinical performance achieved by adding interpretation of Tomosynthesis images to 2D images (hereinafter 2D+Tomo) was studied. 100 cases who gave written informed consent (ST mode: angular range ±7.5deg, 50 cases and HR mode: ±20deg, 50 cases) were obtained and 7 radiologists interpreted all images. In ST, the sensitivity is significantly increased by 15% (P<.01) and specificity is equivalent (P=.73). In HR, sensitivity of 2D+Tomo against 2D alone is significantly increased by 30% (P<.001) and specificity is significantly decreased by 5% (P<.01). ST, which has higher sensitivity and equivalent specificity, can be used for screening, and HR, which can visualize structures such as lesions in details, can be used for diagnosis. Moreover, specificity enhancement due to inhibition of false positive and sensitivity enhancement are confirmed by trial for appropriate segmentation in Japanese category classification C3. Further detailed clinical performance will be studied such as in ROC analysis with more cases.

1 Introduction

Breast cancer is the highest rate of cancer among Japanese women. Early detection and therapy would be the best to reduce the cancer mortality rate. The mammography process is commonly used for the early detection and diagnosis of cancer. However, it is believed that the mammography process may increase the risk of developing cancer due to x-ray irradiations. To prevent this from occurring, processes with lower level of x-ray irradiations and high diagnostic skills are in great demand. As such, in recent years mammography processes with lower x-ray irradiations level, smaller pixel sizes, efficient screening and processing capabilities have been developed [1].

On the other hand, there are many cases of breast cancer in Japan due to the high percentage of dense breast among Japanese women. In comparison to other countries, breast cancer is at its peak in Japan for women from their late 40s to early 50s. It is, therefore, vital that measures be taken to overcome this issue and Tomosynthesis is

H. Fujita, T. Hara, and C. Muramatsu (Eds.): IWDM 2014, LNCS 8539, pp. 536–543, 2014.
© Springer International Publishing Switzerland 2014

being recommended. Tomosynthesis is a technology capable of reducing superimposed structures such as mammary glands. The Tomosynthesis process is able to obtain multiple images from various angles, reconstructs and creates "sliced" images in the human body. In the field of mammography, Tomosynthesis is considered to be a technique which improves diagnostic performance [2,3,4,5,6,7], capable of observing superimposed legions such as tumor and overlapped mammary glands. This would enable easier detection of lesions.

We would now like to discuss the results of the study of the clinical efficacy using the 2-D image of a breast in identical condition as reference and the addition of Tomosynthesis images.

2   Methods and Materials

The study was conducted with the approval of the Institutional Review Board of the National Hospital Organization, Nagoya Medical Center in Japan.

FUJIFILM's AMULET Innovality equipped with Dual Mode Tomosynthesis functionality was used as the mammography device. The Dual Modes are, ST mode which realizes highly efficient workflow and low radiation dose examination with the angular range of ±7.5°, and HR mode which realizes high image quality and high resolution with angular range of ±20°.

The hospital is an institution where patients of breast disease undergo long-term follow-ups, thorough examinations and treatments, and it is not a facility where patients undergo breast screenings. Owing to this, subjects of this study who consented to participate have been selected from patients of the hospital for the purpose of breast diagnosis.

A total of 100 cases in 183 breasts collected from August 19th, 2012 were chosen as the candidates of this study. Among the 100 cases, 50 cases/100 breasts were examined with 2D+ST mode and the other 50 cases/100 breasts were examined with 2D+HR mode. Furthermore, 17 micro-calcifications cases those have less mammary gland and no appearance like masses were excluded from the analysis because additional information could not be obtained though Tomosynthesis image was added to 2D.

In all the cases used for the study in interpretation, the cancer cases confirmed by pathological diagnosis are classified as malignant, no particular findings and mastopathy cases in integrated diagnosis of MMG and US are categorized as normal, and other cases are categorized as benign.

Details of all the cases from the results of this classification are: 43 normal breasts (28 breasts of no particular findings and 15 breasts of mastopathy), 43 benign breasts and 7 malignant breasts in ST mode; and 31 normal breasts (17 breasts of no particular findings and 14 breasts of mastopathy), 50 benign breasts and 9 malignant breasts in HR mode.

Seven radiologists, who are Class A approved radiologists by The Japan Central Institute on Quality Assurance of Breast Cancer Screening, interpreted only 2D and recorded the position of lesions, findings, category classification for Japan and POM

(Probability Of Malignancy). After the interpretation of 2D, the radiologists interpreted 2D with Tomosynthesis images and recorded the same information.

The bases of the category classification for Japan was adapted from BI-RADS (Breast Imaging Reporting and Data System) by ACR (American College of Radiology) and it was optimised to be used in Japan as shown in Table 1. The category 3 or higher needs additional diagnosis such as ultrasound, MRI and biopsy.

Table 1. Category classification for Japan

Category	Class
C1	Negative
C2	Benign
C3	Benign, but malignancy cannot be ruled out
C4	Suspicious abnormality
C5	Highly suggestive of malignancy

POM is a 0 to 100 score assigned by radiologist to each suspicious finding, as their perception of the percentage chance that the suspicious finding might be malignant.

Sensitivities, specificities and AUCs (Area Under the Curve) according to ROC (Receiver Operating Characteristic) analysis [8] (DBM MRMC 2.2 [9]) between 2D alone and 2D+Tomo were compared from the result of the interpretation. Statistical significance tests for the sensitivity and specificity from the results in 2D alone and the results in 2D+Tomo were implemented by McNemar's test.

Discretion flow of positive and negative cases is shown in Figure 1.

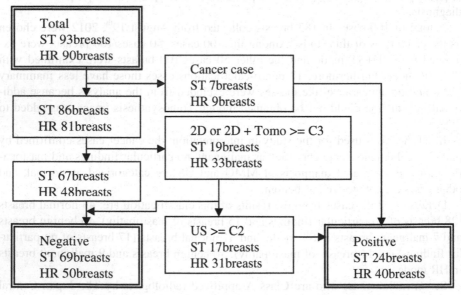

Fig. 1. Discretion flow of positive and negative cases

Mammograpy does not offer a definite diagnosis. Therefore, the purpose of this study is to clarify a detection performance for cases which need additional diagnosis by 2D+Tomo. Now, therefore in this study, the cases other than 'normal' and 'masto-pathy' were considered as Positive, and the rest of the cases were considered as Negative. However, since AUC was calculated by using a probability of malignancy for ROC analysis, only cancer cases were considered as Positive.

3   Results

3.1   Sensitivity

The sensitivity acquired from the result of the interpretations by 2D alone as well as 2D+Tomo, is shown in Table 2. In the interpretations with 2D+Tomo in ST mode, 1.15 times as much as the sensitivity of 2D alone was improved. Moreover, in the interpretations with 2D+Tomo in HR mode, 1.30 times as much as the sensitivity of 2D alone was improved.

Table 2. Sensitivity by all radiologists

Tomo Mode	2D	2D+Tomo	Ratio	P - value
ST mode	64.9%	74.4%	1.15	<.01
HR mode	52.9%	68.9%	1.30	<.001

3.2   Specificity

The specificity acquired from the result of the interpretations by 2D alone as well as 2D+Tomo, is shown in Table 3. There was no significant difference in specificity between the images of the interpretation with 2D+Tomo in ST mode and 2D alone; and the interpretation with 2D+Tomo in HR mode was decreased by 0.95 times as much as the specificity of 2D alone.

Table 3. Specificity by all radiologists

Tomo Mode	2D	2D+Tomo	Ratio	P - value
ST mode	89.4%	89.0%	1.00	.73
HR mode	94.0%	88.9%	0.95	<.01

3.3   ROC Analysis

The value for the AUC from the result of the interpretations by 2D alone as well as 2D+Tomo is shown in Table 4. There was no significant difference between the interpretation with 2D+Tomo (both in ST and HR mode) and 2D alone.

Table 4. Area under the pooled ROC curve

Tomo Mode	2D	2D+Tomo	Difference	P - value
ST mode	0.919	0.963	0.044	0.05
HR mode	0.856	0.875	0.019	0.61

Tomo Mode	95% CI
ST mode	-0.08848 , 0.00006
HR mode	-0.09642 , 0.05800

4   Discussion

4.1   Clinical Performance of Additional Interpretation with HR Images

In interpretations with the HR images added, the specificity decreased though the sensitivity enhancement rate increased compared with the interpretation of 2D alone. This is because the fine lesions such as small tumor and duct ectasis which cannot be visualized in 2D, were visualized as shown in Figure 2. In this way, it is suggested that the interpretations with 2D+Tomo in HR mode is expected to be used for breast diagnosis because it has high sensitivity and structures such as lesion can be visualized in detail.

4.2   Clinical Performance for Additional Interpretation with ST Images

On the other hand, In the interpretations with 2D+Tomo in ST mode, the sensitivity was higher than the 2D alone and the specificity was equivalent though the sensitivity did not increase as much as the interpretation with 2D+Tomo in HR mode. Hence, it is suggested that the interpretations with 2D+Tomo in ST mode is expected to be used for breast screening.

4.3   Opinion: Sensitivity of 2D

Sensitivities acquired from the result of the interpretations of 2D are different between the group of ST and HR mode. The reasons for the difference are considered to be as follows:

1. Numbers of positive cases are biased. (24 breasts in ST mode and 40 breasts in HR mode)
2. Types of positive cases (such as size and form of tumor) are biased.

These reasons should be taken in consideration for future studies.

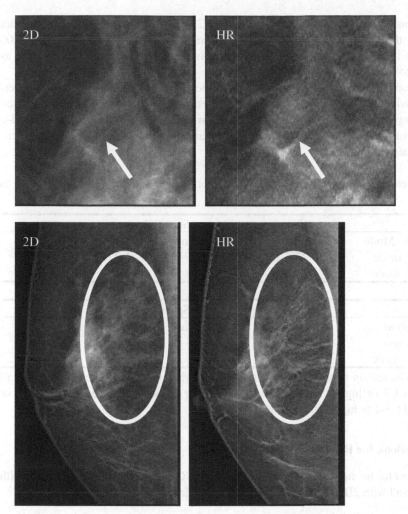

Fig. 2. 2D and HR images of small tumor (arrowed parts in the top images) and duct ectasia (circled in the bottom images)

4.4   Trial for Enhancement of Specificity

In the event the present category classification for Japan of C3 or higher is set as recall, specificity decrease cannot be avoided in the interpretations with 2D+Tomo in HR mode. Therefore, the category C3 was divided into C3-1 (follow-up) and C3-2 (recall), and the sensitivities and specificities of them were compared. The judgment criteria of the division was circumscribed margin, low density and scattered distribution of masses in small quantity. They are categorized based on the experiences of the radiologists. As the result, the specificity, which had been 0.95 times as much as 2D alone in C3, was improved to 0.99 times as much as 2D alone by changing the category to C3-2. It resulted in no significant difference with 2D alone. Moreover, the sensitivity became 1.33

times as much as 2D in C3-2 from 1.30 times in C3. Furthermore, the specificity did not change in the interpretations 2D+Tomo in ST mode compared with 2D alone (1.00 times both in C3 and C3-2); and the sensitivity increased from 1.15 times as much as 2D in C3 to 1.27 times in C-3-2. (Table 5)

Based on the above, it is believed that the specificity which deceased in the interpretation with 2D+Tomo in HR mode could be enhanced with false positive inhibition by dividing the category classification for Japan C3 into C3-1 (follow-up) and C3-2 (recall). In addition, it is believed that the compatibility with the enhancement of sensitivity is also possible.

Table 5. Sensitivity and specificity when the category classification C3-2 or higher is set as recall

	Sensitivity			
Tomo Mode	2D	2D+Tomo	Ratio	P - value
ST mode	43.5%	55.4%	1.27	<.001
HR mode	30.0%	40.0%	1.33	<.001

	Specificity			
Tomo Mode	2D	2D+Tomo	Ratio	P - value
ST mode	94.2%	94.6%	1.00	.64
HR mode	98.3%	97.2%	0.99	.53

Note. The reason why the sensitivity is lower when C3-2 or higher is set as recall than when C3 or higher is set, is that the number of positive cases between C3 or higher and C3-2 or higher are identical.

4.5   Outlook for Results of ROC Analysis

The reasons for no significant difference in the AUC between the interpretations with 2D alone and with 2D+Tomo are likely to be as follow:

1. The number of cancer cases and total cases are insufficient. (6 positive cases out of 43 cases in ST mode and 8 positive cases out of 42 cases in HR mode)
2. The number of cases, which have different results between the interpretation with 2D alone and 2D+Tomo, are extremely rare.

As such, the above should be considered for further studies.

5   Conclusion

Clinical performance that can be achieved from addition of the interpretation of Tomosynthesis images to 2D was studied. The result of this study confirmed that the interpretation with 2D+Tomo in HR mode could have higher sensitivity and the capability of visualizing structures such as lesions in more detail as compared to the interpretation of 2D alone. As such, it is possible to use HR images for breast diagnosis.

In contrast, the interpretation with 2D+Tomo in ST mode has equivalent specificity although it has higher sensitivity compared to the interpretation of 2D alone. Therefore, it is possible to use ST images for screening. Furthermore, the specificity was enhanced due to inhibition of false positive and the sensitivity was enhanced in the interpretation with Tomosynthesis images added to the interpretation of 2D alone by appropriately dividing the Class C3 of the category classification for Japan. More detailed clinical performance studies will be carried out by increasing the number of cases in analyses such as ROC analysis.

References

1. Yoshihiro, O., Keiichiro, S., Takaaki, I., Yuichi, H., Toshirou, H.: A newly developed a-Se mammography flat panel detector with high-sensitivity and low image artifact. In: Proc. of SPIE, vol. 8668, 86685V-1–86685V-9 (2013)
2. Rafferty, E.A., Park, J.M., Philpotts, L.E., Poplack, S.P., Sumkin, J.H., Halpern, E.F., Niklason, L.T.: Assessing Radiologist Performance Using Combined Digital Mammography and Breast Tomosynthesis Compared with Digital Mammography Alone: Results of a Multicenter, Multireader Trial. Radiology 266(1), 104–113 (2013)
3. Rafferty, E.A., Park, J.M., Philpotts, L.E., Poplack, S.P., Sumkin, J.H., Halpern, E.F., Niklason, L.T.: Diagnostic Accuracy and Recall Rates for Digital Mammography and Digital Mammography Combined With One-View and Two-View Tomosynthesis: Results of an Enriched Reader Study. American Journal of Roentgenology 202(2), 273–281 (2014)
4. Wallis, M.G., Moa, E., Zanca, F., Leifland, K., Danielsson, M.: Two-View and Single-View Tomosynthesis versus Full-Field Digital Mammography: High-Resolution X-Ray Imaging Observer Study. Radiology 262(3), 788–796 (2012)
5. Gennaro, G., Toledano, A., di Maggio, C., Baldan, E., Bezzon, E., La Grassa, M., Pescarini, L., Polico, I., Proietti, A., Toffoli, A., Muzzio, P.C.: Digital breast tomosynthesis versus digital mammography: A clinical performance study. European Radiology 20(7), 1545–1553 (2010)
6. Kopans, D.B.: Digital Breast Tomosynthesis From Concept to Clinical Care. American Journal of Roentgenology 202(2), 299–308 (2014)
7. Svahn, T.M., Chakraborty, D.P., Ikeda, D., Zackrisson, S., Do, Y., Mattsson, S., Andersson, I.: Breast tomosynthesis and digital mammography: A comparison of diagnostic accuracy. British Journal of Radiology 85(1019), e1074–e1082 (2012)
8. Hanley, J.A., McNeil, B.: The Meaning and Use of the Area under a Receiver Operating Characteristic (ROC) Cureve. Diagnostic Radiology 143(1), 29–36 (1982)
9. DBM MRMC 2.2 Build 3, http://metz-roc.uchicago.edu/

Image Quality of Thick Average Intensity Pixel Slabs Using Statistical Artifact Reduction in Breast Tomosynthesis[*]

Magnus Dustler[1,*], Pontus Timberg[2], Anders Tingberg[1], and Sophia Zackrisson[2]

[1] Medical Radiation Physics, Department of Clinical Sciences Malmö, Lund University, Malmö
[2] Diagnostic Radiology, Department of Clinical Sciences Malmö, Lund University, Malmö
magnus.dustler@med.lu.se

Abstract. Digital Breast Tomosynthesis (DBT) has the potential to replace or supplement Digital Mammography (DM). Studies have shown that it takes radiologists more time to read DBT examinations compared with DM. The slice separation of image volumes has been set to 1 mm on most systems. By using thicker slices review time could be reduced. This paper investigates the possibility of using 2 mm Average Intensity Pixel (AIP) slabs for image review. The thicker slabs were created using a method based on statistical artifact reduction and super-resolution. Six radiologists were presented with 20 sets of images containing 16 tumor masses and 8 micro-calcification clusters. They ranked 2 mm slabbed sets relative to standard 1 mm. Visibility (P = .0044) of micro-calcifications improved and there was no significant effect on mass visibility (P = .46). The results indicate that it is possible to review DBT-volumes with 2 mm slabs without compromising image quality.

1 Introduction

During recent years, digital breast tomosynthesis, (DBT), has moved from the laboratory to the clinic, with many vendors having developed dedicated systems. Several studies suggest that DBT has the potential to become an important tool in both screening- and clinical settings; showing increased detection rates both in combination with digital mammography (DM) and on its own [1-6]. However, DBT, as an emerging and continuously maturing modality, must adapt and conform to the realities of clinical usage.

Radiologists, especially in a screening setting, prefer novel technologies that decrease, or at least do not increase their workload. If an increase in workload is balanced by corresponding improvements in e.g. patient care this may well be an acceptable tradeoff, but care should be taken to minimize the additional workload required. In the case of DBT, a major negative aspect of the new modality compared to the gold standard of DM is the increased review time [3,4,6,7]. This is a direct consequence of the nature of DBT: sifting through a 3D image volume slice-by-slice

---

* Corresponding author

H. Fujita, T. Hara, and C. Muramatsu (Eds.): IWDM 2014, LNCS 8539, pp. 544–549, 2014.
© Springer International Publishing Switzerland 2014

takes more time than viewing a single 2D mammogram. This is to some extent un-avoidable – especially so in set-ups where DBT images is reviewed in addition to DM images – but optimization of the reviewing of 3D-volumes is important if DBT is to become a screening modality.

Currently, an arbitrarily chosen slice separation of 1 mm has become widely accepted. It is possible to reconstruct at other thicknesses, but this would require the tailoring of filters and parameters to fit the new thickness [8]. In general, tomosynthesis, due to a limited angular range, suffers from relatively substantial out-of-plane artifacts (compared to e.g. CT) which limit the depth resolution, meaning that the size and depth of structures is badly defined [9-12].

This study uses the intuitive method of reducing the amount of images, i.e. using thicker slices. This has been shown to reduce review time, but it remains untested if image quality is adversely affected, which this study seeks to investigate [13].

2   Method

2.1   Slabbing

Combining, or "slabbing", a number of reconstructed slices into a thicker slab has been investigated and is often a standard option on workstations [13-15]. To create slabs, two intuitively simple approaches are standard: average intensity projection (AIP) and maximum intensity projection (MIP). AIP-slabbing smooth images in the z-direction, reducing noise but also reducing contrast of small structures such as micro-calcifications. In MIP-slabs, the noise in each constituent slice will be added together in the z-direction, which can potentially increase the visibility of micro-calcifications by combining vertically separated calcifications into the same slab. Slabs can also be made overlapping, so that each slice is included in more than one slab. This can provide smoother transitions when viewing the volume in a loop or scrolling through it, but has a negative impact on depth resolution if slice number is to be preserved.

To make effective slabs of arbitrary thickness, this study employs a method based on super-resolution and a statistical artifact reduction scheme [16]. In this paper this will be referred to as SRSAR. It bypasses some of the limitations of standard filtered-back projection (FBP) reconstructions by reconstructing very thin slices (0.1 mm) and removes artifacts by an outlier detection algorithm, instead of using a slice-thickness filter. This approach in theory provides better depth resolution by suppressing out-of plane artifacts, but also increases image noise. SRSAR was suitable for the study as the reconstructed thin slices can be collapsed into slabs of suitable thickness, using AIP to limit image noise and preserve depth resolution. In the version we employed, an additional iterative filter was used to reduce image noise. In theory the SRSAR method should yield better soft-tissue contrast and this – along with effective artifact reduction – could offset negative impacts on image quality from slabbing, and thus be a better alternative than simply slabbing standard FBP volumes.

Table 1. Description of grading criteria. All criteria were rated *better*, *equivalent* or *worse* compared to the baseline 1 mm FBP images. It was recognized that increased depth definition may have a negative impact on the detection of calc clusters, so a rating of better in this case is construed to mean more and a rating of worse to mean less.

Tumor masses		Micro-calcifications	
Visibility;	Overall visibility of the structure	*Visibility;*	Overall visibility of the structure
Contrast;	Contrast of the mass compared to immediate surrounding tissue	*In-plane definition;*	Definition and sharpness of micro-calcifications and separation of individual micro-calcifications in clusters
Border;	Definition and sharpness of the mass border and visibility of spiculations	*Depth definition;*	Size and strength of out-of-plane artifacts and separation of clusters into individual slices

2.2   Image Acquisition and Evaluation

All images used in the study were acquired on a MAMMOMAT Inspiration Tomo (Siemens AG, Erlangen, Germany). Unprocessed projection images were extracted from the image database and individually reconstructed. Projection images were reconstructed with standard FBP with 1 mm slice separation, and with SRSAR into 2 mm slabs using no overlap, i.e. each part of the volume was only included once.

20 image volumes were selected from a pool of cases of cancers that had been missed on DM but detected on BT and an additional set of micro-calcification clusters. These cases were considered likely to be subtle and to highlight any differences between 2 mm SRSAR and 1 mm FBP. The images contained a mix of masses – spiculated and non-spiculated, circumscribed and diffuse – and micro-calcifications, both alone and in conjunction with masses. In total, 16 volumes contained masses (biopsy-proven cancers) and 8 contained micro-calcification clusters (both associated with masses and independent of masses).

Evaluation of image quality was carried out using relative visual grading, with image volumes with thicker slabs compared with standard image volumes. Two groups of relevant structures were used: micro-calcifications and tumor masses. For each group three grading criteria were applied (Table 1). Each criterium was graded as better, equivalent or worse than the baseline. ViewDEX [17] was run on a Siemens Syngo MammoReport workstation to display and grade images side-by-side. 6 breast radiologists – all with at least one year of experience of DBT in both clinical and screening settings – were employed to grade the images. A researcher was in attendance during review. Each reader was also asked the subjective question of whether 2 mm SRSAR was, in their opinion, suitable to be used in the clinic.

Friedman's test was used to statistically evaluate the difference between the two sets of images.

3   Results

For masses, 2mm SRSAR had significantly greater contrast (P < .0001), but showed no significant difference in either overall visibility (P = .46) or border definition (P = .77). For micro-calcifications there were significant improvements in visibility (P = .0044), in-plane definition (P < .0001) and depth definition (P <.0001). Results are summarized in Table 2.

Table 2. Results of image quality grading by criteria. All statistically significant differences (according to Friedman's test) are indicated.

	Tumor masses				Micro-calcifications		
	P-value	1 mm FBP	2 mm SRSAR		P-value	1 mm FBP	2 mm SRSAR
Visibility;	.46	Equal	Equal	Visibility;	.0044	Worse	Better
Contrast;	<.0001	Worse	Better	In-plane definition;	<.0001	Worse	Better
Border;	.77	Equal	Equal	Depth definition;	<.0001	Worse	Better

Five out of six readers agreed that the differences between the two sets of images were minor and that the 2 mm SRSAR-images could be used instead of standard 1 mm FBP without impairing image review.

4   Discussion

The SRSAR-images were noted as being somewhat blurred, but with a lower noise level. One reader thought that the blurring would have implications on mass detection. The most notable difference was a perceived greater contrast in the SRSAR volumes, lending the images an appearance closer to DM images. Readers noted that the SRSAR images were more comfortable to read due to both the greater contrast and the lower noise level.

The blurry appearance of masses was noted as a concern by a few radiologists. Although contrast between masses and background was generally improved, especially when masses were located in dense tissue, the definition of edge characteristics suffered in some cases. In the case of spiculated lesions, spiculations were noted by some as sharper and better defined on standard 1mm. On the other hand, it was also noted that the contrast between spiculations and background was better on 2 mm SRSAR. Reviewers were divided as to whether this was an acceptable tradeoff. For circumscribed masses, 2 mm SRSAR was considered to show a greater contrast difference between mass and fibroglandular tissue, with edges more clearly differentiable from the background. Overall, the only statistically significant difference between the two reconstructions is the increased contrast of SRSAR, but there was as noted no statistical differences in either border characteristics or most crucially visibility, meaning that any negative or positive effects on the detection of masses is probably minor.

Calcifications were significantly more visible and better defined on SRSAR, which was reflected in reviewer opinion, with noticeable differences in contrast and sharpness. The radiologists did not view the improved depth definition as advantageous in the detection of calcifications, as clusters were split into separate slices and single calcifications appeared in fewer slices. The exact effects of this on detection is hard to gauge without further investigation. One can either contend that having the structure visible in a large number of slices gives the reader more time to detect it or speculate that having it visible in a single slice will aid detection by a sudden pop-up effect when combined with the higher contrast in SRSAR-images.

Some radiologists noted that very small calcifications seemed to lose contrast on SRSAR compared to FBP though this effect was only present in very small and faint calcifications; other calcifications, as noted, improved in both contrast and definition. The explanation could be that such small structures are interpreted as artifacts and suppressed, or it could be that they are smoothed by the AIP-slabbing.

Our previous work shows that viewing screening volumes at 2 mm rather than 1 mm reduces review times by 20% on normal images [13]. There was no significant change in review time of true positive cases, i.e. cancer. However, as malignant tumors make up only a tiny fraction of the total number of cases, this has little influence on overall workload. As long as there is a non-inferiority in cancer detection between the 2 mm method and the 1 mm method, it is therefore desirable to employ 2mm slices in order to reduce workload.

Five of the six radiologists believed that it would be possible to use 2 mm SRSAR images in screening situations, rating them as either equivalent or superior to 1 mm FBP, while one radiologist believed the new images to be unsuitable due to blurring.

A limitation of the study is that only thick-slice SRSAR was used, and therefore our results cannot separate the effects of SRSAR vs. FBP from 1 mm vs. 2 mm slices. It is plausible that the use of 1 mm SRSAR could provide better detection of lesions, and it is also possible that 2 mm FBP slices or slabs could be non-inferior to 1 mm FBP.

In conclusion, our results support that 2 mm SRSAR images compare well with 1 mm FBP, with a notable improvement in overall image contrast. Contrast and definition of microcalcifications were seen as advantageous for detection, while the overall visibility of masses remained at the same level. In the interest of saving reading time, it would therefore be possible to use 2 mm slices as standard.

Acknowledgments. The authors would like to acknowledge Shiras Abdurahman, Frank Dennerlein, Andreas Fieselmann and Anna Jerebko of Siemens AG Healthcare.

References

[1] Svahn, T., Andersson, I., Chakraborty, D., et al.: The diagnostic accuracy of dual-view digital mammography, single-view breast tomosynthesis and a dual-view combination of breast tomosynthesis and digital mammography in a free-response observer performance study. Rad. Prot. Dos. 139(1-3), 113–117 (2010)

[2] Andersson, I., Ikeda, D.M., Zackrisson, S., et al.: Breast tomosynthesis and digital mammography: A comparison of breast cancer visibility and BIRADS classification in a population of cancers with subtle mammographic findings. Eur. Radiol. 18(12), 2817–2825 (2008)

[3] Gur, D., Abrams, G.S., Chough, D.M., et al.: Digital breast tomosynthesis: Observer performance study. Am. J. Roentgenol. 193(2), 586–591 (2009)

[4] Wallis, M.G., Moa, E., Zanca, F., et al.: Two-view and single-view tomosynthesis versus full-field digital mammography: High-resolution X-ray imaging observer study. Radiology 262(3), 788–796 (2012)

[5] Good, W.F., Abrams, G.S., Catullo, V.J., et al.: Digital breast tomosynthesis: A pilot observer study. Am. J. Roentgenol. 190(4), 865–869 (2008)

[6] Skaane, P., Gullien, R., Bjørndal, H., et al.: Digital breast tomosynthesis (DBT): Initial experience in a clinical setting. Acta Radiol. 53(5), 524–529 (2012)

[7] Good, W.F., Abrams, G.S., Catullo, V.J., et al.: Digital breast tomosynthesis: A pilot observer study. AJR Am. J. Roentgenol. 190(4), 865–869 (2008)

[8] Mertelmeier, T., Orman, J., Haerer, W., et al.: Optimizing filtered backprojection reconstruction for a breast tomosynthesis prototype device. In: Spie Medical Imaging, pp. 61420F-1–61420F-12. International Society for Optics and Photonics, Bellingham (2006)

[9] Wu, T., Moore, R.H., Kopans, D.B.: Voting strategy for artifact reduction in digital breast tomosynthesis. Med. Phys. 33, 2461 (2006)

[10] Wu, T., Moore, R.H., Rafferty, E.A., et al.: A comparison of reconstruction algorithms for breast tomosynthesis. Med. Phys. 31(9), 2636–2647 (2004)

[11] Hu, Y.H., Zhao, B., Zhao, W.: Image artifacts in digital breast tomosynthesis: Investigation of the effects of system geometry and reconstruction parameters using a linear system approach. Med. Phys. 35(12), 5242–5252 (2008)

[12] Zhang, Y., Chan, H.P., Sahiner, B., et al.: Investigation of the Z-axis resolution of breast tomosynthesis mammography systems. In: SPIE Medical Imaging, pp. 65104A-65104A-8. International Society for Optics and Photonics, Bellingham (2007)

[13] Dustler, M., Andersson, I., Förnvik, D., et al.: A Study of the Feasibility of using slabbing to reduce Tomosynthesis Review Time. In: SPIE Medical Imaging, pp. 86731L–86731L. International Society for Optics and Photonics, Bellingham (2013)

[14] Kopans, D., Gavenonis, S., Halpern, E., et al.: Calcifications in the breast and digital breast tomosynthesis. Breast J. 17(6), 638–644 (2011)

[15] Sechopoulos, I., Ghetti, C.: Optimization of the acquisition geometry in digital tomosynthesis of the breast. Med. Phys. 36, 1199 (2009)

[16] Abdurahman, S., Jerebko, A., Mertelmeier, T., Lasser, T., Navab, N.: Out-of-plane artifact reduction in tomosynthesis based on regression modeling and outlier detection. In: Maidment, A.D.A., Bakic, P.R., Gavenonis, S. (eds.) IWDM 2012. LNCS, vol. 7361, pp. 729–736. Springer, Heidelberg (2012)

[17] Håkansson, M., Svensson, S., Zachrisson, S., et al.: ViewDEX: An efficient and easy-to-use software for observer performance studies. Rad. Prot. Dos. 139(1-3), 42–51 (2010)

Detection of Spiculated Lesions in Digital Mammograms Using a Novel Image Analysis Technique

Ashley Seepujak[1], Tomas Adomavicius[1], Sergey Dolgobrodov[1],
Emmanouil Moschidis[2], Xin Chen[2], Anthony Maxwell[3],
Susan M. Astley[2], and Alan M. Roseman[1]

[1] Faculty of Life Sciences, University of Manchester, Oxford Road, Manchester, M13 9PT, UK
[2] Centre for Imaging Sciences, Institute for Population Health,
University of Manchester, Oxford Road, Manchester, M13 9PT, UK
[3] Nightingale Centre and Genesis Prevention Centre, University Hospital of South Manchester,
Manchester M23 9LT, UK
alan.roseman@manchester.ac.uk

Abstract. We have applied novel computational image analysis algorithms to detect malignant masses in mammograms. Our analysis focuses on spiculated lesions, which are particularly challenging for computer-aided detection methods. The algorithm uses the principle of locally-normalised correlation coefficients to identify patterns of motifs representing a spiculated feature. A combination of correlation maps indicating the maximum correlation of the motif at each position relative to the mammogram, and of the pattern of angles for which this maximum is observed, are used to locate spiculated lesions in a verified test dataset. The test set of images has been annotated by an expert reader, and allows objective evaluation of computer-aided detection procedures. In a blind test using an automated procedure our method identified 54% of the lesion locations in the set of test images. This initial blind testing and comparison with expert annotated images, representing a ground truth, indicates feasibility for our approach. Optimisation of the procedure is expected to yield improved performance.

Keywords: Spiculated lesion, mammogram, breast cancer, local correlation.

1 Introduction

Breast cancer represents the most common cancer in women over the age of 50, and in the UK a national mammographic screening programme is in operation for women between the ages of 47 and 73. X-ray mammograms are exceptionally difficult images to interpret owing to the high degree of variability between individuals' breasts, the nature of the projection images, and the variability and subtlety of signs of early cancer. Images are therefore read by two human experts. It has been proposed that should a reliable computer-aided detection (CAD) system be available, it could be used to replace one of the expert reads, thus freeing radiologists for alternative tasks [1]. Current CAD systems do not perform sufficiently well for this at present.

H. Fujita, T. Hara, and C. Muramatsu (Eds.): IWDM 2014, LNCS 8539, pp. 550–557, 2014.
© Springer International Publishing Switzerland 2014

Previously, we developed new pattern-recognition techniques to detect molecular structures in transmission electron cryo-microscopy (cryoEM) images. Radiographs and cryoEM images of biological samples share characteristics which make them challenging for image analysis. This is mainly due to the inherent restrictions presented by the imaging of radiation-sensitive structures, where the radiation dose used to produce the images must be limited, resulting in low contrast and poor signal-to-noise ratio. In this work we describe the application of locally-normalised correlation analysis — a technique developed for cryoEM image analysis — to mammographic imaging.

2 Method

We focus on the detection of spiculated lesions, which have been identified as one of the most challenging types of abnormality for computer-aided detection methods.

The algorithm uses the principle of locally-normalised correlation coefficients to identify patterns of motifs representing a spiculated feature. The local normalisation procedure effectively rescales the motif and the data to minimise the squared differences between equivalent pixels [2,3]. Local normalisation implies that the calculation is performed solely in the region defined by the motif. The calculated correlation coefficient is related to an optimum least squares residual, where the images have been scaled linearly to minimise that residual. This linear scaling optimises two parameters, namely a gain or multiplicative factor, and a constant offset. This allows the procedure to adapt to the arbitrary scaling of the projection images, in which density variations are recorded, but are not calibrated in terms of an absolute mass detected in the path of the imaging beam. The procedure operates in two stages. First, the correlation maps are calculated. The second set of steps consists of identifying peaks in the correlation maps, followed by reliably identifying patterns and peaks located as spiculated lesions.

2.1 Locally Normalised Correlation Coefficients and Correlation Maps

In order to calculate the locally-normalised correlation map, correlation coefficients between a template object and the locally masked area of the mammogram image are determined. An example template is shown in figure 1. A binary mask defines the boundary of the template. Only those points defined by the mask are used in the calculation.

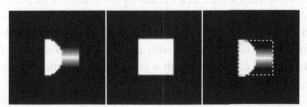

Fig. 1. Left to right: Template image, binary mask, outline of the binary mask on template image indicated by dashed line

The template (and the associated binary mask) is scanned across the images and a normalised correlation coefficient is calculated between the template and the masked image at each position. In order to detect spiculated features in all orientations, the template is rotated through 360 degrees, using a step size of two degrees. The highest correlation coefficient for each position and rotation of the template is stored in a correlation map image. The corresponding angle of rotation of the template at each position is recorded and stored in an image denoted as the omega map. The images were sampled at 94.1 µm per pixel.

2.2   Analysis of Omega Maps

In regions where spiculated features are found, a peak feature is present indicating the radiating nature of the spiculated mass (e.g. figure 2e). This peak appears as geometric sectors ordered around a central origin. This motif resembles a shadowed mountain peak in an aerial photograph. Figure 2f shows one such peak extracted from one of the analysed images. In these regions, when the angles in annuli centred on the peak in the omega map are plotted, they range from 0 to 358 degrees relatively smoothly. Ideally, the relative orientation of the located spiculated features should correspond to a radial progression of orientations which circumscribe the centre of the peak. The slope of a fitted line should be approximately one. In order to reduce noise, a circular trace centred on each point is computed by averaging over several annuli. In order to achieve this, a box drawn around each evaluated peak position is extracted and converted to polar coordinates. Then, radii from 20 to 45 pixels are averaged in order to obtain the trace of the relative rotation of the motif observed, as a function of the orientation around the point. A least square residual was used to score the fit of a line of slope 1 to the points in this calculated profile. The residuals were stored in image maps.

2.3   Lesion Identification

A procedure was devised to calculate a score for the position of identified lesions from the correlation maps and derivatives calculated as described above. The correlation maps were smoothed by convolution with a 2-dimensional Gaussian function with a standard deviation of 10 pixels, and a threshold applied. The residual maps computed from the omega maps (as described in section 2.2) were also thresholded at a set value. Threshold values were determined by optimisation of performance on the training set. Values below the threshold were set to zero. The two thresholded scores were multiplied to obtain scores for positions of lesions. Features in low density regions were removed by multiplication with a third mask. To create this mask, the mammogram image was convoluted with a Gaussian function, as above, to integrate relative density, and a threshold applied at half the maximum value.

2.4   Evaluation of the Procedure

A set of 50 anonymised digital screening mammograms was obtained from the UK National Health Service Breast Screening Programme. These had previously been reviewed by an expert radiologist who marked the positions of all biopsy-proven malignant lesions and verified that no further lesions were present by inspection of subsequent mammograms. 25 of these were classified as spiculated. Ground truth masks identifying the positions of the lesions, as indicated by the clinician, were used in an automated procedure to evaluate the accuracy of lesion detection by our procedure. In the evaluation process the final image indicating the detected peaks is multiplied by the ground truth mask. Peaks are detected and compared to the list obtained before applying the mask. Peaks that match are true positives. Any additional peaks observed which were not within the masked area are false positives. Lack of detection of a peak within the masked area is considered a false negative. The SPIDER[4] image processing suite was used to implement the procedures in section 2.2 and 2.3.

3   Results and Discussion

We tested our method to locate spiculated lesions in craniocaudal (CC) views in this expert-verified test dataset. Figures 2, 3 and 4 illustrate our procedure and show some preliminary results. Correlation maps were computed with the images shown, using the template detailed in figure 1. Two of the 25 images were rejected from the analysis: one because no ground truth was available for the CC image, and one because the lesion was on the very edge. After initial evaluation on a training set of 10 images, blind testing was performed using a further 13 unseen images.

In the first example, figure 2, the lesion appears as a dense mass and is well-defined. A peak in the correlation map clearly indicates its location. The omega map shows a characteristic peak at the identical position, indicative of the detection of radial features. At those locations where the lesion is not present, features in the omega map are less defined and are not as symmetrical.

In the second example, the mass is not as well defined (figure 3). It is not the most dense feature in the image, and there are a number of other regions of high density. Nevertheless, the correlation map indicates a defined peak which coincides with the known lesion position. A distinct peak in the omega map also coincides with this location, and supports this peak detection. The other strong features in the image do not produce well defined peaks in either the correlation map or the omega map. Taken together, these calculations are proving to represent reliable indicators which may be used to detect anomalous masses in the mammogram images.

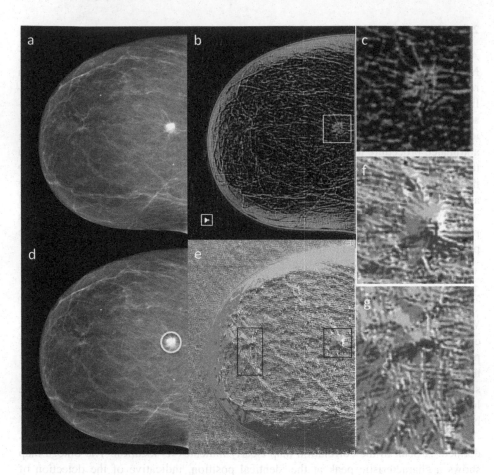

Fig. 2. a. Mammogram processed for display; b. the correlation map of the image with the template (as shown in figure 1) shown as an insert, at 2 times relative scale, bottom left. This map shows the best locally-normalised correlation coefficient at each position, for every orientation of the template. The boxed region identifies a potential hit. The side of the box is 22 mm; c. enlargement of the boxed region shown in b. The peak consists of a ring of high intensity correlation, neither solid nor of Gaussian distribution in form. It is composed of a ring of higher correlation, with a weaker centre, since the template is designed to match features on the periphery of the lesions; d. a mammogram, as in a, with a circle indicating the location of the lesion; e. an image representing the angle of rotation of the template at each position, corresponding to the highest correlation coefficient—the omega map. Rotations in the range 0 to 358 degrees are represented by a scale of black to white. Regions of interest look like mountain peaks, with sectors radiating from a central point; f. an enlarged view of the peak indicated by the square box; g. an enlarged view of the region indicated by the rectangular box (not the lesion region), which contains a less well-defined peak. Enlarged regions are magnified three-fold.

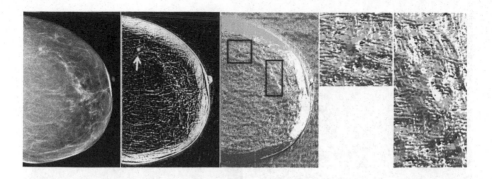

Fig. 3. Left to right: Mammogram, correlation map (lesion indicated by arrow), omega map, enlargement of omega map region indicated by the square box, enlargement of omega map region indicated by the rectangular box. (The rectangular region does not contain the lesion). Enlargements are threefold.

In figure 4 we show the results of the procedure to identify and locate the "mountain peak" motifs introduced in figures 2 and 3. When the map of peak locations (calculated from the minimum residuals, section 2.2) is overlaid on the mammogram, it can been seen that the centres of the peaks identified coincide with globular textured regions. This map is used in conjunction with the correlation maps to identify the cancerous spiculated lesions.

We initially tested our procedure on a set of 10 images in a training stage, and chose suitable values for the thresholds and filters. Evaluation was then performed blindly on a set of 13 unseen images. In this blind test five lesions were identified in images, with zero or one false positive hits. Two more lesions were identified, with four or five false positive hits in addition. For five images the lesion was not detected, but between zero and six false positives (FPs) were returned. No hits were identified in one image. This gives a detection rate of 54%, with a moderately low false positive rate. These initial results demonstrate a proof of principle for our approach. Our procedure is in an early stage of development, and there is potential to improve it by adding additional filters to identify the correct peaks from noise. The parameter settings used here were chosen to yield a relatively low FP rate, however it would be possible to detect a higher number of lesions at the expense of increased FPs, which could then be reduced by further analysis of the properties of the detected regions.

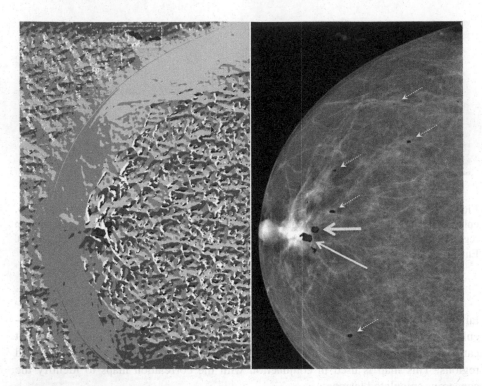

Fig. 4. The peak detection results for one of the omega maps. The map of residuals calculated from the omega map is overlaid on the omega map (left), and on the mammogram image (right). The peaks found in the polar residual analysis are located centrally on the "mountain peak" motifs. The two main peaks are indicated with solid arrows. A few smaller peaks are present, which are more easily seen in the right hand image (indicated by broken line arrows). Simple thresholding to 60% of the maximum peak height eliminated all but the two main peaks indicated by the solid arrows. The correlation map (not shown) is also used to identify the spiculated regions. A threshold is applied to the correlation map and the resultant image is used as a mask to eliminate regions with lower correlation values. This procedure selected only the left hand peak indicated by the long arrow in the images above, which coincides with the region demarcated by the clinician as a spiculated lesion. Two peaks in the background of the image can been seen near the top (indicated by a rectangle on the left panel). Features in regions such as these, outside the breast area, were excluded when the other criteria were applied.

4   Concluding Remarks

We have developed a novel method for detecting spiculated mammographic abnormalities, which in our initial evaluation is robust to other mammographic features. These results are encouraging given that we have not extensively optimised the selection criteria and thresholds. Therefore this preliminary blind testing and comparison with expert annotated images, representing the ground truth, has indicated favourable results. In the future we will optimise the parameters and test our procedure on a larger unseen test set.

Acknowledgements. This work was supported by the Genesis Breast Cancer Prevention Appeal, grant GA 13-001.

References

1. Gilbert, F.J., Astley, S.M., Gillan, M.C., Agbaje, O.F., Wallis, M.G., James, J., Boggis, C.R.M., Duffy, S.W.: Single reading with computer-aided detection for screening mammography. New England Journal of Medicine 359, 1675–1684 (2008)
2. Roseman, A.M.: Particle finding in electron micrographs using a fast local correlation algorithm. Ultramicroscopy 94, 225–236 (2003)
3. Roseman, A.M.: FindEM—A fast, efficient method for particle finding in electron micrographs. Journal of Struct. Biol. 145, 91–99 (2004)
4. Frank, J., Radermacher, M., Penczek, P., Zhu, J., Li, Y., Ladjadj, M., Leith, A.: SPIDER and WEB: Processing and visualization of images in 3D electron microscopy and related fields. J. Struct. Biol. 116, 190–199 (1996)

Spatial Correlation Analysis of Mammograms for Detection of Asymmetric Findings

Paola Casti[1], Arianna Mencattini[1],
Marcello Salmeri[1], and Rangaraj M. Rangayyan[2]

[1] University of Rome Tor Vergata, Department of Electronic Engineering,
00133 Rome, Italy
casti@ing.uniroma2.it
[2] University of Calgary, Department of Electrical and Computer Engineering,
Schulich School of Engineering, Calgary, Alberta, Canada T2N 1N4,
ranga@ucalgary.ca

Abstract. We present a novel method to detect asymmetry in mammograms based upon bilateral analysis of the spatial distribution of density within paired mammographic strips. Various differential measures of spatial correlation of gray-scale values were computed with reference to the position of the nipple for a set of 128 pairs of mammograms from the Digital Database for Screening Mammography (DDSM). Features were selected by stepwise logistic regression and the leave-one-patient-out method was used for cross-validation of results. An area under the receiver operating characteristic curve of 0.87 ($SE = 0.08$) was achieved by using an artificial neural network classifier with radial basis functions.

Keywords: breast cancer, bilateral asymmetry, computer-aided detection, mammography, spatial correlation.

1 Asymmetric Findings in Mammograms

Periodic examination of asymptomatic women via mammographic screening is aimed at early diagnosis of breast cancer and consequent improvement in the prognosis for the patient [1]. Radiologists perform comparative studies of the left and right mammograms of the same patient to prevent missing signs of breast disease. When a greater area of tissue with fibroglandular density is detected in a mammogram relative to the corresponding region in the controlateral breast, it is reported as an asymmetric finding, either local or global [2]. Asymmetric findings on mammograms may indicate a developing or underlying mass. They can be subtle in presentation and hence overlooked or misinterpreted by radiologists.

Several studies have shown the association between mammographic fibroglandular density and the risk of developing breast cancer [3] and substantial effort has been directed to develop methods for quantification of breast density in mammograms [4,5]. In addition to the presence of fibroglandular density, asymmetric fibroglandular findings, which are detected via comparison of the two mammograms of the patient, have proved to be an indicator of increased risk of developing breast cancer [6–8].

H. Fujita, T. Hara, and C. Muramatsu (Eds.): IWDM 2014, LNCS 8539, pp. 558–564, 2014.

The development of automated methods for quantification of asymmetry as part of a computer-aided detection (CADe) system can facilitate more accurate interpretation of mammograms and assist radiologists in the reporting process, so that the efficacy of breast cancer screening and prevention programs can be improved. The complexity of detecting asymmetry in mammograms lies in finding accurate matches between anatomical structures to be compared and in designing measures capable of distinguishing structural asymmetry from physiological or positioning differences between the two breasts of the same patient. Analysis of previous work suggests that automatic detection of asymmetry in mammograms can be achieved [9–15, 18, 19]. However, more effort is needed to devise new methods to increase the performance level and to progress towards clinical application.

2   Dataset of Images

A set of 128 digitized screen-film mammograms, including craniocaudal (CC) and mediolateral-oblique (MLO) projections of the two breasts of each subject, was selected from the Digital Database for Screening Mammography (DDSM) [16]. The images have spatial resolution of 42.5, 43, or 50 μm, and pixel depth of 12 or 16 bits/pixels (bpp). All the asymmetric cases available with proven ground truth, consisting of 16 pairs of focal asymmetry and 16 pairs of global asymmetry, have been included in this study. An additional set of 32 pairs of normal mammograms was randomly selected for the inclusion of control cases [see Figures 1(a) and (c)].

3   Methods for Bilateral Analysis of Spatial Correlation

Bilateral analysis of mammograms was performed via accurate matching of corresponding mammographic strips, and subsequent quantification of differences in the spatial distribution of gray-scale levels, as follows.

1. Each image was downsampled to 600 μm/pixel. Reference anatomical structures, including the breast-skin line, the nipple, and the pectoral muscle (only for MLO views) were extracted by using previously developed methods [17, 20].
2. Two automatic masking procedures were applied to the breast regions of each pair of mammograms: medial and retroglandular for CC views, and milky and retroareolar for MLO views [20, 21], yielding eight paired strips for each masking procedure, as shown in the examples in Figures 1(b) and (d).
3. For each strip, measures of spatial correlation, Sc, were computed with reference to the position of the nipple by comparing a matrix of differences of gray-scale, Δf_{ij}, with a matrix of distances, Δd_{ij}, as follows:

$$Sc = \frac{2}{n(n-1)} \sum_{i=1}^{n} \sum_{j=1}^{n} \Delta f_{ij} \, \Delta d_{ij}, \qquad (1)$$

where n is the number of pixels within each strip. Radial correlation was estimated by assigning $\Delta d_{ij} = |d_i - d_j|$, with d_i, $i = 1, 2, \ldots, n$, equal to the length of the ith pixel's position vector from the nipple. Angular correlation was quantified by assigning $\Delta d_{ij} = \sin \theta_{ij}$, where θ_{ij} is the angle between the position vectors of the ith and the jth pixels. Given the gray-scale level, f_i, of the ith pixel, based on different formulations of Δf_{ij} in Eq. 1, four differential spatial correlation features for both angular and radial correlation were defined as follows:

- $\Delta Sc_1 = |Sc_{dx} - Sc_{sn}|$ with $\Delta f_{ij} = |f_i - f_j|$,
- $\Delta Sc_2 = |Sc_{dx} - Sc_{sn}|$ with $\Delta f_{ij} = |f_i - f_j|/(\max_k f_k + \min_k f_k)$,
- $\Delta Sc_3 = |Sc_{dx} - Sc_{sn}|$ with $\Delta f_{ij} = (|f_i - f_j| - \bar{f})/\sigma_f$,
- $\Delta Sc_4 = |Sc_{dx} - Sc_{sn}|/(Sc_{dx} + Sc_{sn})$ with $\Delta f_{ij} = |f_i - f_j|$,

where dx and sn indicate the right and left mammograms, and $\bar{f}$ and σ_f are the mean and standard deviation of gray-scale values within each strip, respectively. The differential features obtained for each of the eight pairs of

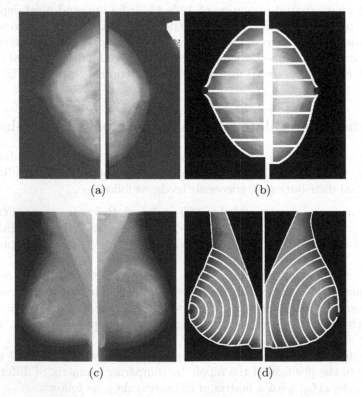

(a)　　　　　　　　(b)

(c)　　　　　　　　(d)

Fig. 1. Pairs of normal CC (a,b) and malignant asymmetric MLO (c,d) views from the DDSM [16] database. (a,c) Original images. (b,d) Bilateral mammographic strips obtained via medial (b) and retroareolar (d) masking procedures.

strips of a given masking procedure were summed, resulting in 32 features for every patient.

4. A threshold of 0.6 on the area under the receiver operating (ROC) characteristic curve, A_z, of the individual features, followed by stepwise logistic regression was applied to the training set of each leave-one-patient-out experiment for automatic selection of features.

5. Three classifiers —linear discriminant analysis (LDA), quadratic discriminant analysis (QDA), and an artificial neural network with radial basis functions (ANN-RBF)— were used for classification of mammograms as normal or asymmetric pairs.

4 Results and Discussion

The results of performance analysis of the individual features are presented in Table 1. The A_z values are reported for the two mammographic projections and the four related masking procedures. The A_z values obtained when the whole breast regions were used for computation of features without using any masking procedure are also reported. The highest A_z of 0.75 was obtained with the ΔSc_3 correlation measure and medial masking of CC views. The results obtained with MLO views are poorer as compared to the results achieved with CC views. Overall, the masking procedures improve the discriminating ability of the features. The combination of features from both CC and MLO views using LDA, QDA, and ANN-RBF classifiers along with automatic feature selection and the leave-one-patient-out cross-validation provided, respectively, A_z (SE) of 0.83 (0.07), 0.72 (0.09), and 0.87 (0.08). The best classification accuracy obtained was 91%, with sensitivity of 1.0 and specificity of 0.81, using the ANN-RBF classifier.

The results achieved in this study are compared in Table 2 with the other results reported in the literature [10,12–15] and in our previous work on detection of asymmetric findings in mammograms [19]. Note that only works with accuracy results and/or ROC analysis are listed. The performance statistics of the selected

Table 1. Classification performance of individual features for spatial pattern analysis of mammograms. Results are given in terms of A_z. Cases with $A_z > 0.7$ are shown in bold.

View	Masking	Radial correlation				Angular correlation			
------	---------	ΔSc_1	ΔSc_2	ΔSc_3	ΔSc_4	ΔSc_1	ΔSc_2	ΔSc_3	ΔSc_4
	Medial	0.67	0.69	**0.75**	0.55	0.60	0.61	0.57	0.68
CC	Retroglandular	0.59	0.47	0.52	0.68	0.47	0.39	0.47	0.54
	None	0.41	0.62	**0.72**	0.43	0.46	0.41	0.50	0.57
	Milky	0.36	0.49	0.50	0.45	0.54	0.63	0.57	0.57
MLO	Retroareolar	0.61	0.61	0.65	0.58	0.55	0.59	0.48	0.57
	None	0.55	0.55	0.50	0.54	0.56	0.47	0.52	0.58

methods show that the results obtained in the present work using, for the first time, all of the available asymmetric cases in DDSM [16], are better than the others reported in the literature. This study indicates that the differences in the spatial distribution of pixel values within paired mammographic strips computed

Table 2. Performance statistics of selected methods for the analysis of asymmetric findings in mammograms. Only works with accuracy results and/or ROC analysis are listed.

Authors	Dataset	Summary of Methods and Results
Miller and Astley [10]	A set of 150 MLO and mediolateral (ML) mammograms including 47 normal and 28 asymmetric pairs.	Six shape, brightness, and topology descriptors from manually marked regions of the fibroglandular components of the breast; LDA classifier and leave-one-out cross-validation: accuracy of 76%.
Ferrari et al. [12]	80 MLO mammograms including 20 normal cases, 14 asymmetric cases, and six architectural distortion cases from the mini-MIAS [22] database.	Gabor wavelets, Karhunen-Loéve transform, Otsu's method, rose diagrams, and three statistical features; Bayesian linear classifier, exhaustive combination technique, and leave-one-out cross-validation: accuracy of 74%.
Rangayyan et al. [13]	88 MLO mammograms including 22 normal cases, 14 asymmetric cases, and eight architectural distortion cases from the mini-MIAS [22] database.	Alignment of the phase responses of Gabor wavelets with reference to the corresponding pectoral muscle edges, 16 directional, morphological, and density features; quadratic Bayesian classifier, exhaustive combination technique, and leave-one-out cross-validation: accuracy rate of 84%.
Tzikopoulos et al. [14]	322 MLO mammograms from the miniMIAS database [22] including 15 asymmetric cases; all the remaining cases treated as symmetric.	Minimum cross-entropy thresholding, 114 differential first-order statistical features; support vector machines, t-test for selection of 18 features, and leave-one-out cross-validation: accuracy of 85%.
Wang et al. [15]	800 full-field digital mammograms, including CC and MLO views of 100 normal cases and 100 verified positive cases for developing breast cancer 6 to 18 months later.	20 features including statistical, textural, and density features from automatically selected regions of interest and the entire segmented breast areas; genetic algorithms, ANN classifier, and leave-one-patient-out cross-validation: area under the ROC curve of 0.78.
Casti et al. [19]	128 images of CC and MLO mammographic projections from the DDSM [16] including 16 pairs of focal asymmetry, 16 pairs of global asymmetry, and 32 randomly selected pairs of normal mammograms.	Multidirectional Gabor filters, automatic masking procedures, rose diagrams, and Moran-like measures of angular similarity; Fisher-LDA, features selection based on A_Z, and leave-one-patient-out cross-validation: $A_Z = 0.84$.
The present study	128 images of CC and MLO mammographic projections from the DDSM [16] including 16 pairs of focal asymmetry, 16 pairs of global asymmetry, and 32 randomly selected pairs of normal mammograms.	Automatic masking procedures, 24 differential measures of spatial correlation of gray-scale values with reference to the position of the nipple; stepwise logistic regression, ANN-RBF classifier, and leave-one-patient-out cross-validation: $A_Z = 0.87$, accuracy of 91%.

with reference to the position of the nipple can be used for detection of bilateral asymmetry.

5   Conclusion and Future Work

Novel methods for the analysis of asymmetry in mammograms have been described in this work that correlate the gray-scale values with relative distances from the nipple in paired strips of bilateral mammograms. Further study will investigate the use of structure functions (e.g., the semivariogram) to characterize the correlation of pixels as a function of distance. The proposed techniques will lead to the development of a robust and comprehensive method to detect asymmetry in mammograms, which may be used as an indicator of increased risk of breast cancer.

References

1. Dowling, E.C., Klabunde, C., Patnick, J., Ballard-Barbash, R.: Breast and cervical cancer screening programme implementation in 16 countries. J. Med. Screen. 17, 139–146 (2010)
2. D'Orsi, C.J., Bassett, L.W., Berg, W.A., Feig, S.A., Jackson, V.P., Kopans, D.B.: BI-RADS: Mammography, 4th edn. American College of Radiology (2003)
3. Oza, A.M., Boyd, N.F.: Mammographic parenchymal patterns: A marker of breast cancer risk. Epidemiologic Rev. 15, 196–208 (1993)
4. Saha, P., Udupa, J., Conant, E., Chakraborty, D., Sullivan, D.: Breast tissue density quantification via digitized mammograms. IEEE Trans. Med. Imag. 20, 792–803 (2001)
5. Jamal, N., Ng, K.H., Looi, L., McLean, D., Zulfiqar, A., Tan, S., Liew, W., Shantini, A., Ranganathan, S.: Quantitative assessment of breast density from digitized mammograms into Tabár's patterns. Phys. Med. Biol. 8, 5843–5857 (2006)
6. Harvey, J., Fajardo, L., Innis, C.: Previous mammograms in patients with impalpable breast carcinoma: Retrospective vs blinded interpretation. Am. J. Roentgenol. 161, 1167–1172 (1993)
7. Scutt, D., Lancaster, G., Manning, J.: Breast asymmetry and predisposition to breast cancer. Breast Cancer Research 8, R14 (2006)
8. Zheng, B., Sumkin, J., Zuley, M., Wang, X., Klym, A., Gur, D.: Bilateral mammographic density asymmetry and breast cancer risk: A preliminary assessment. Eur. J. Radiol. 81, 3222–3228 (2012)
9. Lau, T.K., Bischof, W.F.: Automated detection of breast tumors using the asymmetry approach. Comput. Biomed. Res. 24, 273–295 (1991)
10. Miller, P., Astley, S.: Automated detection of mammographic asymmetry using anatomical features. Int. J. Pattern Recogn. Artif. Intell. 7, 1461–1476 (1993)
11. Karssemeijer, N., Thijssen, M., Hendriks, J., van Erning, L.: Combining single view features and asymmetry for detection of mass lesions. In: 4th International Workshop on Digital Mammography, pp. 95–102 (1998)
12. Ferrari, R.J., Rangayyan, R.M., Desautels, J.E.L., Frère, A.F.: Analysis of asymmetry in mammograms via directional filtering with Gabor wavelets. IEEE Trans. Med. Imag. 20, 953–964 (2001)

13. Rangayyan, R.M., Ferrari, R.J., Frère, A.F.: Analysis of bilateral asymmetry in mammograms using directional, morphological, and density features. J. Electron. Imaging 16, article number 013003 (2007)
14. Tzikopoulos, S.D., Mavroforakis, M.E., Georgiou, H.V., Dimitropoulos, N., Theodoridis, S.: A fully automated scheme for mammographic segmentation and classification based on breast density and asymmetry. Comput. Meth. Prog. Bio. Intell. 102, 47–63 (2011)
15. Wang, X., Lederman, D., Tan, J., Wang, X.H., Zheng, B.: Computerized prediction of risk for developing breast cancer based on bilateral mammographic breast tissue asymmetry. In: 5th International Workshop on Digital Mammography, pp. 934–942 (2011)
16. Heath, M., Bowyer, K., Kopans, D., Moore, R., Kegelmeyer, W.P.: The Digital Database for Screening Mammography, pp. 212–218. Medical Physics Publishing (2001)
17. Casti, P., Mencattini, A., Salmeri, M., Ancona, A., Mangieri, F.F., Pepe, M.L., Rangayyan, R.M.: Automatic detection of the nipple in screen-film and full-field digital mammograms using a novel Hessian-based method. J. Digit. Imaging 26, 948–957 (2013)
18. Mencattini, A., Salmeri, M., Casti, P.: Bilateral asymmetry identification for the early detection of breast cancer. In: 6th IEEE International Workshop on Medical Measurements and Applications, pp. 613–618 (2011)
19. Casti, P., Mencattini, A., Salmeri, M., Rangayyan, R.M.: Masking procedures and measures of angular similarity for detection of bilateral asymmetry in mammograms. In: 10th IEEE International Conference on E-Health and Bioengineering, pp. 1–4 (2013)
20. Casti, P., Mencattini, A., Salmeri, M.: Characterization of the breast region for computer assisted Tabár masking of paired mammographic images. In: 25th IEEE International Symposium on Computer-Based Medical Systems, pp. 1–6 (2012)
21. Tabár, L., Tot, T., Dean, P.B.: Breast cancer, the art and science of early detection with mammography: Perception, interpretation, histopathologic correlation. George Thieme Verlag (2005)
22. Suckling, J., Parker, J., Dance, D., Astley, S., Hutt, I., Boggis, C., Ricketts, I., Stamakis, E., Cerneaz, N., Kok, S., Taylor, P., Betal, D., Savage, J.: The Mammographic Image Analysis Society digital mammogram database Exerpta Medica. International Congress Series 1069, 375–378 (1994)

Temporal Breast Cancer Risk Assessment Based on Higher-Order Textons

Xi-Zhao Li[1], Simon Williams[1], Peter Downey[2] and Murk J. Bottema[1]

[1] School of Computer Science, Engneering and Mathematics,
Flinder University, Bedford Park 5042, SA, Australia
{li0691,s.williams,murk.bottema}@flinders.edu.au
[2] BreastScreen SA, Central Adelaide Local Health Network,
1 Goodwood Road, Wayville, Adelaide, SA, 5034
Peter.Downey@health.sa.gov.au

Abstract. Higher-order texture features from 100 mammographic images with known cancer were compared to texture features from 100 images from women with no known cancer. Texture features from images of the same breasts from screening rounds two and four years previously were also compared. The A_z score for classifying cancer images from non-cancer images was 0.749. The A_z score for classification two years previous to detection of cancer was 0.674 and the score for four years previous was 0.601. There was no signicant difference between classifying images from the round in which cancer was actually detected and the screening rounds two and four years previous. Similar results were obtained if the breast with no known cancer (contralateral breast) was used instead the breast with cancer, leading to the conclusion that texture alone has moderate predictive power regarding breast cancer risk and that this predictive value is roughly constant in the four years prior to mammographically apparent cancer.

Keywords: Temporal, Breast cancer, Risk assessment, Higher-order textons, Texture independent of density.

1 Introduction

Texture analysis plays an important role in image classification. Commonly used texture analysis methods include co-occurrence matrices, run-length statistics, Fourier transforms, Laws texture analysis, fractal dimension analysis, filter banks and so on. Textons were proposed as prototype texture features calculated from the the co-occurrence of filter bank outputs [4]. Textons based on image intensities in $N \times N$ neighborhoods were proposed to replace textons based on filter banks [12]. In breast cancer risk assessment, texture analysis was initially used to classify mammography appearance as in [10].

More recently, breast images were classified into risk groups directly according to different criteria of "true risk". Li et al. [5] computed texture features using co-occurrence matrices, gray-level histograms, fractal analysis, edge frequency analysis and Frourier analysis from central ROIs behind the nipple to

H. Fujita, T. Hara, and C. Muramatsu (Eds.): IWDM 2014, LNCS 8539, pp. 565–572, 2014.

classify high risk group ROIs (BRCA1/BRCA2 gene-mutation carriers) from low risk group ROIs (non BRCA1/BRCA2 carriers). They achieved an A_z score of 0.88. Karamore et al. classified cancer images stratified by estrogen receptor status (high risk) and age-matched control images (low risk) with texture features representing the orientation and heterogeneity of the parenchymal tissues and obtained an A_z score of 0.71 [3]. Keller et al. extracted features from breast metrics such as density features, morphometry features and volumetric features to classify unaffected breast images of cancer cases (high risk) and non-cancer breast images of age-matched control cases (low risk) and achieved a best A_z score of 0.7. Ting et al. studied breast cancer risk associated with longitudinal change in mammographic density in temporal sequences of mammograms [11]. In their study, the time difference between two consecutive screening mammograms for the same woman was around one year and they found that breast cancer risk was associated with increasing density over time for both ipsilateral and contralateral breasts.

The correlation between breast cancer risk and breast density is well-known. The degree to which image texture anomalies correlate to breast cancer risk is less clear. In addition, little is known about changes in texture prior to cancers becoming discernible mammographically. Neither is it clear if changes in texture are restricted to the breast in which cancer will eventually appear or if the changes are bilateral.

Here a temporal study is presented on estimating risk of breast cancer based on higher-order texton texture features which are independent of breast density. Estimates of risk are obtained separately for the breast with cancer and the contralateral breast.

2   Methods

2.1   Data Set

Film mammograms were obtained from the archives of BreastScreen SA (Adelaide, South Australia) and were digitized at 57.0 μm spatial resolution and 12 bit depth. Only CC views were used because previous work found that methods similar to the ones used in this study to classify cases into BI-RADS classes performed better on CC views than on MLO views or the combination of both [7]. Images were collected from three consecutive screening visits, nominally spaced two years apart and with the most recent visit being in 2005 or 2006. Here, a "case" will refer to the collection of images from one woman over all three visits. Cases were designated as cancer if anomalies found at screening during the 2005/6 round were confirmed as cancer by histopathology but no evidence of cancer had been found in previous rounds. Cases were designated as normal if no cancer had been found in any round including at least one screening visit post 2005/6. Evidence of risk was tracked separately in the breast with cancer, referred to as the ipsilateral breast, and the breast without cancer, referred to as the contralateral breast. Thus the study comprised 900 CC images; for each of the three time periods (current, two year previous and four year previous),

Table 1. Illustration of the structure of the data set. n is the number of images in each experimental group for every time period.

		2005, 2006	2003, 2004	2001, 2002
cancer cases	breast with cancer	current ipsilateral high risk $n = 100$	2 year previous ipsilateral high risk $n = 100$	4 year previous ipsilater high risk $n = 100$
	breast without cancer	current contralateral high risk $n = 100$	2 year previous contralateral high risk $n = 100$	4 year previous contralateral high risk $n = 100$
normal cases	random breast	current low risk $n = 100$	2 year previous low risk $n = 100$	4 year previous low risk $n = 100$

there were 100 images in each of the three experimental groups (ipsilateral high risk group, contralateral high risk group, and the low risk group) (Table 1).

For each time period and each experimental group, the 100 available images were divided into two sets of 50 images each; one set of the 50 was used for training and the remaining set was reserved for testing. The 50 cases for each group were selected so as to represent wide mammographic appearance. This was done by informally assigning images to BI-RADS classes and selecting approximately half the images from each BI-RADS class for training.

2.2 Preprocessing

For every image, the breast boundary was drawn manually using *ImageJ* software to remove the non-breast objects such as the labels and the pectoral muscle. Next, an image template was generated according to the breast boundary. The image template was further processed by erosion with 50 pixel radius circular structure element to remove the extreme boundary of the breast. This is necessary because texture properties at the edge of the breast are inconsistent with the rest of the breast due to the geometry of image acquisition.

Images were normalized locally by methods described previously [6] in order to preserve texture and remove background intensity. This was done to separate texture from density before feature extraction and so allow estimates of the potential contribution to risk assessment of pure texture features independent of density. The image template constructed previously was then applied to the normalized images to remove the non-breast objects.

2.3 Experiment Details

Methods similar to these proposed in [8] were used to compute first, second and third-order textons for current, two year previous and four year previous images. However, a variation of the method for generating higher-order textons was applied as follows.

For each pixel, the image intensities of the eight immediate neighbors were used to construct a feature vector of length eight. The total number of these feature vectors was reduced by subsampling by $5 \times 5 \rightarrow 1$ so that every square breast tissue patch of 25 pixels was represented by a single feature vector of length 8.

The feature vectors from the 50 training images in the current ipsilatoral high risk group were accumulated into a feature space. K-means clustering with with $K = 10$ was used to determine cluster centers representing the texture patterns of the ipsilateral high risk group at the current period. The resulting clusters centers are the first-order textons for current ipsilateral high risk group. Similarly, the feature vectors from the 50 training images in the current low risk group were used to determine a separate set of 10 first-order textons for this group. Pixels in each current training and testing image were replaced by the index of the texton that was nearest (among the 20 textons learnt from the two groups) to the first-order feature vector of the pixel according to the Euclidean norm. The resulting images are the first-order texton maps. For each image, the histogram of texton labels of the first-order texton map is the first-order texton representation of the image.

Second-order textons are textons based on the first-order texton map instead of the original image. However, the process for computing second-order textons cannot be exactly the same because the texton map consists of texton labels, which carry no rank information. Consequently, arithmetic operations cannot be applied to the textons labels. Instead, the feature vector associated with a pixel was taken to be the histogram of first-order texton occurrences in the 3×3 neighborhood of the pixel (This step is different from generating feature vectors in [8]). Thus the feature vector associated with each pixel was of length 20, one component representing each of the possible first-order textons. Aside from this change, the process follows that for first-order textons. Feature vectors from 50 training first-order texton maps in the current ipsilateral high risk group and 50 training first-order texton maps in the current low risk group were used to determine a set of 10 second-order textons, respectively. Each pixel in the current training and testing images from these two groups was replaced by a the index of a second-order texton nearest (among the 20 textons learnt from the two groups) to the second-order feature vector of the pixel. Resulting images are second-order texton maps and the histogram of second-order texton labels is the second-order texton representation of the image. Third-order textons, the third-order texton map and the third-order representation of each image were computed exactly the same as their second-order analogs but were based on the second-order texton maps. Together, each image in the current ipsilateral high risk or low risk group was represented by a combined texton histogram of 60 features for classification.

To determine the best feature combination for classifying current ipsilateral high risk from low risk mammograms, sequential feature selection was applied with the A_z score (area under the ROC curve) as the optimisation criterion. The maximum number of features was set at eight. The feature set identified by this process was used to estimate classifier performance on unseen data by using five-fold cross validation (recommended by [2]) on the 100 testing images from the two groups. The average A_z score from the cross validation will be referred to as the current ipsilateral A_z score.

The steps described above were repeated for the 200 two year previous ipsilateral high risk and low risk group images and again for the 200 images from the four year previous period to obtain the previous two year ipsilateral A_z score and the previous four year ipsilateral A_z score.

Finally, the entire process was repeated with the contralateral high risk and low risk group images in current, two and four year previous periods.

All the parameters used in these procedures including the choice of 3×3 neighborhood instead of larger ones, the subsampling factor and the choice of $K = 10$ in K-means clustering were based on previous studies by the authors and other groups [7,8,9,12,1].

3   Results

Table 2. (a) Temporal testing A_z scores of risk classification using 5-fold cross validation; (b) Temporal testing A_z scores of risk classification using 5-fold cross validation with higher-order textons learnt from the current year. In both cases, ± one standard deviation (SD) is shown.

(a)

A_z scores	current year	2 year previous	4 year previous
ipsilateral Vs normal	0.749±0.124	0.674±0.106	0.601±0.154
contralateral Vs normal	0.591±0.128	0.650±0.130	0.682±0.071

(b)

A_z scores	current year	2 year previous	4 year previous
ipsilateral Vs normal	0.749±0.124	0.655±0.066	0.551±0.076
contralateral Vs normal	0.591±0.128	0.601±0.129	0.664±0.059

Classification results for temporal risk assessment using five-fold cross validation are presented in Table 2 (a) and Figure 1. For ipsilateral versus normal, although there was a decrease in classification performance as a function of time prior to the detection of cancer, there was no significant difference between two year previous and current images ($p = 0.2056$, $n = 5$) or between four year previous and current images ($p = 0.0705$, $n = 5$). For contralateral versus normal, again there was no significant difference between two year previous and current images ($p = 0.5363$, $n = 5$) or between four year previous and current images ($p = 0.2855$, $n = 5$) although there was a slight increase in classification performance as a function of time prior to the detection of cancer.

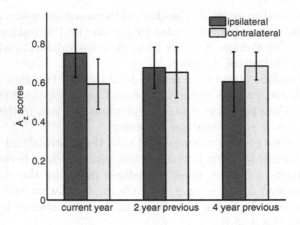

Fig. 1. Temporal A_z scores of risk classification: three dark color bars were the A_z scores of the classification of ipsilateral high risk Vs low risk in current year, previous two years and previous four years; three light color bars were the general A_z scores of the classification of contralateral high risk Vs low risk in the current year, previous two years and previous four years. The error bars show one SD.

In addition, there were no significant differences of classification performance between ipsilateral vs normal and contralateral vs normal A_z scores for current ($p = 0.07257$, $n = 5$), two year previous ($p = 0.7951$, $n = 5$) and four year previous ($p = 0.1135$, $n = 5$) periods.

4   Discussion and Conclusion

Because the focus was on testing the "in principle" information content relevant to breast cancer risk, separate textons and optimal feature sets were found for each time period (current, two year previous and four year previous). This does not yield a practical method for assessing risk clinically since a separate test would be required for estimating risk for different times in the future. Interpreting results would be difficult if, for example, a woman was found to have a high risk of developing cancer in two years time, but a low risk of developing cancer in four years time.

A more practical method would use a single test to estimate risk. This was considered by running a minor variation of the experiments described in Section 2.3. In this variation, the textons and optimal features found using the current images were computed and tested on the images in the two year previous period and the four year previous period. The results (Table 2 (b) and Figure 2) were not substantially different from the original experiment (Table 2 (a) and Figure 1). Accordingly, the methods described here could, in principle, contribute to a clinically useful scheme for estimating breast cancer risk.

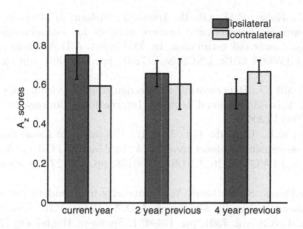

Fig. 2. Temporal A_z scores of risk classification with higher-order textons learnt from the current year. Every single bar represents the same details as in Figure 1.

The results reported here use only texture information and were not combined with other mammographic information such as density or clinical information to provide a comprehensive estimate of breast cancer risk. Thus, it is not yet clear if texture provides information that is complementary to other measures or if it largely reproduces existing measures. This will be the objective for a future study.

The A_z scores for the different groups and times (Table 2 (a) and Figure 1) indicate some trends, but none of the differences are statistically significant. Hence we conclude that texture information relevant to breast cancer risk is not restricted to, or significantly stronger in, the breast destined to develop cancer. Similarly, texture information relevant to breast cancer risk is present at least four years previous to the emergence of mammographically apparent signs of cancer at levels not significantly different from those at the time cancer is detected.

Acknowledgements. We thank BreastScreen SA for providing images for this study.

References

1. Gong, Y.C., Brady, M., Petroudi, S.: Texture based mammogram classification and segmentation. In: Astley, S.M., Brady, M., Rose, C., Zwiggelaar, R. (eds.) IWDM 2006. LNCS, vol. 4046, pp. 616–625. Springer, Heidelberg (2006)
2. Hastie, T., Tibshirani, R., Friedman, J.: The Elements of Statistical Learning: Data Mining, Inference and Prediction, 2nd edn. Springer Series in Statistics. Springer (2008)

3. Karemore, G., Keller, B.M., Oh, H., Tchou, J., Nielsen, M., Conant, E.F., Kontos, D.: Mammographic parenchymal texture analysis for estrogen-receptor subtype specific breast cancer risk estimation. In: Maidment, A.D.A., Bakic, P.R., Gavenonis, S. (eds.) IWDM 2012. LNCS, vol. 7361, pp. 596–603. Springer, Heidelberg (2012)
4. Leung, T., Malik, J.: Representing and recognizing the visual appearance of materials using three-dimensional textons. International Journal of Computer Vision 43(1), 29–44 (2001)
5. Li, H., Giger, M.L., Olopade, O.I., Lan, L.: Validation of mammographic texture analysis for assessment of breast cancer risk. In: Martí, J., Oliver, A., Freixenet, J., Martí, R. (eds.) IWDM 2010. LNCS, vol. 6136, pp. 267–271. Springer, Heidelberg (2010)
6. Li, X.-Z., Williams, S., Bottema, M.J.: Intensity independent texture analysis in screening mammograms. In: Maidment, A.D.A., Bakic, P.R., Gavenonis, S. (eds.) IWDM 2012. LNCS, vol. 7361, pp. 474–481. Springer, Heidelberg (2012)
7. Li, X.-Z., Williams, S., Bottema, M.J.: Background intensity independent texture features for assessing breast cancer risk in screening mammograms. Pattern Recognition Letters 34(9), 1053–1062 (2013)
8. Li, X.-Z., Williams, S., Bottema, M.J.: Constructing and applying higher-order textons: Estimating breast cancer risk. Pattern Recognition 47(3), 1375–1382 (2014)
9. Li, X.-Z., Williams, S., Bottema, M.J.: Texture and region dependent breast cancer risk assessment from screening mammograms. Pattern Recoginition Letters 36(15), 117–124 (2014)
10. Magnin, I.E., Cluzeau, F., Odet, C.L., Bremond, A.: Mammographic texture analysis: An evaluation of risk for developing breast cancer. Optical Engineering 25(6), 780–784 (1986)
11. Ting, C., Astley, S.M., Morris, J., Stavrinos, P., Wilson, M., Barr, N., Boggis, C., Sergeant, J.C.: Longitudinal change in mammographic density and association with breast cancer risk: A case-control study. In: Maidment, A.D.A., Bakic, P.R., Gavenonis, S. (eds.) IWDM 2012. LNCS, vol. 7361, pp. 205–211. Springer, Heidelberg (2012)
12. Varma, M., Zisserman, A.: Texture classification: Are filter banks necessary? In: Proceedings of the 2003 IEEE Computer Society Conference on Computer Vision and Pattern Recognition, vol. 2, pp. 691–698 (2003)

Invariant Features for Discriminating Cysts from Solid Lesions in Mammography

Thijs Kooi and Nico Karssemeijer

Radboud University Medical Center Nijmegen
The Netherlands

Abstract. Feature extraction is an integral of all Computer Aided Diagnosis (CAD) systems. Due to the presence of fibroglandular tissue however, measurements are perturbed by unwanted influences and therefore, the same descriptor will yield different values for different amounts of occluding structures. To aid the statistical learning used for classification, we need to design features that are *invariant* to unwanted influences. In this paper, we propose a simple model of the tumour and its surrounding tissue and show how this model can be used to derive descriptors that are invariant to obscuring tissue, rather than heuristically defining a set of descriptors, which is common practice in many CAD papers. We tailor the descriptors to optimally discriminate between tumours and cysts, by assuming a parametric form of the lesions. Results show a significant discriminative improvement over simple, more commonly used contrast features and we obtained an AUC of 0.77 using both CC and MLO images.

1 Introduction

Research on Computer Aided Detection and diagnosis (CAD) for screening mammography has been fruitful in the past years and as a result systems operating at high sensitivity are ubiquitous. Many CAD systems operate in a two-stage fashion where in the first stage, candidate lesions are detected on a pixel level and in a second stage, the lesions are segmented and new region-based features are computed. The second feature space is subsequently fed to a statistical learning machine, which is expected to give a more accurate estimate of the lesion's nature. The contrast, i.e., the relation between the segmented lesion and its surrounding tissue can tell us something about the disease and is often used as a feature in this stage. Due to the presence of fibroglandular tissue however, measurements are perturbed by unwanted influences and therefore, the same descriptor will yield different values for different amounts of occluding tissue. Given enough training data, we could expect the classification machine to generalise to a sufficient extent. Unfortunately, data is still scarce and therefore we need to aid the learner and design features that are *invariant* [1,2] to unwanted influences, yet covary with the factor we are interested in, i.e., we want descriptors that yield the same value regardless of obscuring structures, yet reliably characterise the nature of the lesion.

H. Fujita, T. Hara, and C. Muramatsu (Eds.): IWDM 2014, LNCS 8539, pp. 573–580, 2014.
© Springer International Publishing Switzerland 2014

In the first part of this paper, we propose a simple model of the tumour and its surrounding tissue by making some assumptions on the tumour growth and segmentation and show how to this model can be used to derive descriptors that are invariant to unwanted influences, rather than heuristically defining a set of descriptors, which is common practice in many CAD papers. In the second part, we tailor the descriptors to optimally discriminate between different geometrical entities, by assuming a parametric form. We apply the descriptors to the problem of discriminating between tumours and cysts: benign fluid-filled sacks exhibiting similar image characteristics to tumours in a mammogram. Experiments are done on simulated lesions, placed in a standard mammography background and on a database of clinical cases with a representative sample of cysts and masses. Results on both sets show a significant discriminative improvement over simple, more commonly used contrast features.

The rest of this paper is organised as follows. In section two, we will describe our model and preprocessing methods, followed by a brief derivation of the features in section 3 and details on the normalisation in section 4. We will present our experiments and discuss results in section 5, followed by a conclusion in section 6.

2   Lesion Model

In order to derive invariant descriptors, we first need a proper definition of invariance. We will call a descriptor D of some signal s invariant to a transformation T if it holds that:

$$D(T(s))) = D(s)$$

In our setting this means that we want to find a descriptor of a tumour (s) is such a way that if the same tumour is found in two different women with different amounts of occluding tissue (T), the descriptor will give the same value. A trivial way to make a descriptor invariant is to simply assign 1 to every exposition of the signal. This however, obliterates all discriminative power and we should therefore aim for an optimum in the trade-off between descriptiveness and invariance.

The first step in our method is to compute a *dense tissue map* of the image [4], which is acquired be means of a physics based image model derived in previous work. We assume the breast is composed of dense and fatty tissue, with corresponding attenuation coefficients. Using empirical data from literature, we get an estimate of the amount of dense and fatty tissue at each pixel, where the former is used in our method. To subsequently derive our descriptors, we propose the following simple model of the lesion f:

$$I(x,y) = \begin{cases} F_z(x,y) + \epsilon & \text{if } (x,y) \text{ lies inside the 2D projection of } f \\ \epsilon & \text{else} \end{cases} \tag{1}$$

where $I(x,y)$ indicates the image value at location (x,y), $\epsilon \sim P(\epsilon)$ is the integral along the z-axis of the nuisance term we are trying to ignore, coming from some undefined distribution and $F_z(x,y) = \int f(x,y,z)dz$ the z-integral of the lesion

f we are trying to describe. The z-axis is chosen to be parallel to the direction of x-ray quanta. This model assumes that the 2D segmentation of the projected lesion is correct and that the tumour grows in such a way that the distribution of tissue in the surrounding region is the same as above and below it. An illustration is provided in figure 1. Using this model, we can not infer anything about the

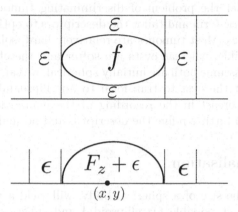

Fig. 1. Illustration of a lateral view of a lesion and its z-integral on the image plane. Here ε indicates the tissue in the breast and ϵ the integral of ε appearing on the image.

exact spatial layout of f, due to the noise term ϵ. However, by looking at the descriptive statistics of the values inside the segmented region ($F_z + \epsilon$) and the values in the surroundings of the region (ϵ), we can still derive descriptors of its shape that are invariant to nuisance ϵ.

3 Moment Invariants

Under the definition of invariance and lesion model we proposed, a descriptor of the mean, invariant to nuisance signal ϵ is given by:

$$\mathbb{E}[F_z] = \mathbb{E}[F_z + \epsilon] - \mathbb{E}[\epsilon] \tag{2}$$

Similar to the mean, the variance will give us an indication of the shape of the z-integral. The sum of variance to two correlated random variables is given by:

$$Var[F_z + \epsilon] = Var[F_z] + Var[\epsilon] + 2Cov[F_z, \epsilon] \tag{3}$$

We can observe $Var[F_z+\epsilon]$ and $Var[\epsilon]$ in our image and are interested in $Var[F_z]$. Unfortunately, we can not observe $Cov[F_z, \epsilon]$. However, by looking at the covariance of $F_z + \epsilon$ and ϵ, we can find an expression for $Var[F_z]$. We can show that the covariance of two correlated random variables X and Y can be written as (a proof of this is left out for brevity)

$$Cov[X, Y] = Cov[X + Y, Y] - Var[Y]$$

Plugging this into equation (3) and rearranging terms, we have that

$$Var[F_z] = Var[F_z + \epsilon] + Var[\epsilon] - 2Cov[F_z + \epsilon, \epsilon] \tag{4}$$

These two features are general descriptors of the z-integral of any geometric body, though in not all situations they may provide useful, discriminative information. We will now consider the problem of discriminating tumours from cysts, by assuming a parametric form and tailor the descriptors to optimally differentiate between these entities. Most tumours are relatively hard, solid objects that are not easily compressible, whereas cysts are softer and therefore more likely to change shape. If we assume both are initially spherical, we can expect the tumour to retain shape, but the cyst to transform to an ellipsoidal form, due to the compression of the breast in the recording of the mammogram. Under these assumptions, we can further refine the descriptor and normalise for scale.

4   Scale Normalisation

Simply increasing the size of a spherical body, will yield a varying feature response. This makes it possible for ellipsoidal and spherical objects to reach similar descriptors, in spite of their apparent disparity. We therefore want to normalise with respect to scale in order to discriminate properly between the two. To this end, we propose the following normalisations. By looking at the z-integral of a sphere

$$F_z = 2\sqrt{(r^2 - x^2 - y^2)}$$

we can see that the expected value as a function of radius r is given by:

$$\mathbb{E}[F_z; r] = \frac{1}{A(r)} \int_{-r}^{r} \int_{-r}^{r} 2\sqrt{(r^2 - x^2 - y^2)} dx\, dy$$

where $A(r)$ indicates the area of the projection of the sphere as a function of its radius. The integral is simply the volume of the sphere, so therefore:

$$\mathbb{E}[F_z; r] = \frac{V(r)}{A(r)} = \frac{1}{\pi r^2} \frac{4}{3} \pi r^3 = r\frac{4}{3}$$

Normalisation by r evidently results in a constant. Using a similar procedure for the second moment descriptor, we will find that a normalisation by r^2 will yield a constant value. The derivation is left out here for brevity. The scale normalised descriptors $\hat{\mathbb{E}}[F_z]$ and $\hat{Var}[F_z]$ are now given by:

$$\hat{\mathbb{E}}[F_z] = \frac{\mathbb{E}[F_z + \epsilon] - \mathbb{E}[\epsilon]}{r} \tag{5}$$

and

$$\hat{Var}[F_z] = \frac{Var[F_z + \epsilon] + Var[\epsilon] - 2Cov[F_z + \epsilon, \epsilon]}{r^2} \tag{6}$$

The following section will present our experimental setup and results acquired when applying this method.

5   Experiments

The experiments are set up to show that each normalisation and both the first and second moment are contributors to the discriminative power of the features. In a first test, we investigated how our model holds in a more or less ideal situation. This way we can see to what extent the assumptions in our model are violated when subsequently testing on real data. We placed masses (z-integrals of spheres) and cysts (z-integrals of ellipsoidal shapes) at random in a mammography background. The parameters of the spheres and ellipsoids were varied at random and the mix between z-integral and mammographic background was also varied randomly, resulting in some clear lesion and some very subtle ones. Examples of simulated lesions are given in 2. In a second test, we applied the

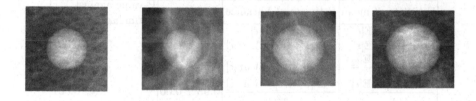

Fig. 2. Illustration of simulated lesions. The left two represent masses and the right two cysts.

methods to real data. Regions were segmented using a dynamic programming algorithm, that has previously been shown to be successful for this task [3]. The data was collected locally from symptomatic women and high risk screening. We removed lesions that were on or close to the pectoralis, because our density algorithm does not support reliable density estimates on the pectoralis yet. A similar thing was done for lesions on or close to the image edge, because we can not reasonably assume to get accurate contrast information from here. Future work will revolve around finding new methods for this. During annotation, all lesions were given a subtlety score by an independent annotator and we remove lesions with extreme subtlety. This left 94 cysts and 173 masses. Images were recorded using a GE mammography machine. Samples were classified by means of a linear logistic regression model, trained using iteratively reweighted least-squares (IRLS). To estimate test performance, we split the train and test data 100 times, resulting in 100 estimates of the ROC and AUC, over which we compute analytical statistics.

5.1   Implementation Details

The computation of covariance assumes an ordered set of pairs and therefore, the use of covariance in (6) requires some elaboration. Considering the fact that the noise we are interested in (the occluding tissue) has some spatial coherence, i.e., the noise between surrounding pixels is strongly correlated, it seems reasonable to assume that points on each side of the acquired segmentation boundary will have roughly the same noise value. Using this intuition, we construct a set of points by taking values along the fitting region on each side of the border and compute the covariance from this set.

The radius parameter we have described before, assumes a circular fitting region, which is in practice never the case. We therefore take the radius as half the maximum diameter of the fitted region. Lastly, the size of the surrounding border (ϵ) is chosen in such a way that the amount of pixels in the lesion and surrounding area are approximately similar if the particular image allows this.

Table 1. Comparison of different feature sets in simulation

Estimate of mean	Estimate of Variance	AUC	P-value against normalised features
$\mathbb{E}[F_z + \epsilon] - \mathbb{E}[\epsilon]$	$Var[F_z + \epsilon]$	0.55 ± 0.01	$\ll 0.001$
$\mathbb{E}[F_z + \epsilon] - \mathbb{E}[\epsilon]$	$Var[F_z + \epsilon] - Var[\epsilon]$	0.58 ± 0.02	$\ll 0.001$
$\dfrac{\mathbb{E}[F_z + \epsilon] - \mathbb{E}[\epsilon]}{r}$	$Var[F_z + \epsilon] - Var[\epsilon]$	0.86 ± 0.07	$\ll 0.001$
$\dfrac{\mathbb{E}[F_z + \epsilon] - \mathbb{E}[\epsilon]}{r}$	$\dfrac{Var[F_z + \epsilon] - Var[\epsilon]}{r^2}$	0.93 ± 0.00	$\ll 0.001$

5.2   Results

On simulated data, our normalised features as described in (5) and (6) gave an average $AUC = 0.95 \pm 0.004$. Table 1 shows the results of a comparison between these and several feature sets that are increasingly similar to our descriptors, thereby proving the value of each step in our methods. The first and second column show the estimate of the first and second moment, the third column the acquired average AUC and the fourth column the P-value tested against our reference features. Significance estimates were acquired by means of a Kruskal-Wallis rank test. On real data, our normalised features as described in (5) and (6) obtained an average AUC of 0.65 +/- 0.07. Table 2 shows results of several other feature sets, in increasing complexity. Again, P-values were computed using a Kruskal-Wallis test.

Table 2. Comparison of different feature sets on our dataset

Estimate of mean	Estimate of Variance	AUC	P-value against normalised features
$\mathbb{E}[F_z + \epsilon] - \mathbb{E}[\epsilon]$	$Var[F_z + \epsilon]$	0.52 ± 0.07	$\ll 0.001$
$\mathbb{E}[F_z + \epsilon] - \mathbb{E}[\epsilon]$	$Var[F_z + \epsilon] - Var[\epsilon]$	0.54 ± 0.01	$\ll 0.001$
$\dfrac{\mathbb{E}[F_z + \epsilon] - \mathbb{E}[\epsilon]}{r}$	$Var[F_z + \epsilon] - Var[\epsilon]$	0.63 ± 0.08	0.006
$\dfrac{\mathbb{E}[F_z + \epsilon] - \mathbb{E}[\epsilon]}{r}$	$\dfrac{Var[F_z + \epsilon] - Var[\epsilon]}{r^2}$	0.62 ± 0.07	0.019

In a third experiment, we averaged the feature output of lesions in CC and MLO images in order to reduce measuring errors. In this setting, our normalised features obtained an AUC of 0.77 ± 0.09, compared to an AUC of 0.66 ± 0.12 using a CC/MLO average of the feature described in the last row of table 1. This was found significant using a Kruskal-Wallis test ($p \ll 0.001$). Illustrations of the final feature spaces of the reference and normalised features are given in figure 3.

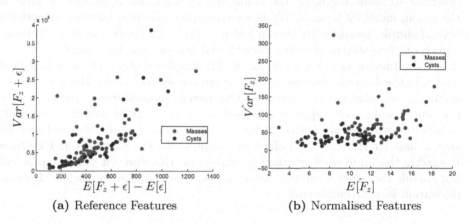

(a) Reference Features   (b) Normalised Features

Fig. 3. Illustration of the Feature Space for Real Data, Averaged between CC and MLO

5.3   Discussion

In an ideal setting, we can see our descriptors fare well and vastly outperform the simple, commonly applied descriptors, described in the first row of table 1. Even though the classification performance on real data is still relatively poor using a single image, we can clearly see an improvement using the proposed descriptors, as is seen from table 2. The progression to more complex descriptors as is presented in the tables, suggests that both a normalisation with respect to the surrounding region and a normalisation with respect to scale are contributors to the improvement and that not only the proposed estimate of the mean, but also the estimate of variance yields useful discriminative information. This can also be seen from the plot of the feature space in figure 3, where two clearer clusters appear in the right image.

To make the estimates less susceptible to outliers, we have tried to replace the regular estimates of location and scale with robust estimates. We tried using the median and winsorising to replace the standard estimate of location and we used the inter quartile range, median absolute difference and Minimum Discriminant Covariance algorithm to generate a robust estimate of the (co)variance. In the case of location, this yielded no difference and in the case of scale, this performed significantly worse. Apart from applying the methods in the density image, we have also tried our method on raw FFDM data, but both methods proved substantially worse in this setting, reaching a classification performance only slightly above what one would expect from a random assignment of labels.

6   Conclusion

In this paper, we showed that by assuming a simple model of a tumour and its surrounding area, lesion features can be derived that in the first place are invariant to tissue occluding the lesion and by assuming a parametric form of the lesion, invariant to scale. We showed our model-derived features outperform several simple, heuristically chosen features, typically applied in other systems. This is our first step on deriving model based descriptors. The model we use, assumes the tumour grows in a specific, highly simplified way and has a simplified shape. In the data we observed so far, the growth seems to hold. However the tumours in our database seem to have a very sharp gradient around the edges, but the centre of the lesion appears flattened. In future work, it may be worthwhile to investigate different parametric forms in the derivation of features. It can be shown that for spherical and ellipsoidal z-integrals, the skewness and kurtosis is exactly the same (and invariant to scale) and therefore for our test problem not useful. For other structures however, these can still prove useful, although derivation is quite cumbersome.

References

1. Geusebroek, J.-M., van den Boomgaard, R., Smeulders, A.W.M., Geerts, H.: Color invariance. IEEE Transactions on Pattern Analysis and Machine Intelligence 23(12), 1338–1350 (2001)
2. Hu, M.-K.: Visual pattern recognition by moment invariants. IRE Transactions on Information Theory 8(2), 179–187 (1962)
3. Timp, S., Karssemeijer, N.: A new 2D segmentation method based on dynamic programming applied to computer aided detection in mammography. Medical Physics 31(5), 958–971 (2004)
4. van Engeland, S., Snoeren, P., Huisman, H.-J., Boetes, C., Karssemeijer, N.: Volumetric breast density estimation from full-field digital mammograms. IEEE Transactions on Medical Imaging 25(3), 273–282 (2006)

Breast Masses Identification through Pixel-Based Texture Classification*

Jordina Torrents-Barrena[1], Domenec Puig[1,**], Maria Ferre[1], Jaime Melendez[2],
Lorena Diez-Presa[3], Meritxell Arenas[3], and Joan Martí[4]

[1] Department of Computer Engineering and Mathematics, University Rovira i Virgili
domenec.puig@urv.cat
[2] Department of Radiology, Radboud University Medical Center
[3] Radiotherapic Oncology Research Group. Hospital Universitari Sant Joan de Reus
[4] Computer Vision and Robotics Research Institute, University of Girona

Abstract. Mammographic image analysis plays an important role in
computer-aided breast cancer diagnosis. To improve the existing knowledge, this paper proposes a new efficient pixel-based methodology for
tumor vs non-tumor classification. The proposed method firstly computes a Gabor feature pool from the mammogram. This feature set is
calculated through multi-sized evaluation windows applied to the probabilistic distribution moments, in order to improve the accuracy of the
whole system. To deal with a high dimensional data space and a large
amount of features, we apply both a linear and non-linear pixel classification stage by using Support Vector Machines (SVMs). The randomness
is encoded when training each SVM using randomly sample sets and, in
consequence, randomly selected features from the whole feature bank obtained in the first stage. The proposed method has been validated using
real mammographic images from well-known databases and its effectiveness is demonstrated in the experimental section.

Keywords: Texture feature extraction, Gabor filters, Support Vector
Machine, mammographic images, pixel-based classification.

1 Introduction

Breast cancer among middle aged women is a significant public health problem in
the world. At present, there are no effective ways to prevent it, because its cause
is not yet fully known. Early detection is the key for improving cancer prognosis
since the death rate can be significantly reduced. Mammography has been one
of the most reliable methods for detecting breast carcinomas [1, 2], in its earliest
and most treatable stage, so it continues to be the primary imaging modality
for breast cancer screening and diagnosis. In addition, it allows the detection of

---

* This work was partly supported by the Spanish Government through projects
TIN2012-37171-C02-01 and TIN2012-37171-C02-02.
** Corresponding author.

H. Fujita, T. Hara, and C. Muramatsu (Eds.): IWDM 2014, LNCS 8539, pp. 581–588, 2014.
© Springer International Publishing Switzerland 2014

other pathologies and may suggest the tumor nature such as normal, benign or malignant.

Nowadays, reading mammograms is a very demanding job for radiologists, who visually examine the images for the presence of deformities that can be associated as cancerous changes. Mammograms are hard to interpret because of the complex tissue morphology of the breast and the number of imaging parameters that affect its acquisition. For this reason, the radiologists judgments depend on their training, experience and subjective criteria. There are several lesions that are characteristics of breast cancer such as microcalcifications, masses, architectural distortions and bilateral asymmetry. Since some lesions are often indistinguishable, because they have similar features to normal mammary tissue, automated detection and classification is even more difficult.

Furthermore, some other diseases have similar patterns to the breast cancer, which challenges the diagnosis. Manual readings may result misdiagnosis due to human errors caused by visual fatigue. To improve accuracy and efficiency of screening mammography, computer aided techniques are introduced. Therefore, CAD systems have been shown to be a helpful tool [3]. They can provide an important contribution for breast cancer control by marking suspicious regions and detecting abnormalities, to decrease the death rate among women with this disease.

This paper presents a framework for tumor vs non-tumor identification founded on a pixel-based texture classification approach, which is broadly divided in two stages. In the first stage, texture features are extracted from both tumor and normal regions by using a Gabor filter bank. In the second stage, a pixel-based texture classification strategy by using SVMs is applied [4], which provides the probability of each pixel in the mammogram to belong to a tumor region.

The rest of the paper is organized as follows. In Section 2, we present the proposed methodology. First, we describe the feature extraction step and then, the pixel-based classification algorithm. Experiments are shown and discussed in Section 3. Finally, conclusions and further tasks are given in Section 4.

2   Proposed Methodology

The texture classification methodology proposed in this work is as follows. During an initial training stage, a set of prototype features is computed at every texture pattern of interest (normal/tumor). The training images associated with each pattern are first filtered by applying a multichannel Gabor filter bank, obtaining a cloud of texture feature vectors for every pattern [5–7]. A set of prototypes is then extracted in order to represent that cloud. During the evaluation stage of the classifier, a given test image is processed in order to identify the texture pattern corresponding to each of its pixels. This is done by first applying the multichannel Gabor filter bank to the test image. A feature vector is thus obtained for every pixel. Each vector is classified into one of the given texture patterns by a SVM-based classifier fed with the prototypes extracted during the training stage. The stages involved in this scheme are detailed below.

2.1 Texture Feature Extraction

Textural properties in an image can be used to detect different types of information such as edges, lines, spots, flat areas and other local patterns. Some of these properties can be observed in mammograms at different scales and orientations. For this reason, we define a Gabor filter bank in order to capture texture patterns in mammograms, as it has been shown to be optimal in the sense of minimizing the joint two-dimensional uncertainty in space and frequency.

Gabor Filters. A wide variety of texture feature extraction methods have been proposed in the literature. Among them, multichannel filtering techniques based on Gabor filters have received considerable attention. The texture feature extraction stage of this work is based on the optimized multichannel Gabor wavelet filters. The next paragraphs give a brief overview about them.

Gabor filters are biologically motivated convolution kernels that have enjoyed wide usage in a myriad of applications in the field of computer vision and image processing. In order to extract local spatial textural micro-patterns in mammogram ROIs, Gabor filters can be tuned with different orientations and scales, and thus provide powerful statistics which could be very useful for breast cancer detection.

A two-dimensional Gabor filter defined as a Gaussian kernel modulated by an oriented complex sinusoidal wave can be described as follows [5, 8, 6]:

$$g(x, y) = \frac{1}{2\pi\sigma_x\sigma_y} \exp^{-\frac{1}{2}(\frac{\tilde{x}^2}{\sigma_x^2} + \frac{\tilde{y}^2}{\sigma_y^2})} \exp^{2\pi j W \tilde{x}} \tag{1}$$

$$\tilde{x} = x \cdot \cos\theta + y \cdot \sin\theta \quad \text{and} \quad \tilde{y} = -x \cdot \sin\theta + y \cdot \cos\theta \tag{2}$$

where σ_x and σ_y are the scaling parameters of the filter and describe the neighborhood of a pixel where weighted summation takes place, W is the central frequency of the complex sinusoidal and $\theta \in [0, \pi)$ is the orientation of the normal to the parallel stripes of the Gabor function.

Evaluation of Texture Methods over Multisized Windows. The texture features that characterize each pixel and its surrounding neighborhood (window) are both the mean and standard deviation of the module of the Gabor wavelet coefficients. The Gabor filter bank has been configured with four scales and six orientations, and a range of frequencies between 0.05 and 0.4. The orientations and frequencies for a bank are calculated using the following equations:

$$orientation(i) = \frac{(i-1)\pi}{m} \quad \text{where} \quad i = 1, 2, ..., m \tag{3}$$

$$frequency(i) = \frac{f_{max=0.4}}{(\sqrt{2}^{i-1})} \quad \text{where} \quad i = 1, 2, ..., n \tag{4}$$

where m is the total number of orientations and n is the total number of frequencies. Therefore, every feature vector is composed by a total of 48 dimensions: $6(scales) \times 4(orientations) \times 2(mean, stdev)$.

The means and stdevs mentioned above are computed for W different window sizes. W is set to 3 in this case: 1×1, 33×33 and 51×51. Thus, W sets of feature vectors are generated for each pixel of the given texture patterns during the training stage, as well as for each pixel of the test image during the classification stage.

2.2   Supervised Pixel-Based Classification

Once the features characterizing both normal and tumor tissue have been extracted, the goal of this stage is to classify the pixels of an input test mammogram into one of the two patterns of interest (normal/tumor).

Support Vector Machine-Based Classifier. A classification problem encompasses the assignment of an unseen pattern to a predefined class, according to the characteristics of the pattern, presented in the form of a feature vector. However, a classifier needs to be trained in order to perform this task.

A way to efficiently summarize and learn all the available information obtained from the training set is through SVMs, since they are the most advanced ones, generally, designed to solve binary classification problems. SVM formulation is based on statistical learning theory [9, 10] and has attractive generalization capabilities in linear and non-linear decision problems. The classifier maps an M-dimensional data point into a class label based on an aggregating decision function. A supervised classification task involves separating data into training and test sets. Each instance in the training set contains the class label and the features. The goal of the SVM is to produce a model, based on the training data, which predicts the target values of the test data given only the test data features. Given a training set of instance-label pairs (x_i, y_i), $i = 1, ..., l$, where $x_i \in R^n$ and $y \in \{1, -1\}^l$, the SVM casts the classification problem into an optimization problem. The training vectors x_i are mapped into a higher or infinite dimensional space. The SVM finds a linear separating hyperplane with the maximal margin in this higher dimensional space by using what is called the kernel trick.

The four basic kernel functions are linear, polynomial, sigmoid and radial, from which we only use two of them (linear and radial). For linearly separable problems, kernel function is simply the dot product of the two given points in the input space:

$$k(x_i, x) = x_i \cdot x \tag{5}$$

However, for non-linear problems, the original input space is mapped through a non-linear function, possibly making the data linearly separable, using different suitable kernels (for computational efficiency). In our experiments, RBF (radial basis function) kernel is used as given by:

$$k(x_i, x) = \exp^{(-\gamma\|x_i-x\|^2)}, \gamma > 0 \tag{6}$$

There are two parameters now tied with the RBF kernel: γ that represents the width of the kernel function, and C (a regularization parameter) who controls the trade-off between error of SVM and margin maximization [9].

2.3   Breast Masses Identification System

The block diagram of the breast cancer identification system is detailed below (see Fig. 1). The proposed system is composed of four main stages: pre-processing, feature extraction, feature selection and classification. Various existing approaches differ in the choice of techniques for these stages. Our proposed approach for feature extraction is robust against noise (this method has been described in detail in subsection 2.1). Then, we apply a significant selection of the features extracted. In the training mode we choose all the pixels inside the tumor region, by contrast, when the classifier is in the prediction phase, a random selection is applied in order to choose both some normal pixels and also pixels affected by the disease. In this way, the next step will use both types of information.

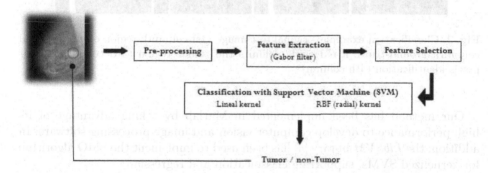

Fig. 1. Breast Masses Detection System

3   Experimentation

This section describes the materials used for the development and validation of the proposed technique, as well as the experimental results obtained through the application of the proposed methodology to a well-known mammogram database.

3.1   Materials

The algorithm proposed in this paper has been evaluated on the mammograms of the mini-MIAS database [11] that comprises 322 images of 1024×1024 pixels (e.g., Fig. 2, 1st column). Every image includes information about the existing anomalies: it comprises the location of the lesion and the radius of the circle that roughly delimits the lesion (e.g., Fig. 2, 3rd column). We randomly selected several cases from this database which contain true and false masses (but with suspicious tissues). These ROIs are used for training and testing.

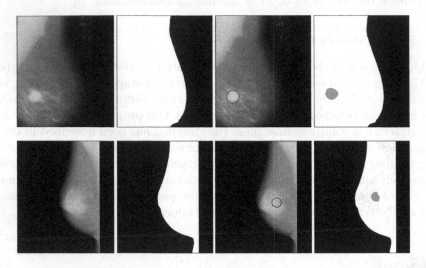

Fig. 2. Classification example: original test image (1st column), region of interest (2nd column), ground-truth: a red circle delimits the tumor region (3rd column), tumor pixels identification (4th column)

Our method has been implemented in Matlab by taking advantage of its high performance to develop computer vision and image processing software. In addition, the *LibSVM* library [4] has been used to implement the SMO algorithm for kernelized SVMs, supporting classification and regression.

3.2   Experimental Results

The convenient values of the SVM parameters to reach good accuracy ratios for discrimination between tumor and normal regions were found by means of an iterative procedure. Furthermore, our algorithm removes the background regions in the mammogram and focusses the tumor search in the breast region (e.g., Fig. 2, 2nd column). Finally, each pixel in the test mammogram is classified as belonging to tumor or normal region (e.g., grey pixels have been classified as belonging to a tumor in Fig. 2, 4th column).

Commonly used evaluation measures of the predictive ability of the breast cancer detection systems are *sensitivity* (a measure of true positive rate) and *specificity* (a measure of true negative rate) under *ROC curve*. In addition, the *F1* score also helps to determinate the effectiveness of our pixel-based classifier. We adopt these performance measures to evaluate the proposed system.

First of all, *F1* score can measure the discrimination capability of the classifier between the cancerous and normal regions (the closer the *F1* to 1, the better the tumor identification). The *F1* score is defined as: $F1 = 2TP/2TP + FN + FP$, where *TP*, *FN* and *FP* are the number of true positives, false negatives and false positives respectively. The average results corresponding to the mini-MIAS database [11] classification are shown in Table 1. Notice that, especially the SVM classifier based on the radial kernel produces good identification ratios for the tumor pixels (TP ratio), and relatively low false detections (FP ratio).

A second analysis is based on the *ROC curve* and a complete sensitivity/specificity report, a fundamental tool for diagnostic test evaluation. Fig. 3 shows the *ROC curves* corresponding to both SVM classifiers, where the true positive rate (Sensitivity) is plotted in function of the false positive rate (Specificity) for different cut-off points of a parameter. Each point on the *ROC curve* represents a sensitivity/specificity pair corresponding to a particular decision threshold. The area under the *ROC curve* (AUC) is a measure of how well a parameter can distinguish between two diagnostic groups (tumor/non-tumor).

Table 1. Quality scores corresponding to different configurations of the SVM classifier. All the ratios are shown between 0 and 1.

Classifier	Window-size	TP	FP	TN	FN	*F1*	*Overall Accuracy*
SVM (linear)	1x1	0.88	0.66	0.34	0.12	*0.66*	*0.80*
	33x33	0.83	0.66	0.34	0.17	*0.57*	*0.77*
	51x51	0.76	0.67	0.33	0.24	*0.54*	*0.73*
SVM (radial)	1x1	0.91	0.56	0.44	0.09	*0.59*	*0.79*
	33x33	0.89	0.59	0.40	0.11	*0.58*	*0.79*
	51x51	0.93	0.33	0.67	0.07	*0.33*	*0.72*

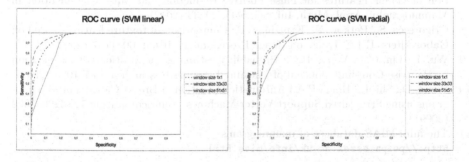

Fig. 3. ROC curves for the different configurations of the SVM classifier

4 Conclusions

This paper proposes a new pixel-based texture classification method for tumor region identification in mammograms. The proposed method firstly computes Gabor based features from the mammograms by means of multi-sized evaluation windows applied to the probabilistic distribution moments. Then, the identification of tumor regions is performed through a pixel-based classification scheme by using SVMs, which is able to deal with a high dimensional data space and a large amount of features. Promising results have been obtained for the identification of tumor regions on the mammograms of the mini-MIAS database. Further work will consist of combining new statistical texture features extracted from the Gabor filters and applying optimization methods to determine the optimal parameters of the SVM.

References

1. Yufeng, Z.: Breast Cancer Detection with Gabor Features from Digital Mammograms. Algorithms 3, 44–62 (2010)
2. Ioan, B., Gacsadi, A.: Directional Features for Automatic Tumor Classification of Mammogram Images. Biomedical Signal Processing and Control 6(4), 370–378 (2011)
3. Tang, J., Rangayyan, R.M., Xu, J., El Naqa, I.: Computer-Aided Detection and Diagnosis of Breast Cancer with Mammography: Recent Advances. IEEE Trans. Information Technology in Biomedicine 13(2), 236–251 (2009)
4. Chang, C.C., Lin, C.J.: LIBSVM: A Library for Support Vector Machines. ACM Transactions on Intelligent Systems and Technology 2(3), Article 27 (2011)
5. Manjunath, B.S., Ma, W.Y.: Texture Features for Browsing and Retrieval of Image Data. IEEE Trans. on Pattern Analysis and Machine Intelligence 18(8), 837–842 (1996)
6. Hussain, M., Khan, S., Muhammad, G., Berbar, M., Bebis, G.: Mass Detection in Digital Mammograms Using Gabor Filter Bank. In: Proc. IET Image Processing, July 2-3, pp. 1–6 (2012)
7. Hussain, M., Khan, S., Muhammad, G., Ahmad, I., Bebis, G.: Effective Extraction of Gabor Features for False Positive Reduction and Mass Classification in Mammography. Appl. Math. Inf. Sci. 6(1), 29–33 (2012)
8. Grigorescu, S., Petkov, N., Kruizinga, P.: Comparison of texture features based on Gabor filters. IEEE Trans. on Image Processing 11(10), 1160–1167 (2002)
9. Wu, T., Lin, C.J., Weng, R.C.: Probability estimates for Multiclass Classification by Pairwise Coupling. Journal of Machine Learning Research 5, 975–1005 (2003)
10. Wang, D., Shi, L., Heng, P.A.: Automatic Detection of Breast Cancers in Mammograms using Structured Support Vector Machines. Neurocomputing 72, 3296–3302 (2009)
11. The mini-MIAS database of mammograms:
    http://peipa.essex.ac.uk/info/mias.html

Automated Labeling of Screening Mammograms with Arterial Calcifications

Jan-Jurre Mordang[1], Jakob Hauth[1],
Gerard J. den Heeten[2,3], and Nico Karssemeijer[1]

[1] Department of Radiology, Radboud University Medical Center, Nijmegen,
The Netherlands
[2] The National Expert and Training Centre for Breast Cancer Screening, Nijmegen,
The Netherlands
[3] Department of Radiology, Academic Medical Center, Amsterdam, The Netherlands

Abstract. For the automatic detection of malignant microcalcification clusters in screening mammograms a computer aided detection (CADe) system has been developed. The most frequent false positives of this system are breast arterial calcifications (BACs). The purpose of this study was to construct a method for selecting cases with BACs in mammographic screening data as part of a procedure to reduce false positives of the CADe system. To automatically select cases containing BACs, a GentleBoost classifier was trained. For composing the training set, the CADe system was applied on 10,000 normal cases. From these cases, 400 cases with the most significant false positives were included in the training set and an additional 200 cases with less obvious false positives. For testing, an independent test set was created by cluster detection of 1,000 normal cases and 95 malignant cases. After cluster detection 342 normal cases contained false positives and in 93 malignant cases true positive clusters were detected. In the training set, 244 cases showed signs of BACs and in the test set 95 cases. A total of 102 case-based features were calculated to train the classifier. A ROC curve was calculated of the classification of the test set bootstrapped 5000 times. The area under the curve of the ROC was 0.92 and already 44% of the cases with BACs were detected without any false positives. Furthermore, 90% of the cases with BACs were detected at a false positive rate of 20%. The performance of the proposed selection method implies a good feasibility to classify cases with BACs at high specificity. By using this selection we will be able to apply dedicated methods for false positive reduction due to BACs.

Keywords: Mammography, calcifications, arterial, pattern recognition, computer aided detection.

1 Introduction

Microcalcification clusters in the breast are a biomarker for breast cancer. For the purpose of automatic detection of these malignant clusters a computer aided detection (CADe) system has been developed. However, not all microcalcifications

H. Fujita, T. Hara, and C. Muramatsu (Eds.): IWDM 2014, LNCS 8539, pp. 589–596, 2014.
© Springer International Publishing Switzerland 2014

in the breast are malignant as benign calcifications can be observed in mammograms as well. The most frequent benign calcification clusters that are marked with a high malignancy likelihood by the current CADe system are breast arterial calcifications (BACs) (example shown in Figure 1). Therefore, by adding an additional false positive removal classification to our CADe system, specified on detecting BACs, might improve the system. Selecting cases with BACs and removal of false positive clusters in only these cases can prevent the removal of malignant clusters and ultimately lead to a more specific system for the detection of malignant microcalcification clusters. Therefore, the purpose of this study was to construct a method for selecting cases with BACs in mammographic screening data.

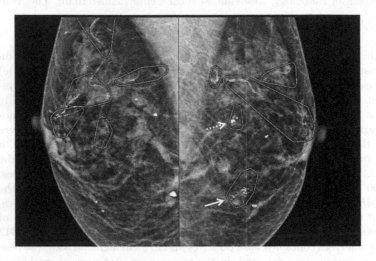

Fig. 1. Example of microcalcification cluster detection in 2 mammograms containing BACs, macrocalcifications and a malignant microcalcification cluster. The malignant cluster is denoted with the solid arrow. A false positive due to a macrocalcification is denoted with the dashed arrow. All other annotations are false positives due to BACs.

2   Methods

The framework for the selection of cases with BACs consists of four stages. The first stage is the selection of the microcalcification candidates in raw screening mammograms with a cascade classification scheme. In the next stage, the selected microcalcification candidates are clustered. And in the third stage, false positive clusters are removed with a trained classifier. The last stage consists of a case-based approach for the selection of cases with BACs. The first three stages are based on the work of Bria et al[1]. Therefore, these stages will only be touched very briefly in the next section. The fourth stage will be discussed in more detail in the subsequent section. A full flowchart of the framework is visualized in Figure 2.

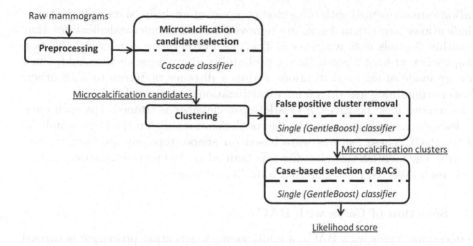

Fig. 2. Flowchart of the whole framework. There are 4 main stages: i) microcalcification candidate selection, ii) clustering, iii) false positive cluster removal, and iv) classification of cases with BACs. Type of classification is denoted in *italic* and (intermediate) results are underlined.

2.1   Microcalcification Cluster Detection

For the detection of microcalcifications in raw mammograms, a cascade classifier is trained[13]. After preprocessing, for each pixel in the mammogram a patch is made with a dimensions of 13 x 13 pixels where the pixel lies in the center of the patch. This patch goes through 4 stages where in each stage the patch is classified by a GentleBoost classifier[11]. Features for each stage are determined during training from a total of 8 groups of Haar-like features[8]. These feature groups are be scaled and translated within the patch. Examples of these groups are shown in Figure 3. Patches classified as negative in one of the first three stages are removed and the remaining patches obtain a probability score in the last classification stage. For the four stages 3, 6, 11, and 51 haar-like features were calculated, respectively.

Microcalcification candidate classification in a mammogram leads to an image where each pixel corresponds to a probability score or zero if the patch is removed in an early stage of the cascade classifier. In these probability images, microcalci-

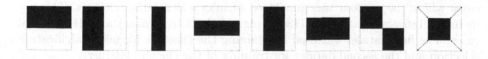

Fig. 3. Examples of the haar-like features groups

fications are segmented with connected component analysis. Macrocalcifications, calcifications larger than $1mm$, are removed as well as microcalcifications that lie within 2 pixels from a macrocalcification. Furthermore, a microcalcification is kept when at least 2 pixels have a probability above a preset threshold. Clusters are made of microcalcifications within a distance of $10mm$ to each other. Clusters containing less than 3 microcalcifications are discarded.

To remove false positives, a GentleBoost classifier is trained. For each cluster, features are calculated on the microcalcifications within the cluster and the cluster itself. These features ware based on shape, topology, probability, and texture. The GentleBoost classifier was trained on 100 regression stumps. As a result each detected cluster obtains a likelihood score.

2.2   Selection of Cases with BACs

To determine cases with BACs, a multi-view classification procedure is carried out. In this procedure, all views of a case are analyzed, i.e. medio-lateral oblique and cranio-caudal views of the right and left breast. In these views, the microcalcification cluster detection is performed resulting in detected clusters with a likelihood score. For the multi-view analysis only likelihood scores above a specified threshold are considered. This threshold is set a the highest case-based sensitivity for malignant cases in the microcalcification cluster detection (100% detection rate at 33% false positive rate).

Features are calculated on a case level. These features are based on shape, topology, probability, texture, and vesselness[7]. For each cluster in each view a total of 24 cluster features are calculated. For each case (containing 2 or 4 views) the mean, standard deviation, maximum and minimum of all cluster features in each view are taken. Additionally, 6 case-based features are calculated based on the number of clusters in each view and the number of views. This leads to a total of 102 features per case. Table 1 shows the whole list of features for training of the classifier. On these features a GentleBoost classifier is trained using 50 regression stumps as weak learners. The output of the classifier is a probability score for the presence of BACs in the case.

2.3   Performance Evaluation

Several datasets were obtained from the Dutch Breast Cancer Screening Program (Bevolkings Onderzoek Midden-West, The Netherlands). For the microcalcification candidate selection and cluster detection, 2 datasets were composed. One dataset where individual microcalcification centers were annotated containing 129 abnormal cases (70 benign and 59 malignant). The second dataset contained cases where the contour was annotated of microcalcification clusters. This set included 186 abnormal cases (134 benign and 52 malignant) and 315 normal cases. The first dataset was used for training the classifier for microcalcification selection and the second dataset for training of the cluster classifier.

Two datasets were composed for the selection of cases with BACs. For the training set, cluster classification was carried out on 10,000 normal cases. From

Table 1. Features for classifier training for the case-based selection of cases with BACs

Cluster features	
cls Area	The area of the cluster.
cls Eccentricity	$\frac{I_{xx}+I_{yy}-\sqrt{(I_{xx}-I_{yy})^2+4I_{xy}^2}}{I_{xx}+I_{yy}+\sqrt{(I_{xx}-I_{yy})^2+4I_{xy}^2}}$ where I_{xx}, I_{yy} and I_{xy} are the moments of inertia.
cls Ellipse	The ratio between the long axis and the short axis of a fitted ellipse.
cls Number	The number of microcalcifications in the cluster.
cls Coverage	$\sum_{i=1}^{n} \frac{A_{mC_i}}{A_{cls}}$ where A_{mC_i} is the area of the microcalcification i, n the number of microcalcifications within A_{cls}, the cluster area.
cls Density	$\frac{2|E|}{n(n-1)}$ where E is the number of edges of the graph.
cls Orientation	The orientation of the cluster with respect to the xy-plane.
cls Distance to skin/air	The distance of the center of the cluster to the skin air boundary.
cls Probability	Cluster probability from the cluster detection.
cls Hessian (5)	The Hessian-based vesselness filtered image at varying scale ($0.2 \leq \sigma \leq 1.0$, steps of 0.2)
cls Tubeness (5)	$k_{line}(\lambda_1, \lambda_2) = \frac{\lambda_2-\lambda_1}{\lambda_2}$ where $\lambda_1 \leq \lambda_2$, the absolute eigenvalues calculated at varying scale ($0.2 \leq \sigma \leq 1.0$, steps of 0.2)
cls Lambda (5)	The highest absolute eigenvalue λ_2 at varying scale ($0.2 \leq \sigma \leq 1.0$, steps of 0.2)
Case features	
Case total cls	The number of clusters in the case.
Case cls per view (4)	The number of clusters per view. (Mean, standard deviation, maximum and minimum)
Case number of views	The number of views.

these cases a group of 400 normal cases with the most significant false positives and a group of 200 normal cases with less obvious false positives were included. In this training set, a researcher experienced in reading mammograms labeled each case if it contained BACs. The test set consisted of 1,000 normal and 95 malignant cases. In this set, cases with BACs were labeled by a resident of the radiology department. The normal cases in the training and test set were randomly selected from a database containing over 50,000 normal cases.

To evaluate the performance of the selection of cases with BACs, the trained classifier, trained on the training set, was tested on the test set. After classification, each case obtained a probability score. Of the classified dataset a Receiver Operating Characteristic (ROC) curve was made. The sensitivity is calculated by determining the number of cases with BACs labeled as positive divided by the total number of cases with BACs. The specificity is calculated by dividing the number of cases without BACs labeled as negative by the total number cases without BACs. The ROC curve was generated by bootstrapping the test set 5000 times.

3 Results

In the training set, 208 of the 400 cases with the most significant false positives showed signs of BACs and 36 cases in 200 cases with less obvious false positives. The test set contained 10 malignant and 98 normal cases with BACs. And after cluster detection, 342 normal cases were left over in the test set of which 87 cases contained BACs. From the 95 malignant cases in the test set 93 cases were detected of which 8 cases contained BACs.

Figure 4 shows the ROC curve of the selection of cases with BACs plotted with 95% confidence intervals. The area under the curve of the ROC was 0.92. Furthermore, these results show that a sensitivity 0.44 is reached with no false positives up to a sensitivity of 0.90 at a specificity of 0.80.

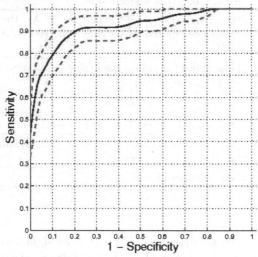

Fig. 4. ROC curve of the classification of cases with BACs, bootstrapped 5000 times. 95% confidence intervals are plotted with the dashed lines.

4 Discussion

The percentage of cases with BACs found by the resident in the test set (9.7%) corresponds with the percentages found in literature[6,9,12]. Although BACs are of no interest in breast cancer screening, the presence of BACs is associated with atherosclerosis and cardiovascular disease[3,5,10]. Selection of these cases with the proposed method can also be used for the detection of diseases other than breast cancer.

Analysis of the 400 selected cases with the most significant false positives in the training set resulted in 32 cases (8%) with true false positives (e.g. obvious detection errors), 109 cases with calcifications (27%), 51 cases with macrocalcifications (13%), and 208 cases with BACs (52%). Showing that BACs are the most frequent false positives in our CADe system.

Several studies are done on automatic detection of vascular calcifications in the breast[2,4]. However, these studies are evaluated on the individually detecteded BAC clusters. While the proposed method is based on the case-based selection method. This makes it difficult to compare the different methods. Nonetheless, false positive reduction in the cases with BACs, selected by the proposed system, still has to be done as a future work. An example of the flowchart for future work is shown in Figure 5.

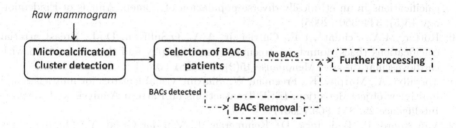

Fig. 5. Flowchart of the framework for future work. The solid blocks and arrows are proposed in this study, The dashed blocks and arrows will be done in future studies.

The proposed framework shows a good performance for the selection of cases with breast arterial calcifications. By using this selection we will be able to apply dedicated methods for false positive reduction due to BACs while minimizing the risk of removing relevant true positive microcalcification clusters.

References

1. Bria, A., Karssemeijer, N., Tortorella, F.: Learning from unbalanced data: A cascade-based approach for detecting clustered microcalcifications. Medical Image Analysis 18(2), 241–252 (2013)
2. Cheng, J.Z., Cole, E.B., Pisano, E.D., Shen, D.: Detection of arterial calcification in mammograms by random walks. In: Information Processing in Medical Imaging, Wiliamsburgh, VA, pp. 713–724 (2009)
3. Crystal, P., Crystal, E., Leor, J., Friger, M., Katzinovitch, G., Strano, S.: Breast artery calcium on routine mammography as a potential marker for increased risk of cardiovascular disease. The American journal of cardiology 86(2), 216–217 (2000)

4. Ge, J., Chan, H.P., Sahiner, B., Zhou, C., Helvie, M.A., Wei, J., Hadjiiski, L.M., Zhang, Y., Wu, Y.T., Shi, J.: Automated detection of breast vascular calcification on full-field digital mammograms. In: Proceedings of the SPIE, vol. 6915, pp. 691517-691517-7 (2008)
5. Kataoka, M., Warren, R., Luben, R., Camus, J., Denton, E., Sala, E., Day, N., Khaw, K.T.: How predictive is breast arterial calcification of cardiovascular disease and risk factors when found at screening mammography? American Journal of Roentgenology 187(1), 73–80 (2006)
6. Kemmeren, J.M., van Noord, P.A., Beijerinck, D., Fracheboud, J., Banga, J.D., van der Graaf, Y.: Arterial calcification found on breast cancer screening mammograms and cardiovascular mortality in women the dom project. American Journal of Epidemiology 147(4), 333–341 (1998)
7. Li, Q., Sone, S., Doi, K.: Selective enhancement filters for nodules, vessels, and airway walls in two- and three-dimensional CT scans. Medical Physics 30, 2040–2051 (2003)
8. Papageorgiou, C.P., Oren, M., Poggio, T.: A general framework for object detection. In: IEEE Sixth International Conference on Computer Vision, pp. 555–562. IEEE (1998)
9. Reddy, J., Son, H., Smith, S.J., Paultre, F., Mosca, L.: Prevalence of breast arterial calcifications in an ethnically diverse population of women. Annals of Epidemiology 15(5), 344–350 (2005)
10. Rotter, M.A., Schnatz, P.F., Currier Jr, A.A., O'Sullivan, D.M.: Breast arterial calcifications (bacs) found on screening mammography and their association with cardiovascular disease. Menopause 15(2), 276–281 (2008)
11. Torralba, A., Murphy, K., Freeman, W.: Sharing visual features for multiclass and multiview object detection. IEEE Transactions on Pattern Analysis and Machine Intelligence 29, 854–869 (2007)
12. Van Noord, P., Beijerinck, D., Kemmeren, J., Van der Graaf, Y.: Mammograms may convey more than breast cancer risk: Breast arterial calcification and arteriosclerotic related diseases in women of the dom cohort. European Journal of Cancer Prevention: The Official Journal of the European Cancer Prevention Organisation (ECP) 5(6), 483 (1996)
13. Viola, P., Jones, M.: Rapid object detection using a boosted cascade of simple features. In: Proceedings IEEE Conf. on Computer Vision and Pattern Recognition, vol. 1, pp. I-511 – I-518 (2001)

False Positive Reduction in CADe Using Diffusing Scale Space

Faraz Janan[1], Sir Michael Brady[2], and Ralph Highnam[1]

[1] Volpara Solutions Ltd.
(faraz.janan,ralph.highnam@volparasolutions.com)
[2] University of Oxford, UK
mike.brady@oncology.ox.ac.uk

Abstract. Segmentation is typically the first step in computer-aided-detection (CADe). The second step is false positive reduction which usually involves computing a large number of features with thresholds set by training over excessive data set. The number of false positives can, in principle, be reduced by extensive noise removal and other forms of image enhancement prior to segmentation. However, this can drastically affect the true positive results and their boundaries. We present a post-segmentation method to reduce the number of false positives by using a diffusion scale space. The method is illustrated using Integral Invariant scale space, though this is not a requirement. It is quite general, does not require any prior information, is fast and easy to compute, and gives very encouraging results. Experiments are performed both on intensity mammograms as well as on Volpara® density maps.

Keywords: False positive reduction, mammograms, mammographic density maps, Integral Invariants, scale space, Fast Marching Algorithm.

1   Introduction

Breast cancer is the most common type of cancers, with over 55000 cases reported annually and over 12000 deaths in the UK alone. In most cases, mammography is the first step towards diagnosing breast cancer where a radiologist tries to find abnormalities, which are mostly masses, microcalcification, architectural dissertation or breast asymmetry, in an x-ray mammogram. A number of approaches have been proposed over the past decade to detect masses in mammograms. Nevertheless, the high number of false positives poses a major challenge for relying on the segmentation accuracy, in clinical use and thus robustness of these computers aided detection (CADe) systems [1]. However, its use can significantly reduce the false negative errors and could improve individual performance of the radiologist to potentially eliminate the need of double reading [2]. False positive reduction (FPR) methods try to improve CADe performance by purging the number of candidate regions which may be suspicious of abnormality. Various approaches exist in literature, ranging from texture features [3] to shape [4], from simple thresholding [5] to expensive computational methods [6], [7]. Here we propose a simple and robust method based on Integral Invariant kernel [8], [9] to detect masses in mammograms, while highlighting a few

H. Fujita, T. Hara, and C. Muramatsu (Eds.): IWDM 2014, LNCS 8539, pp. 597–605, 2014.

potential candidates. Additionally, it can suggest their ordering in a mammogram for likelihood to be a mass. It should be noted that this is not a classification method to detect cancers, but in essence, it reduces the pool of candidate regions post-segmentation.

Here, we have applied Integral Invariants scale space [9] to reduce the number of false positives in mammograms. Integral invariants have been previously applied to mammograms for mass detection, segmentation and feature enhancement [9]–[13]. As the integral invariants retain causality at increasing scales for salient regions in 2D shapes; they also retain causality when applied to a surface, which is a 3D embedding of a 2D image. An x-ray image is an example of such an embedding in which 'interesting regions' appear brighter (and denser) than normal breast tissue and form causal peaks. These peaks maintain causality in response to integral invariant diffusion. Here, we show that this could be applied to the scale space of segmented regions in order to evaluate their saliency, and consequently to reduce the number of false positives in mammograms. Most of the mass segmentation algorithms segments three types of regions inside a breast, which are: 1) a masses 2) fibro-glandular tissues or stroma and 3) regions of light intensity and homogeneous texture surrounded by higher intensity and heterogeneous textures. The number of false positives could be reduced by extensive noise removal; linear/non-linear filtering, however, this drastically affects the true positive results and its boundaries. We have devised a mechanism to restrict the selection of fibro-glandular tissues and lighter homogeneous regions. Simulations are performed on synthetic images and density & intensity mammograms.

2   Methodology

Suppose that a region R_i in a mammogram has an intensity/density profile C_i^k extracted across it at k spatial scales, such that $C_i^k(p) \in R_i$ where $i = 1,..,n$; $r = 1,..,k$, and $p = II_k(x,y) \in \Omega_i$. Here II_k is the Integral Invariant function at the pixel location (x,y) in a diffused domain Ω_i at kth scale for the region R_i. However, we contend that the saliency of region should also depend upon the overall density of the breast. For example, a dense region of a certain volumetric density that is certainly salient in a fatty breast may not be regarded as evidently salient or suspicious inside a very dense breast. As explained in Fig 1, we define a cost function T_i to determine the saliency of the region R_i in a Volpara® density map [14] by:

$$T_i = \left(\sum_{p=1}^{l} \left(\frac{C_i^1(p) - C_i^k(p)}{length\ of\ C_i^1} \right) \right) * \frac{\overline{D}_i}{D_B} \quad (1)$$

$\overline{D}_i$ is the average volumetric density of a region R_i, and D_B is the overall volumetric density of the breast. For intensity images it will be the ratio of average intensity in the region versus the maximum intensity inside the breast. The other point is that the height of density/intensity profile for a mass is greater (almost double) than that of the fibroglandular tissue or locally low intensity homogeneous regions. This means that a mass will have a relatively higher peak than that of the 'non-interesting' regions. This is one of the reasons to include the difference between the peaks of maximum and minimum intensity/density scale profile, as illustrated in Fig 1.

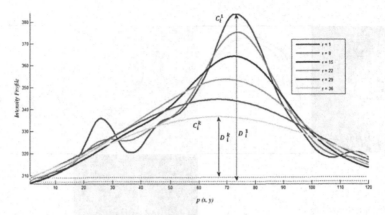

Fig. 1. Intensity profile scale space of a region

With this in mind, we modify the cost function as follows:

$$T_i = \left(\sum_{p=1}^{l} \left(\frac{C_i^1(p) - C_i^k(p)}{length\ of\ C_i^1} \right) \right) * \frac{\overline{D}_i}{D_B} * \left(D_i^1 - D_i^k \right) \quad (2)$$

$$where\ D_i^r = abs(\ \max\ (C_i^r) - \min(C_i^r)\ )\ ;\ r = 1,..,k$$

T is negative for low intensity locally homogeneous regions. Regions may be ranked on the basis of their costs to provide likelihood ordering for being a mass. We have found that a true mass will yield a tight and regular pattern of intensity/density profile from the Integral Invariant scale space, dissected along it. Conversely, it will be more distributed and haphazard for false positives. This can be seen in the Fig 3. The intensity/density profile is extracted using the gradient descent method on distance maps generated by the Fast Marching Algorithm (FMA) as in Fig 2. To understand how the method works, we simulated a surface which has peaks and dips of various amplitudes, as shown in the Fig 4. The surface given in Fig 4 is segmented in Fig 5, and FPR is applied to it.

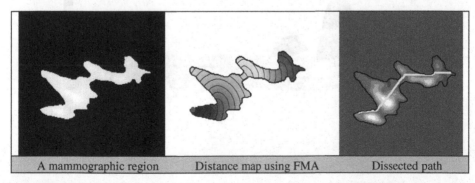

| A mammographic region | Distance map using FMA | Dissected path |

Fig. 2. Dissection of a mammographic region to extract intensity/density profile. The path is labelled in yellow figure, approaching from green to red spot in the rightmost images. The distance map is calculated using FMA in the middle figure, whereas the dissected path is computed using gradient decent method.

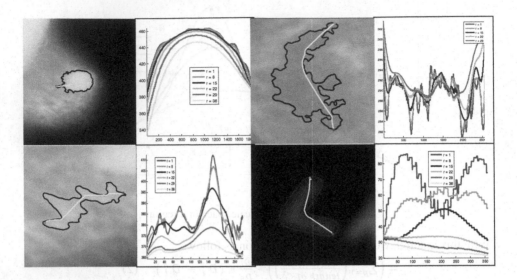

Fig. 3. Various mammographic regions along with the corresponding II scale space. The mass in the top left gives a high value of T for compact intensity profiles across all given scales.

It can be seen that both, less bright and all dark regions, are eliminated by this process. Based on the T values, the method can grade regions based on the probability of its likelihood of being of interest. This grading and selection of very bright to less bright regions is dependent on the threshold, which is user defined and is application specific.

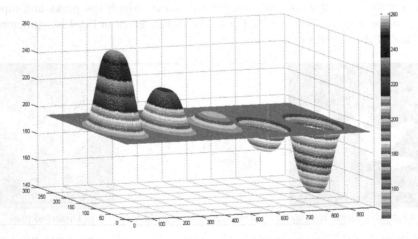

Fig. 4. A simulation surface in a false colour model

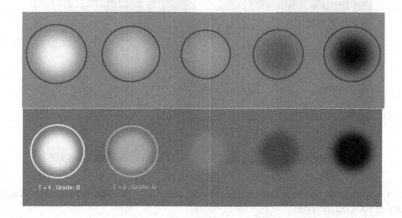

Fig. 5. (Top) segmented regions from Fig 4, final results from FPR method (bottom)

3   Results

The method has been applied to both Volpara® density maps and intensity images from USF database, with very encouraging results. The ground truth for the USF database was crudely delineated to highlight location of abnormality rather than its precise boundary, whereas only laterality was known for Volpara® density maps.

For Volpara® images, the method has also been applied to density maps obtained from 'Manchester 50/50 dataset', which includes 50 screen detected cancers and an equal number of normals, anonymised, each with LCC, LMLO, RCC and RMLO views. These comprise FFDM raw images from a GE Senographe Essential system. FPR was applied to all segmented regions in mammograms and regions of interest were identified. 100% accuracy for true positives was noticed where a grading scheme was applied to grade candidate regions with a T_i beyond a certain threshold. If a false positive is counted for all those mammograms where true positives did not get the highest score after applying FPR method for likelihood of being a mass, despite those true positives survived it, the false positive rate is 0.24 per image. Fig 6 shows a mammogram where false positives are removed and the true positive is retained well within accurate margins.

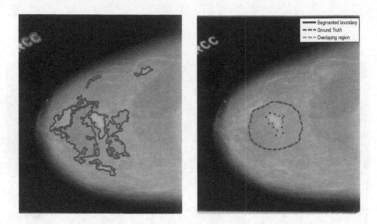

Fig. 6. A segmented mammogram on the left, whereas the ground truth and the segmented boundary of ROI on the right

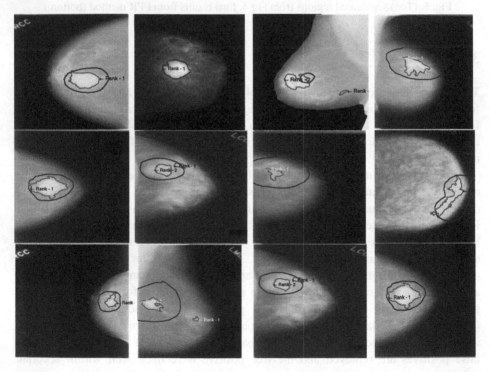

Fig. 7. Examples of segmented mammograms from USF database using the illustrated FPR method

Fig 7 and Fig 8 shows a few examples of segmented masses in intensity and density images from USF and Manchester 50/50 database respectively.

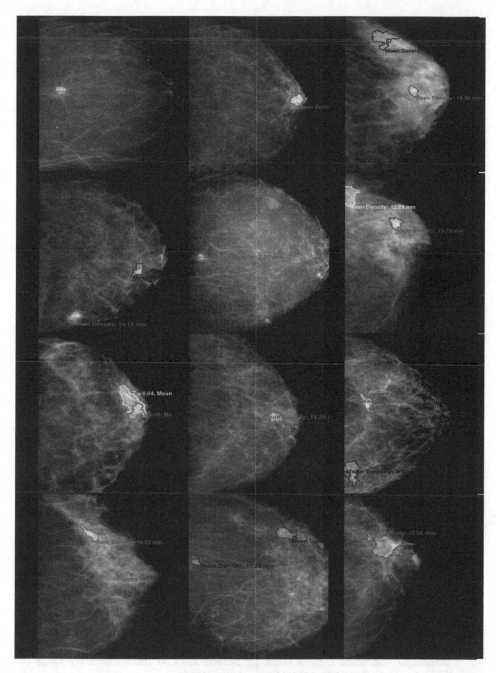

Fig. 8. Cancers retained on the density maps. Regions highlighted in red ($T_i \geq T$) are most likely to be masses, followed by yellow ($T > T_i \geq \frac{3T}{5}$) and blue ($\frac{3T}{5} > T_i \geq \frac{T}{2}$) respectively

4   Discussion

We have presented a false positives reduction method to detect regions of interests in mammograms. FPR typically involves the processing of a large pool of features in a computational training framework or by extensive noise removal. However, aggressive denoising can adversely affect the true positive results. We have developed a method using diffusion scale space, with Integral Invariants as an example, to reduce post-segmentation candidate regions. The method is based on the premise that diffusion scale space of a mass yields a high peaked compact set of density/intensity |profile over a range of scales, unlike false positives. The method is applied to both density and intensity images with very encouraging results. The major limitation is threshold selection, which is not unique to this method, and can be estimated empirically. Setting up a criterion for dynamic thresholding for this method will highly improve its effectiveness.

References

[1] Nishikawa, R.M., Kallergi, M.: 6.3. Computer-aided detection, in its present form, is not an effective aid for screening mammography (2008) Colin, G.-T., Hend, W.R.:

[2] Astley, S.M., Gilbert, F.J.: Computer-aided detection in mammography. Clin. Radiol. 59, 390–399 (2004)

[3] Lladó, X., Oliver, A., Freixenet, J., Martí, R., Martí, J.: A textural approach for mass false positive reduction in mammography. Comput. Med. Imaging Graph. 33, 415–422 (2009)

[4] Mudigonda, N.R., Rangayyan, R.M., Leo Desautels, J.E.: Detection of breast masses in mammograms by density slicing and texture flow-field analysis. IEEE Trans. Med. Imaging 20, 1215–1227 (2001)

[5] Rangayyan, R.M.: Biomedical image analysis. CRC press (2004)

[6] Li, L., Zheng, Y., Zhang, L., Clark, R.A.: False-positive reduction in CAD mass detection using a competitive classification strategy. Med. Phys. 28, 250–258 (2001)

[7] Truong, Q.D., Nguyen, M.P., Hoang, V.T., Nguyen, H.T., Nguyen, D.T., Nguyen, T.D., Nguyen, V.D.: Feature Extraction and Support Vector Machine Based Classification for False Positive Reduction in Mammographic Images. In: Li, S., Jin, Q., Jiang, X., Park, J.J.(J.H.) (eds.) Frontier and Future Development of Information Technology in Medicine and Education. LNEE, pp. 921–929. Springer, Heidelberg (2014)

[8] Manay, S., Hong, B.-W., Yezzi, A.J., Soatto, S.: Integral invariant signatures. In: Pajdla, T., Matas, J(G.) (eds.) ECCV 2004. LNCS, vol. 3024, pp. 87–99. Springer, Heidelberg (2004)

[9] Janan, F., Brady, S.M.: Integral invariants for image enhancement. In: 2013 35th Annual International Conference of the IEEE Engineering in Medicine and Biology Society (EMBC), pp. 4018–4021 (2013)

[10] Janan, F., Brady, M., Tromans, C., Highnam, R.: Standard Attenuation Rate and Volpara(R) Volumetric Density Maps. In: Second MICCAI International Workshop on Breast Image Analysis, BIA 2013, Nagoya, Japan (2013)

[11] Janan, F., Brady, M.: Shape matching by integral invariants on eccentricity transformed images. In: 2013 35th Annual International Conference of the IEEE Engineering in Medicine and Biology Society (EMBC), pp. 5099–5102 (2013)

[12] Janan, F., Brady, S.M.: Region matching in the temporal study of mammograms using integral invariant scale-space. In: Maidment, A.D.A., Bakic, P.R., Gavenonis, S. (eds.) IWDM 2012. LNCS, vol. 7361, pp. 173–180. Springer, Heidelberg (2012)

[13] Hong, B.-W., Brady, M.: Segmentation of mammograms in topographic approach (2003)

[14] Highnam, R., Brady, S.M., Yaffe, M.J., Karssemeijer, N., Harvey, J.: Robust breast composition measurement-volparaTM. In: Martí, J., Oliver, A., Freixenet, J., Martí, R. (eds.) IWDM 2010. LNCS, vol. 6136, pp. 342–349. Springer, Heidelberg (2010)

Automated Detection of Architectural Distortion Using Improved Adaptive Gabor Filter

Ruriha Yoshikawa[1], Atsushi Teramoto[1], Tomoko Matsubara[2], and Hiroshi Fujita[3]

[1] Graduate School of Health Sciences, Fujita Health University, Aichi, Japan
82012315@fujita-hu.ac.jp
[2] Nagoya Bunri University, Aichi, Japan
[3] Graduate School of Medicine, Gifu University, Gifu, Japan

Abstract. Architectural distortion in mammography is the most missing finding for radiologists, despite high malignancy. Many research groups have developed methods for automated detection of architectural distortion. However, improvement of their detection performance is desired. In this study, we developed a novel method for automated detection of architectural distortion in mammograms. To detect the mammary gland structure, we used an adaptive Gabor filter, whichconsists of three Gabor filters created by changing the combination of parameters. The filter that is best matched to the mammary gland structure pixel by pixel in the mammogram is selected. After detecting the mammary gland, enhancement of the concentrated region and false positive reduction are performed. In the experiments, we verified the detection performance of our method using 50 mammograms. The true positive rate was found to be 82.45%, and the number of false positive per image was 1.06. These results are similar to or better than those of existing methods. Therefore, the proposed method may be useful for detecting architectural distortion in mammograms.

Keywords: Mammography, CAD, architectural distortion, Gabor filter.

1 Introduction

Mammography screening is carried out for detecting breast cancer early. The findings obtained from mammography are mass, micro-calcification, and architectural distortion. Among them, architectural distortion is the most elusive finding for doctors. Moreover, it is classified as having a high malignancy in breast cancer. Therefore, it is important to detect and treat architectural distortion at an early stage. Many research groups have developed automated detection methods for architectural distortion[1–3]subsequent to two other findings [4,5].However, conventional methods failed to produce acceptably low false positive and high true positive rates [1–3]. Therefore, further improvement of the detection rate is desired. In order to improve the detection performance, it is essential to analyze the mammary gland structure more accurately. In this study, we propose an improved detection method for architectural distortion using an adaptive Gabor filter, which uses three Gabor filters, and we evaluated its detection performance.

H. Fujita, T. Hara, and C. Muramatsu (Eds.): IWDM 2014, LNCS 8539, pp. 606–611, 2014.
© Springer International Publishing Switzerland 2014

2   Methods

The proposed method consists of 6 steps: pre-processing, detection of mammary gland structure, extraction of primary mammary glands, calculation of the degree of concentration, segmentation, and false positive reduction.

2.1   Pre-processing

Images of the breast area are extracted by automated thresholding and labeling. In order to emphasize the line patterns, trend removal using a top-hat filter and gamma correction is performed.

2.2   Detection of Mammary Gland Structure

In order to detect the mammary gland structure, a Gabor filter[6] is introduced. A Gabor filter [Fig. 1;Eqs.(1) and (2)] is a type of line detection filter. The maximum value of $h(x,y)$ is obtained at an angle that line structures of mammary gland and filter shape is matched.

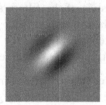

Fig. 1. Gabor filter function

$$h(x, y) = f(x, y) \otimes g(x, y) \tag{1}$$

$$g(x, y) = \exp\left(-\frac{x'^2 + \gamma^2 y'^2}{2\sigma^2}\right) \cos\left(2\pi \frac{x'}{\lambda} + \varphi\right), \tag{2}$$

$$x' = x\cos\theta + y\sin\theta, y' = -x\sin\theta + y\cos\theta, \tag{3}$$

where λ is the wavelength of the filter function, γ is the aspect ratio, σ is the deviation of the Gaussian factor that determines the effective size of filtering, φ is the phase, and θ represents an direction of Gabor filter.

In this study, mammary gland structure is extracted using the adaptive Gabor filter as shown in Fig.2 [7].

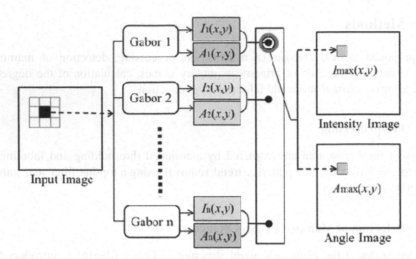

Fig. 2. Schematic of the adaptive Gabor filter

The n types of Gabor filter functions $g_i(x,y)$ ($i=1,2...n$) have different characteristics. The intensity image $I_i(x,y)$ and the angle image $A_i(x,y)$ are obtained by filtering the target pixel. Here, the characteristics of the filters are determined by changing λ, γ, and σ. From prepared filters, the best-matched filter g_i is selected such that $I_i(x,y)$ has the highest value among all intensity images for each pixel; the intensity image $I_{max}(x,y)$ and angle output image $A_{max}(x,y)$ are obtained.

In this study, we introduced three Gabor filters ($n=3$) and selectively and locally applied the filter most appropriate for the mammary gland structure.

2.3   Extraction of Primary Mammary Glands

The mammary gland structure involved in the formation of the architectural distortion (hereafter referred to as the primary mammary gland structure) is extracted in three steps in order to simplify the angle image. The steps are: (1) thresholding for narrowing the mammary gland region, (2) removal of non-primary line components, and (3) removal of mammary glands that have an anatomical normal orientation.

2.4   Calculation of the Degree of Concentration

A finding named spicula specific to architectural distortion indicates concentration and distortion of the mammary gland structure. Thus, the degree of concentration is calculated using the post-processed angle image $A_{max}(x,y)$. The concentration index $C(P)$ is defined as described in Fig.3 and Eq.(4) [8].

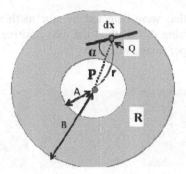

Fig. 3. Schematic of concentration index

$$C(P) = \sum_{R} \frac{dx \mid \cos \alpha \mid}{r}, \tag{4}$$

Where R is the range of processing coverage, dx is the length of a line element, Q is center of dx, r is the distance of line segment PQ, α is the angle between dx and PQ, and A and B are the inner and outer diameters of the region of interest, respectively.

2.5   Segmentation

The initial candidate regions of architectural distortion are identified by performing thresholding and are determined on the basis of individual breast density.

2.6   False-Positive Reduction

In order to reduce false positives, 23 types of characteristic features are calculated using the three images: the original image, intensity image, and concentration image. We calculated the following characteristic features: (1)area, (2)concordance rate of the filter, (3) density of the mammary gland, (4)position of the candidate region, (5) minimum pixel value, (6)maximum pixel value, (7)kurtosis of the pixel value, (8)skewness of the pixel value, and (9)standard deviation depending on the characteristics of each image. Finally, true positives and false positives are classified using a support vector machine [9,10]and these characteristic features.

3   Experiments

In order to evaluate the effectiveness of the proposed method, we evaluated its detection performance using 50 mammograms(200images),of which 20 were normal and 30 contained architectural distortion. These images were obtained from the digital database of screening mammography [11].

Figure 4 shows images that were detected by our method. Spicula and retraction findings were detected. Using this method the true positive rate was 82.45%,and the number of false positives per image was 1.06.

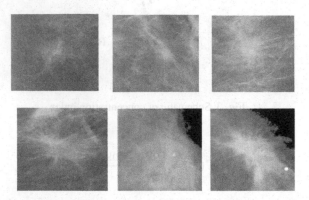

Fig. 4. Architectural distortions detected by the proposed method

4   Conclusion

We investigated an automated scheme for detecting architectural distortion (spicula) using an adaptive Gabor filter. We evaluated this method using 50 clinical mammograms (200 images).The true positive rate was 82.45%, and the number of false positives per image was 1.06. These results are similar to or better than those of existing methods. Therefore, the proposed method may be useful as an automatic method for detecting architectural distortion.

Acknowledgment. This work was supported in part by "Computational Anatomy for Computer-aided Diagnosis and Therapy: Frontiers of Medical Image Sciences," funded by a Grant-in-Aid for Scientific Research in Innovative Areas, MEXT, Japan.

References

1. Matsubara, T., Fukuoka, D., Yagi, N., et al.: Detection method for architectural distortion based on analysis of structure of mammary gland on mammograms. International Congress Series: Computer Assisted Radiology and Surgery 1281, 1036–1040 (2005)
2. Rangayyan, R.M., Shantaun, B., Jayasree, C., et al.: Measure of divergence of oriented patterns for the detection of architectural distortion in prior mammograms. International Journal of Computer Assisted Radiological Surgery 8(4), 527–545 (2013)
3. Nemoto, M., Honmaru, S., Shimizu, A., et al.: A pilot study of architectural distortion detection in mammograms based on characteristics of line shadows. International Journal of Computer Assisted Radiology and Surgery 4(1), 27–36 (2009)
4. Jiang, Y., Nishikawa, R.M., Schmidt, R.A., et al.: Improving breast cancer diagnosis with computer- aided diagnosis. Academic Radiology 6(1), 22–33 (1999)

5. Giger, M.L., Huo, Z., Kupinski, M.A., et al.: Computer-aided diagnosis inmammography. In: Fitzpatrick, J.M., Sonka, M. (eds.) The Handbook of Medical Imaging(2), Medical Imaging Processing and Analysis. SPIE, 915-1004 (2000)
6. Gabor filter for image processing and computer version: http://matlabserver.cs.rug.nl/edgedetectionweb/web/edgedetection_examples.html
7. Yoshikawa, R., Teramoto, A., Matsubara, T., Fujita, H.: Detection of Architectural Distortion and Analysis of Mammary Gland Structure in Mammograms Using Multiple Gabor Filters. Medical Imaging Technology 30(5), 287–292 (2012) (in Japanese)
8. Mekada, Y., Oza, K., Hasegawa, J., et al.: Features of Local Concentration Patterns in Line Figures and TheirApplications. IEICE, D-II, J77-D-2(9), 1788–1796 (1994) (in Japanese)
9. Cristianini, N., Shawe-Taylor, J.: An introduction to support vector machine and other kernel-based leaning methods. Cambridge University Press, Cambridge (2000)
10. Corinna, C., Vladimir, V.: Support-Vector Networks. Machine Learning 20(3), 273–297 (1995)
11. University for South Florida Digital Database Mammography Home Page: http://marathon.csee.usf.edu/Mammography/Database.html

Detecting Abnormal Mammographic Cases in Temporal Studies Using Image Registration Features

Robert Martí[1], Yago Díez[1], Arnau Oliver[1], Meritxell Tortajada[1],
Reyer Zwiggelaar[2], and Xavier Lladó[1]

[1] Computer Vision and Robotics Group, University of Girona,
Av. Lluís Santaló 17071, Spain
{marly,yago,aoliver,txell,llado}@atc.udg.edu
http://atc.udg.edu/~marly
[2] Department of Computer Science, Aberystwyth University,
Ceredigion, SY23 3DB, Wales, UK
rrz@aber.ac.uk

Abstract. Image registration is increasingly being used to help radiologists when comparing temporal mammograms for lesion detection and classification. This paper evaluates the use of image and deformation features extracted from image registration results in order to detect abnormal cases with masses. Using a dataset of 264 mammographic images from 66 patients (33 normals and 33 with masses) results show that the use of a non-rigid registration method clearly improves detection results compared to no registration (AUC: 0.76 compared to 0.69). Moreover, feature combination using left and right breasts further improves the performance (AUC to 0.88) compared to single image features.

1 Introduction

The detection of abnormalities in mammographic images is an important research topic in breast image analysis. Initial approaches found in the literature [1] were based on the analysis of individual images alone in order to detect (CADe) and classifiy (CADx) microcalcificacions and masses. While microcalcification detection has achieved a sufficient maturity for clinical (and commercial) CAD systems, mass detection still has to improve in terms of specificity and sensitivity. This is mainly due to a larger shape variability and the intensity inhomogeneity of the lesion itself but also of the surrounding tissue which often hinders the detection and segmentation steps.

A way of improving abnormality detection performance is the use of various images from the same patient, similar to radiologists when reading mammographic cases. This has already been approached using contralateral (comparing left and right breasts), ipsilateral (CC and MLO) [2] or temporal [3,4] (same view at different time intervals) studies. Common approaches to compare various images are based on image registration to spatially correlate the images

H. Fujita, T. Hara, and C. Muramatsu (Eds.): IWDM 2014, LNCS 8539, pp. 612–619, 2014.

or to extract and match image features (i.e. nipple position, principal axes or salient regions). This paper belongs to the former set of approaches. The aim of this work is to investigate whether image registration results can be used for the detection of malignant cases in temporal images of the same patient. Temporal comparison has been chosen rather than contralateral or ipsilateral assuming that radiological findings are better detected by analysing breast evolution over time. Note that the aim is not to obtain a particular lesion detection or segmentation but to classify cases as normal or abnormal using solely image registration results. This is of particular interest for CAD systems as a pre-sorting step (classification of normal and abnormal cases) or as prior information for subsequent processing.

The image registration algorithm used in this paper is similar to the work in [5]. The algorithm is based on combining an affine transformation maximising a mutual information similarity measure with a non-rigid point correspondence approach based on a robust point matching algorithm. Intensity and deformation based features obtained from the registration are subsequently used in a machine learning framework to detect abnormal cases with lesions. The contribution of the paper is two-fold: the application of a non-rigid point based image registration algorithm to temporal full-field digital mammographic (FFDM) images, and the use of a machine learning framework with features extracted from the registration results for evaluating detection of malignant cases in temporal images.

2   Image Database

A total of 264 full-field digital (FFD) mammograms were used from 66 different women randomly chosen from a screening population. From those, 33 were normal, while 33 suffered from breast cancer with a visible malignant mass in one of the breasts. Mass area size ranged from 8 to 356 mm^2 with a median area of 64.12 mm^2. Each woman had two mammographic studies (acquired 1-2 years apart) and each study contained two medio-lateral oblique images. Craniocaudal views were also available but were not used in this study (will be used in future work). Mammograms were acquired using a Selenia FFD mammography system, with resolution 70 micron per pixel, size 4096x3328 or 2560x3328, and 12-bit depth. As the aim is the temporal comparison of mammograms, each mammogram image was registered to its homonymous mammogram from the posterior studies, performing 132 registrations. The presence of masses was annotated by expert radiologists. This allowed us to distinguish between those registration instances containing masses from those not containing them. Hence, for a woman diagnosed with breast cancer we had a registration of the breast with the mass, referred to as *Abnormal with Lesion* (AL), and the registration of the breast without the lesion (healthy breast), referred to as *Abnormal* (A). For a normal case, both registrations were considered as *Normal* (N).

3   Methodology

The main goal here is to investigate whether image registration results can provide significant information in order to help detecting abnormal cases. The overall methodology includes an initial image pre-processing step, registration of temporal images, and mammogram (or patient) classification based on features extracted from the registration results. Figure 1 shows the general framework of the methodology used, while the following subsections provide more details on each step.

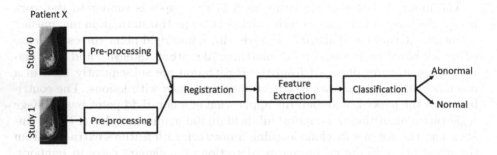

Fig. 1. Overview of the proposed methodology

3.1   Image Pre-processing

Image pre-processing is performed to minimise mammogram and breast variability and to facilitate the subsequent registration step. In that sense, the breast area is automatically segmented using simple thresholding and the pectoral muscle is removed [6]. In addition, a peripheral enhancement method is applied to compensate thickness variations in the breast periphery based on Tortajada et al. [7]. The method automatically restores the overexposed area by equalising the image using information from the intensity of non-overexposed neighbour pixels. The correction is based on a multiplicative model and on the computation of the distance map from the breast boundary. Finally, images are downsampled to half the size using bilinear interpolation in order to reduce computational cost. Figure 2 shows an example of the pre-processing steps described.

3.2   Image Registration

The registration methodology is based on robustly matching interest points in two mammographic images of the same view type. After an initial affine registration maximised by a mutual information metric, the registration algorithm

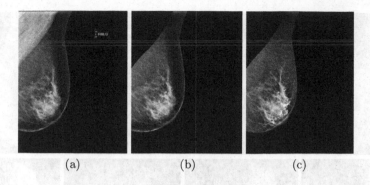

(a) (b) (c)

Fig. 2. Pre-processing: (a) Original mammogram (b) pectoral muscle removal, and (c) peripheral enhancement

extracts interest points found in the boundary and applies a robust point matching approach obtaining a non-linear transformation [5]. Salient points are defined by computing a maximal local curvature measure in the breast boundary. The point matching approach used here is based on the work of Zheng et al. [8], which uses shape contexts as the measure of point similarity and a graph matching formulation followed by relaxation labelling for obtaining the final point matches.

Point Matching. The robust point correspondence method is based on an iterative graph matching process in order to minimise correspondence errors [8]. Those errors are related to a cost matrix (C_{ij}) which describes the cost of matching one point i in one image (row i) with a point j in the second image (column j). The elements of this cost matrix are obtained using shape contexts [9]. Relaxation labelling is applied to the cost matrix in order to minimise ambiguous matchings. The optimal assignment of the points in the cost matrix is obtained using the Hungarian method, as in [9]. At the end of each iteration, the matched points are used for transforming one point set (p) in order to match the other (q). This transformation is based on a Thin-Plate Splines (TPS) transform, obtaining a smooth transformation between matched points. The transformed points p and q are used for building the cost matrix for the next iteration. The stopping criteria of the iterative process is usually stated in terms of a maximum number of iterations or when the number of matches does not change with respect to the last iteration.

Figure 3 shows an example of image registration of a normal and abnormal case, with the transformed moving image, the difference image and the deformation field magnitude. While differences in the deformation field are difficult to appreciate, structural dissimilarities in the difference image are highlighted, including the lesion in the abnormal case.

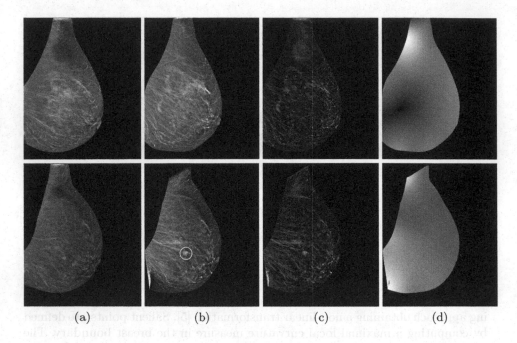

| (a) | (b) | (c) | (d) |

Fig. 3. Image Registration: (a) Fixed and (b) transformed moving mammograms, (c) image difference and (d) deformation field magnitude (brighter areas denote larger deformation). Top row shows a normal mammogram and bottom a mammogram with a lesion (white circle).

3.3   Image Features

From the registration results we extract three sets of features which are then used to classify a patient into normal or abnormal. The first feature set is computed from the difference image while the second set is extracted from the deformation field (the displacement experienced by each pixel normalised by the image size). In these two sets (difference image and deformation field) the features computed are the first five statistical moments of the intensity or deformation distribution. Finally, the third set of features is composed of various similarity measures commonly used in image registration computed between the fixed and moving images: root mean squared error, cross-correlation, entropy of the difference image and mutual information [10], having a total of 14 features.

Feature Combination. The above described features are computed for each single temporal registration. As we are registering left and right temporal mammograms of the same patient independently, we also study the effect of combining the features hence obtaining a unique feature vector for each woman. The hypothesis is that this combination can help towards the classification as in normal cases those features are likely to be more stable compared to abnormal cases due to the development of breast cancer. Various simple combinations have been tested: mean, signed and absolute differences, and minimum and maximum. Experimental results evaluating the different combination approaches have shown that combining using the maximum value obtained the best results.

3.4 Classification

Features have been used in a Random Forest (RF) classifier in order to differentiate between normal and abnormal cases containing a mass. The parameters were experimentally set to 500 decision trees and a feature subset size of 3 features for each tree. Although other classifiers (such as SVM, Adaboost and KNN) and feature selection methods have been tested, RF obtained the best results overall. PRTools software has been used for the implementation [11]. All features have been normalised to a zero mean and unit standard deviation. A leave-one-woman-out validation approach has been used for testing.

4   Results

Figure 4 and Table 1 show classification results in terms of ROC curve (true positive rate (TPR) against false positive rate (FPR)) and area under the curve (AUC) when using the proposed algorithm (robust point matching (RPM)) compared to no registration (No Reg), and affine transformation using mutual information (Aff). Features are computed for two cases: for a single registration (*Single*) or combining left and right temporal features using the maximum of both features (*Combined*). For the single case, only one mammogram is used for feature extraction: the one with the mass for abnormal cases and left or right randomly selected for normal ones.

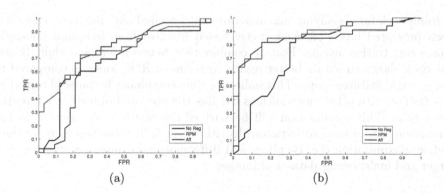

(a)   (b)

Fig. 4. Abnormal classification ROC curves using features from robust point matching of the boundary points (RPM) and Affine algorithms also compared to no registration. (a) Single features; (b) combination using the maximum operation

Table 1. AUC for classification of abnormal cases. Features used in the classifier are obtained after no registration (No Reg), affine registration (Aff) or robust point matching of the boundary points (RPM). Single features are compared to their combination using the maximum operation.

	No Reg	RPM	Aff
Single	0.69	0.76	0.71
Combined	0.76	0.88	0.84

Regarding the ROC curves with single features, the use of RPM shows a clear improvement compared to no registration or even affine registration. This is also reflected in the AUC values (0.69 and 0.71 for No Reg and Aff compared to 0.76 for the RPM).

Regarding feature combination, it is also clear that results improve in all cases, including the no registration case. Differences are relevant with respect to the use of registration algorithms compared to no registration, although between Aff and RPM (0.84 vs 0.88) this difference is not that evident. This indicates that non-rigid registration improves classification results, however, further investigation should be carried out including other non-rigid algorithms. Regarding feature analysis it has been observed that features based on the intensity similarity (moments of the difference image and mutual information) show better discriminant properties than the rest of the features. However, with the inclusion of other registration algorithms this could change in favour of other features such as the deformation field.

5   Conclusions

A framework for classifying mammograms into normal and abnormal cases has been presented based on using image based features from temporal non-rigid image registration results. Feature combination between left and right breast has been shown to obtain better results in terms of ROC analysis compared to using single features alone. This indicates that combining features obtained in this fashion with other views such as CC has the potential of further improving the results. This combination will be part of the future work, as well as the evaluation of additional registration algorithms specially those based on intensity metric maximisation (i.e. B-splines and diffeomorphic demons) or the use of a larger and multi-center dataset of images.

Acknowledgements. The research leading to these results has been supported by the Spanish Science and Innovation grant no. TIN2012-37171-C02-01.

References

1. Oliver, A., Freixenet, J., Marti, J., Perez, E., Pont, J., Denton, E.R., Zwiggelaar, R.: A review of automatic mass detection and segmentation in mammographic images. Medical Image Analysis 14(2), 87–110 (2010)
2. Samulski, M., Karssemeijer, N.: Optimizing case-based detection performance in a multiview CAD system for mammography. IEEE Transactions on Medical Imaging 30(4), 1001–1009 (2011)
3. Marias, K., Behrenbruch, C.P., Parbhoo, S., Seifalian, A., Brady, M.: A registration framework for the comparison of mammogram sequences. IEEE Transactions on Medical Imaging 24(6), 782–790 (2005)
4. Díez, Y., Oliver, A., Lladó, X., Freixenet, J., Martí, J., Vilanova, J., Martí, R.: Revisiting intensity-based image registration applied to mammography. IEEE Transactions on Information Technology in Biomedicine 15(5), 716–725 (2011)
5. Martí, R., Raba, D., Oliver, A., Zwiggelaar, R.: Mammographic registration: Proposal and evaluation of a new approach. In: Astley, S.M., Brady, M., Rose, C., Zwiggelaar, R. (eds.) IWDM 2006. LNCS, vol. 4046, pp. 213–220. Springer, Heidelberg (2006)
6. Kwok, S.M., Chandrasekhar, R., Attikiouzel, Y., Rickard, M.: Automatic pectoral muscle segmentation on mediolateral oblique view mammograms. IEEE Transactions on Medical Imaging 23(9), 1129–1140 (2004)
7. Tortajada, M., Oliver, A., Martí, R., Vilagran, M., Ganau, S., Tortajada, L., Sentís, M., Freixenet, J.: Adapting breast density classification from digitized to full-field digital mammograms. In: Maidment, A.D.A., Bakic, P.R., Gavenonis, S. (eds.) IWDM 2012. LNCS, vol. 7361, pp. 561–568. Springer, Heidelberg (2012)
8. Zheng, Y., Doermann, D.: Robust point matching for nonrigid shapes by preserving local neighborhood structures. PAMI 28(4), 643–649 (2006)
9. Belongie, S., Malik, J., Puzicha, J.: Shape matching and object recognition using shape contexts. IEEE Transactions on Pattern Analysis and Machine Intelligence 24(4), 509–522 (2002)
10. Zitova, B.: Image registration methods: A survey. Image and Vision Computing 21(11), 977–1000 (2003)
11. Duin, R., Juszczack, P., Paclik, P., Pekalska, E., de Ridderand, D.M.J., Tax, D.: PRTools4, A Matlab Toolbox for Pattern Recognition. Delft University of Technology (2004)

Analysis of Mammographic Microcalcification Clusters Using Topological Features

Zhili Chen[1,*], Harry Strange[2], Erika Denton[3], and Reyer Zwiggelaar[2]

[1] Faculty of Information and Control Engineering,
Shenyang Jianzhu University, Shenyang, 110168, China
zzc@sjzu.edu.cn
[2] Department of Computer Science,
Aberystwyth University, Aberystwyth, SY23 3DB, UK
{hgs08,rrz}@aber.ac.uk
[3] Department of Radiology,
Norfolk and Norwich University Hospital, Norwich, NR4 7UY, UK
erika.denton@nnuh.nhs.uk

Abstract. In mammographic images, the presence of microcalcification clusters is a primary indicator of breast cancer. However, not all microcalcification clusters are malignant and it is difficult and time consuming for radiologists to discriminate between malignant and benign microcalcification clusters. In this paper, a novel method for classifying microcalcification clusters in mammograms is presented. The topology/connectivity of microcalcification clusters is analysed by representing their topological structure over a range of scales in graphical form. Graph theoretical features are extracted from microcalcification graphs to constitute the topological feature space of microcalcification clusters. This idea is distinct from existing approaches that tend to concentrate on the morphology of individual microcalcifications and/or global (statistical) cluster features. The validity of the proposed method is evaluated using two well-known digitised datasets (MIAS and DDSM) and a full-field digital dataset. High classification accuracies (up to 96%) and good ROC results (area under the ROC curve up to 0.96) are achieved. In addition, a full comparison with state-of-the-art methods is provided.

1 Introduction

Microcalcifications are small deposits of calcium in breast tissue that appear as small bright spots in mammograms [1–4]. The presence of microcalcification clusters is a primary sign of breast cancer. The radiological definition of microcalcification clusters is that at least three microcalcifications are present within a 1 cm^2 region [4, 5]. The spatial resolution of mammography is very high (normally in the range of $40-100\mu m$ per pixel) and therefore mammography enables the detection of microcalcifications at an early stage. However, not all microcalcification clusters necessarily indicate the presence of cancer, only certain kinds

---

* This work is partially funded by Science & Research Project of Liaoning Province Eduction Deparatment, China (No. L2013225).

H. Fujita, T. Hara, and C. Muramatsu (Eds.): IWDM 2014, LNCS 8539, pp. 620–627, 2014.
© Springer International Publishing Switzerland 2014

of microcalcifications are associated with a high probability of malignancy [6, 7]. In clinical practice, it is difficult and time consuming for radiologists to interpret mammograms and distinguish malignant from benign microcalcifications. This results in a high rate of unnecessary biopsy examinations [3, 5]. To improve diagnosis accuracy of radiologists, computer-aided diagnosis (CAD) systems have been applied to reduce the false positive rate while maintaining sensitivity [3, 8].

Various automatic approaches have been proposed to characterise and classify microcalcifications into malignant and benign [3, 9]. These methods use such features as shape, morphology, cluster based features, intensity and texture [3, 9]. Many of these methods describe the shape and morphology of individual microcalcifications [1, 4], however, there are a range of techniques that concentrate on global (statistical) features of microcalcification clusters [2, 8, 11, 13]. In addition, a variety of classifiers, such as k-Nearest Neighbours (kNN) [1, 5, 11], Artificial Neural Networks [2, 12–16] and Support Vector Machines (SVM) [8, 15, 17], have been employed to build classifier models using the extracted feature sets. The performance of ANN and SVM in classifying malignant and benign microcalcifiation clusters was compared in [15]. For the classification of malignant and benign microcalcifications, the values of the area under the ROC curve achieved by all of the discussed publications range from 0.74 to 0.98.

However, most of existing approaches have their own disadvantages. Firstly, for the approaches based on the shape/morphology of individual microcalcifications, informative features cannot be attained when microcalcifications are very small (occupying only a few pixels). Secondly, microcalcifications may have very low contrast with respect to the surrounding tissue especially when microcalcifications form within dense tissue which has high and homogeneous intensity, and as such the performance of the approaches based on the intensity variations and texture features may be affected. In addition, for the approaches describing the spatial distribution of microcalcifications within a cluster, the global cluster features were computed based on a fixed resolution and the distance-based features rely on the original spatial resolution of mammography. This results in a lack of robustness and adaptiveness to different spatial resolutions of mammograms in particular screen-film mammograms acquired by different digitisers.

According to some studies on the evaluation of breast microcalcifications, malignant microcalcifications tend to be small, numerous (> 5 per focus within 1 cm^2) and densely distributed because they lie within the milk ducts and associated structures in the breast and follow the ductal anatomy [6, 7, 18]. However, benign microcalcifications are generally larger, smaller in number ($< 4 - 5$ per 1 cm^2) and more diffusely distributed as these microcalcifications arise within the breast stroma, benign cysts or benign masses [6, 7, 18]. These differences result in variations in the distribution and closeness of microcalcifications within the clusters and provide radiologists with information which enables decisions regarding the need for further assessment and possible breast biopsy. Hence, we propose a novel method for modelling and classifying microcalcification clusters in mammograms based on their topological properties. The topology of microcalcification clusters is analysed at multiple scales using a graphical representation

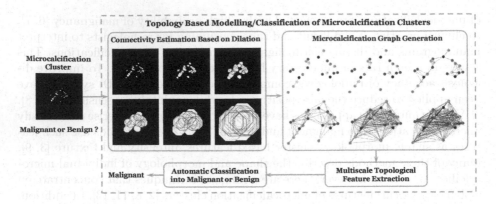

Fig. 1. Methodology workflow for topology based modelling and classifying malignant and benign microcalcification clusters in mammograms

of their topological structure. This method is distinct from existing cluster-based analysis approaches that compute the distance-based cluster features at a fixed scale. In this method, a set of topological features are extracted from microcalcification graphs at multiple scales and a multiscale topological feature vector is subsequently generated to discriminate between malignant and benign cases.

2   Data and Method

The data used in the experiments consists of three datasets. The first dataset was taken from the Mammographic Image Analysis Society (MIAS) database, containing 20 image patches with the same size of 512×512 pixels. The spatial resolution is $50\mu m \times 50\mu m$ per pixel. The second dataset was extracted from the Digital Database for Screening Mammography (DDSM) database, containing 80 image patches with varied sizes (the average size of these image patches is 487×447 pixels). The mammograms in DDSM were digitised by four scanners and the spatial resolution ranges from 42 to 50 microns per pixel. In contrast to the first two datasets, the third dataset contains 25 full-field digital image patches extracted from a non-public mammographic database. These mammograms were acquired using a Hologic Selenia mammography unit, with a resolution of 70 microns per pixel. The average size is 352×301 pixels. All image patches were taken from different mammograms, each containing a microcalcification cluster. The diagnostic gold standard (benign or malignant) of all microcalcification clusters in this study has been provided by biopsy: there are 9 malignant and 11 benign clusters in the MIAS dataset, 36 malignant and 44 benign clusters in the DDSM dataset, and 14 malignant and 11 benign clusters in the Digital dataset.

The proposed method works on binary microcalcifications which were detected using an automatic detection approach developed in [19]. Fig. 1 illustrates the workflow of our methodology. Firstly, we estimate the connectivity between microcalcifications within a cluster using morphological dilation, which

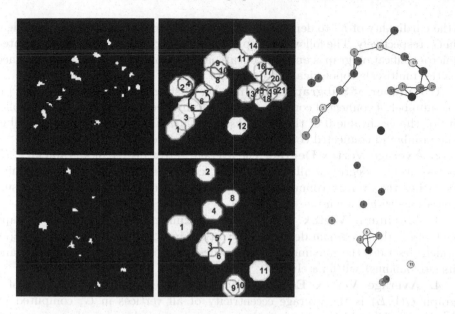

Fig. 2. Example microcalcification clusters: malignant (top row) and benign (bottom row). First column: binary microcalcifications (cluster region is zoomed and microcalcification No. 12 for benign falls outside the displayed region); second column: dilated microcalcifications at scale 8; third column: microcalcification graphs.

is performed on each individual microcalcification using a disk-shaped structuring element over a range of scales. Here, the scale corresponds to the radius of the structuring element measured in pixels. The dilation results of two example clusters are shown in Fig. 2. The boundaries of dilated microcalcifications are displayed using different colours and each individual microcalcification is labelled with a sequential number which is ordered according to the spatial location of the corresponding microcalcification in the image patch.

We represent the topology of microcalcification clusters in the form of graphs. A microcalcification graph is generated based on the spatial connectivity relationship between microcalcifications within a cluster, where each node represents an individual microcalcification and an edge between two nodes is created if the two corresponding microcalcifications are connected or overlap in the 2D image plane. The microcalcification graphs corresponding to the two examples of malignant and benign clusters are shown in the third column of Fig. 2. The node locations in the two graphs are in accordance with the original spatial distribution of microcalcifications within the two clusters.

For each microcalcification cluster, we generate a series of microcalcification graphs over a range of scales and extract a set of graph theoretical features. These features constitute the topological feature space for the classification of malignant and benign clusters. Here, we use $G(V, E)$ to represent a graph where V is the vertex set and E is the edge set, and use $|V|$ (the cardinality of V) and $|E|$

(the cardinality of E) to denote the number of vertices and the number of edges in G, respectively. The following graph metrics are extracted from the generated microcalcification graphs and are concatenated to form a feature vector, termed as the multiscale topological feature vector.

1. Number of Subgraphs. The number of subgraphs of a graph $G(V, E)$ is the number of connected components in G, computed by counting the multiplicity of the eigenvalue 0 of the *normalised Laplacian matrix* $\mathcal{L}$, which describes the number of connected components within a microcalcification cluster.

2. Average Vertex Degree. The average vertex degree of a graph $G(V, E)$ is the average degree of all vertices in G, computed by $\sum_{i \in V} d(i)/|V|$, which describes the average connectedness between a microcalcification and its surroundings within a cluster.

3. Maximum Vertex Degree. The maximum vertex degree of a graph $G(V, E)$ is the maximum degree of all vertices in G, computed by $\max_{i \in V} d(i)$, which describes the maximum connectedness between a microcalcification and its surroundings within a cluster.

4. Average Vertex Eccentricity. The average vertex eccentricity of a graph $G(V, E)$ is the average eccentricity of all vertices in G, computed by $\sum_{i \in V} e(i)/|V|$, which represents the average longest distance of a microcalcification to other reachable microcalcifications in a connected component.

5. Diameter. The diameter of a graph $G(V, E)$ is the maximum eccentricity of all vertices in G, computed by $\max_{i \in V} e(i)$, which indicates the longest distance between two microcalcifications in a connected component.

6. Average Clustering Coefficient. The average clustering coefficient of a graph $G(V, E)$ is the average clustering coefficient of all vertices in G, computed by $\sum_{i \in V} c(i)/|V|$, which indicates how concentrated a microcalcification's neighbourhood is and how close it is from being a clique.

7. Giant Connected Component Ratio. The giant connected component of a graph $G(V, E)$ is the largest set of vertices that are reachable from each other. The giant connected component ratio is the ratio of the number of vertices in the giant connected component to the number of vertices in G, which shows the percentage of microcalcifications in the largest connected component with respect to all microcalcifications in a cluster.

8. Percentage of Isolated Points. The percentage of isolated points of a graph $G(V, E)$ is the ratio of the number of isolated points (vertices with degree equal to 0) to the number of vertices in G, which provides the percentage of isolated microcalcifications in a cluster.

After generating the multiscale topological features, a k-Nearest Neighbours based classifier is used for classifying microcalcification clusters into malignant and benign. The kNN classification is based on a simple majority vote, unless equal class probability is indicated, in which case a Euclidean weighted approach is adopted. A range of values for k are employed when generating the experimental results which are documented in the following section.

Table 1. Our results and a comparison with those achieved by related work

Method	Database	Case	Feature	Classifier	Result
[1]	unknown	18	shape	kNN	CA = 100%
[4]	DDSM	183	shape	thresholding	$A_z = 0.96$
[2]	unknown	191	texture&cluster	ANN	$A_z = 0.86$
[8]	MIAS	25	cluster	SVM	$A_z = 0.81$
[12]	unknown	54	texture	ANN	$A_z = 0.88$
[5]	Nijmegen	103	multiwavelet	kNN	$A_z = 0.89$
[11]	Liverpool	38	shape/cluster	kNN	$A_z = 0.79, A_z = 0.84$
[13]	University of Chicago Hospitals	49	morphology	ANN	$A_z = 0.80$
[17]	University of Chicago	104	cluster&morphology	Ada-/Cas-SVM	$A_z = 0.81, A_z = 0.82$
[14]	DDSM	150	varied features	ANN	$A_z = 0.98$
[15]	DDSM	150	varied features	ANN/SVM	$A_z = 0.93, A_z = 0.94$
Ours	MIAS	20	topology	kNN	CA = 95%, $A_z = 0.96$
Ours	Digital	25	topology	kNN	CA = 96%, $A_z = 0.96$
Ours	DDSM	80	topology	kNN	CA = 95%, $A_z = 0.96$

3 Experimental Set-Up and Results

To evaluate the performance of the classifier models built by using the multiscale topological features, a leave-one-out cross-validation scheme was employed for all datasets. Two evaluation metrics were used for this work. The first was overall classification accuracy (CA), which provides a summary of the performance for balanced datasets (such as the datasets used here). ROC analysis was employed as the second evaluation approach to assess the predictive ability of a classifier by using the area under the ROC curve denoted by A_z. The details about the construction of the ROC curve by defining a malignancy measure based on the kNN classifier can be found in [10].

We investigated a range of scales up to 64 and as such the dimensionality of the multiscale topological feature space was up to $8 \times 65 = 520$ (8 graph based features were extracted at each scale and scale 0 was included as well). The bottom part of Table 1 shows the best classification results achieved over 65 scales for the three datasets. The number of scales used for generating the results shown in Table 1 was 9, 43 and 12 for MIAS, DDSM and Digital, respectively. Fig. 3 shows the classification results with respect to variation in the value of k for the three datasets. As shown in Fig. 3, small variations in k provided similar results in most cases. For the two smaller datasets, MIAS and Digital, the kNN classifier produced slightly better performance when using smaller k values; while for DDSM, relatively stable results were indicated for larger k values.

4 Discussion and Conclusions

As described above, good classification results have been obtained for all the three datasets. The Digital dataset provided slightly better results than those of MIAS and DDSM, which might be due to the more accurate detection of microcalcifications using digital mammography. As stated in [19], the detection approach indicates the best performance when using the Digital dataset. In addition, we compared our method with state-of-the-art approaches in the literature.

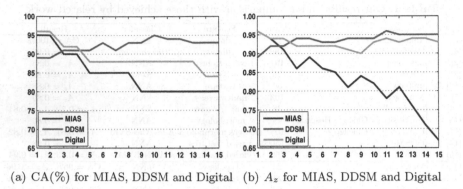

(a) CA(%) for MIAS, DDSM and Digital   (b) A_z for MIAS, DDSM and Digital

Fig. 3. The classification results with respect to different k values for the three datasets. Note that some curves for different datasets are overlapped.

A summary of the comparison is also provided in Table 1. It should be noted that the various approaches in Table 1 use different images taken from different databases, and therefore it is a qualitative comparison. As shown in Table 1, our method produced comparable results to the various approaches.

One inherent limitation of the developed method is that it cannot provide a reliable classification for the case where the cluster is structureless or few microcalcifications are segmented within the cluster. Another concern of the proposed method is that its performance might depend on the performance of the previous microcalcification detection approach. False negatives or false positives may affect the global topology/connectivity of microcalcification clusters. However, the experimental results demonstrate the robustness and effectiveness of the developed method when combined with automatic microcalcification detection. This indicates its potential application in conjunction with automatic detection approaches in CAD systems.

In summary, we have presented a novel approach to analyse microcalcifications in terms of the connectivity and topology for classifying malignant and benign clusters. Unlike most features (e.g. shape/morphological features) in previous publications extracted at a single scale, a graphical representation of microcalcification clusters describing the multiscale topological characteristics was developed in this paper. Eight graph metrics were extracted and constituted the multiscale topological feature vector, which has been used to classify microcalcification clusters into malignant and benign. The proposed method has been evaluated using three datasets: MIAS, DDSM and Digital. Good classification results have been obtained for all the datasets. This demonstrates the capability of our method in dealing with two categories of mammograms, which allows it to be applied in both film and digital mammography. Future work will concentrate on evaluating the stability of the proposed method against the size of the evaluation dataset. In addition, the most significant microcalcification graph metrics for malignancy analysis will be investigated by performing feature selection.

References

1. Shen, L., et al.: Application of Shape Analysis to Mammographic Calcifications. IEEE Transactions on Medical Imaging 13(2), 263–274 (1994)
2. Dhawan, A.P., et al.: Analysis of Mammographic Microcalcifications Using Gray-level Image Structure Features. IEEE Transactions on Medical Imaging 15(3), 246–259 (1996)
3. Cheng, H.D., et al.: Computer-Aided Detection and Classification of Microcalcifications in Mammograms: A Survey. Pattern Recognition 36(12), 2967–2991 (2003)
4. Ma, Y., et al.: A Novel Shape Feature to Classify Microcalcifications. In: IEEE 17th International Conference on Image Processing, pp. 2265–2268 (2010)
5. Soltanian-Zadeh, H., et al.: Comparison of Multiwavelet, Wavelet, Haralick, and Shape Features for Microcalcification Classification in Mammograms. Pattern Recognition 37(10), 1973–1986 (2004)
6. Sickles, E.A.: Breast Calcifications: Mammographic Evaluation. Radiology 160(2), 289–293 (1986)
7. Dähnert, W.: Radiology Review Manual, 6th edn. Lippincott Williams & Wilkins, Philadelphia (2007)
8. Papadopoulos, A., et al.: Characterization of Clustered Microcalcifications in Digitized Mammograms Using Neural Networks and Support Vector Machines. Artificial Intelligence in Medicine 34(2), 141–150 (2005)
9. Elter, M., Horsch, A.: CADx of mammographic masses and clustered microcalcifications: A review. Medical Physics 36, 2052–2068 (2009)
10. Chen, Z., Denton, E.R.E., Zwiggelaar, R.: Classification of Microcalcification Clusters Based on Morphological Topology Analysis. In: Maidment, A.D.A., Bakic, P.R., Gavenonis, S. (eds.) IWDM 2012. LNCS, vol. 7361, pp. 521–528. Springer, Heidelberg (2012)
11. Betal, D., et al.: Segmentation and numerical analysis of microcalcifications on mammograms using mathematical morphology. British Journal of Radiology 70, 903–917 (1997)
12. Chan, H.P., et al.: Computerized classification of malignant and benign microcalcifications on mammograms: Texture analysis using an artificial neural network. Physics in Medicine and Biology 42, 549–567 (1997)
13. Rana, R.S., et al.: Independent evaluation of computer classification of malignant and benign calcifications in full-field digital mammograms1. Academic Radiology 14, 363–370 (2007)
14. Ren, J., et al.: Effective recognition of MCCs in mammograms using an improved neural classifier. Engineering Applications of Artificial Intelligence 24, 638–645 (2011)
15. Ren, J.: ANN vs. SVM: Which one performs better in classification of MCCs in mammogram imaging. Knowledge-Based Systems 26, 144–153 (2012)
16. Dheeba, J., Selvi, S.T.: A Swarm Optimized Neural Network System for Classification of Microcalcification in Mammograms. Journal of Medical Systems 36, 3051–3061 (2012)
17. Wei, L., et al.: Microcalcification classification assisted by content-based image retrieval for breast cancer diagnosis. Pattern Recognition 42, 1126–1132 (2009)
18. Feig, S.A., et al.: Evaluation of breast microcalcifications by means of optically magnified tissue specimen radiographs. Recent Results in Cancer Research 105, 111–123 (1987)
19. Oliver, A., et al.: Automatic microcalcification and cluster detection for digital and digitised mammograms. Knowledge-Based Systems 28, 68–75 (2012)

Differentiation of Malignant and Benign Masses on Mammograms Using Radial Local Ternary Pattern

Chisako Muramatsu[1], Min Zhang[1], Takeshi Hara[1], Tokiko Endo[2,3], and Hiroshi Fujita[1]

[1] Department of Intelligent Image Information, Gifu University, Gifu, Japan
{chisa,min,hara,fujita}@fjt.info.gifu-u.ac.jp
[2] Department of Radiology, Nagoya Medical Center, Nagoya, Japan
[3] Department of Radiology, Higashi Nagoya National Hospital, Nagoya, Japan
endot@nnh.hosp.go.jp

Abstract. Texture information of breast masses may be useful in differentiating malignant from benign masses on digital mammograms. Our previous mass classification scheme relied on shape and margin features based on manual contours of masses. In this study, we investigated the texture features that were determined in regions automatically selected from square regions of interest (ROIs) including masses. As a preliminary investigation, 149 ROIs including 91 malignant and 58 benign masses were used for evaluation by a leave-one-out cross validation. The local ternary pattern and local variance were determined in sub regions with the high contrast and a core region. Using an artificial neural network, the classification performance of 0.848 in terms of the area under the receiver operating characteristic curve was obtained.

Keywords: Breast masses, mammograms, computer-aided diagnosis, classification, texture feature, local ternary pattern.

1 Introduction

Distinction between benign and malignant lesions on mammograms can be difficult. We have been investigating a computerized image analysis method for assisting radiologists' diagnosis of breast images. In our previous studies [1-4], determination of similarity measures was investigated for retrieval of reference images that are similar to a new case to be diagnosed. Some characteristics of breast masses that radiologists may consider during the mammography reading include the mass shapes, e.g., round or irregular, the margin characteristics, e.g., circumscribed or spiculated, and the density, whether it is higher than that of the surrounding fibrograndular tissue or isodense. The image features determined for the similarity measures included such features characterizing the shape, density and margin. However, in our previous methods, it has been found that the shape and margin features are predominantly useful, and the density features, such as the contrast and standard deviation in pixel values, were considered not very useful. This fact indicates that the characteristics that radiologists find for diagnosis might not be fully reflected in our previous features. Other features such as textural features may represent mass density characteristic and be useful in the distinction between benign and malignant masses.

H. Fujita, T. Hara, and C. Muramatsu (Eds.): IWDM 2014, LNCS 8539, pp. 628–634, 2014.
© Springer International Publishing Switzerland 2014

In addition, the shape and margin features were determined on the basis of the manual outline of a mass in our previous study. However, obtaining the detailed contour of a mass from practitioners is not practical, and automatic delineation is not easy. In this study, we investigated new textural features, namely, modified local ternary patterns (LTP) [5], determined in regions automatically selected from a square region of interest (ROI) including masses for classification between benign and malignant masses.

2   Materials and Methods

2.1   Database

Digital mammograms used in this study were obtained at Nagoya Medical Center, Nagoya, Japan, with either the phase contrast mammography (PCM) units (Mermaid/Pureview, Konica Minolta, Inc.) or computer radiography (CR) system (Mammomat 3000, Siemens and C-Plate, Konica Minolta). This study was approved by the institutional review board. The pixel sizes of the images are 25 (PCM) and 43.75 (CR) microns and the gray level is 12 bits. For image processing, the pixel size and gray scale were unified to 50 microns and 10 bits by linear interpolation. All the mammograms were retrospectively reviewed by one of two radiologists with the diagnostic report and the corresponding ultrasonography images, if available, and the square ROIs including masses were obtained. In this study, 149 ROIs, including 91 malignant and 58 benign masses were used. The malignant masses were confirmed by biopsy or surgery, while benign masses were diagnosed by biopsy or follow-ups with other image modalities. The average and standard deviation of mass diameters are 35 $\pm$ 18 mm, and the size of ROIs ranged from 250 x 250 to 1758 x 1758 pixels.

2.2   Methods

Modified Local Ternary Pattern. Local ternary pattern (LTP) [5] is a variant of the local binary pattern (LBP) [6], which is a sequence of binarized information of the pixels surrounding the pixel of interest. Assuming there is a slope or an edge around the pixel of interest, such as in Fig. 1(a), the surrounding pixels are compared with the pixel of interest and binarized to have 1 or 0 depending on the superiority of the pixel value, as in Fig. 1(b). LBP takes the parameters of R and P, which are the radius and the number, respectively, of the surrounding pixels for comparison and 1 and 8, respectively, for the above example. Starting arbitrarily from the pixel on the right in clockwise, the pattern for this pixel of interest will be 00011110. For an ROI, the histogram of patterns is built and used for the subsequent process of classification.

Because actual images include some noise, LTP was proposed to include a margin on the threshold, and the output became three values as -1, 0, and 1, corresponding to the surrounding pixel values smaller than that of the pixel of interest minus a threshold, within the threshold, and larger than that plus threshold, respectively. If we set the threshold to 3 in the same example above, the output becomes as in Fig. 1(c). These values can be separated by the positive and negative values to two binary patterns of 00011100 and 11000001 and handled as the regular LBP. The histograms of the positive and negative patterns are concatenated.

In LBP with $P=8$, the number of possible patterns, which is also the number of histogram bins, will be $2^8 = 256$. Ojala et al. [6] found that the majority of the meaningful patterns can be represented by the basic patterns and, therefore, proposed the "uniform" patterns, which include at most two transitions between 0 and 1. All the other patterns are grouped into the non-uniform pattern. The pattern in Fig. 1(b) is the uniform pattern. This reduces the number of patterns to 59. In addition, they proposed the rotation invariance by disregarding the directionality of the patterns. As a result, the number of patterns could be further reduced to 10 for $P=8$.

In the classification of benign and malignant masses, however, the direction of the edges at margin is an important characteristic. Therefore, we employed the uniform patterns but also considered the direction of the patterns. Instead of the regular rotation variant patterns, we rotated the patterns with reference to the direction of mass center. By assuming the center of ROI as the center of a mass, the patterns are rotated so that the binary sequence always starts from the pixel closest to the center of an ROI. In order to reduce the number of bins, we summed the fractions of patterns corresponding to the positive and negative patterns.

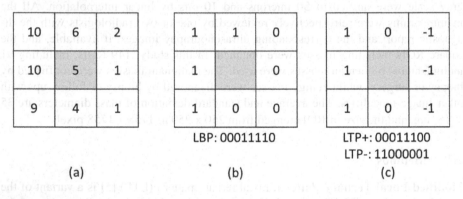

LBP: 00011110

LTP+: 00011100
LTP-: 11000001

(a)   (b)   (c)

Fig. 1. An example of LBP and LTP determination. (a) The pixel of interest (shaded) and the surrounding pixels, (b) LBP values, (c) LTP values with the threshold set to 3.

Overall Classification Method. For determination of the LTP, the images were first down sized to ¼ (by half in each direction) by pixel averaging, and the gray scale was reduced to 8 bits. From the square ROIs, most descriptive sub-ROIs of 50 x 50 pixels in size based on the histogram were selected. The histograms of sub-ROIs were obtained for all pixels, except the ones on edges, by scanning the 50 x 50 pixel window. The sub-ROIs with the largest histogram widths were consecutively selected without allowing the overlap. The maximum number of sub-ROIs was varied on the basis of the size of the original square ROIs. Figure 2 shows the locations of the selected sub-ROIs for a malignant ROI and a benign ROI. The squares in the figure are 10 x 10 pixels and not the actual size of sub-ROIs (50 x 50 pixels). Note that the contrast of the original images was lowered in this figure for presentation purpose. The LTP was determined at each pixel in these sub-ROIs and the combined histogram was obtained for the case.

By selecting the sub-ROIs with the high contrast, the regions around the margin of a mass are likely selected as in Fig. 2. However, the texture characteristic of the core region is also important. In addition to the high contrast sub-ROIs, an LTP histogram for a core sub-ROI of 50 x 50 pixels placed in the center of the square ROI was also obtained. For the core ROI, the rotation invariant LTP was determined. In this study, the threshold for LTP was set to 5 and the R and P parameters were set to 2 and 8, respectively. As the supplemental information, the histograms of variances in pixel values were obtained in both selected sub-ROIs and the core sub-ROI [6]. The variance for each pixel was determined in the 7 x 7 pixel area, and the number of bins was set to 10. Therefore, the total number of the features (concatenated histogram bins) was 89.

For classification of benign and malignant ROIs, an artificial neural network (ANN) was used. The feed forward ANN with a backpropagation algorithm was employed. The ANN was trained and evaluated by a leave-one-out cross validation method. Because of the large number of features relative to the number of training cases, the feature reduction was performed by a forward feature selection. The result was evaluated by the area under the receiver operating characteristic curve (AUC). The parameters of ANN were selected experimentally on the basis of the AUC.

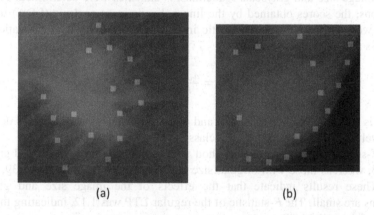

(a)   (b)

Fig. 2. Locations of selected sub-ROIs specified by small squares. (a) A malignant ROI of 392 x 392 pixels, and (b) a benign ROI of 276 x 276 pixels.

3   Results

With the forward feature selection, 6 features were selected. Four were from the radial LTP in the selected sub-ROIs and two were from the rotation invariant LTP in the core ROI. No feature was selected from the variance histograms in this study. Figure 3 shows the change in classification performance in terms of AUC with the number of features selected. For each number of features, at least 3 different numbers of hidden units were tested. The selected numbers of hidden units and training iterations were 5 and 200, respectively. The classification performance was 0.848 in terms of AUC.

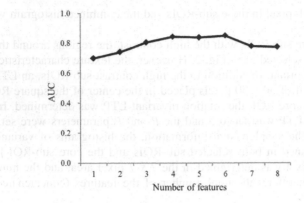

Fig. 3. Change in AUC with the number of features selected

4   Discussion

For evaluation of the effectiveness of the radial LTP to the regular LTP and the effects of image size and grayscale reductions, *F*-statistics were determined. For these evaluations, the scores obtained by the linear discriminant analysis (LDA) using all features were employed. The *F*-statistic in this study is defined as the ratio of the inter-class and intra-class variances by

$$F = \frac{S_b}{S_w} = \frac{n_1 n_2}{n} \cdot \frac{(m_1 - m_2)^2}{n_1 \sigma_1^2 + n_2 \sigma_2^2},$$

where *n* is the number of cases and m and σ are the mean and the standard deviation, respectively, of   LDA scores for each class.

The *F*-statistic of the proposed method with the reduced image size and grayscale was 1.73, whereas those with original size and grayscale were 1.56 and 1.39, respectively. These results indicate that the effects of the image size and grayscale reductions are small. The *F*-statistic of the regular LTP was 1.12, indicating the effectiveness of the radial LTP.

In this study, descriptive sub-ROIs were selected automatically on the basis of the histogram of pixel values. In the previous studies for classification of textural patterns, LBP or LTP was determined at all pixels within the images to be classified. However, for the classification of lesions like breast masses, unrelated information could be included by using all pixels which might affect the classification. On the other hand, by automatically selecting sub-ROIs, some were placed at regions unrelated to the mass, such as at the breast margin, as shown in Fig. 4. Sampling method should be investigated further in the future.

For reducing the number of features, a forward selection method was employed in this study. Liao et al. [7] proposed the selection of dominant patterns for reduction of the numbers of bins. Nanni et al. [8] selected the useful patterns on the basis of the variances of the training cases. The number of features was further reduced by the principal component analysis. They applied the method for classification of benign and malignant masses and obtained the high classification performance. Although the performances of their method and our proposed method cannot be directly compared because of the different databases used, it is possible that some useful information may have been lost by selecting a small number of features. The feature reduction method must be investigated in the future study.

In this study, we investigated the usefulness of texture features, i.e., modified LTP, for classification between benign and malignant masses on mammograms. The LTP was determined in sub-ROIs that were automatically selected from a square ROI including a mass so that no precise segmentation of the mass was required. As a preliminary investigation, the classification performance was relatively well using only texture features without using contour information.

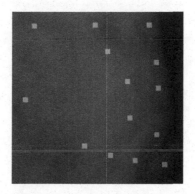

Fig. 4. Selected sub-ROIs at the breast margin

Acknowledgment. This study was partly supported by the Grants-in-Aid for Scientific Research for Young Scientists (No. 21791179) by Japan Society for the Promotion of Science and by a Grant-in-Aid for Scientific Research on Innovative Areas (No. 21103004), MEXT, Japan. Authors are grateful to Mikinao Oiwa, MD, and Misaki Shiraiwa, MD, for their contribution in this study.

References

1. Muramatsu, C., Li, Q., Schmidt, R.A., Shiraishi, J., Doi, K.: Determination of similarity measures for pairs of mass lesions on mammograms by use of BI-RADS lesion descriptors and image features. Acad. Radiol. 16, 443–449 (2009)
2. Muramatsu, C., Nishimura, K., Oiwa, M., Shiraiwa, M., Endo, T., Doi, K., Fujita, H.: Correspondence among subjective and objective similarities and pathologic types of breast masses on digital mammography. In: Maidment, A.D.A., Bakic, P.R., Gavenonis, S. (eds.) IWDM 2012. LNCS, vol. 7361, pp. 450–457. Springer, Heidelberg (2012)
3. Muramatsu, C., Nishimura, K., Endo, T., Oiwa, M., Shiraiwa, M., Doi, K., Fujita, H.: Represenattion of lesion similarity by use of multidimensional scaling for breast masses on mammograms. J. Digit. Imaging. 26, 740–747 (2013)

4. Nishimura, K., Muramatsu, C., Oiwa, M., Shiraiwa, M., Endo, T., Doi, K., Fujita, H.: Psychophysical similarity measure based on multi-dimensional scaling for retrieval of similar images of breast masses on mammograms. In: Novak, C.L., Aylward, S. (eds.) Proc. of SPIE Med. Imaging, vol. 8670, pp. 86701R1–R6 (2013)
5. Tan, X., Triggs, B.: Enhanced local texture feature sets for face recognition under difficult lighting conditions. IEEE Trans. Image Processing 19, 1635–1650 (2009)
6. Ojala, T., Pietikainen, M., Maenpaa, T.: Multiresolution gray-scale and rotation invariant texture classification with local binary patterns. IEEE Trans. Pattern Anal. Mach. Intel. 24, 971–987 (2002)
7. Liao, S., Law, M.W.K., Chung, A.C.S.: Dominant local binary patterns for texture classification. IEEE Trans. Image Processing 18, 1107–1118 (2009)
8. Nanni, L., Brahnam, S., Lumini, A.: A very high performing system to discriminate tissues in mammograms as benign and malignant. Expert Systems with Applications 39, 1968–1971 (2012)

Statistical Temporal Changes for Breast Cancer Detection: A Preliminary Study

Gobert N. Lee and Mariusz Bajger

Medical Device Research Institute
School of Computer Science, Engineering and Mathematics,
Flinders University, PO Box 2100
Adelaide SA 5001, Australia
{gobert.lee,mariusz.bajger}@finders.edu.au

Abstract. In this paper, we propose a statistical temporal change scheme for early breast cancer detection. Temporal mammographic data have been found useful to detect changes in the breasts of women. Many temporal analysis approaches require temporal image registration. Variations in patient positioning, changes in the field of view and natural changes in the breasts over time pose significant challenges. Our proposed scheme, on the other hand, does not depend on image registration. Instead, the temporal statistical region merging technqiue was used to find homogeneous breast regions over time. Changes identified are then assessed for abnormality by a rule-based classifier. Using a small temporal dataset of 10 women (5 cancerous and 5 normal), the detection rate was found to be 100% with a 0.1 false positive per case (that is, only one false positive was found in the entire dataset of 10 cases). These preliminary results show that the proposed temporal changes detection scheme has a great potential in providing clinical assistance in early breast cancer detection. The results, however, need to be further verified with a larger dataset.

Keywords: temporal analysis, temporal change detection, statistical region merging, computer-aided detection, mammography.

1 Aim and Background

Mammograms are commonly used for breast cancer screening and detection. The application of computer algorithms to aid the detection of breast cancer in mammograms and other breast imaging modalities is an important and ongoing research area (see [5,24,8,7,11,10] for example). In order for a computer algorithm to be of any clinical use, not only the detection rate needs to be high, but also the number of false positive needs to be low. The literature shows that many computer-aided detection (CAD) schemes enjoy high detection rates but the number of false positives remains a challenge. In order to improve the accuracy of computer-aided detection and diagnosis systems, attention has been drawn to the use of multiple mammograms (as opposed to single mammogram). Bilateral comparison techniques compare the left and right mammograms acquired in

H. Fujita, T. Hara, and C. Muramatsu (Eds.): IWDM 2014, LNCS 8539, pp. 635–642, 2014.

the same mammographic examination/screening round. A significant asymetry in the left and right breasts may be a key mammographic finding towards the detection of breast cancer. Temporal mammographic analysis reveals changes in the breast over time. It identifies the development of lesions in the current mammograms with respect to the previously taken mammograms for the same women.

When processing multiple mammographic images (bilateral comparison or temporal analysis), image registration is typically required [24,25,17,19,20,8,4,23,14,12]. Studies show that CAD systems using multiple-images perform better than those employing single-image only [24,25,19,20,26,21]. The techniques of medical image registration has been reviewed in a number of publications (see [13,16,18,27] for example). In particular, [6] reviews image registration techniques related to the inter- and intra-modality breast images including mammogram-to-mammogram while [22] reviews four methods specifically for mammogram registration. The matching of multiple mammographic images is not trivial. Variations in patient positioning, changes in the field of view, and differences in x-ray exposure observed from one mammogram to another make the registration of mammographic data challenging. In addition, natural changes in the composition of the breast over time further complicate the matter.

This study focuses on temporal mammographic data analysis. Temporal mammographic data have been found useful in literature to detect changes in women's breasts but a moderate success in the image registration pre-processing step can limit the success in the overall temporal analysis. In this paper, we propose a statistical temporal change detection scheme for breast cancer detection. The scheme detects temporal changes in (statistical) homogeneous local breast regions in screening mammograms. A key feature of this method is that rigorous image registration was not required although general good practice in patient positioning was assumed.

2   Dataset

Temporal mammographic images retrieved from the archives of BreastScreen SA were used in this retrospective study. Criteria for case inclusion were as follow. For cancer cases: (1) malignant mass was found at current screening and was verified by histopathology, and (2) mammograms from two immediate previous screening rounds were available and were found normal. For normal cases: (1) the result of the current screening was found normal, (2) mammograms from two immediate previous screening rounds were available and were also found normal.

Ten sets of temporal screening mammograms were selected from the archives randomly. Each set contained mammograms pertaining to the same woman acquired from three consecutive screening rounds at a two year interval. Of the ten women, five of them were diagnosed with breast cancer in the most recent (current) screening round while the other five were normal. Each cancer case contained only one lesion, located in either the right or the left breast. Sizes of the lesions ranged from $7mm$ to $20mm$ ($7mm$, $20mm$, $7mm$, $10mm$ and $11mm$). The lesions were observed in both the craniocaudal and the mediolateral views. The average age of the women in the cancer group at the time of diagnosis was 62 (65, 57, 65, 64 and 57, respectively). For the normal group, the average age at current screening round was 60 (60, 63, 59, 61 and 58).

The selected film-screen mammograms were digitized at 48 μm spatial resolution and 12 bit depth using a Vidar Diagnostic Pro Advantage film digitizer. The digitized screening mammograms were then annotated by an experienced radiologist specializing in mammography.

3   Method

In the pre-processing stage, the breast region was first extracted in each mammogram. The extracted breast regions were then standardized, cropped and subsampled to a size of about 250×350 (depending on the original size of the breast). No rigorous temporal image registration was required. However, general good practice in patient positioning was assumed.

3.1   Statistical Region Merging

The statistical region merging (SRM) technique by Nock and Nielsen [15] was originally proposed for the segmentation of natural scene images. We had previously applied the technique in medical image segmentation with satisfactory results [3,9,1,2]. The technique is based on probability theory and comprises of two components: a merging predicate and the order of testing the predicate for growing regions. Considering two regions R and R' in an image I, based on the concentration theory, the probability of

$$|(\bar{R} - \bar{R}') - \mathbb{E}(\bar{R} - \bar{R}')| \geq g\sqrt{\frac{1}{2Q}\left(\frac{1}{|R|} + \frac{1}{|R'|}\right)\ln\frac{2}{\delta}}, \qquad (1)$$

is smaller than δ ($0 < \delta \leq 1$) where $\bar{R}$ denotes the average intensity across the region R, $\bar{R}'$ denotes the average intensity across the region R', g denotes the gray scale of the image, $\mathbb{E}(\cdot)$ denotes the expectation operator, $|\cdot|$ denotes cardinality, and Q denotes the number of random variables that each image pixel is modeled with.

For regions R, R' to be merged, $\mathbb{E}(\bar{R} - \bar{R}') = 0$, hence formula (1) yields the merging predicate

$$P(R, R') = \begin{cases} true & \text{if } |\bar{R} - \bar{R}'| \leq \sqrt{b^2(R) + b^2(R')} \\ false & \text{otherwise} \end{cases} \qquad (2)$$

where

$$b(R) = g\sqrt{\frac{1}{2Q|R|}\ln\frac{2}{\delta}}. \qquad (3)$$

The order of testing the predicate is based on the function

$$f(p, p') = |I(p) - I(p')|, \tag{4}$$

where p and p' are image pixels, $I(.)$ is the intensity function, and $| \cdot |$ is the absolute value function.

Based on the above, a mammogram can be segmented into statistically homogeneous regions. Our implementation of the SRM algorithm was graph-based. That is, an image was transformed into a four-connected graph $G = (V, E)$ such that each pixel in the image was associated with a vertex in the graph. The gray value associated with an image pixel was considered as an attribute of a vertex.

3.2   Temporal SRM

The SRM technique, described in Section 3.1, applies to a single mammogram. The image pixels that have the same expected intensity are grouped together as homogeneous regions. For temporal analysis of the breast, a sequence of mammograms over time was considered. Image pixels of all available mammograms in the sequence were considered simultaneously. Our graph-based implementation of the SRM in Section 3.1 was extended to *temporal SRM*. Grouping of the image pixels into homogeneous regions was based on the same predicate. The constructed graph had a connectivity of 6 for temporal SRM. In this setting, to alleviate the influence of noise, intensities of pixels in equation (4) were replaced

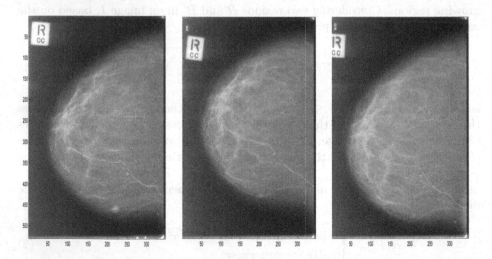

Fig. 1. An example of temporal mammographic data of a cancer case (c1462rc). The images shown are (from left) current screening mammogram on which cancer was detected and previous screening mammogram from 2 and 4 years ago. The images were subsampled by 10 for illustration purpose.

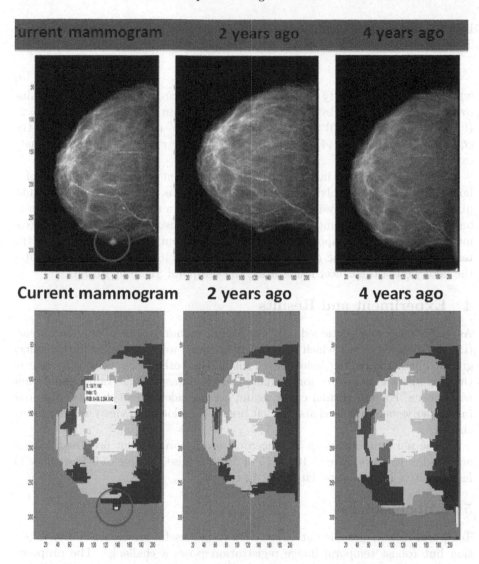

Fig. 2. Temporal cancer detection (cancer case c1462rc) : (Top panel) Temporal screening mammograms (enhanced, standardised and subsampled pre-processed) of a woman. (From left) Current screening mammogram (mammogram of interest for cancer detection); screening mammogram obtained 2 years prior (normal with no call back); 4 years prior (normal with no call back). The cancer lesion is circled in red in the current mammogram. (Bottom panel) Mammograms processed with the temporal statistical region merging algorithm (from left) current; 2years prior; 4 years prior. Statistical homogeneous breast regions over time are marked with the same (false) color in the bottom three images.

by a moving average over a region defining a neighbourhood around the pixel. That is,

$$f(p, p') = |\bar{N}_{p,p'} - \bar{N}_{p',p}|, \tag{5}$$

where $I(.)$ is the intensity function and $\bar{N}_{p,p'}$ indicates the average pixel value over the region defined by the pixels that are within Euclidean distance $\leq 2r$ (for some integer $r \geq 0$) and that are closer to p' than to p. Note that the equation (5) reduces to (4) for $r = 0$. In this study $r = 5$ was found adequate experimentally.

Image pixels/regions in the current mammogram that were not part of a homogeneous region involving the immediate previous mammogram were scrutinized. Abnormality analysis was then performed by a rule-based classifier based on a number of measurements including image intensity, contrast, size and geometrical properties. Temporal changes were then identified. Figure 1 depicts the temporal mammographic data of a cancer case (c1462rc). Figure 2 illustrates the detection of the cancer lesion using the temporal SRM algorithm.

4   Experiment and Results

As each cancer case contained only one lesion, mammograms of only one breast (i.e. the diseased breast which may be left or right) were of interest in the cancer group. Furthermore, the lesions were visible in both views, thus, only one of the two views is necessary for an independent dataset. The craniocaudal view was chosen. For the normal cases, again, for an independent dataset, only one breast per woman was used and the left breast (craniocaudal view) was randomly chosen.

Of the ten temporal cases (5 cancerous and 5 normal), our proposed scheme achieved a detection rate of 100 % (5 of 5) at a false positive of 0.1 per case (1 false positive in the entire dataset of 10 cases).

5   Conclusion

Temporal mammographic data have been found useful for breast cancer detection but robust temporal image registration poses a challenge. The proposed statistical temporal change detection scheme tracks homogenous local breast tissues over time without the need for rigorous temporal image registration. Together with a rule-based classifier, the scheme achieved superior results of 100 percent detection with just one false positive among the entire dataset set of 10 cases. These preliminary findings are very promising. However, more studies with larger datasets would be needed to verify the method robustness.

References

1. Bajger, M., Lee, G., Caon, M.: Full-body CT segmentation using 3D extension of two graph-based methods: A feasibility study. In: Proc. of the IASTED International Conference on Signal Processing, Pattern Recognition and Applications (SPPRA 2012), Crete, Greece, pp. 43–50 (2012)

2. Bajger, M., Lee, G., Caon, M.: 3D segmentation for multi-organs in CT images. Electronic Letters on Computer Vision and Image Analysis 12(2), 13–27 (2013)
3. Bajger, M., Ma, F., Williams, S., Bottema, M.: Mammographic mass detection with Statistical Region Merging. In: Proc. of DICTA 2010 Digital Image Computing: Techniques and Applications, Sydney, Australia, pp. 27–32 (2010)
4. Filev, P., Hadjiiski, L., Chan, H.-P., Sahiner, B., Ge, J., Helvie, M.A., Roubidoux, M., Zhou, C.: Automated regional registration and characterization of corresponding microcalcificaiton clusters on temporal pairs of mammograms for interval change analysis. Medical Physics 35, 5340 (2008)
5. Giger, M.L., Chan, H.-P., Boone, J.: History and status of cad and quantitative image analysis: The role of medical physics and aapm. Medical Physics 35, 5799 (2008)
6. Guo, Y., Sivaramakrishna, R., Lu, C.-C., Suri, J.S., Laxminarayan, S.: Breast image registration techniques: A survey. Med. Biol. Eng. Comput. 44, 15–26 (2006)
7. Horsch, K., Giger, M.L., Venta, L.A., Vyborny, C.J.: Computerized diagnosis of breast lesions on ultrasound. Medical Physics, 157–164 (2002)
8. Karssemeijer, N., te Brake, G.: Combining single view features and asymmetry for detection of mass lesions. In: Digital Mammography, pp. 95–102 (1998)
9. Lee, G., Bajger, M., Caon, M.: Multi-organ segmentation of CT images using statistical region merging. In: Proc. of the IASTED International Conference on Biomedical Engineering (BioMed 2012), Innsbruck, Austria, pp. 199–206 (2012)
10. Lee, G.N., Fukuoka, D., Ikedo, Y., Hara, T., Fujita, H., Takada, E., Endo, T., Morita, T.: Classification of benign and malignant masses in ultrasound breast image based on geometric and echo features. In: Krupinski, E.A. (ed.) IWDM 2008. LNCS, vol. 5116, pp. 433–439. Springer, Heidelberg (2008)
11. Lee, G.N., et al.: Classifying breast masses in volumetric whole breast ultrasound data: A 2.5-dimensional approach. In: Martí, J., Oliver, A., Freixenet, J., Martí, R. (eds.) IWDM 2010. LNCS, vol. 6136, pp. 636–642. Springer, Heidelberg (2010)
12. Linguraru, M.G., Marias, K., Brady, J.M.: Temporal mass detection. In: International Workshop on Digital Mammography, pp. 347–350 (2002)
13. Maintz, J.B., Viergever, M.A.: A survey of medical image registration. Medical Image Analysis 2(1), 1–36 (1998)
14. Marias, K., Brady, J.M., Highnam, R.P., Parbhoo, S., Seifalian, A.M.: Registration and matching of temporal mammograms for detecting abnormalities. In: Proceedings of Medical Image Understanding and Analysis (British Machine Vision Association), pp. 97–100 (1999)
15. Nock, R., Nielsen, F.: Statistical Region Merging. IEEE Trans. Pattern Anal. Mach. Intell. 26(11), 1452–1458 (2004)
16. Pluim, J.P.W., Maintz, J.B.A., Viergever, M.A.: Mutual-information-based registration of medical images: A survey. IEEE Transactions on Medical Imaging 22(8), 986–1004 (2003)
17. Rueckert, D., Sonoda, L.I., Hayes, C., Hill, D.L.G., Leach, M.O., Hawkes, D.J.: Nonrigid registration using free-form deformations: Application to breast mr images. IEEE Transactions on Medical Imaging 18(8), 712–720 (1999)
18. Sotiras, A., Davatzikos, C., Paragios, N.: Deformable medical image registration: A survey. IEEE Transactions on Medical Imaging 32(7), 1153–1190 (2013)
19. Timp, S., Karssemeijer, N.: Interval change analysis to improve computer aided detection in mammography. Medical Image Analysis 10, 82–95 (2006)
20. Timp, S., Varela, C., Karssemeijer, N.: Temporal change analysis for characterization of mass lesions in mammography. IEEE Transactions on Medical Imaging 26(7), 945–953 (2007)

21. van Engeland, S., Karssemeijer, N., Hendriks, J.: Using information from two mammographic views to improve computer-aided detection of mass lesions. In: Digital Mammography, pp. 377–381 (2003)
22. van Engeland, S., Snoeren, P., Hendriks, J., Karssemeijer, N.: A comparison of methods for mammogram registration. IEEE Transactions on Medical Imaging 22(11), 1436–1444 (2003)
23. Wei, J., Chan, H.-P., Zhou, C., Wu, Y.-T., Sahiner, B., Hadjiiski, L.M., Roubidoux, M.A., Helvie, M.A.: Computer-aided detection of breast masses: Four-view strategy for screening mammography. Medical Physics 38(4), 1867–1876 (2011)
24. Yin, F.-F., Giger, M.L., Doi, K., Vyborny, C.J., Schmidt, R.A.: Computerized detection of masses in digital mammograms: automated alignment of breast images and its effect on bilateral-subtraction technique. Medical Physics 21, 445 (1994)
25. Yin, F.-F., Giger, M.L., Vyborny, C.J., Doi, K., Schmidt, R.A.: Comparison of bilateral-subtraction and single-image processing techniques in the computerized detection of mammographic masses. Investigative Radiology 28(6), 473–481 (1993)
26. Zheng, B., Chang, Y.-H., Gur, D.: Computerized detection of massess from digitized mammograms: Comparison of single-image segmentation and bilateral-image subtraction. Radiat. Prot. Dsimetry. 124(2), 130–136 (2007)
27. Zitova, B., Flusser, J.: Image registration methods: A survey. Image and Vision Computing 21, 977–1000 (2003)

Comparison of Calcification Cluster Detection by CAD and Human Observers at Different Image Quality Levels

Pádraig T. Looney[1], Lucy M. Warren[1,2], Susan M. Astley[3], and Kenneth C. Young[1,2]

[1] National Coordinating Centre for the Physics of Mammography,
Royal Surrey County Hospital NHS Foundation Trust, Guildford, UK
[2] Department of Physics, University of Surrey, Guildford, UK
[3] Centre for Imaging Sciences, Institute of Population Health, Faculty of Medical and Human Sciences, Manchester Academic Health Science Centre, University of Manchester, Oxford Road, Manchester M13 9PT, UK

Abstract. Previous studies have compared the performance of human observers to the performance of human observers using CAD. Here we compare the performance of human observers to Hologic's ImageChecker CAD system using a set of 162 images with simulated calcification clusters. The quality of the images was reduced to create four other image sets at different image qualities. These were analysed by the CAD system and the relevant information from the resulting DICOM structured reports was parsed. At the highest image quality level the figure of merit for the CAD was 0.82 and 0.84 for the humans. At the lowest image quality level the figure of merit for the CAD and humans were 0.62 and 0.55 respectively. At each image quality level there was no significant difference (p>0.05). The effect of changes in image quality on calcification detection was similar for human observers and the CAD system.

Keywords: CAD, JAFROC, Image Perception, Python.

1   Introduction

The aim of this study was to compare the performance of the Hologic (Hologic Inc, Bedford) ImageChecker CAD system to the performance of human readers detecting calcification clusters in digital mammograms at different image quality levels. There have been comparisons of the performance of human observers using CAD to human observers without CAD [1]. However, relatively little previous work has compared CAD to human observers, as performed in this work. Since CAD systems are developed using images from particular systems operating at specific image quality levels it was expected that CAD may be sensitive to changes in image quality.

2   Method

2.1   Human Observer Study and Image Sets

A previous study investigated whether detector type, dose level or image processing significantly affected the detection of calcification clusters by expert mammographers

H. Fujita, T. Hara, and C. Muramatsu (Eds.): IWDM 2014, LNCS 8539, pp. 643–649, 2014.
© Springer International Publishing Switzerland 2014

[2]. In that study 162 cases, read as normal, were collected from a Hologic Selenia digital mammography system. Patients aged 47-73 years had been referred for a mammography examination as they were either symptomatic or high risk. Women with mammograms containing extensive vascular or benign calcification (over large portions of the breast) were excluded from the study. A single view (CC or MLO) from a single breast (left or right) was randomly selected from each case. The average glandular dose for a 50-60mm breast was 2.09mGy. Between one and three simulated calcification clusters were inserted into 81 of the 162 images using a published and validated method [3].

These images were transformed to produce four other sets of 162 images at different levels of image quality: CR images at the same dose level as the normal dose DR images ("normal dose CR") and at half this dose level ("half dose CR"), and DR images at half and quarter the original dose level ("half dose DR" and "quarter dose DR," respectively). Seven observers viewed the images on calibrated 5 megapixel monitors (BARCO Model: MDMG-5121) and were asked to mark regions they suspected to be a calcification cluster. They were asked to ignore single calcification or vascular calcification. The observers marked the location of the suspected cluster and assigned a score from 1-5 according to their confidence that the suspicious region was a cluster (5 being highest confidence).

Image quality was measured for each image set using the CDMAM test object (Artinis, Netherlands) in terms of threshold gold thickness for different detail diameters. The results of this previous study using human observers are compared to the CAD output on the same image sets.

2.2   CAD Analysis

The human observers had been shown processed images, however CAD operates on the unprocessed (raw) digital data. The 810 unprocessed images were sent to the Hologic R2Server and the CAD results were received as a DICOM structured report at a DICOM SCP created using DCM4CHE 2.7. Using the Python DICOM library PyDICOM [4] scripts and modules were written to decode the structured reports. A graphical user interface was created using the user interface libraries PyQT and QT to display the structured report and processed images with the CAD marks overlying (figure 1) [5]. Visual inspection of the structured reports allowed automated Python scripts to be developed to process the structure reports.

ImageChecker provides three types of CAD marks – Calc (indicates a cluster of calcifications), Mass (indicates a mass or an architectural distortion) and Malc (indicates a region where a mass and one or more clusters of calcifications are present). Since, in this study, we are only concerned with calcifications we restricted our attention to CAD marks of type Calc and Malc. Each CAD mark has a 'certainty of finding' item in the structured report. The certainty of finding is a value between zero and one hundred and was used as the confidence level in the JAFROC analysis. In our analysis the CAD system acts as another observer. The observers in the observer study were asked to mark a single point in the centre of the suspected cluster. Hence, we use the centre point of the calcification cluster in our statistical analysis and do not use the outline of the cluster. In the case of a Calc CAD mark the centre of

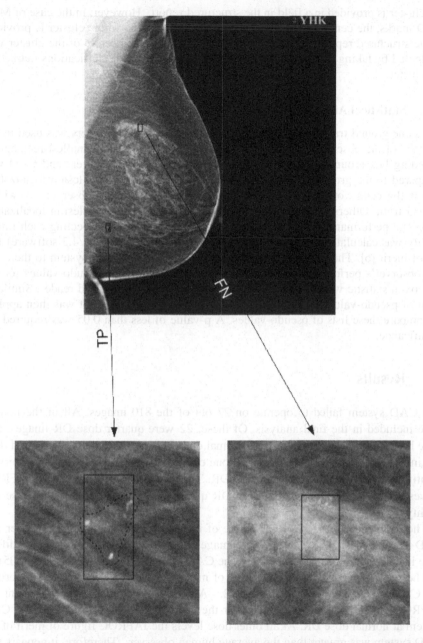

Fig. 1. Sample image with a correctly located calcification cluster (TP) and a calcification cluster that was not located by the CAD system. The CAD mark is shown with the dashed black line and the ground truth location is the solid black rectangle. The observers correctly localised both clusters. At normal dose DR image quality the cluster on the left was marked by 6 out of 7 observers and the cluster on the right was marked by all 7 observers.

the cluster is provided in a field in the structured report. However, in the case of Malc CAD marks, the centre of each calcification rather than the whole cluster is provided in the structured report. Therefore for Malc CAD marks the centre of the cluster was computed by taking the geometric mean of the centres of the calcifications marked in the cluster.

2.3   Statistical Analysis

The same ground truth location of the simulated calcification clusters was used in the analysis of the observer and CAD marks. This consisted of the smallest rectangular bounding box around the cluster. The performance of the observers and CAD was compared to the ground truth and was recorded as being correct (lesion localization LL) if the centre of the cluster as marked by the CAD or an observer lay within ground truth. Otherwise the mark was recorded as incorrect (non-lesion localization NL). The performance of each observer and the CAD system inspecting each image quality was calculated as the JAFROC (performed using JAFROC 4.2 software) figure of merit [6]. The comparison of the performance of the CAD system to the average observer's performance was made using a t-test. A list of pseudo-values for the Wilcoxon statistic was calculated by jackknifing over each case and reader. Similarly a list of pseudo-values was calculated for the CAD system. A t-test was then applied to compare these lists of pseudo-values. A p-value of less than 0.05 was required for significance.

3   Results

The CAD system failed to operate on 27 out of the 810 images. All of the images were included in the final analysis. Of these, 22 were quarter dose DR images, two were half dose DR images, two were normal dose DR images and one was a half dose CR image. The CAD system identified one cluster that none of the human observers identified in normal dose and half dose DR. The CAD and average observer AFROC curves are shown for the normal dose DR quality in figure 2 and the half dose DR quality in figure 3.

The difference in the JAFROC figure of merit between the average observer and CAD is given in Table 1. For all of the image qualities there was no significant difference in calcification detection between the CAD and the human observers (p>0.05).

The reader-averaged JAFROC figure of merit and the JAFROC figure of merit of the CAD system are shown in Table 2. Although not statistically significant the JAFROC figure of merit was greater for the average human observer than the CAD system at normal dose DR. At all other dose levels the JAFROC figure of merit of the CAD system was greater than the average human observer. Therefore, it appears that the area under the curve decreases at a greater rate for the human observers than the CAD system with change in detector and dose. The threshold gold thickness had a negative correlation with both human ($R^2=0.86$) and CAD ($R^2=0.92$) figures of merit since higher thresholds indicate poorer image quality (figure 4).

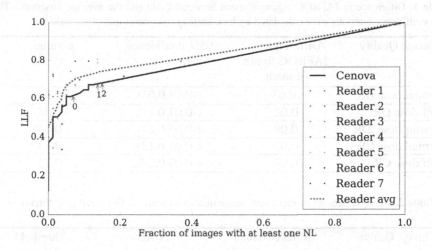

Fig. 2. AFROC curves of human and CAD system at normal dose DR. The reader average AFROC curve (dashed line) and the CAD AFROC curve (solid line) are shown. The operating points of the CAD system are shown by the points labeled lines labeled '0', '1' and '2'. The individual reader results are also shown.

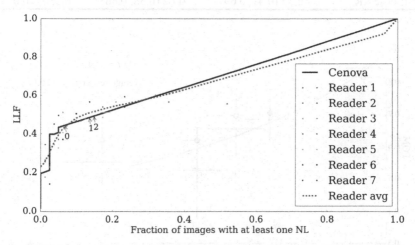

Fig. 3. AFROC curves of human and CAD system at half dose DR. The reader average AFROC curve (dashed line) and the CAD AFROC curve (solid line) are shown. The operating points of the CAD system are shown by the points labeled lines labeled '0', '1' and '2'. The individual reader results are also shown.

Table 1. Difference in JAFROC figure of merit between CAD and the average observer. The 95% confidence intervals were calculated by jack-knifing over cases and observers.

Image Quality	Difference in JAFROC figure of merit	95% confidence interval	p-value
Normal dose DR	-0.03	(-0.08,0.03)	0.70
Half dose DR	0.02	(-0.07,0.11)	0.88
Quarter dose DR	0.09	(-0.05,0.24)	0.63
Normal dose CR	0.04	(-0.04,0.12)	0.73
Half dose CR	0.07	(-0.07,0.20)	0.72

Table 2. JAFROC figures of merit and image quality in terms of threshold gold thickness

Image Quality	Average Human	CAD	Threshold gold thickness for 0.25mm detail (μm)
Normal dose DR	0.84 (0.80, 0.90)	0.82 (0.76, 0.87)	0.167 ± 0.012
Half dose DR	0.68 (0.59, 0.78)	0.70 (0.65, 0.76)	0.233 ± 0.017
Quarter dose DR	0.53 (0.38, 0.67)	0.62 (0.57, 0.66)	0.284 ± 0.021
Normal dose CR	0.66 (0.57, 0.74)	0.70 (0.64, 0.75)	0.257 ± 0.02
Half dose CR	0.55 (0.41, 0.69)	0.62 (0.58, 0.66)	0.350 ± 0.027

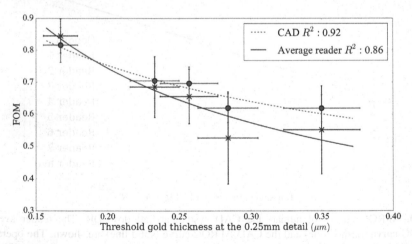

Fig. 4. The figure of merit of the average reader and CAD are plotted against the threshold gold thickness for the 0.25mm detail found from a CDMAM. The error in the FOM is taken from the 95% confidence interval and the error in the threshold gold thickness is taken to be twice the standard error in the mean.

4   Discussion and Conclusions

We have compared the performance of a CAD system to human observers. Our analysis has shown that for the particular set of mammography images used in this study there was no significant difference in calcification detection between the CAD algorithm and the performance of the human observers. Thus changes in image quality due to dose and detector design had a similar effect on the performance of the human observers and the CAD system. Both degraded rapidly with a reduction in image quality. If anything there was a tendency for the CAD system to be less affected by the changes in image quality than the human observers. This suggests that the CAD algorithm was relatively robust for the large differences in image quality used in this study. This result gives reassurance that the wide range in doses and image qualities encountered in screening programs is not more of a problem for CAD systems than human observers at least in terms of calcification detection. However maintaining high image quality is important for both CAD and human observers.

Acknowledgements. This work is part of the OPTIMAM project and is supported by CR-UK & EPSRC Cancer Imaging Programme in Surrey, in association with the MRC and Department of Health (England). We would also like to thank Hologic for the use of their CAD system

References

1. Fenton, J.J., Abraham, L., Taplin, S.H., Geller, B.M., Carney, P.A., D'Orsi, C., Elmore, J.G., Barlow, W.E.: Effectiveness of computer-aided detection in community mammography practice. Journal of the National Cancer Institute 103(15), 1152–1161 (2011)
2. Warren, L.M., Mackenzie, A., Cooke, J., Given-Wilson, R.M., Wallis, M.G., Chakraborty, D.P., Dance, D.R., Bosmans, H., Young, K.C.: Effect of image quality on calcification detection in digital mammography. Med. Phys. 39, 3202–3213 (2012)
3. Warren, L.M., Green, F.H., Shrestha, L., Mackenzie, A., Dance, D.R., Young, K.C.: Validation of simulation of calcifications for observer studies in digital mammography. Phys. Med. Biol. 58, N217–N228 (2013)
4. Mason, D.: SU-E-T-33: Pydicom: An Open Source DICOM Library. Medical Physics 38, 3493–3493 (2011)
5. Hunter, J.D.: Matplotlib: A 2D graphics environment. Computing in Science & Engineering 9, 90–95 (2007)
6. Chakraborty, D.P.: Analysis of location specific observer performance data: Validated extensions of the jackknife free-response (JAFROC) method. Academic Radiology 13, 1187–1193 (2006)

A Novel Image Enhancement Methodology for Full Field Digital Mammography

Wenda He[1], Minnie Kibiro[2], Arne Juette[2],
Erika R.E. Denton[2], Peter Hogg[3], and Reyer Zwiggelaar[1]

[1] Department of Computer Science,
Aberystwyth University, Aberystwyth, SY23 3DB, UK
{weh,rrz}@aber.ac.uk
[2] Department of Radiology,
Norfolk & Norwich University Hospital, Norwich, NR4 7UY, UK
{minnie.kibiro,arne.juette,erika.denton}@nnuh.nhs.uk
[3] School of Health Sciences,
Salford & University of Salford, Salford, M5 4WT, UK
p.hogg@salford.ac.uk

Abstract. During breast screening it is necessary and essential to compress the breast with a compression paddle, in order to obtain a clear mammographic image. The quality of the image has a direct correlation with the accuracy of mammogram reading, which in turn could affect radiologist's interpretation. Clinical observation has indicated that breast compression may have a side effect on image quality during the image acquisition and can result in unexpected variations in texture and intensity appearances, between breast tissue near the skinline and the rest of the breast. Within computer aided mammography, such variations increase the difficulty in breast tissue modelling and can be detrimental to image analysis, leading to incorrect prompts which can have an impact on sensitivity and specificity of screening mammography. We present an automatic image enhancement approach, in which both Cranio Caudal and Medio-Lateral Oblique views are utilised. We estimate the relative breast thickness ratio at a given projection location in order to alter/correct an inconsistent intensity distribution as a means of improving mammographic image quality. Our dataset consists of 360 full field digital mammographic images was used in a quantitative and qualitative evaluation. Visual assessment indicated good and consistent intensity variation over the processed images, whilst texture information (breast parenchymal patterns) was preserved and/or enhanced. By improving the consistency of the intensity distribution on the mammographic images, the developed method has demonstrated a potential benefit in density based mammographic segmentation and risk assessment. This in turn can be found useful in computer aided mammography, and is beneficial in a clinical setting by aiding screening radiologists in the process of decision making.

Keywords: digital mammography, peripheral enhancement, compression paddle.

H. Fujita, T. Hara, and C. Muramatsu (Eds.): IWDM 2014, LNCS 8539, pp. 650–657, 2014.
© Springer International Publishing Switzerland 2014

1 Introduction

According to the American College of Radiology's Breast Imaging Reporting and Data System (Birads) [1], the mammographic breast composition is categorised into four patterns: 1) Birads I, the breast is almost entirely fat (< 25% glandular); 2) Birads II, the breast has scattered fibroglandular densities (25% − 50%); 3) Birads III, the breast consists of heterogeneously dense breast tissue (51% − 75%); and 4) Birads IV, the breast is extremely dense (> 75% glandular).

During screening a breast is subjected to compression, which can affect the image quality across the mammogram. Clinical observations have shown that the peripheral area may not be compressed due to reduce of breast thickness, and cause a breast tissue bulge with possible air gaps above and under the bulge. This may lead to x-ray scattering which can affect image quality and limits the quantitative usefulness of the image [2]. For a breast, the attenuation difference between glandular and adipose (fatty) tissue is not large and relatively small residual scatter signals can cause large errors when estimating tissue thickness [2]. Therefore, it is necessary to develop an image processing method to improve the visibility of the peripheral uncompressed area and reduce variations in the compressed area of the projected breast, which facilities presentation and can be beneficial to follow up analysis [3]. Enhancement methods developed to deal with issues related to uneven breast thickness can be categorised into two groups as parametric [3, 4] and non-parametric [5].

Byng et al. [3] developed an non-parametric filter based algorithm to tackle uneven breast thickness related effect as seen in the peripheral areas of the mammograms. To identify the large change in digital·signal and equalise the intensity change, the mammographic image is isotropically blurred to represent tissue thickness with smoother variations, instead of using tissue density to achieve the similar results directly. The average intensity of a small region around the border pixels is calculated for each row, and the value is used in a conventional threshold process to separate the peripheral area from the rest of the breast. The equalised image is obtained by multiplying the pixel values in the periphery by a correction function. The method is only applied in the peripheral area; it is simple and can be effective. However, breast parencyma can be very different from case to case with intricate texture, whilst the isotropic filter may overly blur structures at certain orientations, leading to less desirable results. Snoeren and Karssemeijer [4] investigated an anisotropic filtering approach (direction parallel to the skin edge), the processed images show 'hidden' details behind the nipple which may not be perceived on the original mammograms. The method processes the entire breast within the interior part; breast parenchyma remain unchanged but may display higher contrast after correction. This is due to the thickness variations are much stronger in the direction perpendicular to the sinkline, and the thickness decreases from the chest wall outwards. Prior to the correction, a breast is segmented into fatty and dense areas using an interactive method. Then a linear interpolation is used to replace all the dense tissue with nearby fatty tissue. Binary Otsu thresholding [6] is employed to better identify the peripheral area. The enhancement is performed by adding correction terms to pixel values in the peripheral area. This approach has improved peripheral texture appearances for those structural texture with orientations (e.g. blood vessels). However, the interactive dense tissue segmentation and fatty tissue replacement via interpolation can potentially compound errors through the process, leading to incorrect enhancement. At the same time, it can be time consuming and subjective.

As a non-parametric peripheral enhancement method, Snoeren and Karssemeijer [5] proposed a technique that can only be applied to unprocessed digital mammograms (before logarithmic transformation) with a linear relationship between exposure and grey value. A geometric model of the three-dimensional shape of the breast is used for correction, instead of using filtered images. The interior (fully/mostly compressed area without air gaps) is modelled by two non-parametric planes which requires three degrees of freedom, one for the onset and two for the slops. The exterior (not fully compressed breast periphery with air gaps) is modelled by bands of semi-circles and determined by the breast outline. Once the parameters of the geometric model are obtained, the correction process is performed similar to [4] where dense tissue is separated and interpolated with fatty tissue. After the dense tissue replacement, the grey values of a breast that only consists of fatty tissue is then modelled. The process assumes a linear relationship between tissue thickness and log-exposure (Beer's law of attenuation). Both methods (i.e. [4] and [5]) are critically depends on accurate segmentation of the breast, and [5] is limited to unprocessed digital mammograms. In the case of large cysts deposited in the peripheral areas, the correction process may distort the tissue appearances; this also applies to dense abnormalities (e.g. tumours).

This paper presents a parametric based enhancement method, which estimates/approximates the breast thickness ratios using both Mediolateral Oblique (MLO) and Cranio-Caudal (CC) views, without using an interactive dense tissue segmentation nor fatty tissue interpolation [5]. The correction process is partially similar to the processes in [7, 8], with additional features to balance intensity not only in peripheral areas but also in breast interiors. An automatic selection method is incorporated in order to better target those mammograms requiring enhancement in a systematic way.

2 Data and Method

The dataset consists of 360 mammographic images processed for optimal visual appearance to radiologists, in which a total of 56, 120, 120 and 64 images are associated with Birads density categories I to IV, respectively. The number of images which do and do not require enhancement are 148 and 212, respectively. Note that the images were assessed visually. Despite that the categorisation was performed subjectively, the problematic images were easy to identify and in-between cases are relatively small. However, an objective method would be good to use and is considered as future work.

The developed methodology starts off with an automatic image selection, and the main process can be broken down into four steps: 1) x-ray penetration weighting map generation, 2) intensity balancing, 3) intensity ratio propagation, and 4) boundary stitching.

It is assumed that the automatic calibrated parameters, i.e. compression force (CF), breast thickness (BT) and peak kilovoltage (KVP), follow a normal distribution; see Table 1 shows the statistical values calculated for all three calibrated parameters. Based on our experimental observations, a mammographic image should be processed if its calibrated parameters are less than the mean values. The robustness of using the calibrated parameters as constrains was limited due to large breast tissue density, composition and size variations and additional conditions based on prior knowledge were incorporated. Specifically, the Otsu algorithm was used to generate a binary image separating the peripheral area (PA) and breast interior (BI). Three properties were calculated: total peripheral area (TPA), vertical peripheral area coverage ($VPAC$) in image rows and pectoral coverage (PC) in image rows. Note that the PA may extend to the BI after the binary segmentation. Therefore, a mammographic image (img) needs to be processed if $CF_{img} <= \overline{CF}$ & $BT_{img} <= \overline{BT}$ & $KVP_{img} <= \overline{KVP}$ & $15\% < TPA_{img} < 50\%$ & $VPAC_{img} > 75\%$ & $PC_{img} < 30\%$; the threshold values were empirically defined through trail and error. It should be noted that not all the mammographic images need to be enhanced, some of them are of superb quality; such as soft and/or median size breasts which have automatic calibration parameters in line with optimum settings for the optimum photon energy (e.g. ~30 kVp). Therefore, the automatic selection method is only applied to problematic mammographic images.

Table 1. Statistical values calculated for all three calibrated parameters

	Maximum	Minimum	Median	Standard deviation
CF	249.1	44.5	103.5	34.5
BT	104.0	29.0	61.7	14.8
KVP	35.0	24.0	30.3	2.2

The x-ray penetration probability has a direct correlation with breast thickness (e.g. the thicker the breast the harder to penetrate it). In principle, there are many attributes (e.g. dosage, filter, anode) which should be taken into account when modelling the x-ray penetration probability. However, due to physical complexity (e.g. unknown combination factors in x-ray bean spectrum and breast tissue composition), the x-ray penetration probability was modelled in a simplified way, by wrapping up all other elements in a "black box" and only consider it as inversely proportional to the breast thickness. Note that the developed methodology does not require the absolute correct measurement for the breast thickness. A x-ray penetration probability weighting map was generated for each image, by calculating and propagating the relative breast thickness ratios based on the CC/MLO pair; e.g. to a CC view the relative breast thickness ratio (r) can be estimated based on the projected physical contour of the compressed breast as seen on MLO view; in particular, the skinline was firstly extracted from the MLO view, and split in two at the furthest pixel to the chest wall to form the upper and lower skinlines (e.g. blue and green lines in Fig. 1 (c)). For each pixel on the top skinline, a corresponding pixel was sought on the lower skinline, to form a parallel line (*p-line*) (e.g. red line in Fig. 1 (d)) to the chest wall by linking the two pixels. This process was repeated for all the pixels on the top skinline, and resulting in a series of parallel lines (e.g. Fig. 1 (d)(e)). In the CC view, the r at a given point (p) (e.g. 'A' in Fig. 1 (a)) is calculated based on the boundary pixel (p_{base}) (e.g. 'B' in Fig. 1 (a)) which separates PA and BI as

$$r = \frac{p - line(p)}{p - line(p_{base})},$$ (1)

where both pixels are on the thickest projected section (e.g. blue lines in Fig. 1 (a)(b)) in the CC view. The x-ray penetration probability weighting map for the CC view was completed, by assigning the rest of the pixels on the thickest projected section with the estimated breast thickness ratios in the same way, and propagating the calculated ratios to the pixels have the same distance to the skinline (e.g. pixels on the yellow lines in Fig. 1 (a)(b)) .

To reduce the intensity distribution variation, a base weight (w_{base}) was firstly calculated as

$$w_{base} = \frac{\sum_{i=0}^{N} W_i(x, y)}{N}, \forall\, W_i(x, y) \in S,$$ (2)

where W and S denote the weighting map and the boundary between PA and BI. For each pixel within the BI, the intensity value $P(x, y)$ was altered to

$$P'(x, y) = \frac{w_{base}}{W(x, y)} P(x, y).$$ (3)

After the intensity balancing, the local intensity ratio was propagated as a means of improving tissue appearance in PA (similar to the process described in [8]). From pixels at the boundary S to the skinline within the PA, the intensity value was altered by calculating the propagation ratio (pr) for each pixel $P(x, y)$ with distance to the skinline $D(x, y)$ and within an empirically defined 17×17 neighbourhood (see Section 3 for the effects of using different neighbourhood sizes) as

$$I_{avgP_1} = \frac{\sum_{j=0}^{M} P_j(x, y)}{M}, \forall\, P_j(x, y) = D(x, y) + 1,$$

$$I_{avgP_2} = \frac{\sum_{i=0}^{N} P_i(x, y)}{N}, \forall\, P_i(x, y) = D(x, y) + 2,$$ (4)

$$pr = \frac{I_{avgP_2}}{I_{avgP_1}},$$

$$P'(x, y) = pr \times P(x, y);$$

where $D(x, y) + 1$ and $D(x, y) + 2$ are pixel distances to skinline 1 and 2 steps further away from the observed pixel.

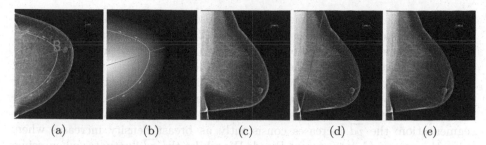

$\quad$(a)$\qquad\qquad$(b)$\qquad\qquad$(c)$\qquad\qquad$(d)$\qquad\qquad$(e)

Fig. 1. Image illustration, from left to right, a CC view, its distance map, the paired MLO view, parallel lines near the pectoral muscle and near the nipple

Finally, boundary stitching (local normalisation) was applied to seamlessly normalise pixels intensity within the boundary S, thickened to a 5 pixels band, in order to gradually smooth the transition from BI to PA. The maximum and minimum intensity values were determined within an empirically defined 7×7 neighbourhood (see Section 3 for the effects of using different neighbourhood sizes).

3   Results and Discussion

The automatic image selection achieved 86.5% and 93.9% accuracies in choosing images which do and do not require enhancement, respectively.

Visual assessment was conducted to assess the images quality after enhancement. For the majority of the cases, the processed images have shown improvement in texture appearances and contrast in the peripheral areas. However, intensity within BI can be over or under balanced if PA and BI were not separated correctly, or the breast thickness ratios were wrongly estimated. Experimental results indicated that a larger neighbourhood may result in unwanted artefacts, due to incorrect local intensity alternation which affects texture appearance and can be perceived as artefacts, but the processed images seem to have minimum texture distortion, and were suitable for the follow up image analysis. It should be noted that the enhanced mammographic images are currently used as pre-processed images prior to further analysis, and not for presentation purpose which would require additional validations (e.g. in a clinical environment) which is outside the scope of the current study, but it is considered as future work.

To assess the usefulness of the developed method as a form of pre-processing, a k-means clustering based mammographic segmentation was conducted. The hypothesis is that the average percent density $(\overline{pd} = \frac{\sum_{img=0}^{n} pd_i}{n}$ where n denote the number of Birads I/II/III/IV images) derived from the segmented processed images should be better in line or closer to Birads density models, compared to the $\overline{pd}$ derived from the segmented original images. Only the pixel intensity was considered in the feature space, in order to focus on the intensity aspect and to eliminate statistical variations when incorporating other features (e.g. texture and geometric features). Each mammographic image was segmented into three classes (k = 3 in the k-means), 'non-dense', 'semi-dense' and 'dense'; the later two were considered 'dense tissue'. Fig. 2 shows segmentation examples. Note that segmentation based on two classes (e.g. 'non-dense' and 'dense') was performed; however, the obtained results were less satisfactory when compared to the segmentation based on three classes. Visual assessment indicated that the segmentation for the processed images are anatomically more accurate and consistent over the breast parenchyma. Table 2 shows the derived $\overline{pd}$ after the segmentation; the $\overline{pd}$ increases consistently as breast density increases when using the processed data, except Birads IV; whilst the $\overline{pd}$ fluctuates when using the original data. For Birads I, the derived $\overline{pd}$ are much closer to the density model when using the processed data; for Birads II and III, the $\overline{pd}$ are within or in line with the density models when using the processed data, whilst the results for the original images are less accurate; and for Birads IV, it is difficult to determine the impact due to the lack of samples, but visual assessment indicated that the developed method may cause more harm to the image segmentation quality in Birads IV, leading to incorrect segmentation and percent density measurement.

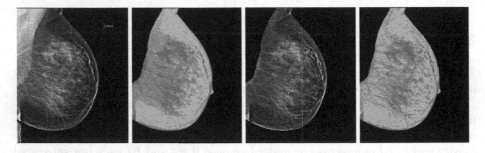

Fig. 2. From left to right, the original image, its segmentation, the processed image, and its segmentation. The processed data shows more segmented blood vessels in the peripheral areas, glandular tissue segmentation are realistic as they are grouped towards the centre or nipple areas, and more correctly identified fatty tissue.

Table 2. Average percent density derived after the segmentation based on all the images in the dataset. 'O' and 'P' denote the original and processed data, respectively. 'Automatic', 'Manual' and 'All' indicate the processed images were selected automatically, manually and using the entire dataset, respectively.

	Birads	Automatic O	Automatic P	Manual O	Manual P	All O	All P
I	< 25%	60.0%±4%	40.3%±7%	60.0%±6	40.2%±7	60.2%±7	40.9%±9
II	25% − 50%	59.6%±13%	47.1%±11%	59.2%±12	46.2%±11	56.6%±11	47.9%±10
III	50% − 75%	53.8%±3%	50.8%±6%	54.6%±2	51.5%±3	52.7%±11	49.4%±9
IV	> 75%	52.8%±0%	49.2%±3%	45.4%±0	57.0%±0	56.2%±7	42.5%±6

4   Conclusions

The developed mammographic image enhancement can be used to improve image appearance and is robust in dealing with inter and intra class variation. The segmentation results for the processed images are anatomically more accurate and consistent over the breast parenchyma. Clear improvements can be seen in the derived average percent density in all Birads density categories, except in Birads IV. The developed methodology can be used as a form of pre-processing before mammographic segmentation. Such a method can be found useful in quantification of change of relative proportion of dense tissue, as a means of aiding radiologists' estimation in mammographic risk assessment.

References

1. American College of Radiology. Breast Imaging Reporting and Data System BI-RADS, 4th edn. American College of Radiology, Reston (2004)
2. Ducote, J.L., Molloi, S.: Scatter correction in digital mammography based on image deconvolution. Physics in Medicine and Biology 55, 1295–1309 (2010)
3. Byng, J.W., Critten, J.P., Yaffe, M.J.: Thickness-equalization processing for mammographic images. Radiology 203(2), 564–568 (1997)
4. Snoeren, P.R., Karssemeijer, N.: Thickness correction of mammographic images by means of a global parameter model of the compressed breast. IEEE Transactions on Medical Imaging 23(7), 799–806 (2004)
5. Snoeren, P.R., Karssemeijer, N.: Thickness correction of mammographic images by anisotropic filtering and interpolation of dense tissue, vol. 5747, pp. 1521–1527. SPIE (2005)
6. Sezgin, M., Sankur, B.: Survey over image thresholding techniques and quantitative performance evaluation. Journal of Electronic Imaging 13, 146–165 (2004)
7. Karssemeijer, N., Te Brake, G.: Combining single view features and asymmetry for detection of mass lesions. In: Karssemeijer, N., Thijssen, M., Hendriks, J., Erning, L. (eds.) Digital Mammography. Computational Imaging and Vision, vol. 13, pp. 95–102. Springer, Netherlands (1998)
8. Tortajada, M., Oliver, A., Martí, R., Vilagran, M., Ganau, S., Tortajada, L., Sentís, M., Freixenet, J.: Adapting breast density classification from digitized to full-field digital mammograms. In: Maidment, A.D.A., Bakic, P.R., Gavenonis, S. (eds.) IWDM 2012. LNCS, vol. 7361, pp. 561–568. Springer, Heidelberg (2012)

Correlation between Topological Descriptors of the Breast Ductal Network from Clinical Galactograms and Texture Features of Corresponding Mammograms

Predrag R. Bakic[1], David D. Pokrajac[2], Mathew Thomas[1], Angeliki Skoura[3], Tatyana Nuzhnaya[4], Vasileios Megalooikonomou[3,4], Brad Keller[1], Yuanjie Zheng[1], Despina Kontos[1], James C. Gee[1], Gilda Cardenosa[5], and Andrew D.A. Maidment[1]

[1] Dept. of Radiology, University of Pennsylvania, Philadelphia, PA, USA
[2] Computer and Information Sciences Dept., Delaware State University, Dover, DE, USA
[3] Computer Engineering and Informatics Dept., University of Patras, Greece
[4] Computer and Information Science Dept., Temple University, Philadelphia, PA, USA
[5] Dept. of Radiology, Virginia Commonwealth University, Richmond, VA, USA
Predrag.Bakic@uphs.upenn.edu

Abstract. Mammographic texture has been reported as a biomarker of cancer risk. Recent publications also suggest correlation between the topology of the breast ductal network and risk of cancer. The ductal network can be visualized by galactography, the preferred imaging technique for nipple discharge. We present current results about the correlation between topological and textural properties of clinical breast images. This correlation was assessed for 41 galactograms and 56 mammograms from 13 patients. Topology was characterized using feature extraction techniques arising from text-mining, validated previously in the classification of normal, benign, and malignant galactograms. In addition, we calculated 26 texture descriptors using an automated breast image analysis pipeline. Regression analysis was performed between texture and topological descriptors averaged over all images of the same patient. These data demonstrate a correlation between topology and a subset of texture features with borderline statistical significance due to the limited sample size.

Keywords: Texture analysis, topology descriptors, galactograms, mammograms.

1 Introduction

Previously, we analysed the topological properties of the branching network of breast ducts as visualized by galactography, an x-ray imaging procedure of the contrast-enhanced breast ductal network (1-3). That analysis suggested a correlation between cancer risk and ductal network topology; this correlation also has been supported by evidence from murine cancer models (4). Clinical visualization of breast ducts is, however, not routinely performed; galactography is indicated infrequently, and it mostly commonly reveals benign findings (5, 6).

H. Fujita, T. Hara, and C. Muramatsu (Eds.): IWDM 2014, LNCS 8539, pp. 658–665, 2014.
© Springer International Publishing Switzerland 2014

On the other hand, texture descriptors of breast parenchyma are known to correlate with cancer risk (7-9). Our work is motivated by a desire to determine whether there is an association between parenchymal texture descriptors and ductal topology. Such an analysis would lead to improved models of breast anatomy, and may lead to a better understanding of breast cancer risk. Currently, breast cancer risk is estimated using patient demographic information and parenchymal texture features extracted from 2D mammograms. The spatial arrangement of breast tissue is, however, three-dimensional, stressing the need to understand the relationship between parenchymal structure and image texture.

The UPenn X-ray Physics Lab has extensive experience with the simulation of breast anatomy and imaging (10, 11). The development of the UPenn breast phantom is predicated upon a set of anatomically justified elements. To that end, we have chosen not to model the parenchymal texture by a random field with statistical properties similar to clinical data. This development process has been incremental, and continues to this day. For example, we have just recently begun to model the hierarchical organization of Cooper's ligaments seen in breast histology slices. A preliminary validation of a model of this small scale tissue detail, published separately in this proceedings, indicates good agreement with clinically estimated texture (12).

This paper presents our current results about the correlation between the ductal topology of clinical galactograms and the parenchymal textural properties of clinical mammograms from the same group of women. Understanding the relationship between mammographic texture and spatial distribution of breast anatomy will help optimize and extend our fully automated software pipeline for breast anatomy and imaging simulation; ultimately, we would like to be able to simulate specific cohorts of women, stratified by age, risk, and other factors.

2   Methods

2.1   Topological Analysis of Galactograms

In this paper, we analysed images of existing, anonymized clinical galactograms of 49 women, obtained from Virginia Commonwealth University. The data collection was performed after IRB review and was HIPAA compliant. Clinical galactograms were digitized from film, and categorized based upon the visibility of the ductal network. Ductal trees were traced manually from galactograms, followed by Prufer encoding of the breadth-first labelled ductal tree nodes (3). Then tf-idf significance weighting (3), originally used in text mining, was performed on the traced and encoded ductal trees. After manually tracing the ductal networks, a subset of 41 galactograms from 13 patients with well-defined ductal trees was selected for further processing and testing.

2.2   Texture Analysis of Mammograms

We measured 26 texture features in 56 digitized mammograms from the 13 selected patients imaged at Virginia Commonwealth University. Texture analysis was performed using a fully automated software pipeline which extracted a large set of image features from the digitized mammograms (13). The pipeline calculates texture feature maps at points on a regular spatial lattice, determined by two parameters: the window size and the lattice distance. Here we use a window size of 63 pixels, and a lattice distance of 31 pixels. The analysed features are organized into three groups, including (i) descriptors of grey-level histograms, (ii) co-occurrence features, and (iii) run length features. These texture features have been used previously in breast cancer risk assessment studies (9). For the correlation analysis, the texture feature maps were averaged over the whole breast region (excluding the pectoral muscle and air).

2.3   Hypothesis Testing

We tested the hypothesis that there is a correlation between mammographic texture features and ductal topology descriptors. To that end, we have calculated the linear regression (14). The goal was to predict values of texture features averaged over all mammograms of the same patient as a function of the topological properties estimated from the corresponding manually-traced ductal networks, averaged over all galactograms of the same patient. Prior to the regression analysis, we combined the tf-idf topological descriptors via principal component analysis (PCA). The regression model considered the first 13 PCA components and the 26 texture features.

2.4   Power Calculations

It can be demonstrated that a small sample size (in this case 13 patients), could lead to large estimated p-values and hence rejection of valid linear regression models (large Type II error). To demonstrate the effect of sample size, we simulated an augmented dataset by bootstrapping (15). The bootstrapping was performed by replicating data records, with added Gaussian noise, for each PCA attribute and response variable. The standard deviation of the noise was 50% of the estimated standard deviation of the attributes or response variables.

3   Results and Discussion

Fig. 1 shows an example of a clinical galactogram used in this study (Fig. 1(a)), and the corresponding manually-traced ductal tree (Fig. 1(b)). The Prufer encoding and the tf-idf weights corresponding to the traced tree is also given (Fig. 1(c-d)). The example shown illustrates a breast with a malignant finding. Fig. 2 shows an example of a clinical mammogram from the same woman (Fig. 2(a)) and the corresponding texture feature map (Fig. 2(b)). Shown in this example, is a map of the entropy texture feature.

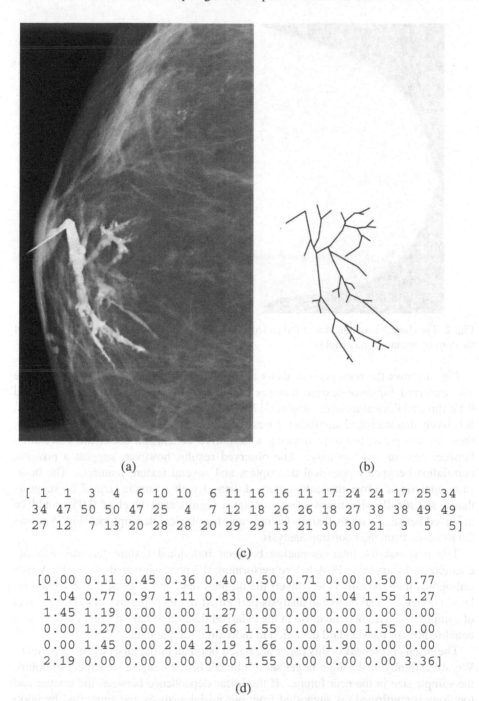

(a)

(b)

[1   1   3   4   6 10 10   6 11 16 16 11 17 24 24 17 25 34
 34 47 50 50 47 25   4   7 12 18 26 26 18 27 38 38 49 49
 27 12   7 13 20 28 28 20 29 29 13 21 30 30 21   3   5   5]

(c)

[0.00 0.11 0.45 0.36 0.40 0.50 0.71 0.00 0.50 0.77
 1.04 0.77 0.97 1.11 0.83 0.00 0.00 1.04 1.55 1.27
 1.45 1.19 0.00 0.00 1.27 0.00 0.00 0.00 0.00 0.00
 0.00 1.27 0.00 0.00 1.66 1.55 0.00 0.00 1.55 0.00
 0.00 1.45 0.00 2.04 2.19 1.66 0.00 1.90 0.00 0.00
 2.19 0.00 0.00 0.00 0.00 1.55 0.00 0.00 0.00 3.36]

(d)

Fig. 1. Illustration of the topological descriptors of the breast ductal network. Shown are: (a) a clinical galactogram with malignant finding; (b) the corresponding manually-traced ductal tree; (c) the Prufer encoding; and (d) the tf-idf weights corresponding to the ductal tree.

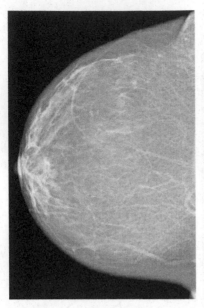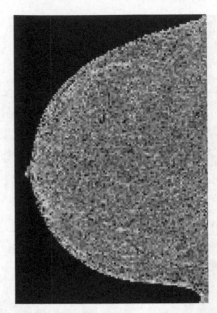

Fig. 2. The clinical mammogram of the patient from Fig. 1 (left) and the corresponding map of the entropy texture feature (right)

Fig. 3 shows the regression analysis results. A borderline statistical significance was observed for three texture features (features 9-11, p-values between 0.05 and 0.1); three additional features (features 17, 20, 24) had p-values between 0.1 and 0.15. It is likely that statistical significance was not achieved due to the limited sample size; thus, we are prevented from drawing a definitive conclusion about the correlation between texture and topology. The observed results, however, suggest a possible correlation between topological descriptors and several texture features. The bootstrap analysis of a hypothetically enlarged dataset with a sample size of 26 suggests that a statistically significant regression (at a significance level of 0.05) could be achieved between various texture features and topological descriptors. Fig. 3 shows the p-values from the bootstrap analysis.

The potential for inter-correlation between individual texture features was accounted for by applying PCA before performing the regression analysis, as PCA uses orthogonal transformations to convert the original data into a set of linearly uncorrelated variables. The bootstrap analysis performed in this paper to estimate the effect of sample size, assumed the noise in the enlarged data set to have a standard deviation equal to 50% of the standard deviation in individual sample data.

The results presented in this paper are based upon an initial analysis of 13 patients. We are currently analysing a larger set of clinical breast images; we expect to double the sample size in the near future. If the linear dependence between the texture and topology is confirmed (as suggested from our initial analysis and supported by bootstrapping), texture descriptors could be used as a proxy for topology, since the ductal network is not routinely visible in clinical images. Identifying texture features, or combinations of texture features, which have the strongest correlation with topology could improve the understanding of texture-based risk biomarkers.

If, however, the increased sample size does not confirm the correlation between topology and texture, it could suggest that topology may carry risk-related information independent from texture descriptors. This could potentially lead to an improvement in the accuracy of breast cancer risk estimation techniques, assuming a clinically feasible method for the visualization and characterization of breast ducts (e.g., MRI or tomosynthesis) is available.

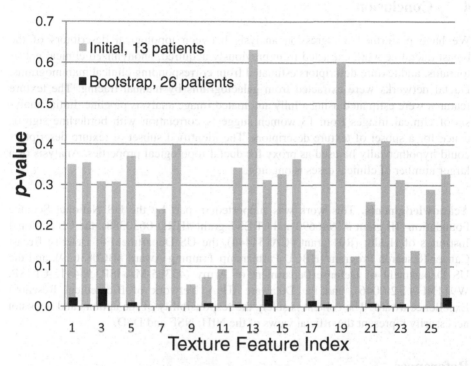

Fig. 3. p-value for the regression of individual texture features (averaged over all mammograms of the same patient) as a function of principal component analysis (PCA) components for the topological descriptors (tf-idf weights, averaged of all the traced ductal networks of the same patient). Shown are the results of the initial analysis of 13 patients, as well as the bootstrap results modelling a dataset of 26 cases.

It is worth noting the limitations of the current study. First, the ductal trees analysed in this paper were manually-traced from digitized galactograms. The manual tracing was performed by one person (a third-year medical student with experience in breast imaging). We believe that manual tracing did not compromise the analysis. In our previous study of ductal topology, we observed relatively low variations (a root-mean-square fractional error on the order of 2%) in estimated topological features due to manual tracing (2).

Additional potential limitations include the use of average texture descriptors, and the inter-correlation between individual descriptors of texture (or topology). In this paper, the regression analysis was performed using texture features averaged over the breast region in each mammographic image. These average values may suppress the differences in feature histograms calculated over mammographic images. In the future, we may repeat the analysis based upon other histogram moments, or using the full histogram as the texture descriptor.

4   Conclusion

We have performed a regression analysis between topological descriptors of the breast ductal network extracted from previously acquired, anonymized clinical galactograms, and texture descriptors estimated from corresponding clinical mammograms. Ductal networks were extracted from galactograms by manual tracing. The texture features were estimated using a fully automated image analysis pipeline. Initial analysis of clinical images from 13 women suggests correlation with borderline significance for a subset of texture descriptors. The identified subset of texture descriptors could hypothetically be used as proxy for ductal topological properties. Analysis of a larger number of clinical cases is ongoing.

Acknowledgments. This work was supported in part by the US National Science Foundation (III grant # 0916690 and CREST grant #HRD-0630388), the US National Institutes of Health (R01 grant #CA154444), the US Department of Defense Breast Cancer Research Program (HBCU Partnership Training Award #BC083639), and the US Department of Defense/Department of Army (45395-MA-ISP, #54412-CI-ISP, W911NF-11-2-0046), and the Delaware IDeA Network of Biomedical Research Excellence award. The content is solely the responsibility of the authors and does not necessarily represent the official views of the NIH, NSF and DoD.

References

[1] Bakic, P.R., Albert, M., Maidment, A.D.: Classification of galactograms with ramification matrices: Preliminary results. Academic Radiology 10(2), 198–204 (2003)
[2] Bakic, P.R., Albert, M., Brzakovic, D., Maidment, A.: Mammogram synthesis using a three-dimensional simulation. III. Modeling and evaluation of the breast ductal network. Medical Physics 30(7), 25–1914 (2003)
[3] Megalooikonomou, V., Barnathan, M., Kontos, D., Bakic, P.R., Maidment, A.D.A.: A Representation and Classification Scheme for Tree-Like Structures in Medical Images: Analyzing the Branching Pattern of Ductal Trees in X-ray Galactograms. IEEE Transactions on Medical Imaging 28(4), 93–487 (2009)
[4] Atwood, C.S., Hovey, R.C., Glover, J.P., Chepko, G., Ginsburg, E., Robison, W.G., et al.: Progesterone induces side-branching of the ductal epithelium in the mammary glands of peripubertal mice. Journal of Endocrinology 167(1), 39–52 (2000)

[5] Dinkel, H.P., Trusen, A., Gassel, A.M., Rominger, M., Lourens, S., Muller, T., et al.: Predictive value of galactographic patterns for benign and malignant neoplasms of the breast in patients with nipple discharge. British Journal of Radiology 73(871), 14–706 (2000)

[6] Cardenosa, G., Doudna, C., Eklund, G.: Ductography of the breast: technique and findings. America Journal of Roentgenology 162, 7–1081 (1994)

[7] Wolfe, J.N.: Breast patterns as an index of risk for developing breast cancer. American Journal of Roentgenology 126(6), 7–1130 (1976)

[8] Li, H., Giger, M.L., Huo, Z., Olopade, O.I., Lan, L., Weber, B.L., et al.: Computerized analysis of mammographic parenchymal patterns for assessing breast cancer risk: Effect of ROI size and location. Medical Physics 31(3), 55–549 (2004)

[9] Kontos, D., Bakic, P.R., Carton, A.-K., Troxel, A.B., Conant, E.F., Maidment, A.D.A.: Parenchymal Pattern Analysis in Digital Breast Tomosynthesis: Towards Developing Imaging Biomarkers of Breast Cancer Risk. Academic Radiology 16(3), 98–283 (2008)

[10] Bakic, P.R., Albert, M., Brzakovic, D., Maidment, A.D.A.: Mammogram synthesis using a 3D simulation. I. Breast tissue model and image acquisition simulation. Medical Physics 29(9), 9–2131 (2002)

[11] Pokrajac, D.D., Maidment, A.D.A., Bakic, P.R.: Optimized generation of high resolution breast anthropomorphic software phantoms. Medical Physics 39(4), 302–2290 (2012)

[12] Abbey, C.K., Bakic, P.R., Pokrajac, D.D., Maidment, A.D.A., Eckstein, M.P., Boone, J.: Non-Gaussian Statistical Properties of Virtual Breast Phantoms. In: Mello-Thoms, C.R., Kupinski, M.A. (eds.) SPIE Image Processing, Observer Performance, and Technology Assessment, vol. 9037. SPIE, San Diego (2014)

[13] Zheng, Y., Wang, Y., Keller, B.M., Conant, E.F., Gee, J.C., Kontos, D.: A fully-automated software pipeline for integrating breast density and parenchymal texture analysis for digital mammograms: Parameter optimization in a case-control breast cancer risk assessment study. In: Novak, C.L., Aylward, S. (eds.) SPIE Computer-Aided Diagnosis, vol. 8670. SPIE, Lake Buena Vista (2013)

[14] Devore, J.: Probability and Statistics for Engineering and the Sciences. Brooks/Cole, Belmont (2008)

[15] Efron, B.: The jackknife, the bootstrap and other resampling plans, Philadelphia, PA (1982)

Breast Volume Measurement Using a Games Console Input Device

Stefanie T.L. Pöhlmann[1], Jeremy Hewes[2], Andrew I. Williamson[3],
Jamie C. Sergeant[4,5], Alan Hufton[1], Ashu Gandhi[6],
Christopher J. Taylor[1], and Susan M. Astley[1]

[1] Centre for Imaging Sciences, Institute of Population Health,
University of Manchester, UK
stefanie.pohlmann@postgrad.manchester.ac.uk
[2] School of Physics and Astronomy, University of Manchester, Manchester, UK
[3] The Photon Science Institute, School of Physics and Astronomy, University of
Manchester, Manchester, UK
[4] Arthritis Research UK Centre for Epidemiology, Institute of Inflammation and
Repair, Faculty of Medical and Human Sciences, Manchester Academic Health
Science Centre, University of Manchester, Manchester, UK
[5] NIHR Manchester Musculoskeletal Biomedical Research Unit, Central Manchester
NHS Foundation Trust, Manchester Academic Health Science Centre
[6] University of Manchester, Manchester Academic Health Sciences Centre, University
Hospital of South Manchester, Manchester, UK

Abstract. The automated measurement of breast volume has applications both in facilitating the decisions made by surgeons prior to breast reconstruction and in improving density estimation. We describe a novel approach to volume measurement for surgical planning, using a games console input device - the Microsoft Kinect. We have explored the ability of the device to measure surface depth for a range of distances and angles, demonstrating a mean depth error of below 1.5 mm for a distance range of interest (0.5 - 0.8 m). We have also validated the use of the system for volume measurement using a full-sized model female torso. The Kinect-based result is in good agreement with the volume measured by filling a mould of the breast with water (225.5 ± 8.7 ml, 229.4 ± 9.7 ml respectively). The method has the potential to provide convenient, cost- and time-effective measurement of breast volume in clinical practice.

Keywords: breast volume, breast surgery, breast density, Microsoft Kinect.

1 Introduction

Measuring breast volume is crucial for planning breast surgery - whether to predict the cosmetic outcome or to choose an appropriate surgical strategy [1]. Knowledge of the shape and the volume of the breast can also contribute to more accurate assessment of breast density (measured as the proportion of dense glandular tissue in the breast volume). Nevertheless there is no standard method for

H. Fujita, T. Hara, and C. Muramatsu (Eds.): IWDM 2014, LNCS 8539, pp. 666–673, 2014.
© Springer International Publishing Switzerland 2014

measuring breast volume [2]. When measuring breast density, the use of two-dimensional mammographic images to derive volume measurement suffers from the ambiguity of estimating a three-dimensional (3D) shape from its planar representation [3]. Techniques used for surgical planning include anthropomorphic (anatomic) measurements, moulding, the Grossmann device and measurements based on Archimedes principle. None of these is well established clinically due to lack of reliability or inconvenience [1, 4]. More recent techniques like stereophotogrammetry (using a stereo camera array) [5], laser scanning [2] breast CT or MRI describe the 3D shape of the breast accurately but their use is restricted by high complexity and cost. Those automated or semi-automated methods use complex imaging equipment, which needs stationary installation, maintenance and trained staff. This paper proposes the use of a games console input device for automated measurement of breast volume.

It is aimed to provide a convenient, fast and inexpensive method that allows non-contact measurement and uses small, transportable equipment which is ready for use without time and labour intense installation and calibration. The definition of the region of interest, the portion of the breast for calculating the volume can be indicated by markings on the patients skin and is therefore flexible and adaptable to different tasks.

The Microsoft Kinect for Xbox 360 input device (Kinect) is a relatively cheap, small sensor based on infra-red light triangulation. It is an optical device, which projects a speckle pattern onto a scene within its field of view and evaluates how this pattern is distorted by the objects in the scene. By comparing the original to the distorted pattern it measures the location and shape of objects without contact, working at ambient indoor light conditions [6]. It was originally designed for computer gaming and human interaction in a virtual environment, but has found wide application in research including medical applications such as patient size measurement [7] and respiratory motion tracking [8]. Recently published papers have demonstrated the feasibility of using the Kinect for breast imaging. In one application, two Kinect sensors were used to map the breast surface [9, 10] whereas others use a single Kinect to assess the aesthetic aspects of breast-conserving cancer treatment [11] or breast surgery in general [12].

2   Methods

The Kinect sensor has two outputs: a depth image, generated with the help of laser triangulation and an RGB image of the field of view. The depth image is presented as a cloud of points representing the location of objects within the sensor field of view. All experiments were performed using the KinectFusion mode, which sums multiple frames and combines them independently of sensor movement [13]. This mode was chosen as the field of view of the sensor can be enlarged and parts of the breast, which can not be evaluated in a "single shot" can be resolved by slow movement of the sensor. Also blank spots in the depth image e.g. due to reflection can be covered by a slightly different viewing angle.

In the following section two experiments are described. A feasibility study evaluating the suitability of the sensor using a simple index card model was performed before using the Kinect for automated measurement of breast volume and validating this method.

Feasibility Study: The Effect of Distance and Angle on Performance. The suitability of the Kinect to capture the shape of the female breast with adequate precision is demonstrated using a simple index card model. In contrast to other studies [6, 8, 14], our experiments focus on distances appropriate for imaging the human body. Due to the curved nature of the breast, and the fact that not all portions of skin directly face the sensor, the performance of the method was evaluated at a range of angles.

A plain index card (7.5 cm x 12.5 cm) was mounted on an optical rail in the centre of the Kinect's field of view at distances of 0.5 (nearest distance assessable with the Kinect), 0.6, 0.8, 1.0 and 1.2 meters, facing directly towards the Kinect (0 degrees) and at 15, 30, 45 and 60 degrees from the Kinect. In total 25 configurations were evaluated (see Fig. 1a). The Kinect remained static during image acquisition.

Depth images were stored and close measurement points (less than 0.1 mm apart) were merged using Meshlab. As sharp edges cannot be well resolved by the Kinect [14], points at the edges of the index card were excluded from the measurements (see Fig. 1b). However this weakness is not relevant for the application in breast imaging as the curved shape of the breast does not exhibit such behaviour. It is therefore feasible to limit the assessment of performance to a central 5 cm x 5 cm region covering about 2000 measurement points.

The ground truth for the evaluation of measurement accuracy was the distance of the cards from the sensor which was determined to a mm using the optical rail. For the assessment of precision it was assumed that the index cards are flat and can be described by a plane.

A plane was fitted onto the resulting point cloud. Precision was evaluated by calculating the point-to-plane error using Matlab. To evaluate accuracy the measured mean distances were normalized to the 0.5 meter distance, as the exact location of the focus point within the sensor is not known.

Feasibility Study: Automated Measurement of Breast Volume. In order to assess the feasibility of the method to measure breast volume, we performed an experiment using a model female torso, comparing breast volume measured with Kinect against breast volume calculated from a mould of the breast. Three small beads were attached to the torso, one below the nipple at the inframammary fold, one on the sternum between the two nipples, and one at the lateral border; these were used to define the chest wall and orient the mould. To acquire Kinect images, the torso was placed on a level surface; the Kinect was slowly turned and tilted to obtain a point cloud without gaps describing the entire breast surface. The resulting point cloud was preprocessed using Meshlab merging all measurement points closer than 0.1 mm.

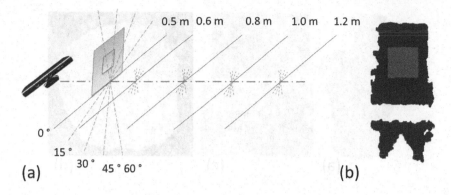

Fig. 1. (a): Feasibility study: Index cards are placed at the indicated locations and angles; (b): one of the point clouds showing the index card on top of the sledge of the optical rail, 5 cm x 5 cm region evaluated for the study highlighted

Fig. 2a shows the depth image with the underlying point cloud obtained from the Kinect sensor. The beads can be seen in Fig. 2b in which RGB colour data from the Kinect are displayed in conjunction with the Kinect depth image.

The volume calculation was performed using Matlab. In order to separate the breast volume from the torso, a plane was fitted onto the chest wall as defined by the position of the three beads. The point cloud was rotated and translated to align the chest wall plane with the global coordinate system (Fig. 3a). The volume enclosed by the x-y plane of the coordinate system and the point cloud was calculated by double integration (Fig. 3b).

The ground truth against which the Kinect-based volume was assessed was obtained by filling a clay mould of the breast with liquid (Fig. 2d). The results were also compared to anthropomorphic (anatomic) measurement of the breast using the formula proposed by Qiao [15] (Fig. 2c):

$$V = 1/3 \times \Pi \times MP^2 \times (MR + LR + IR - MP)$$

For all three methods, measurements were repeated ten times to assess the associated error.

3   Results

Feasibility Study: The Effect of Distance and Angle on Performance.
For measurement accuracy the point clouds of the cards directly facing the sensor were evaluated. For all cards the mean distance from the sensor is within the accuracy of distance measurement on the optical rail.

The precision of depth measurement is influenced by the distance of the object from the sensor and the angle to the sensor. For the shorter distances evaluated (0.5, 0.6 and 0.8 m) at the complete angular range the mean point-to-plane error

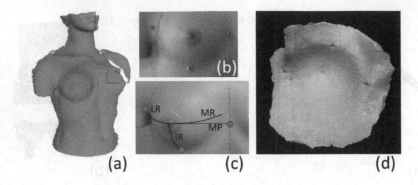

Fig. 2. (a): Depth image with underlying point cloud obtained from the Kinect sensor; (b): Detail of the same image conjoined with RGB colour; (c): Distances used for anthropomorphic measurement and placements of the beads: MR - distance between nipple and medial border, IR -distance between nipple and inframammary fold, LR - distance between nipple and lateral border, MP - mammary projection; (d): Mould of the breast of the torso

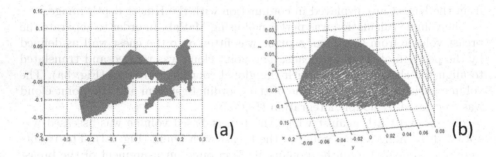

Fig. 3. (a): Point cloud of the torso, rotated and translated so that the chest wall plane aligns with the x-y plane of the global coordinate system; (b): Resulting point cloud above the x-y plane for calculating the breast volume

was below 1.5 mm as depicted in table 1. Even the challenging configurations featuring large angles of 45 degrees or above can be resolved with adequate precision. In contrast to this, for objects located further from the sensor (at 1.0 and 1.2 m), larger angles showed a mean point-to-plane error above 1.5 mm.

For the more favourable, nearer distances (0.5, 0.6 and 0.8 m), all card positions yielded a point-to-plane-error of less than 2 mm for over 80% of the evaluated points (Fig. 5). Small angles towards the sensor resulted in a higher proportion of points less than 2 mm from the fitted plane.

Table 1. Mean point-to-plane error (in mm) dependent on distance to object (in m) and angle (degrees)

distance from the sensor	angle facing the sensor				
	0	15	30	45	60
0.5	0.45 ±0.37	0.54 ±0.41	0.49 ±0.38	0.58 ±0.67	0.71 ±0.56
0.6	0.44 ±0.38	0.47 ±0.33	0.46 ±0.33	0.87 ±1.15	0.81 ±0.74
0.8	0.68 ±0.51	0.67 ±0.48	0.71 ±0.50	1.06 ±1.07	1.39 ±1.41
1.0	1.64 ±1.06	1.19 ±1.14	1.20 ±0.84	1.93 ±2.25	1.57 ±1.35
1.2	1.10 ±0.88	2.19 ±2.27	1.31 ±1.58	2.91 ±2.65	3.73 ±2.21

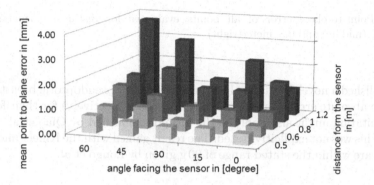

Fig. 4. Relationship of distance, angle and mean point-to-plane error

Feasibility Study: Automated Measurement of Breast Volume. The markers placed on the torso were clearly visible in both the Kinect image and within the mould. Therefore it was possible to automatically align a plane which separates the breast from the chest wall (Fig. 3a). Results obtained using the three different measurement methods are depicted in table 2.

Table 2. Measured volume (in ml) using the Kinect approach, mould filling and an anthropometric formula

	Measured volume		
	mean	standard deviation	standard error
Kinect method	225.5	8.7	2.8
Mould filling	229.4	9.7	3.0
Anthropomorphic formula	136.6	7.3	2.3

The volume measured using the Kinect approach lies within of our validation approach using the mould. The anthropomorphic measurement resulted in a smaller volume. The absence of folds around the breast for a non-ptotic breast complicates the localisation of characteristic anatomical landmarks. For example, Longo et al.

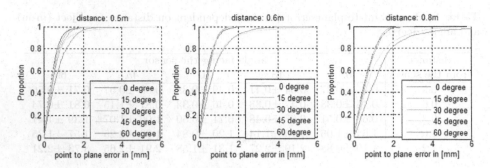

Fig. 5. Point-to-plane error of all points evaluated for distance 0.5 meter (left), 0.6 meter (middle) and 0.8 meter(right)

[16] published a novel formula only for use in ptotic or pseudoptotic breasts. They claim an absolute error of approximately 90 g (ml respectively) for their formula. This limitation might also apply to the formula published by Qiao et al. [15], although this was not explicitly stated. The result gained with the Kinect and mould method are within the stated range of 90 g given by Longo et al.

4   Discussion

We have shown that automated breast volume measurement using the Kinect is feasible and a relevant work-flow could be established.

The performance of depth measurement was shown using plain index cards at know positions on a optical rail. To evaluate precision the point-to-plane error was evaluated. Within a distance window of 0.5 to 0.8 m, the Kinect allows depth measurements with a mean error of less than 1.5 mm.

Angles up to 60 degrees can still be evaluated without limitations. This shows the suitability of the Kinect for breast imaging.

The presented method has the potential to provide convenient, cost/time-effective measurement of breast volume in clinical practice. Its reliability was validated with the help of a water filled mould. Volume obtained with anthropomorphic measurement does not back up the gained results but might be less appropriate in the absence of ptotic breasts.

Acknowledgements. The authors are grateful to the Breast Cancer Campaign for funding this work.

References

[1] Kayar, R., Civelek, S., Cobanoglu, M., Gungor, O., Catal, H., Emiroglu, M.: Five methods of breast volume measurement: A comparative study of measurements of specimen volume in 30 mastectomy cases. Breast Cancer: Basic and Clinical Research 5, 43–52 (2011)

[2] Kovacs, L., Eder, M., Hollweck, R., Zimmermann, A., Settles, M., Schneider, A., Endlich, M., Mueller, A., Schwenzer-Zimmerer, K., Papadopulos, N.A., Biemer, E.: Comparison between breast volume measurement using 3D surface imaging and classical techniques. Breast 16(2), 137–145 (2007)

[3] Katariya, R., Forrest, A., Gravelle, I.: Breast volumes in cancer of the breast. British Journal of Cancer 975, 270–273 (1974)

[4] Bulstrode, N., Bellamy, E., Shrotria, S.: Breast volume assessment: Comparing five different techniques. Breast 10(2), 117–123 (2001)

[5] Henseler, H., Smith, J., Bowman, A., Khambay, B.S., Ju, X., Ayoub, A., Ray, A.K.: Investigation into variation and errors of a three-dimensional breast imaging system using multiple stereo cameras. Journal of Plastic, Reconstructive & Aesthetic Surgery: JPRAS 65(12), 332–337 (2012)

[6] Khoshelham, K., Elberink, S.O.: Accuracy and resolution of Kinect depth data for indoor mapping applications. Sensors 12(2), 1437–1454 (2012)

[7] Cook, T.S., Couch, G., Couch, T.J., Kim, W., Boonn, W.W.: Using the Microsoft Kinect for patient size estimation and radiation dose normalization: Proof of concept and initial validation. Journal of Digital Imaging 26(4), 657–662 (2013)

[8] Alnowami, M., Alnwaimi, B., Tahavori, F., Copland, M., Wells, K.: A quantitative assessment of using the Kinect for Xbox360 for respiratory surface motion tracking. In: Proceedings of SPIE: Medical Imaging 2012, vol. 8316, pp. 1T1–10 (2012)

[9] Choppin, S.B., Probst, H., Goyal, A., Clarkson, S., Wheat, J., Hospitals, D.: Breast volume calculation using a low-cost scanning system. In: 4th International Conference Exhibition on 3D Body Scanning, pp. 11–14 (2013)

[10] Wheat, J., Choppin, S., Goyal, A.: Development and assessment of a Microsoft Kinect based system for imaging the breast in three dimensions. Medical Engineering & Physics (in press, February 2014)

[11] Oliveira, H.P., Cardoso, J.S., Magalhães, A.T., Cardoso, M.J.: A 3D low-cost solution for the aesthetic evaluation of breast cancer conservative treatment. Computer Methods in Biomechanics and Biomedical Engineering: Imaging & Visualization, 1–17 (December 2013)

[12] Henseler, H., Kuznetsova, A., Vogt, P., Rosenhahn, B.: Validation of the Kinect device as a new portable imaging system for three-dimensional breast assessment. Journal of Plastic, Reconstructive & Aesthetic Surgery: JPRAS (in press, January 2014)

[13] Newcombe, R.A., Davison, A.J., Izadi, S., Kohli, P., Hilliges, O., Shotton, J., Molyneaux, D., Hodges, S., Kim, D., Fitzgibbon, A.: KinectFusion: Real-time dense surface mapping and tracking. In: 10th IEEE International Symposium on Mixed and Augmented Reality, pp. 127–136 (October 2011)

[14] Meister, S., Izadi, S., Kohli, P.: When can we use KinectFusion for ground truth acquisition? In: Proceedings Workshop Color-Depth Camera Fusion Robot, pp. 3–8 (2012)

[15] Qiao, Q., Zhou, G., Ling, Y.: Breast volume measurement in young Chinese women and clinical applications. Aesthetic Plastic Surgery 21(5), 362–368 (1997)

[16] Longo, B., Farcomeni, A., Ferri, G., Campanale, A., Sorotos, M., Santanelli, F.: The BREAST-V: A unifying predictive formula for volume assessment in small, medium, and large breasts. Plastic and Reconstructive Surgery 132(1), 1e–7e (2013)

Towards Spatial Correspondence between Specimen and In-vivo Breast Imaging

Thomy Mertzanidou[1], John Hipwell[1], Mehmet Dalmis[2], Bram Platel[2],
Jeroen van der Laak[2], Ritse Mann[3], Nico Karssemeijer[2],
Peter Bult[4], and David Hawkes[1]

[1] Centre for Medical Image Computing, University College London,
Gower Street, WC1E 6BT London, UK
[2] Diagnostic Image Analysis Group, Radboud University Medical Centre,
P.O. Box 9101, 6500 HB Nijmegen, The Netherlands
[3] Department of Radiology, Radboud University Medical Centre,
P.O. Box 9101, 6500 HB Nijmegen, The Netherlands
[4] Department of Pathology, Radboud University Medical Centre,
P.O. Box 9101, 6500 HB Nijmegen, The Netherlands
t.mertzanidou@cs.ucl.ac.uk

Abstract. Radiological in-vivo imaging, such as X-ray mammography and Magnetic Resonance Imaging (MRI), is used for tumour detection, diagnosis and size determination. After tumour excision, histopathological imaging of the stained specimen is used as the gold standard for characterisation of the tumour and surrounding tissue. Relating the information available at the micro and macroscopic scales could lead to a better understanding of the in-vivo radiological imaging. This in turn has potential to improve therapeutic decision making and, ultimately, patient prognosis and treatment outcomes. Accurate alignment of data, necessary to maximise information retrieval from the different scales, can be problematic however, due to the large deformation that the breast tissue undergoes after surgery. In this work we present a methodology to reconstruct a 3D volume from multiple X-ray breast specimen images. The reconstructed volume can be used to bridge the gap between histopathological and in-vivo radiological images. We demonstrate the use of this algorithm on four mastectomy samples. For one of these cases, a specimen MRI was also available and was used to provide an assessment of the performance of the reconstruction technique.

Keywords: breast histology-radiology registration, 3D volume reconstruction.

1 Introduction

Radiological images (for example X-ray mammography, DCE-MRI and ultrasound) are routinely used for detection, diagnosis, tumour size determination, therapy planning and treatment monitoring. The image resolution is limited however, ranging from approximately 0.1 mm for X-ray mammography to 1 mm for

H. Fujita, T. Hara, and C. Muramatsu (Eds.): IWDM 2014, LNCS 8539, pp. 674–680, 2014.
© Springer International Publishing Switzerland 2014

MRI. Histopathological analysis of excised tissue provides high resolution images (less than 1 μm) and is used as the gold standard for tumour characterisation: for example to differentiate between benign and malignant lesions, to define the tumour grade and to determine whether all the cancerous tissue has been successfully removed at surgery. Establishing spatial correspondences between histopathological and radiological images could improve our understanding of the relationship between these types of images. Accurate alignment of the tissue microstructure to the in-vivo imaging could potentially be used to predict tumour invasiveness and indicate whether any features extracted from clinical images are linked to pathological outcomes.

There are various techniques that have been proposed in the literature to align histological slides to in-vivo imaging. These are mainly focused on animal brain and human prostate data, for which the deformation after excision is less than that exhibited by mastectomy and breast lumpectomy samples. Existing approaches often require either manual interaction [1,2] or the acquisition of additional images of the whole ex-vivo specimens before cutting and further slicing with the microtome; such as a specimen MRI [3,4] or block-face photographs of the sectioning process [3,5].

As breast is a highly deformable organ, aligning the in-vivo to specimen imaging is a difficult task. Firstly, the breast positioning varies between different radiological acquisitions and surgery. In addition, after excision the breast undergoes further complex deformations due to slicing, cutting, fixing and sectioning with the microtome. A reconstructed volume from whole-mount serial breast section images was previously proposed [6], where pair-wise manual registrations were employed for an initial alignment between slices and point-based linear affine registrations followed for refinement. Another attempt to align breast histological to radiological images was proposed for the interpretation of ultrasound (US) elastography images [7], where the pathology slides were warped to the US image based on manually defined landmarks on the boundaries of a tumour.

This work describes a 3D volume reconstruction methodology that can be used to compose a 3D specimen image of the breast, from multiple X-ray images of specimen slices. The methodology employs two automated approaches that were previously proposed for the 3D volume reconstruction of brain images [8,9]. This volume can be used as an intermediate image in order to bridge the gap between histological and in-vivo radiological images. To demonstrate the methodology we have reconstructed 3D volumes from four mastectomy cases. For one case, a specimen MRI was also used in order to visually assess the quality of the reconstructed volume and demonstrate that this could be useful for mapping to the in-vivo MRI of the patient.

2   Methodology

2.1   Data Acquisition Protocol

The data used in this work were acquired in the Radboud University Medical Centre, where the specimen handling is as follows: the excised mastectomy specimens are inked, vacuum-packed and refrigerated to preserve and stiffen the tissue. Then, the specimen is sliced axially using a meat slicing machine in 4-5 mm thick slices. Digital X-ray images of the slices are acquired and the tissue is later sampled, put into cassettes and further processed into paraffin blocks. The approximate position of the tissue parts, that are sampled for further processing and staining, is annotated on the digital X-ray images of the slices. Details of the complete protocol can be found in [10].

The goal of this work is to produce a 3D volume reconstructed from the X-ray images of the specimen slices. The link between this volume and the histology slides can be provided via the annotations on the digital X-ray specimen slice images, while the link to pre-operative imaging (such as MRI) could be achieved via a 3D registration algorithm between in-vivo and ex-vivo imaging.

2.2   Pre-processing

The slices obtained from a given specimen appear in sequence, in a number of X-ray images, with each image typically comprising 3 to 6 slices. Before registration, the slices are segmented from the background using thresholding and a hole filling algorithm. Manual interaction is required for cases when the slices are touching with no clear boundary between them. A histogram matching technique is used for intensity normalisation of the segmented slices, as intensity ranges vary between different X-ray acquisitions. For this task, the slice in the middle of the stack is used as a reference image.

2.3   3D Volume Reconstruction

Pair-wise registrations To reconstruct a 3D volume, the individual slices are initially registered using pair-wise registrations of the serial slices. For this task we use an intensity-based approach with a rigid-body block-matching transformation [8] that was first proposed for the registration of serial histological sections from animal brain data. The advantage of the block-matching technique is that it only assumes local similarities between sequential slices, rather than assuming that the anatomy is related across the whole image. Local rigid transformations are initially computed across local areas (blocks) and the final transformation is estimated using the most closely matching block-pairs.

In our experiments, we use an implementation with a multi-resolution scheme consisting of six levels. As in the original reference [8] the similarity measure is the correlation coefficient and the final transformation is computed using the L_1 estimator, rather than least squares regression. As in the pre-processing step, the slice in the middle of the stack is used as a reference image.

Global energy optimisation. To avoid the propagation of registration errors across slices and the dependency of the registration result on the chosen reference slice, we add a second, subsequent registration scheme, where each slice I_i is simultaneously aligned to both neighbouring images I_{i-1} and I_{i+1}. This approach was initially proposed for a 3D volume reconstruction from serial au-toradiographic sections of a rat's brain [9].

For N slices, the parameters that are estimated are:

$$\Theta = \{\Theta_1, ..., \Theta_{r-1}, \Theta_{r+1}, ..., \Theta_N\}, \tag{1}$$

where I_r is the reference image and $\Theta_i = \{t_x^i, t_y^i, \theta^i\}$ for a 2D rigid transforma-tion. Considering the similarity, S, across all slices, the optimisation problem of the global energy function $E(\Theta)$ can be defined as:

$$\Theta = \underset{\Theta}{\mathrm{argmax}}(E(\Theta)) = \sum_{i=1}^{N-1} E_i(\Theta_i) = \sum_{i=1}^{N-1} \sum_{j \in R_i} (S(T_{\theta_i}(I_i(x)), T_{\theta_j}(I_j(x))) : x \in \Omega)$$

$$\tag{2}$$

where R_i is the neighbourhood of, i.e. adjacent slices to, image I_i. Instead of optimising the global energy directly across all images, the local energy E_i is optimised sequentially for all the slices. We use two neighbouring slices in our implementation ($R_i = [i-1, i+1]$), as their thickness is 4-5 mm and are therefore less likely to influence the registration of slices that are further away.

The similarity measure that we use for this registration step is normalised cross correlation and the optimisation scheme is gradient descent.

3   Experiments

To demonstrate the quality of the reconstructed volumes, we have applied the proposed method to four mastectomy samples. The number of slices was 39-43 per case and their thickness was 4 mm. Figures 1 and 2 show examples for three of the reconstructed volumes.

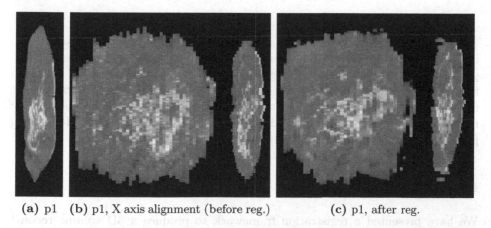

(a) p1   (b) p1, X axis alignment (before reg.)   (c) p1, after reg.

Fig. 1. Results of the reconstructed volume for patient 1. (a) Axial plane (this is the high resolution image where annotations of the tissue sampling are made), (b) coronal and sagittal planes using an alignment of the X axis according to centres of mass of the slices (initial position before registration) and (c) after registration.

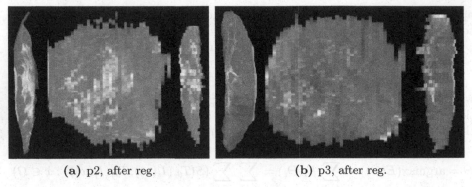

(a) p2, after reg. (b) p3, after reg.

Fig. 2. Results of the reconstructed volumes for patients 2 and 3. From left to right: axial, coronal and sagittal planes after registration for (a) patient 2 and (b) patient 3.

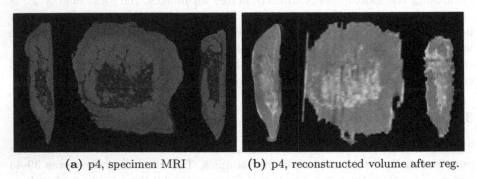

(a) p4, specimen MRI (b) p4, reconstructed volume after reg.

Fig. 3. Patient 4, from left to right: axial, coronal and sagittal planes of (a) the specimen MRI and (b) the registered reconstructed volume

For one of the cases, there was a specimen T1-weighted MRI acquired using a clinical breast scanner, although this is not typically part of the clinical protocol. We have applied a 3D rigid block-matching registration [8] between the reconstructed volume and the specimen MRI, in order to illustrate that the reconstructed volume produces a reasonable result and can subsequently be mapped, initially to the specimen MRI, and in future to the in-vivo MRI of the patient. The registration result is shown in Figure 3.

4   Conclusion

We have presented a registration framework to produce a 3D volume reconstructed from multiple X-ray breast specimen images. The proposed algorithm was applied to four mastectomy cases. For one case this volume was subsequently registered to a specimen MRI. The results show that this technique produces 3D volumes, where the anatomical structures appear to have continuity across slices.

Also, corresponding structures can be seen between the reconstructed volume and the specimen MRI.

This framework can be used in future work to provide a link between the histopathology slides and the in-vivo MRI of the patient. The clinical protocol described here [10] is particularly suited for this purpose, as the slicing process produces slices of approximately the same thickness, due to the specimen being cooled and sliced with a meat slicer. Moreover, the annotation protocol on the digitally acquired X-ray images that identifies the approximate position of the histology slide, is invaluable for the link to histology. For the link to radiological imaging, a challenging registration task between the specimen and the in-vivo MRI will need to be tackled.

Further developments include the use of a more flexible transformation model than the rigid transformation used here, that would be better able to capture the complex transformation that the slices undergo. Finally, the reconstructed volume will be tested for subsequent mapping of histological features to in-vivo radiological imaging using the process described above.

Acknowledgements. This work was funded by the European 7th Framework Program grant VPH-PRISM (FP7-ICT-2011-9, 601040) and the Engineering and Physical Sciences Research Council grant MIMIC (EP/K020439/1).

References

1. Mazaheri, Y., Bokacheva, L., Kroon, D., Akin, O., Hricak, H., Chamudot, D., Fine, S., Koutcher, J.: Semi-automatic deformable re gistration of prostate MR images to pathological slices. Journal of Magnetic Resonance Imaging 32(5), 1149–1157 (2010)
2. Chappelow, J., Bloch, N., Rofsky, N., Genega, E., Lenkinski, R., DeWolf, W., Madabhushi, A.: Elastic registration of multimodal prostate MRI and histology via multiattribute combined mutual information. Medical Physics 38(4), 2005–2018 (2011)
3. Park, H., Piert, M., Khan, A., Shah, R., Hussain, H., Siddiqui, J., Chenevert, T., Meyer, C.: Registration methodology for histological sections and in vivo imaging of human prostate. Academic radiology 15(8), 1027–1039 (2008)
4. Alic, L., Haeck, J., Bol, K., Klein, S., van Tiel, S., Wielepolski, P., de Jong, M., Niessen, W., Bernsen, M.E., Veenland, J.: Facilitating tumor functional assessment by spatially relating 3D tumor histology and in vivo MRI: Image registration approach. PloS One 22835, e22835 (2011)
5. Dauguet, J., Delzescaux, T., Condé, F., Mangin, J., Ayache, N., Hantraye, P., Frouin, V.: Three-dimensional reconstruction of stained histological slices and 3D non-linear registration with in-vivo MRI for whole baboon brain. Journal of Neuroscience Methods 164(1), 191–204 (2007)
6. Clarke, G., Murray, M., Holloway, C., Liu, K., Zubovits, J., Yaffe, M.: 3d pathology volumetric technique: A method for calculating breast tumour volume from whole-mount serial section images. International Journal of Breast Cancer 2012, 691205–691205 (2012)

7. Chuang, B., Myronenko, A., English, R., Noble, A.: Interpreting ultrasound elastography: Image registration of breast cancer ultrasound elastography to histopathology images. In: 2010 IEEE International Symposium on Biomedical Imaging: From Nano to Macro, pp. 181–184. IEEE (2010)
8. Ourselin, S., Roche, A., Subsol, G., Pennec, X., Ayache, N.: Reconstructing a 3D structure from serial histological sections. Image and Vision Computing 19(1), 25–31 (2001)
9. Nikou, C., Heitz, F., Nehlig, A., Namer, I., Armspach, J.: A robust statistics-based global energy function for the alignment of serially acquired autoradiographic sections. Journal of Neuroscience Methods 124(1), 93–102 (2003)
10. Bult, P., Hoogerbrugge, N.: Familial breast cancer: Detection of prevalent high-risk epithelial lesions. In: Methods of Cancer Diagnosis, Therapy and Prognosis, pp. 61–71. Springer, Heidelberg (2008)

SIFT Texture Description for Understanding Breast Ultrasound Images

Joan Massich[12,*], Fabrice Meriaudeau[2], Melcior Sentís[3], Sergi Ganau[3], Elsa Pérez[4], Domenec Puig[5], Robert Martí[1], Arnau Oliver[1], and Joan Martí[1]

[1] Computer Vision and Robotics Group, University of Girona, Spain
jmassich@atc.udg.edu
[2] Laboratoire Le2i-UMR CNRS, University of Burgundy, Le Creusot, France
[3] Department of Breast and Gynecological Radiology, UDIAT-Diagnostic Center,
Parc Taulí Corporation, Sabadell, Spain
[4] Department of Radiology, Hospital Josep Trueta of Girona, Spain
[5] Department of Computer Engineering and Mathematics, University Rovira i
Virgili, Tarragona, Spain

Abstract. Texture is a powerful cue for describing structures that show a high degree of similarity in their image intensity patterns. This paper describes the use of Self-Invariant Feature Transform (SIFT), both as low-level and high-level descriptors, applied to differentiate the tissues present in breast US images. For the low-level texture descriptors case, SIFT descriptors are extracted from a regular grid. The high-level texture descriptor is build as a Bag-of-Features (BoF) of SIFT descriptors. Experimental results are provided showing the validity of the proposed approach for describing the tissues in breast US images.

Keywords: breast cancer, ultrasound, texture, SIFT.

1 Introduction

Breast cancer is the second most common cancer (1.4 million cases per year, 10.9% of diagnosed cancers) after lung cancer, followed by colorectal, stomach, prostate and liver cancers. In terms of mortality, breast cancer is the fifth most common cause of cancer death. However, it places as the leading cause of cancer death among females both in western countries and in economically developing countries [3].

Medical imaging plays an important role in breast cancer mortality reduction, contributing to its early detection through screening, diagnosis, image-guided biopsy, treatment follow-up and suchlike procedures [5]. Despite Digital Mammography (DM) still remains as the image modality of reference for diagnose purposes, Ultra-Sound (US) offers useful complementary diagnose information due to its capabilities for differentiating between solid lesions that are benign or

---

* This work was partially supported by the Spanish Science and Innovation grant nb. TIN2012-37171-C02-01 and TTIN2012-37171-C02-02 and the Regional Council of Burgundy.

H. Fujita, T. Hara, and C. Muramatsu (Eds.): IWDM 2014, LNCS 8539, pp. 681–688, 2014.

malignant [6]. It is estimated that between 65 ~ 85% of the biopsies prescribed using only mammography imaging could be avoided if US information had been taken into account while issuing the diagnose [7].

In US images, texture is a major characteristic to distinguish between different breast tissues, which also allows assessing of the lesion's pathology [6]. Thus, the importance of incorporating texture data from US images into Computer Aided Diagnosis (CAD) systems. A comprehensive list of texture descriptors used for detection, segmentation or diagnose tasks applied to US breast images is given in Cheng et al. [1], where most of the descriptors are ad-hoc descriptors or based on well-known texture descriptors such as co-occurrence matrices, wavelet coefficients or Gray-Level Difference Method (GLDM).

This article explores the usage of Self-Invariant Feature Transform (SIFT) descriptors for encoding the US characteristic texture produced by the speckle noise present within the images. Its performance is evaluated using a multi-label annotated dataset.

2   Material and Methods

In order to develop segmentation methodologies applied to delineate breast lesions in US data, a set of 700 US images was acquired at the *UDIAT Diagnostic Centre of Parc Tauli* in Sabadell (Catalunya), between 2010 and 2012. All the images were provided with accompanying Ground Truth (GT) delineation of the lesions present in the image. From this image database, a reduced dataset of 16 images corresponding to different patients was selected and complemented with multi-label GT in order to evaluate the texture description of the observable tissues in the breast.

Figure 1 illustrates a breast image from the dataset with its associated GT.

3   Using SIFT as a Low-level Texture Descriptor in Order to Differentiate the Tissues Present in Breast US Images

Self-Invariant Feature Transform (SIFT) [4] transforms key-points into scale and rotation invariant coordinates relative to local features. The SIFT descriptor at

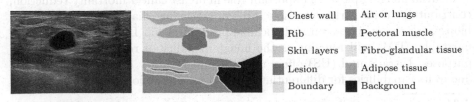

Fig. 1. Dataset sample. From left to right: image sample, accompanying multi-label GT, tissue label GT color-coding.

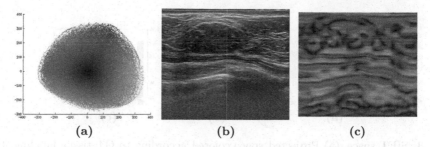

(a)   (b)   (c)

Fig. 2. Low level SIFT descriptor example. (a) Arbitrary coloring of the projected SIFT space. (b) Original image. (c) Recoding of the extracted SIFT descriptors using the color coding in (a).

a particular key-point, samples the magnitude and orientation of the gradients surrounding this key-point to generate a 128-element feature. When setting up SIFT as a texture descriptor, the key-points are considered to be a regular grid in order to generate evenly sparse SIFT descriptors.

The usage of SIFT descriptor brings invariability to scale, rotation and minor affine transformations along with robustness to illumination changes [4], which allows to characterize the tissues despite the variability from US acquisition.

In order to analyze the US images, a SIFT descriptor is extracted at every pixel position and them mapped into the SIFT space. The 128-dimension feature is projected into a two dimensional space using Principal Component Analysis (PCA). When combining features using PCA is convenient to know the ratio known as explained variation, which in this case is given by $\frac{\lambda_1+\lambda_2}{\sum_{i=1}^{128}\lambda_i} = 21.6\%$. For the remaining of the article all the calculations are carried out directly in the projected space. However, it should be assumed that in a higher space with greater explained variation, better separability could be achieved. Figure 2 offers a visual interpretation of a breast US image in terms of low-level SIFT descriptors, where the extracted SIFT descriptors from all the images in the dataset have been projected into the 2D principal component space (Figure 2a). These SIFT descriptors have been arbitrary colored in order to visually assess the descriptors (the more similar the colors, the closer the SIFT descriptors).

Thus, the analysis of the tissue distribution is performed in the texture space defined by the SIFT descriptors by means of the Maximum A Posteriori (MAP) estimator, as described in equation 1.

$$P(\omega|\bar{x}_a) = \frac{P(\bar{x}_a|\omega) \cdot P(\omega)}{P(\bar{x}_a)} \tag{1}$$

Where $P(\omega|\bar{x}_a)$ is the probability that the sample a belongs to class $\omega \in W$ (see fig. 1b as a reminder of the GT available classes) where $\bar{x}_a$ is the feature vector representing the sample a, such that x_a^i is the ith feature. $P(\bar{x}_a|\omega)$ corresponds to the Maximum Likelihood (ML) of the feature distribution for a particular class ω, while $P(\omega)$ and $P(\bar{x}_a)$ are the priors for the class and feature respectively.

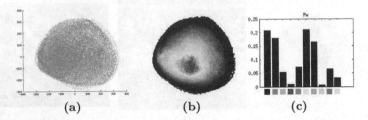

<table>
</table>

(a)   (b)   (c)

Fig. 3. SIFT space. (a) Projected space colored according to GT tissue labeling. (b) $P(\bar{x}_a)$. (c) $P(\omega)$

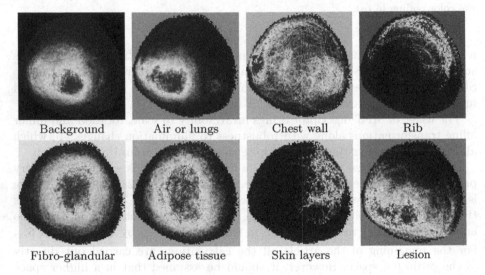

Background	Air or lungs	Chest wall	Rib
Fibro-glandular	Adipose tissue	Skin layers	Lesion

Fig. 4. Distribution of the SIFT descriptors for some classes in the GT

Figure 3 uses the entire dataset to illustrate the underlying problem and the priors extracted from the same dataset. Fig. 3a shows a scatter plot where every sample has been colored according to its GT. Fig. 3b shows an occurrence study of the samples carried out in a discretization of the SIFT space. Fig. 3c illustrates the class prior $P(\omega)$ corresponding to the proportion of samples present in the dataset for each class.

Figure 4 shows the feature distribution study for every class, corresponding to the $P(\bar{x}_a|\omega)$ in eq. 1. Similarities and dissimilarities between classes can be observed through the tendencies within the features representing each class. To illustrate that, it can be observed in figure 1 that the adipose tissue class contains Cooper's ligaments which are highly dense fibers, and fibro-glandular tissue is made of dense fibers and unstructured fat. Or, the difficulty to produce accurate GT delineations, which often happens for those regions where the structures are not clear enough to the user (i.e. the background class in fig. 1).

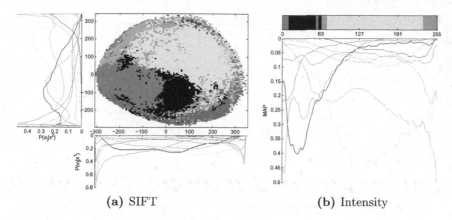

(a) SIFT   (b) Intensity

Fig. 5. Qualitative evaluation of the MAP labeling of the feature space

Equation 2 illustrates how to produce the preferred labeling of the space, as is illustrated in fig. 5a. On it, the marginals $P(\omega_i|x^j)$ where $j \in \{1,2\}$ are also represented to obtain a deeper understanding of the MAP.

$$labeling(\bar{x}) = \underset{i}{\arg\max} \quad P(\omega_i|\bar{x}) \quad \text{where } i \in [1..|W|] \qquad (2)$$

For comparison purposes, the labeling process has been carried out on the SIFT space as well as on the intensity space to analyze the tissue characterization. Figure 5 shows the qualitative evaluation of the MAP labeling for both spaces. From this results, the SIFT feature space is preferred since when using intensity some of the classes has no mode.

In order to generate cross-validated quantitative results, the descriptors have been randomly sampled as follows: (10.000 samples×10 classes)×5 folds. At each round 4 folds have been used for training the ML term in eq. 1 ($P(\bar{x}_a|\omega)$) and the remaining fold has been used for testing. The labeling results are provided in figure 6 as boxplots representing the confusion matrices distribution across the folds. In the figure, the samples are grouped by the actual class of the sample and distributed by the predicted classes. The top label represents the samples' actual class, whereas the predicted class is color coded at the bottom. Boxplots in blue represent the results of classifying the samples using intensity, whereas the bloxpots in red represent the results obtained when using SIFT. The lack of variability within the boxplots illustrates a repeatability of the results across the samples, which gets accentuated when using SIFT. The results show that the preferred labels which cover larger portion of the feature space achieve better results than the other classes. This is more clear for the intensity case since there are classes with no mode and therefore all the samples of this class are misclassified (see fig. 5). The sensitivity or True-Positive Ratio (TPR) allows to obtain a general sense of performance across all the labels. The TPR value obtained for the intensity case is $16.6 \pm 27.5\%$, whereas for the SIFT case is $18.8 \pm 17.2\%$ which show that both feature spaces produce similar results. Notice

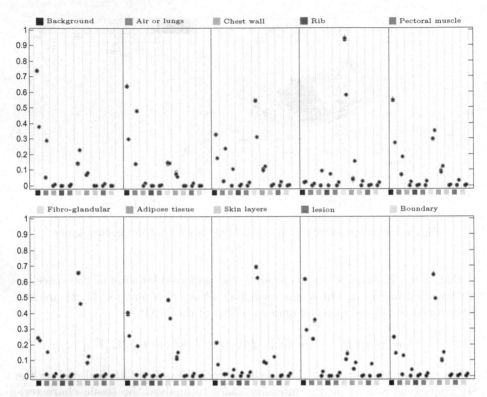

Fig. 6. Confusion matrices results distribution represented as boxplots. The results are grouped by actual class of the samples and distributed by the predicted label.

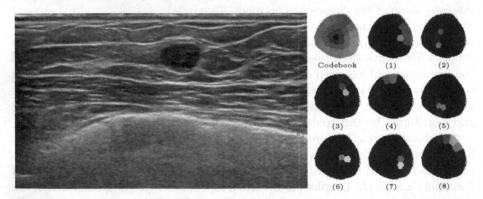

Fig. 7. SIFT-BoF descriptors qualitative analysis. (Left) image example. (Right) Dictionary representation colored using the location of the keypoint location in fig. 3a space. (1-8) Occurrence of the dictionary's key-points associated to each region highlighted in the original image.

that the large variability reported is due to missclassification of the labels with no mode, as can be observed in figure 5.

4   High-Level Texture Descriptor Using Bag-of-Features (BoF) and SIFT Descriptors

Texture is an area property related to spatial repetition of structures, similar statistical properties of the area or both. A technique to embed statistical properties of a low level descriptor is Bag-of-Features (BoF) which analyses the occurrence of a set of keywords (or key-points) within a particular region [2].

In our proposal, the words or features representing the images are SIFT descriptors. In order to determine the words forming the dictionary or codebook needed to generate the BoF descriptors, the space of SIFT descriptors is clustered in order to produce a hard quantification of this space. In this case, a k-means procedure with $k = 36$ is used to generate the codebook. To generate the BoF-SIFT feature, all the SIFT descriptors are substituted for the closest SIFT descriptor in the codebook. Finally the texture description from a particular area is expressed as the keywords' occurrence in this area. The descriptor is normalized so that the sum of all the occurrences is 1.

In our application, the areas used for extracting BoF descriptors are determined by using Quick-Shift (QS) super-pixels, as is shown in figure 7. The figure shows a codebook partitioning the feature space into 36 groups along with the BoF descriptors for the 8 highlighted super-pixels. For the visualization of the BoF features a heat color coding has been used to represent the occurrence of each word within the codebook.

In order to quantitatively assess the performance of SIFT embedded within a high-level feature descriptor such as BoF, a dataset of super-pixels with its associated GT and BoF-SIFT descriptor has been build up. At this point a super-pixel is eligible if it is larger than 50 pixels and is fully contained within the same GT label. This second constrain has been relaxed for skin and rib classes allowing super-pixels with 75% label contained to be eligible. The study has been carried out only for all the tissue classes, thus excluding background and boundary classes. To perform the evaluation 20 folds of 8 super-pixels (one per class) have been selected forming a set of 152 samples for training and 8 samples for testing at each round. The experiments have been repeated under the same conditions with 3 different codebooks in order to take into account the variability introduced by the codebook building. Again, for comparison purposes the experiment has been repeated using both intensity and SIFT. The classification has been carried out using Support Vector Machine (SVM). The TPR results achieved are $29 \pm 3.6\%$ for the case of intensity and $33.5 \pm 2.3\%$ for the case of SIFT, showing their similar performance and the improvement from using high-level texture descriptor over the low-level texture descriptor.

5   Conclusions

The present study was designed to explore the usage of SIFT feature space as a texture for characterizing the different tissues present in a breast US image. During the study, SIFT information have been used both as a low-level texture descriptor and encoded within a high-level texture descriptor using BoF. Performance of using the SIFT space has been evaluated by comparison with intensity. The results show that both performances are equivalent.

One of the limitaitons of this work is that all the calculations have been performed using the 2D PCA projected space which does not include all the variability of the data.

Despite these limitations, SIFT and intensity spaces produce similar results, which encourage further studies on using SIFT texture descriptors characterizing breast tissues in US images.

References

1. Cheng, H.D., Shan, J., Ju, W., Guo, Y., Zhang, L.: Automated breast cancer detection and classification using ultrasound images: A survey. Pattern Recognition 43(1), 299–317 (2009)
2. Csurka, G., Dance, C., Fan, L., Willamowski, J., Bray, C.: Visual categorization with bags of keypoints. In: Workshop on Statistical Learning in Computer Vision, ECCV, vol. 1, p. 22 (2004)
3. Jemal, A., Bray, F., Center, M.M., Ferlay, J., Ward, E., Forman, D.: Global cancer statistics. CA: A Cancer Journal for Clinicians 61(2), 69–90 (2011)
4. Lowe, D.G.: Distinctive image features from scale-invariant keypoints. International Journal of Computer Vision 60(2), 91–110 (2004)
5. Smith, R.A., Saslow, D., Sawyer, K.A., Burke, W., Costanza, M.E., Evans, W., Foster, R.S., Hendrick, E., Eyre, H.J., Sener, S.: American cancer society guidelines for breast cancer screening: Update 2003. CA: A Cancer Journal for Clinicians 53(3), 141–169 (2003)
6. Thomas Stavros, A.: Breast ultrasound. Lippincott Williams & Wilkins (2004)
7. Yuan, Y., Giger, M.L., Li, H., Bhooshan, N., Sennett, C.A.: Multimodality computer-aided breast cancer diagnosis with ffdm and dcemri. Academic Radiology 17(9), 1158 (2010)

Comparison of Methods for Current-to-Prior Registration of Breast DCE-MRI

Yago Díez[1], Albert Gubern-Mérida[1,2], Lei Wang[3], Susanne Diekmann[3],
Joan Martí[1], Bram Platel[2], Johanna Kramme[3], and Robert Martí[1]

[1] Dept. Computer Architecture and Technology, University of Girona, Girona, Spain
[2] Dept. Radiology, Radboud University Medical Center, Nijmegen, The Netherlands
[3] Fraunhofer MEVIS - Institute for Medical Image Computing, Bremen, Germany

Abstract. The use of prior studies to complement the information in
Breast Dynamic Contrast-Enhanced Magnetic Resonance Imaging
(DCE-MRI) can help to reduce the currently high false positive ratios.
Registration is a fundamental part of this process, as registration algorithms provide automatic correspondences between current and prior studies. The deformable nature of the breast and differences in acquisition
protocols make this a particularly challenging problem. In this paper we
study three registration algorithms (Affine, SyN and Demons) applied to
DCE-MRI images obtained from clinical practice. The methodology followed for this study included using segmentation algorithms in order to
focus on the area of the breast. Anatomical landmarks were also added by
an expert for evaluation purposes. This allowed us to use an anatomical-
landmark-based measure in order to evaluate the quality of registration.
Additionally, an image metric was also used for the same purpose. Results,
shown to be statistically significant indicate how SyN obtains the best results in terms of the two measures considered.

1 Introduction

Breast Dynamic Contrast-Enhanced Magnetic Resonance Imaging (DCE-MRI)
is recommended for breast cancer screening in women with cumulative lifetime
breast cancer risk of more than 20-25% (US and EU guidelines [5]). This modality presents high sensitivity and low to moderate specificity, which can lead to
a substantial amount of false positives. Having prior studies taken into account
by clinicians during the assessment of new exams can help to circumvent this
problem. Direct comparison of breast DCE-MRI scans taken over time is required in clinical practice but is often time consuming and lacks accuracy due
to limitations of commercially available viewers.

A novel software work-flow to compare current and prior exams should provide
automatic linkage of findings in prior and current images, extract clinically assessable parameters maps [6] and offer user friendly informative viewing solutions
for reading these images and maps. In order to perform these tasks, temporal
registration is required to align current and prior studies of the same patient.
However, registration of breast DCE-MRI exams acquired at different times is

H. Fujita, T. Hara, and C. Muramatsu (Eds.): IWDM 2014, LNCS 8539, pp. 689–695, 2014.
© Springer International Publishing Switzerland 2014

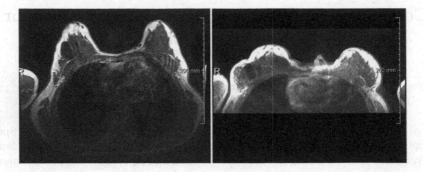

Fig. 1. These two axial slices acquired with one year difference from the same patient exemplify the difficulties registration algorithms may encounter in this registration scenario: Positioning problems (supine versus prone), technical problems (breast coil versus body phased array) and physiological changes (cysts of different sizes).

a challenging problem. Differences on breast compression and positioning have a strong influence on images due to the deformable nature of the breast as well as variability of breast tissue due to cycle and external effects (see example of Fig. 1). Moreover, image acquisition protocols may also vary producing different signal intensity values and different field of views.

In this work we evaluate three registration algorithms available in literature to align and compensate deformations between current and prior DCE-MRI studies: Affine, SyN [1] and Demons [8] registration. Distances between anatomical landmarks placed by an expert as well as global image metrics are used to evaluate the results.

2   Materials and Methods

2.1   Study Dataset

18 breast T1-weighted DCE-MRI studies from 9 patients were collected in the Radboud University Nijmegen Medical Centre. For each patient, a pair of DCE-MRI studies was available: a DCE-MRI exam acquired in 2011 (current) and a DCE-MRI exam acquired in 2010 (prior). Breast MRI examinations were performed in coronal or transverse orientation on either a 1.5 or 3 Tesla Siemens scanner (Magnetom Avanto, Magnetom Skyra or Magnetom Trio).

2.2   Preprocessing

Before being able to use the images for registration certain preprocessing steps are necessary. We provide some details in this section and Figure 2 presents an overview of all the steps (preprocessing, registration and evaluation) used in this study.

The involuntary motions and muscle relaxation during the image acquisition of DCE-MRI result in motion artifacts, which need to be corrected for better lesion reading. The first post-contrast image is commonly chosen as the reference image. The pre-contrast and other post-contrast images are then registered to the reference. Thus, only the registration between two pre-contrast images in the current and prior DCE-MRI studies is necessary in the follow-up temporal registration task. In this work, we used the method proposed by Böehler et al. to compensate motions in each DCE-MRI study [2].

In order to focus on breast structures, a breast segmentation algorithm was run on all patients. The method used for this [9] used a dedicated Hessian-based sheetness filter to enhance and segment the pectoralis muscle and breast-air boundaries simultaneously. Subsequently, the algorithm extracts a binary mask indicating breast regions. Consequently, for each patient we obtained two images (for left and right breast) per study which were registered independently.

For evaluation purposes, landmarks were placed in all pairs of DCE-MRI volumes by a radiologist with expertise in breast imaging. Each annotation consisted of two corresponding points, each of which was placed on each of the volumes composing the DCE-MRI pair. Notice how correspondence of landmarks is a key factor, so if a particular anatomical structure was only visible in one of the scans it was not used for landmark placement. Annotations were manually performed by comparing time points, subtracted and MIPS images and were visually validated on axial, sagittal and coronal planes. This process already yielded some insight in the difficulties faced by registration methods. For example, differences in the position of patients during image acquisition (prone or supine) made the placing of landmarks challenging. Technical differences in the acquisition process or physiological changes also added to these problems. See figure 1 for an example. Concerning the anatomical landmarks used for landmark placement, nipples were marked in all cases. Vessels and fat/glandular tissue margins were also placed whenever possible. A total of 10 pairs of corresponding landmarks were set for each DCE-MRI pair.

2.3   Registration Methods

Three registration methods were evaluated in this work. First of all, we considered Affine registration. This method provides comparison grounds for other registration results and is also used as an initialization step by the two non-rigid methods evaluated. This method was implemented using the Insight Toolkit (ITK) libraries[1]. Affine (and in some cases Rigid) registration methods are used because they are fast and produce images that are artifact-free [3]. Although these methods are very convenient for some applications, they are global in nature (a single affine motion is applied to the whole of the image). This characteristic makes it difficult for them to account for local variations [4].

The second registration method studied in this work is SyN, which is part of the Advanced Normalization Tools (ANTs) package[2] and uses bi-directional

---

[1] Insight Segmentation and Registration Toolkit webpage, http://www.itk.org/.
[2] Advanced Normalization Tools webpage,
http://www.picsl.upenn.edu/ANTS/download.php.

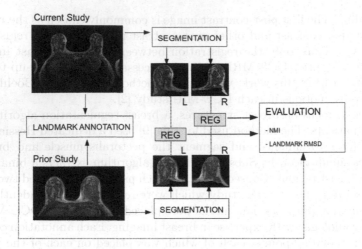

Fig. 2. Overview of the validation of process for current-to-prior registration in breast DCE-MRI: (1) landmark annotation on current and prior studies, (2) segmentation of left and right breasts, (3) current-to-prior registration for each breast and (4) evaluation based on Normalized Mutual Information (NMI) metric and distances between landmarks

diffeomorphism [1]. These bidirectional diffeomorphisms do not need to distinguish between target and source images thus enhancing their application scenarios. The third evaluated registration algorithm was Demons registration method based on Thirion's demons [3] [8]. All registration algorithms were independently applied to each breast using automatic breast segmentation masks.

2.4   Evaluation

Evaluating the quality of a registration method is a challenging problem. Even assessing how much two given images resemble each other is still an open problem. Image metrics exist, and play an important role in registration methods. Registration is often viewed as an optimization process and these measures are used to drive this optimization. Additionally, these metrics are also used to evaluate the performance of image registration. This is done under the assumption that an improvement in the similarity metric between images after registration means better alignment. However, this is not always the case. Specifically some studies showed how some registration results, although better in terms of Mutual Information, were deemed as "unrealistic and containing many image artifacts" by experts [3]. Furthermore, Rohlfing [7] showed that it is possible to design a method that obtains the best results in terms of image metrics while making

---

[3] We used an ITK implementations see "the itk programming guide" (http://www.itk.org/ItkSoftwareGuide.pdf) for details on how to download the code for classical itk demons.

absolutely no sense in medical terms. Hence, although we consider that image metric results have to be reported due to their role in optimization part of registration, alternative evaluation strategies must be prioritized.

Consequently, we computed Root-Mean-Square (RMS) distance between landmarks points of each DCE-MRI pair before and after registration. This type of measure agrees with recent trends on evaluation of registration algorithms [7] and is the main quality criterion used in this work. Additionally, results on Normalised Mutual Information (NMI) are also reported. NMI is chosen assuming a non fully linear intensity relationship between images. Concerning the statistical significance of results, Kolmogorov-Smirnov tests were run in order to ensure the normality of data. After that, one-tailed difference of means Student t-tests ($\alpha = 0.05$) were computed to see whether significant improvements in means were observed.

3   Results

Figure 3 summarises the obtained results. Two boxplots are presented corresponding to (a) RMS landmark-based metric (in mm) and (b) NMI image metric. Affine registration yielded ($mean \pm stdev$) 95.73 ± 60.32 mm and 1.11 ± 0.04, for RMS and NMI respectively. Values of RMS and NMI were, for the SyN algorithm, 72.89 ± 36.77 mm and 1.21 ± 0.04. Demons registration obtained 91.82 ± 52.07 mm and 1.12 ± 0.07, respectively. Improvements respect to the state prior to registration were observed to be statistically significant for all methods and criteria. Concerning results after registration, non-rigid methods performed better than Affine registration for the NMI criterion. For the landmark distance criterion, a statistically significant difference was only observed when comparing Affine and SyN (p-value = 0.025). Figure 4 shows visual examples for two registration cases. Note how the second row presents a more challenging case where SyN registration (Figure 4 (d)) is able to produce a noticeably better registration.

4   Discussion

In this work, we compared three registration methods to align and compensate deformations between current and prior DCE-MRI exams of the same patient. Temporal registration is the basis of a clinical software workflow to compare current and prior exams and reduce the number of false positive findings in DCE-MRI screening. Landmark-based and image-based metrics were used as evaluation measures.

Best results overall were obtained with SyN registration for the two measures studied. These results were shown to be statistically significant. Visual inspection of individual results showed that cases perceived to be more difficult (due to the differences in acquisition making the images less similar) coincided with those were higher landmark-based errors were observed.

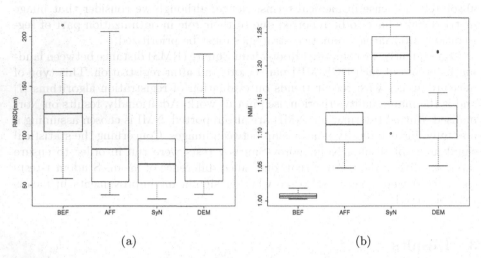

(a)   (b)

Fig. 3. Evaluation of prior-to-current breast DCE-MRI registration: (a) landmark-based (RMS) and (b) image-based (NMI) metric results before (BEF) and after Affine (AFF), SyN (SyN) and Demons (DEM) registration. Note that, for NMI, high positive values represent better registration results.

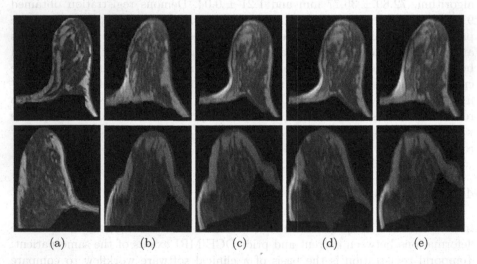

(a)   (b)   (c)   (d)   (e)

Fig. 4. Two registration examples. First row registration of a left breast, second row, registration of a right breast. Columns: (a) target and (b) source images and output images using (c) Affine, (d) SyN and (e) Demons algorithms.

In future work, we will increase the number of DCE-MRI studies in the dataset and more non-rigid registration algorithms will be evaluated. We will also focus on clinical application of registration. Specifically, parameter maps including morphology and kinetic information will be calculated and compared.

Acknowledgements. The research leading to these results has received funding from the European Unions Seventh Framework Programme FP7 under grant agreement no 306088 and has been supported by the Spanish Science and Innovation grant nb. TIN2012-37171-C02-01.

References

1. Avants, B., et al.: Symmetric diffeomorphic image registration with cross-correlation: Evaluating automated labeling of elderly and neurodegenerative brain. Medical Image Analysis 12(1), 26–41 (2008)
2. Böehler, T.: A combined algorithm for breast MRI motion correction. SPIE Medical Imaging 6514, 65141R–65141R–10 (2007)
3. Diez, Y., Oliver, A., Lladó, X., Freixenet, J., Martí, J., Vilanova, J.C., Martí, R.: Revisiting intensity-based image registration appplied to mammography. IEEE Transactions on Information Technology in BioMedicine 15(5), 716–725 (2011)
4. Diez, Y., Oliver, A., Cabezas, M., Valverde, S., Martí, R., Vilanova, J., Ramió-Torrentà, L., Rovira, A., Lladó, X.: Intensity Based Methods for Brain MRI Longitudinal Registration. A Study on Multiple Sclerosis Patients. Neuroinformatics, PMID:24338728 (to appear 2014)
5. Mann, R.M., Kuhl, C.K., Kinkel, K., Boetes, C.: Breast MRI: guidelines from the european society of breast imaging. Eur. Radiol. 18, 1307–1318 (2008)
6. Platel, B., Mus, R., Welte, T., Karssemeijer, N., Mann, R.: Automated Characterization of Breast Lesions Imaged with an Ultrafast DCE-MR Protocol. IEEE Transactions on Medical Imaging, PMID 24058020 (to appear 2014)
7. Rohlfing, T.: Image similarity and tissue overlaps as surrogates for image registration accuracy: Widely used but unreliable. IEEE Transactions on Medical Imaging 31(2), 153–163 (2012)
8. Thirion, J.P.: Non-rigid matching using demons. In: Proc. IEEE Conf. on Computer Vision and Pattern Recognition, pp. 245–261 (1996)
9. Wang, L., et al.: Fully automatic breast segmentation in 3D breast MRI. IEEE International Symposium on Biomedical Imaging, 1024–1027 (2012)

A Study on Mammographic Image Modelling and Classification Using Multiple Databases

Wenda He[1], Erika R.E. Denton[2], and Reyer Zwiggelaar[1]

[1] Department of Computer Science,
Aberystwyth University, Aberystwyth, SY23 3DB, UK
{weh,rrz}@aber.ac.uk
[2] Department of Radiology,
Norfolk & Norwich University Hospital, Norwich, NR4 7UY, UK
erika.denton@nnuh.nhs.uk

Abstract. Within computer aided mammography, there are many image analysis methods have been developed for mammographic image classification. Some of these were developed and validated using well known publicly available databases, and others may have chosen to use independent/private databases for their investigations. Often, despite the promising results described in the literature, it is not unusual to see when adapting an established method with the recommended configurations for a different database, the obtained results are not in line with expectation. This paper presents results of a study with respect to the implications of mammographic image classification using different classifiers trained with variations, such as differences in parameter settings, classifiers, using single databases, combined and across databases. The results indicated that it is unlikely to have an universal parameter settings and classifiers, which can be used to achieve the best classification without tuning. Additional databases used at the training stages do not necessarily lead to more accurate density classifications; whilst classifiers trained with images obtained using one type of image acquisition are not ideal for classifying images obtained using different image acquisition. The related issues of optimal parameter configuration, classifier selection, and utilising single or multiple databases at the training stage are discussed.

Keywords: Birads, computer aided mammography, mammographic density classification.

1   Introduction

Computer-aided diagnosis/detection (CAD) has been widely used in clinical practices to aid radiologists in interpretation of screening mammograms. Within computer aided mammography, the likelihood of a woman developing breast cancer can be determined through mammoraphic risk assessment [1]. To standardise mammography reporting and reduce confusion in breast imaging interpretations, Birads (American College of Radiology's Breast Imaging Reporting and Data

H. Fujita, T. Hara, and C. Muramatsu (Eds.): IWDM 2014, LNCS 8539, pp. 696–701, 2014.
© Springer International Publishing Switzerland 2014

System) [2] was developed as a quality assurance tool and covers the significant relationship between increased breast density and decreased mammographic sensitivity in detecting cancer [3]. Each mammography report starts with a breast density description which is used to inform the clinician about the possible effect on the sensitivity of the examination due to the mammographic density of the patient [4]. Mammographic breast composition is categorised into four classes: Birads 1, the breast is almost entirely fat ($< 25\%$ glandular); Birads 2, the breast has scattered fibroglandular densities ($25\% - 50\%$); Birads 3, the breast consists of heterogeneously dense breast tissue ($51\% - 75\%$); and Birads 4, the breast is extremely dense ($> 75\%$ glandular). Such a quantitative measure suggests the use of an accurate and repeatable computational method to perform automatic mammographic density classification. There are many image analysis methods suitable and/or have been purposely developed for mammographic density classification. Some of the methods were developed and validated using publicly available databases and others may have used independent/private databases for their investigations. It is not unusual to see when adapting an established method with the recommended configurations for a different database, that the obtained results are not in line with expectation; despite the promising results described in the literature.

The conducted study investigated the implications of applying a well known texture analysis method to mammographic density classification, using models and classifiers trained with variations in the parameter settings and use of databases (i.e. single, multiple and across databases). The aim and objective of the study is to find out: 1) whether there is an universal parameter setting and classifier to achieve consistent classification results, and 2) how does the use of different databases effect the discrimination power of the trained classifiers and subsequent results. This paper presents the study findings, issues of optimal parameter configuration, classifier selection, and utilising multi-databases at the training stage are discussed.

2   Data and Method

Two publicly available databases were used in the study, one is the Mammographic Image Analysis Society (MIAS) database, and the other is the Digital Database for Screening Mammography (DDSM) database; the image acquisition methods used for the two databases were distinctively different. The MIAS database consists of 322 images, only 320 are usable (files mdb296rl and mdb295ll are excluded due to historical reasons); with respect to Birads ('B') density categories, the numbers of B_1 to B_4 images are 87, 103, 94 and 37, respectively. The second database used is a subset of the full DDSM database which consists of 831 images and has been used in other publications (e.g. [5,6]); the numbers of B_1 to B_4 images are 106, 336, 255 and 134, respectively. It should be noted that currently there is no publicly available full-field digital mammography database; therefore only digitised databases were used; so further experiments could be directly compared with our findings. To keep the image resolutions more or less consistent, each of the images from the MIAS and DDSM was resized to 500 pixels across, and the orthogonal size was adjusted accordingly based on the original image size; see Fig. 1 for examples. Ground truth for both databases were obtained as consensus ground truth based on three independent radiologists with different mammographic reading experience.

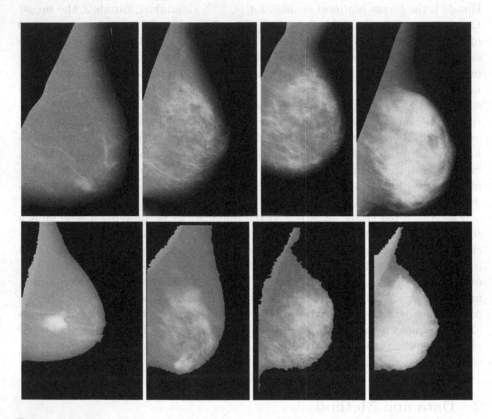

Fig. 1. Example mammographic image from MIAS (top row) and DDSM (bottom row) databases; images from left to right represent Birads density categories from low to high (i.e. Birads 1 to 4). Note that different pectoral/background segmentation methods were used for the databases.

Each database was split (randomly with an equal distribution in Birads densities) into three subsets, for training (40%), validation (20%) and evaluation (40%). Noted that the random image selection based experiment was performed five times. A well established multi-resolution grey-scale and rotation invariant local binary pattern (LBP) was employed [7] in the study. Each of the experiments consists of three stages: 1) generating mammographic image LBP representation, 2) optimal parameter and classifier selection, and 3) mammograhpic density classification.

LBP is computational simple yet an efficient approach to texture analysis for its uniformity, non-parametric discrimination of samples and prototype distribution [7]. It is assumed that breast parenchymal patterns associated with Birads densities can be modelled using LBP distributions. A generalised grey-scale and rotation invariant operator $LBP_{P,R}$ was used to detect 'uniform' patterns, in a circular symmetric neighbourhood P of any quantisation of the angular space, and at any spatial resolution which was determined by a circle of radius R [7]. The operator responses are expected to be independent in multi-resolution analysis, and the responses over different resolutions can be combined with a rotation invariant variance measure $VAR_{P,R}$ (characterises local texture contrast). The joint distribution $LBP_{P,R}/VAR_{P,R}$ is assumed to be able to incorporate both breast parenchymal texture (*e.g.* orientation and coarseness) and density variations in the derived feature vectors, which can be used to train a classifier for mammographic density classification. The reader is referred to [7] for the methodology details.

For mammographic images associated with the same Birads density category and with similar texture appearance, it is expected that the joint distributions (feature vectors) are correlated and closely clustered in the feature space. Different LBP parameter configurations result in the joint distributions for a mammograhic image with different feature dimensions. Therefore a classifier trained using a particular LBP configuration can be used for a breast density classification, and the resultant classification accuracy can be used as an indicator, to determine the discriminative power of the derived feature vectors with respect to the used LBP configuration. An automatic parameter selection scheme was employed to choose the optimal parameters (i.e. P and R) for the LBP approach. A set of neighbourhoods (i.e. {7, 17, 27, 37, 47, 57, 67}) and corresponding radii (i.e. {2, 4, 7, 9, 12, 14, 18}) covering small to large breast anatomical structures were predefined. The total number of combinations ($C(n,r) = n!$ / $(r!(n-r)!)$), where n = 7, r ={1, 2, ..., 7}) for the multi-resolution configuration is 127. A collection of 57 classifiers available in Weka [8] (*e.g.* trees (12), bayes (6), functions (5), lazy (1), meta (25), misc (1) and rules (7)) was used. Each classifier was trained using the 127 sets of feature vectors derived from the randomly selected training set for each Birads density class, and the classifier was validated using the validation set. It is expected that different classifiers behave differently, and the optimal LBP configuration varies from one classifier to another. Therefore, the optimal parameter configuration reflects the discriminative power and statistical variations of the feature vectors, and was determined based on a total of 57 (classifiers) × 127 (combinations) = 7239 tests. Note that the time complexity and number of resolutions used were assessed, and the choices were made in favour of configurations that used less time to process and less resolutions needed.

All the images from the remaining evaluation sets were used in the risk classification, with the optimal parameter configuration and associated classifier. The density classifications were performed in the Weka environment which includes: 1) base line density classification (i.e. training and testing images are from the same database), 2) classification using the classifier trained with a native and an additional different database (e.g. training using MIAS + DDSM and testing on MIAS), and 3) classification using the classifier trained with a different database (e.g. training using MIAS and testing on DDSM).

3   Results and Discussion

Table 1 shows the density classification accuracies are the same or marginally improved when using an additional database at the training stages; the classification accuracies are significantly reduced when only using a different databases at the training stages. Through thousands of tests, SMO (sequential minimal optimisation) seems to produce more best classification cases in different test categories. Table 1 indicates that it is essential to cover anatomical structures at all sizes, in order to achieve good risk classification results; however, the best combination seems to vary from case to case. In addition, when not taking the rotation invariant variance measure $VAR_{P,R}$ into account to characterise local texture contrast, for 67% of the cases, there is on average 2.4% decrease in the density classification accuracies, and 1.9% increase in the density classification accuracies for the rest of 33% of the cases. This indicates that overall it is beneficial to use rotation invariant variance measure, but the effects are not consistent for all the cases. The average standard deviation for the classification accuracies is ± 3.7% for the random image selection based experiment (repeated five times); alternative cross-validation based evaluations are considered as future work. In

Table 1. Birads density classification accuracies (the best in the five repeated experiments) when using different training schemes; SMO, LMT, NNge, LADTree denote sequential minimal optimisation, logistic model trees, non-nested generalised exemplars and decision trees with LogitBoost strategy, respectively.

Training	Testing	Accuracy	Best classifier	Neighbourhoods (windows)
MIAS	MIAS	79%	SMO	27 37 47
MIAS+DDSM	MIAS	81%	LMT	7 27 47 57 67
DDSM	MIAS	69%	NNge	7 17 27 37 47 57
DDSM	DDSM	63%	SMO	7 17 27 47 67
MIAS+DDSM	DDSM	63%	SMO	7 37 57 67
MIAS	DDSM	53%	LADTree	7 17 37 57

terms of the use of a multi-resolution approach, the results indicate that it does not seem to have an universal setting, even when the image resolutions are more or less the same; the best parameter settings seem to vary based on the classifiers used. Therefore, it may be beneficial to perform similar validation tests before applying a methodology to novel experiments (e.g. mammographic image modelling and density classification using other databases), in order to achieve the best classification results with the optimal pair of parameter setting and classifier. The experimental results also indicate that there is not much value for adding an additional database at the training stage, when the mammograhic images were obtained using (very) different image acquisition methods; unless the images need to be classified were obtained using the same methods. It should be noted that when image normalisation was used as a means of pre-processing, the obtained results indicated similar findings with lower density classification results. It appears that the standard normalisation technique used may alter breast parenchymal appearances (e.g. intensity distribution), which can significantly affect the density based image classification and should be used carefully.

4 Conclusions

The conducted novel experiment used two publicly available databases and a well known texture analysis method from the literature. Based on the results, it is concluded that: 1) optimal parameter and classifier selection can be beneficial in adapting a methodology to mammographic image analysis, 2) using an additional database at the training stage does not necessarily show great improvements in the density classification, and 3) it may not be ideal to train a classifier using mammographic images obtained under one type of image acquisition, and use for classifying images obtained under a different acquisition process.

References

1. Wei, J., Chan, H.P., Wu, Y.T., Zhou, C., Helvie, M.A., Tsodikov, A., Hadjiiski, L.M., Sahiner, B.: Association of computerized mammographic parenchymal pattern measure with breast cancer risk: A pilot case-control study. Radiology 260(1), 42–49 (2011)
2. American College of Radiology, Breast Imaging Reporting and Data System BI-RADS, 4th edn. American College of Radiology, Reston (2004)
3. Sickles, E.A.: Wolfe mammographic parenchymal patterns and breast cancer risk. American Journal of Roentgenology 188(2), 301–303 (2007)
4. Gram, I.T., Bremnes, Y., Ursin, G., Maskarinec, G., Bjurstam, N., Lund, E.: Percentage density, Wolfe's and Tabár's mammographic patterns: Agreement and association with risk factors for breast cancer. Breast Cancer Res. 7, 854–861 (2005)
5. Tortajada, M., Oliver, A., Martí, R., Vilagran, M., Ganau, S., Tortajada, L., Sentís, M., Freixenet, J.: Adapting breast density classification from digitized to full-field digital mammograms. In: Maidment, A.D.A., Bakic, P.R., Gavenonis, S. (eds.) IWDM 2012. LNCS, vol. 7361, pp. 561–568. Springer, Heidelberg (2012)
6. Chen, Z., Arnau, O., Denton, E.R.E., Zwiggelaar, R.: A multiscale blob representation of mammographic parenchymal patterns and mammographic risk assessment. International Conference on Computer Analysis of Images and Patterns 12(8), 3838–3850 (2013)
7. Ojala, T., Pietikainen, M., Maenpaa, T.: Multiresolution gray-scale and rotation invariant texture classification with local binary patterns. IEEE Transactions on Pattern Analysis and Machine Intelligence 24(7), 971–987 (2002)
8. Frank, E., Witten, I.H., Hall, M.A.: Data Mining: Practical machine learning tools and techniques, 3rd edn. Morgan Kaufmann, San Francisco (2011)

Quasi-3D Display of Lesion Locations Simulated by Two Views of Digital Mammography

Yu Narita[1], Noritaka Higashi[2], Yoshikazu Uchiyama[3], and Junji Shiraishi[3]

[1] Graduate School of Health Sciences,
Kumamoto University, Kumamoto, Japan
`109m7020@st.kumamoto-u.ac.jp`
[2] Kumamoto Health Care Center,
Japanese Red Cross Society, Kumamoto, Japan
`nonta4511@yahoo.co.jp`
[3] Faculty of Life Sciences,
Kumamoto University, Kumamoto, Japan
`{y_uchi,j2s}@kumamoto-u.ac.jp`

Abstract. In the interpretation of digital mammography, intuitive recognition of the spatial location of a lesion projected on the images requires considerable experience for radiologist or radiological technologist. In order to support radiologists and radiological technologists to reading mammography, we have developed a computerized scheme to produce a simulated three-dimensional (3D) display of lesion locations by using craniocaudal (CC) and mediolateral-oblique (MLO) views of digital mammography. In the preliminary results obtained from 20 cases with lesions, 100% of lesions were correctly displayed on the simulated 3D image in which locations were verified by the certificated breast radiological technologist.

Keywords: digital mammography, three-dimension, simulation.

1 Introduction

In the interpretation of digital mammography, because of two-dimensional nature of craniocaudal (CC) and mediolateral-oblique (MLO) views of digital mammography, intuitive recognition of the spatial location of a lesion projected on the images requires considerable experience for radiologist or radiological technologist. In case of ultrasound examination following to mammography, identification of spatial location of lesions on the mammography is important for accurate and prompt procedure. Therefore, if the lesion location is displayed on the three-dimensional (3D) image, it would be useful for radiologists and/or radiological technologists to identifying lesions intuitively.

The purpose of this study is to display a spatial location of the lesion on the simulated 3D breast image which is produced by using CC and MLO views of digital mammography.

H. Fujita, T. Hara, and C. Muramatsu (Eds.): IWDM 2014, LNCS 8539, pp. 702–706, 2014.
© Springer International Publishing Switzerland 2014

2   Materials and Methods

2.1   Estimation of a Lesion Location in 3D Space

In this study, we defined a location of the top of nipple for CC and MLO views, cc(xc0, yc0) and mlo(xm0, ym0), respectively, as the origin of 3D space for simulated 3D breast images ($3d$(0, 0, 0)). The spatial location of a lesion ($3d$(x, y, z)) was estimated from the 2D lesion location on CC (cc(xc, yc)), and on MLO (mlo(xm, ym)) (Fig.1). The z coordinate of a lesion center in quasi-3D volume could be determined by averaging two distances in x coordinates between top of the nipple and the center of lesion on CC and MLO views as follows;

$$z = [(xm - xm0) + (xc - xc0)] / 2 \qquad (1)$$

and the x coordinate of a lesion center in quasi-3D volume could be determined by the distance in y coordinate between the top of nipple and the lesion center on CC view.

$$x = yc0 - yc \qquad (2)$$

The y coordinate of a lesion center in quasi-3D volume could be determined by use of an angle θ of X ray tube for MLO view, the x coordinate determined, and the distance in y coordinate between the top of nipple and the lesion center on MLO view.

$$y = \tan(90 - \theta)x + (ym0 - ym) / \sin\theta \qquad (3)$$

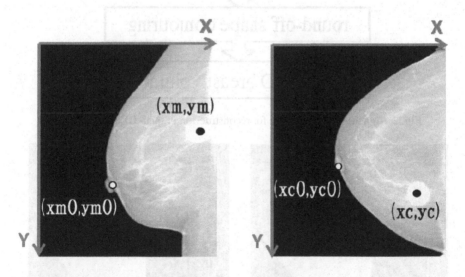

Fig. 1. The x, y coordinates of the top of nipple and lesion center on CC and MLO views

2.2   Image Database

We used 154 cases with 308 pairs of digital mammography which were examined in our university hospital between February 2010 and February 2011. The use of those cases was approved by the IRB and all images were anonymized for this study. All digital mammography were obtained with full field digital mammography system(Senographe 2000-DS, GE), and have 1914x2294 matrix size with 0.1mm pixel size (16bit grayscale). The reference standard of the lesion location was determined by consensus of two certificated breast radiological technologists.

2.3 Computerized Scheme for Reconstructing Quasi-3D Breast Volume

The quasi-3D volume was produced by use of two views of digital mammography. Initially, the original size of CC and MLO image was reduced into 287 x 344 matrix size, because the high resolution property was not necessary for displaying lesion locations.

The outline of the computerized scheme was indicated in Fig. 2.

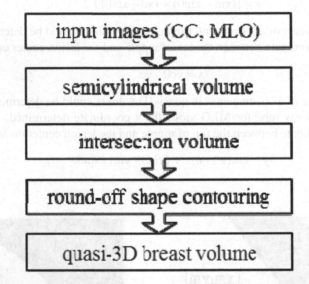

Fig. 2. Computerized procedure for reconstruction of quai-3D breast volume

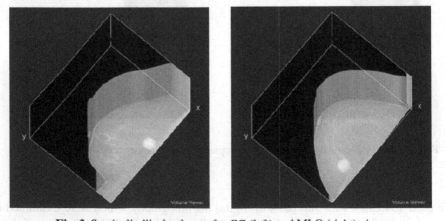

Fig. 3. Semicylindlical volumes for CC (left) and MLO (right) views

The first step for producing quai-3D volume, the semicylindrical volume was reconstructed simply by integrating 2D image for CC and MLO views (Fig. 3.). The intersection of semicylindrical volumes for two views was then produced by matching the CC plane along the perpendicular line from the top of nipple to chest wall on MLO view (Fig. 4.).

In order to make quasi-3D breast volume realistic, we applied round-off shape contouring (Fig. 5.).

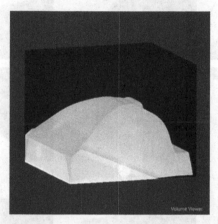

Fig. 4. Intersection of semicylindrical volumes for two views

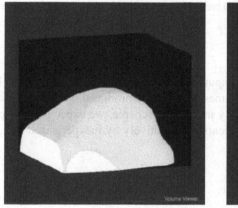 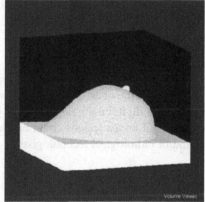

Fig. 5 Round-off shape contouring for intersection volume (left) to produce quasi-3D breast volume (right)

3 Results and Discussion

Preliminary result obtained from 50 cases with 56 malignant and benign lesions, lesion locations were correctly displayed on the quasi-3D breast volume in terms of 100% agreement with the locations determined by the certificate radiological radiologists. Figure 5 illustrates examples of CC/MLO views and their quasi-3D breast volumes obtained by this study.

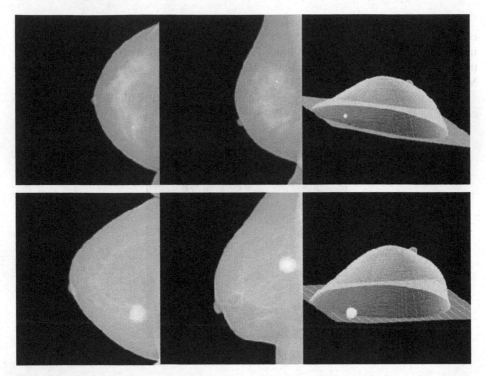

Fig. 5. Examples of CC,MLO and their quasi-3D breast volume with lesion location (white sphere)

4   Conclusions

In conclusion, we developed a novel computerized scheme for displaying spatial lesion locations in the quasi-3D breast volumes which were produced by using CC and MLO views of digital mammography. By use of this scheme, we expected that spatial locations of breast lesions could be identified intuitively by inexperienced radiologists and/or radiological technologists.

References

1. Tse, G., Tan, P.H., Fernando: SchmittAnatomy and Physiology of the Breast. In: Fine Needle Aspiration Cytology of the Breast, pp. 1–5 (2008)
2. Tanaka, A., et al.: Effectiveness of the comprehensive evaluation based on the combinatorial analysis using mammography and ultrasonography in breast cancer screening. In: Health Care Center, Kusatsu General Hospital,
   http://www.shigamed.ac.jp/education/ejournal/contrib/
   26-05paper.pdf (accessed November 08, 2013)
3. Saito, T., Toriwaki, J.: Euclidean Distance Transformation for Three Dimensional Digital Images. The Transactions of the Institute of Electronics, Information and Communication Engineers D-II, J76-D-II(3), 445–453 (1993)

A Shearlet-Based Filter for Low-Dose Mammography

Huiqin Jiang[1,*], Yunyi Zhang[1,*], Ling Ma[2], Xiaopeng Yang[3], and Yumin Liu[1]

[1] School of Information Engineering of Zhengzhou University and Zhengzhou Engineering Technology Research Center for Medical Informatization, 100 Science Road, High-tech Development Zone, Zhengzhou City, Henan Province, 450001, China
[2] Fast Corporation 2791-5 Shimoturuma Yamoto, Kanagawa Japan
[3] Department of Equipment of the First Affiliated Hospital of Zhengzhou University and Zhengzhou Engineering Technology Research Center for Medical Informatization
iehqjiang@zzu.edu.cn

Abstract. To improve image quality of low-dose mammography images, we study a new approach of removing Poisson noise from a degraded image in shearlet domain. We first transform Poisson noise into a near Gaussian noise by a shearlet-based multiply variance stabilizing transform (VST). Second, the initial positions of ideal shearlet coefficients are found by thresholding Gaussian noise coefficients. Third, an iterative scheme is proposed to estimate non-noise coefficients from the found initial ideal shearlet coefficients. Finally, the reduced noise image is obtained by the inverse shearlet transform on the estimated coefficients. The main contribution is to combine thresholding and the iterative scheme. A range of experiments demonstrate that the proposed method outperforms the traditional shearlet-based method.

Keywords: Low-dose mammography, De-noising, Shearlet Transform, Multiply VST, Poisson noise.

1 Introduction

Mammography is the first line to defense against breast cancers. Low dose mammography scanning has been gradually used to lower the radiation exposure for care of patients. However, down scaling the radiation intensities results in increased quantum noise, affecting diagnostic accuracy [1]. The quantum noise can be simulated by Poisson processes [2]. Therefore, our research purpose is to eliminate the Poisson noise from the low-dose mammography images.

Wavelet transform is a powerful tool for image denoising [3, 4]. However, most of the previously developed wavelet-based denoising algorithms assume a Gaussian noise for the data and estimate the local statistics of image pixels, which is not valid for the low-dose mammography images. Recent years, some algorithms have been proposed for denoising Poisson count data [5, 6]. The main scheme is first to turn Poisson noise to a near Gaussian noise using Variance stabilization transform (VST). Second, the

---

* Corresponding authors.

H. Fujita, T. Hara, and C. Muramatsu (Eds.): IWDM 2014, LNCS 8539, pp. 707–714, 2014.

noise is removed using a conventional denoising algorithm for Gaussian noise. Then, the reduced noise image is obtained using an inverse transformation. For example, B.Zhang et al. proposed to combine VST with Wavelet, Ridgelet and Curvelet, leading to MS-VST, which has good performance in low-count situation [5]. Markku Mäkitalo et al. proposed the optimal inversion of the anscombe transformation and have demonstrated that the proposed method is a very efficient filtering solution compared to with some of the best existing methods for Poisson image denoising [6], Moreover, some studies have shown that the traditional wavelets are not very effective in dealing with multidimensional signals containing distributed discontinuities.

Shearlets have been mathematically proven to represent distributed discontinuities such as edges better than the traditional wavelets [7]. In this paper, a shearlet-based method to reduce Poisson noise is presented. A shearlet-based multiply VST is proposed to transform Poisson noise to Gaussian distribution. Then, we estimate non-noise coefficients by combining thresholding and the iterative scheme developed. Finally, the reduced noise image is obtained by the inverse shearlet transform on the estimated coefficients. The computer simulations were performed to show the potential of the presented method for reduction of Poisson noise in low-dose mammography images.

2   A Shearlet-Based Multiply VST

In this section, we present a shearlet-based multiply variance stabilizing transform (SMVST) by combining Nonsubsampled Shearlet Transform (NSST) [8] with VST. As shown in Fig1, the SMVST can be described as following:

Firstly, we calculate the stabilized coefficients at scale j using Equation (1)

Where, $f_a^{\ j}$ denotes the approximation at level j, (j =0,1,2). $f_a^{\ 0}$ denotes the input image. c^j is calculated using Equation (2).

$$Z_j(f_a^{\ j}) = \text{sgn}(f_a^{\ j} + c^j)\sqrt{\left| f_a^{\ j} + c^j \right|} \tag{1}$$

$$c^j = \frac{7t_2^j}{8t_1^j} - \frac{t_3^j}{2t_2^j} \tag{2}$$

$t_k = \sum_i (H^{\ j}(i))^k, (k = 1,2,3), H^j = H^{\uparrow 1} * H^{\uparrow 2}... * H^{\uparrow j}, i$ is the length of H^j, $H^{\uparrow j}$ and $G^{\uparrow j}$ denote the low pass filter and the high pass filter at level j, respectively.

Secondly, NSST is performed to decompose the image into next level

The NSST includes two parts: multiscale decomposition and the localization of direction. We choose the Nonsubsampled Laplacian pyramid scheme for multiscale decomposition. By this method, $Z_j(f_a^{\ j})$ can be decomposed into the approximation f_a^{j+1} and the high frequency components f_d^{j+1} at level $j+1$. Then, we implement

the localization of direction on f_d^{j+1} to generate k directional sub-bands at level $j+1$:

$f_d^{j+1,1}, f_d^{j+1,2}, \ldots\ldots f_d^{j+1,k}$.

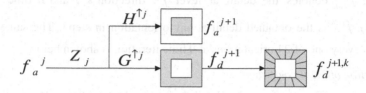

Fig. 1. The flow diagram of the shearlet-based multiply VST

Using SMVST, Poisson noise can be transformed into a near Gaussian process with asymptotic constant variance in shearlet domain. Then, we can estimate the threshold using the designed method for Gaussian noise.

3 Proposed Method

A shearlet-based method for denoising Poisson noise is developed in the following manner. There are five steps.

Step1: Decomposing the noisy image to some sub-band images using SMVST
Choosing $k=16$ at level $j=1$ and $k=8$ at level $j=2$, respectively, we decompose the noisy image to the approximation and the details in 24 orientations using the above description SMVST.

Step2: Find the initial position of ideal shearlet coefficients
For each orientation, we calculated the threshold [9] at the corresponding sub-band and select the position of ideal coefficients $M_{j,k}$ using Equation (3) and Equation (4), respectively.

$$T = \sigma\sqrt{2\ln N} \tag{3}$$

$$M_{j,k} = \left\{(x, y)/f_d^{j,k}(x, y) \geq T\right\} \tag{4}$$

Where, N is the size of the image, $\sigma \approx Median(|f_d^{j,k}|)/0.6745$ is the estimated noise variance.

Step 3: Apply NSST to noisy mammography image
Choosing $k=16$ at level $j=1$ and $k=8$ at level $j=2$, respectively, we decompose the noisy image to the approximation f_a and the details in 24 orientations using the above description NSST.

Step4: Estimate non-noise coefficients using the iterative algorithm

We construct a iterative algorithm shown in Equation (5).

$$f_{d,n}^{j,k+1} = P_M f_{d,n}^{j,k} - b_n \, \text{sgn}(P_M f_{d,n}^{j,k}) \qquad (5)$$

Where, $f_{d,n}^{j,k}$ denotes the detail at level j, direction k, and n time iteration ($n=1,2,3$). $f_{d,1}^{j,k}$ is the obtained detail at any orientation in step3. The same process applied to every one of 24 orientations at n time iteration is shown below:

(1) Selection of ideal coefficient

Select ideal coefficients from the detail $f_{d,n}^{j,k}$ according to the index of the found $M_{j,k}$ by the description method in step2. P_M denotes the operator of selection of ideal coefficients at every iteration.

(2) Shrinkage of coefficients

We apply threshold method to coefficients $P_M f_{d,n}^{j,k}$ by soft threshold as shown in Equation (5). $b_n = \sigma_n \cdot (N-n)/(N-1)$ is threshold, $\sigma_n \approx Median(|f_{d,n}^{j,k}|)/0.6745$ is the estimated variance of $f_{d,n}^{j,k}$. This step adopted to smooth the selected ideal coefficients removes artificial noise caused by P_M.

Step5: Apply inverse NSST

We reconstruct the final reduced noise image with $f_{d,4}^{j,k}$ at each orientation and f_a in step3 by inverse NSST.

4   Experiment and Results

To validate the efficiency of the proposed method, the experiments were conducted on the real 25 mammography images come from the First Affiliated Hospital of Zhengzhou University and 8 mammography images with different amount of Poisson noise. Both visual and quantitative evaluations are presented with implementation of the proposed method in a series of mammography images.

4.1   Visual Evaluation

In this subsection, the experiments are conducted on real low-dose mammography images. The obtained experiment results are shown in Fig.2. Fig.2 (a) shows the example of standard-dose mammography image using the tube voltage (29 kVp), the tube current (61 mAs), and the exposure time (1143 mAs). Fig.2 (b) shows the example of reduced-dose mammography image using the tube voltage (25 kVp), the tube current (62 mAs), and the exposure time (402 mAs). Fig.2 (c) and Fig.2 (d) are the region of interest (ROI) chosen from Fig.2 (a) and Fig.2 (b). The processed images by literature method and proposed method are shown in Fig.2 (e) and Fig.2 (f), respectively.

Even if the x- ray dose reduced by 30% as shown in Fig.2 (b), the visual quality of the processed image using the proposed method is improved clearly in comparison with the literature method [10] and is almost the same as the standard-dose image.

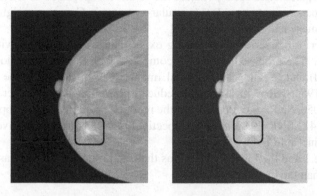

(a)The standard-dose image(5.8680mGy)   (b)The reduced-dose image(1.3240mGy)

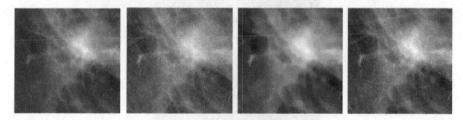

(c) ROI in image (a)   (d) ROI in image (b)   (e)Literature method   (f)Proposed method

Fig. 2. The obtained experiment results

4.2   Quantitative Evaluation

The Signal to Noise Ratio (SNR) of an image and a Mean Structure Similarity (MSSIM) between the reference X and the processed images Y are measured for image quality assessment. The MSSIM [11] is defined using Equation (6) and (7).

$$MSSIM(X,Y) = \frac{1}{M} \sum_{j=1}^{M} SSIM(x_j, y_j) \qquad (6)$$

Where, x_j and y_j are the image contents at the $j-th$ local window and M is the number of local windows in the image.

$$SSIM\,(x,\,y) = [l(x,\,y)]^{\alpha} \cdot [c(x,\,y)]^{\beta} \cdot [s(x,\,y)]^{\gamma} \qquad (7)$$

x and y are the reference and the reduced noise image. The three components $l(x,\,y)$, $c(x,\,y)$ and $s(x,\,y)$ denote the luminance comparison function, the contrast comparison function and the structure comparison function, respectively. $\alpha,\,\beta$ and γ are parameters used to adjust the relative importance of the three components. In this paper, we use a 11×11 circular-symmetric Gaussian weighting window scanning the image and set $\alpha = \beta = \gamma = 1$.

We also perform a series of denoising experiments using images with controlled noise amounts. The proposed method is compared with literature method [10]. Fig.3 (a), (b), (c) (d) and (e) show the original image, ROI in Fig.3 (a), the noisy image (MSSIM=0.7195, SNR=7.8186dB), the reduced noise image by the literature method (MSSIM=0.8050, SNR= 9.6706dB), and the reduced noise image by proposed method (MSSIM= 0.8417, SNR= 9.9668 dB), respectively. Results of quantitative evaluations are presented in Table.1.

From Table.1 and the Fig3, it is obvious that the proposed method has higher SNR and MSSIM than the literature method.

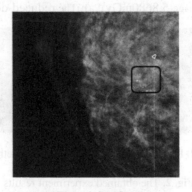

(a)The original image

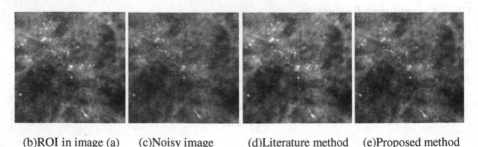

(b)ROI in image (a)   (c)Noisy image   (d)Literature method   (e)Proposed method

Fig. 3. Noise reduced result of ROI in mammography image

Table 1. The quantitative evaluation of noise remove for ROI images

Image	Noise Image		Literature Method		Proposed method	
	MSSIM	SNR/dB	MSSIM	SNR/dB	MSSIM	SNR/dB
1	0.7195	7.8186	0.8050	9.6706	0.8417	9.9668
2	0.7695	8.7110	0.8126	10.0157	0.8571	10.4645
3	0.8388	12.0709	0.8245	12.8045	0.8818	14.1780
4	0.6970	6.1969	0.7934	7.5354	0.8279	7.7103
5	0.7846	8.6281	0.8121	9.5984	0.8606	10.0920
6	0.8364	8.7589	0.8137	8.9315	0.8713	9.4700
7	0.7981	9.2574	0.8531	10.6499	0.8707	10.7503
8	0.8467	9.3846	0.8564	9.8965	0.8869	10.1838

5   Conclusions

In this paper, a shearlet-based filter for removal of Poisson noise is proposed. Experimental results show that the proposed method not only has a higher SNR than the literature method , but also the Mean Structure Similarity of reduced noise image obtained by the proposed method increased by 5% compared to the literature method. In the future work, we will study the adaptive algorithm for accurately separating the high-frequency of image and noise.

Acknowledgments. The research work was supported by National Natural Science Foundation of China (No.61271146), Projects of technological innovation of SMEs in Henan Province (No. 132203210030) and Projects of science and technology innovation team of Zhengzhou (No.131PCXTD630).

References

1. Sperl, J., Bequé, D., Claus, B., De Man, B., Senzig, B., Brokate, M.: Computer-Assisted Scan Protocol and Reconstruction (CASPAR) —Reduction of Image Noise and Patient Dose. IEEE Transactions on Medical Imaging 29(3), 724–732 (2010)
2. Jiang, H., Li, W., Liu, Y., Wang, Z., Ma, L.: Comparison Study of Filters for Poisson Noise Removal. In: 2011 RISP International Workshop on Nonlinear Circuits, Communications and Signal Processing, Tianjin, China, March 1-3, pp. 171–174 (2011)
3. Wang, J., Lu, H., Wen, J., Liang, Z.: Multiscale Penalized Weighted Least-Squares Sinogram Restoration for Low-Dose X-Ray Computed Tomography. IEEE Transsactions on Biomedical Enineering 55(3), 1022–1031 (2008)
4. Jiang, H., Wang, Z., Ma, L., Liu, Y., Li, P.: A Novel Method to Improve the Visual Quality of X-ray CR Images. International Journal of Image, Graphics and Signal Processing (IJIGSP) 3(4), 25–31 (2011)
5. Zhang, B., Fadili, J.M., Starck, J.-L.: Wavelets, Ridgelets, and Curvelets for Poisson Noise Removal. IEEE Trans. Image Process. 17(7), 1108–1903 (2008)
6. Mäkitalo, M., Foi, A.: Optimal Inversion of the Anscombe Transformation in Low-Count Poisson Image Denoising. IEEE Transactions on Image Processing 20(1), 99–109 (2011)

7. Easley, G.R., Labate, D., Colonna, F.: Shearlet Based Total Variation for Denoising. IEEE Trans. Image Process. 18(2), 260–268 (2009)
8. Easley, G.R., Labate, D., Lim, W.-Q.: Sparse directional image representations using the discrete shearlet transform. Applied and Computational Harmonic Analysis 25, 25–46 (2008)
9. Donoho, D.L., Johnston, I.M.: Ideal spatial adaptive via wavelet shrinkage. Biometrika 81, 425–455 (1994)
10. Haizhi, H., Hui, S., Chengzhi, D.: Shearlet shrinkage denoising based total variation regularization'. Journal of Image and Graphics 16(2), 168–173 (2011)
11. Wang, Z., Bovik, A.C., Sheikh, H.R., et al.: Image quality assessment: From error visibility to structural similarity. IEEE Transactions on Image Processing 13(4), 600–612 (2004)

Evaluation of Human Contrast Sensitivity Functions Used in the Nonprewhitening Model Observer with Eye Filter

Ramona W. Bouwman[1], Ruben E. van Engen[1], David R. Dance[2],
Kenneth C. Young[2], and Wouter J.H. Veldkamp[1,3]

[1] Dutch Reference Centre for Screening, Radboud University Nijmegen Medical Centre
(LRCB), P.O. Box 6873, 6503 GJ Nijmegen, The Netherlands
r.bouwman@lrcb.nl
[2] National Coordinating Centre for the Physics in Mammography (NCCPM),
Royal Surrey County Hospital, Guildford GU2 7XX, United Kingdom and Department of
Physics, University of Surrey, Guildford, GU2 7XH, UK
[3] Department of Radiology, Leiden University Medical Centre,
Albunisdreef 2, 2333 ZA Leiden, The Netherlands

Abstract. Model observers which can serve as surrogates for human observers
could be valuable for the assessment of image quality. For this purpose, a good
correlation between human and model observer is a prerequisite. The nonprewhitening model observer with eye filter (NPWE) is an example of such a model
observer. The eye filter is a mathematical approximation of the human contrast
sensitivity function (CSF) and is included to correct for the response of the human eye. In the literature several approximations of the human CSF were
found. In this study the relation between human and NPWE observer performance using seven eye filters is evaluated in two-alternative-forced-choice (2-
AFC) detection experiments involving disks of varying diameter and signal
energy and two background types. The results show that the shape of the CSF
has an impact on the correlation between human and model observer. The inclusion of a CSF may indeed improve the relation between human and model
observer. However, we did not find an eye filter which is optimal in both backgrounds.

Keywords: model observers, image quality, NPWE, eye filter, contrast sensitivity.

1 Introduction

In general, image quality analysis and system optimization studies in full field digital
mammography (FFDM) are performed using contrast detail analysis or linear system
metrics like DQE and NEQ. The limitations of both approaches is the use of uniform
backgrounds where quantum noise is dominating. Furthermore the pixel values must
have a known relationship with entrance air kerma on the image receptor (like in unprocessed images), whereas for clinical images this relation might not be known due
to (non-linear) processing. Furthermore, the radiological task is often dominated by

H. Fujita, T. Hara, and C. Muramatsu (Eds.): IWDM 2014, LNCS 8539, pp. 715–722, 2014.

anatomical structures rather than quantum noise. Statistical anthropomorphic model observers (model observers acting as human observers) use the image statistics to determine the detectability without the assumption of linearity or the assumption that quantum noise is dominating. Therefore statistical anthropomorphic model observers might be used for the assessment of image quality in clinical images.

Acceptance of anthropomorphic model observers for image quality assessment strongly depends on the relation between model and human observer. Rolland and Barrett [1] have investigated this using two different model observers: a pre- and a nonprewhitening matched filter (PW and NPW) and concluded that the NPW model observer fails to predict human observer performance in lumpy backgrounds. Burgess et al [2] subsequently demonstrated that the NPW model observer can predict the human response if a spatial frequency filter is included which mimics the contrast sensitivity function (CSF) of the human eye. This was followed by several studies where the NPWE (NPW eye) model observer was applied. In the literature several approximations of the human CSF can be found. The origin of these approximations varied from fitting experimental data to applied research in the field of human vision. The aim of this paper is to investigate the detection of a NPWE model observer using different eye filters compared with the detection of human observers. This has been studied by performing a two-alternative-forced-choice experiment (2-AFC) using simulated white noise backgrounds (WN), representing an ideal quantum noise limited system and clustered lumpy backgrounds (CLB), simulating clinical breast structures [3].

2   Method

The NPWE model observer correlates the signal template and the image after convolution with an eye filter. This means that the NPWE model observer only takes the signal template into account and does not incorporate background statistics. For an image g_n (with n = 1 (object absent) or 2 (object present)) the decision variable (T) of the NPWE model observer can be estimated using:

$$T(g_n) = [E^t \cdot E \cdot (B \cdot s_2)]^t \cdot g_n \tag{1}$$

where t is the matrix transpose, B the imaging system blur, s_2 the signal template and E the eye filter which is defined in the spatial frequency domain and is assumed to be radially symmetric. The decision variable (T) is subsequently used to estimate a detectability index d' by:

$$d'_{NPWE} = \frac{\langle T \rangle_1 - \langle T \rangle_2}{\sqrt{\frac{1}{2}\sigma_1^2 + \frac{1}{2}\sigma_2^2}} \tag{2}$$

where $\langle T \rangle$ is the mean and σ the standard deviation of the decision variable T. In a 2-AFC experiment with normally distributed test statistics, d' is related to the fraction of correct response in the experiment (proportion correct, PC) by:

$$PC = \frac{1}{2} + \frac{1}{2} \cdot erf\left(\frac{d'}{2}\right) \tag{3}$$

where erf is the Gaussian error function: $erf(x) = \frac{2}{\sqrt{\pi}} \cdot \int_0^x e^{-t^2} dt$.

In 1994 Burgess [2] argued that the human CSF could be mathematically expressed using the following formula (eye filter 1) in equation 4:

$$E(f) = f^{1.3} \cdot e^{-bf^2} \tag{4}$$

where f is the spatial frequency (lp/degree) and b is chosen to obtain E_{max} at 4 lp/degree. In his study images of 128x128 pixels (54 mm^2) were displayed on a monitor with a mean luminance of 60 cd/m^2 with an average viewing distance of 0.5 m. In two subsequent papers of Burgess [4-5] a simple approximation of the Barten model of human contrast sensitivity was used to mathematically express the human CSF [6] (eye filter 2) in equation 5:

$$E(f) = f \cdot e^{-bf} \tag{5}$$

where f is the spatial frequency (lp/degree) and b is chosen to obtain E_{max} at 4 lp/degree. For these experiments images were evaluated at several viewing distances between 0.5 and 2.5 m and a mean luminance of 150 cd/m^2. In addition to the eye filters used in the work of Burgess, two other eye filters were found in combination with the NPWE model observer [7-8] (eye filters 3 and 4) in equations 6 and 7:

$$E(f) = f^{1.9} \cdot e^{-2f^{0.5}} \tag{6}$$

$$E(f) = 0.605f^2 \cdot e^{-f/1.748} \tag{7}$$

where equation 6 is the result of a fit to experimental data from the field of natural imaging. In this study images were displayed on a monitor with a mean luminance between 12 and 30 cd/m^2 with an average viewing distance of 2.0 m [9]. Equation 7 is the result of a best fit from experiments conducted in the field of human vision by Kelly [10] in which the visibility of sine-wave gratings were scored. This equation was subsequently used for the evaluation of image quality of flat panel detectors used in radiography. The images were evaluated on a monitor with a mean luminance of 180 cd/m^2 and a viewing distance of 0.4 m.

With the purpose of evaluating the perceived image quality on monitor display devices, Barten proposed the following equation [6] (eye filter 5) in equation 8:

$$E(f) = af \cdot e^{-bf} \sqrt{(1 + 0.06 \cdot e^{bf})} \tag{8}$$

where, $a = \dfrac{540 \cdot (1 + 0.7/L)^{-0.2}}{1 + \frac{12}{w \cdot (1 + f/3)^2}}$, $b = 0.3 \cdot \left(1 + 100/L\right)^{0.15}$, L is the luminance in cd/m^2

and w the angular display size in degrees. In subsequent work, Barten [11] developed a model of the human CSF which was implemented as a filter for the evaluation of the image quality using a channelized Hotelling observer by Park [12] (eye filter 6) which is given in equation 9:

$$E(f) = \cfrac{M_{opt}(f)}{k\sqrt{\cfrac{2}{T}\left(\cfrac{1}{x_0^2}+\cfrac{1}{x_{max}^2}+\cfrac{f^2}{N_{max}^2}\right)}\cdot\left(\cfrac{1}{\eta\cdot p\cdot E}\cfrac{\Phi_0}{1-e^{-(f/f_0)^2}}\right)} \qquad (9)$$

Explanation of the parameters can be found in the work by Park et al [12].

In work by Watson and Ahumada [13] a standard method for foveal contrast detection was proposed which includes the following specific CSF formula (eye filter 7) in equation 10:

$$E(f) = sech\left(\frac{f}{f_0}^p\right) - a\cdot sech\left(\frac{f}{f_1}\right) \qquad (10)$$

where f is again the spatial frequency and f_0=4.3469, f_1=1.4476, a=0.8514 and p=0.7929. It must be noted that this CSF was part of the model proposed for foveal contrast detection and will be implemented in this study as an eye filter on its own. The parameters used in this formula were based on the best fit for their experiments. In these experiments monochrome images with different stimuli were viewed with a total angular span of 2.133 degrees and a mean luminance of 30 cd/m^2.

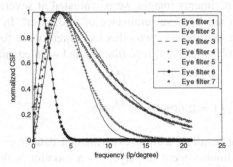

Fig. 1. The eye-filters (normalized to their peak frequency) used in this study. For eye filters 5 and 6 a mean luminance of 80 cd/m^2 is used for display purposes.

The seven different eye filters described above are shown in fig. 1. In our study the impact of the eye filter on the human-model comparison has been investigated. To evaluate the correlation between the NPWE model observer and human observer a 2-AFC experiment was conducted using computer generated WN and CLB images [3]. For each 2-AFC test a set of paired images with 256x256 pixels was generated, one image with and one without a disk shaped object. The objects were generated from a high resolution disk which was down scaled to 6, 12, 18, 30 and 60 pixels in diameter. For each diameter three signal energies (SE) were chosen such that human observers were expected to score 65 to 95 percent correctly. Since the CLB images were optimized to simulate mammographic backgrounds as obtained from a GE FFDM unit [3], objects used for the CLB images were blurred using the system MTF of a GE Essential X-ray unit.

Four human observers (physicists who are trained in image quality aspects in mammography) were asked to score 300 images for each background, object SE and diameter. The images were scored in a clinical reading environment using a DICOM calibrated 5 MP mammography monitor with a pixel size of 165 μm. The images were displayed 1-to-1 and zooming and leveling were not allowed. The observers were asked to keep their viewing distance constant at approximately 0.4 m. All sets were scored by human and model observers whereby the signal present and signal absent images were shown to the human observers as pairs. For some eye filters monitor luminance needs to be known. For these eye-filters the mean luminance is estimated based on the distribution of pixel values in the image resulting in a mean luminance of 20-180 cd/m^2 for CLB images and 40-80 cd/m^2 for the WN images.

To investigate the significance of the eye filter used on the human-model comparison a trend analysis is performed by fitting a straight line between human and model observer detectability (d') using mixed effect models to estimate the population mean and to include random effects for the individual observers. For each eye filter the goodness of fit was evaluated by comparing r^2 [14] and the residuals, difference between measured and predicted d', for each diameter.

3   Results

In fig. 2 and fig. 3 the resulting eye filter with the largest r^2 are shown. In fig. 2a-d the d'$_{human}$ versus d'$_{NPWE}$ graphs for eye filter 4 with CLB images are shown for each observer with the resulting fit for the population (solid line) and the individual observers (dashed line). In fig. 2e the residuals to the population are shown. In fig. 3 similar plots can be found for WN images in combination with eye filter 6. For each eye filter and background the same set of graphs were evaluated. Findings for all eye filters and both backgrounds are summarized in table 1.

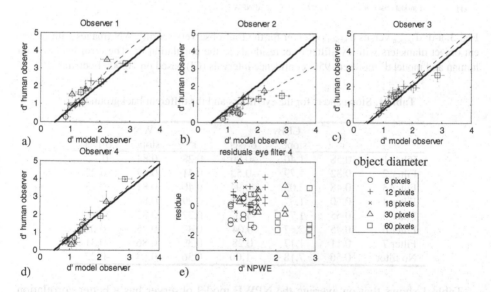

Fig. 2. a-d: d'$_{human}$ versus d'$_{model}$ observer for the four observers scoring WN images with different object diameters (eye-filter 4). e: residuals to the population fit. The error bars of both human and model d' represent 95% confidence intervals (CI) based on 10.000 bootstraps.

Comparing the data of each observer (fig. 2 and 3) a large spread in performance between observers is noted. Nevertheless, individual observer performance can be predicted using the simple linear model. From the residual plots of the population it is observed that there is no strong correlation for either diameter or d'_{NPWE} for CLB images while there might be a small dependence with diameter for WN images. By comparing all residuals with and without eye filter, it is suggest that inclusion of an eye filter may result in a smaller diameter dependency for CLB however this change in diameter dependency is not that obvious for WN images.

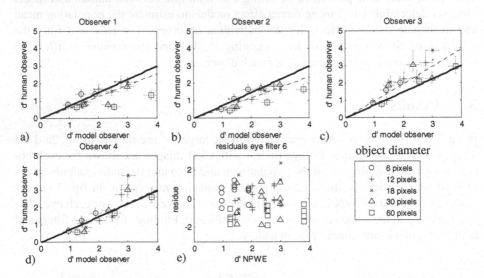

Fig. 3. a-d: d'_{human} versus d'_{model} observer for the four observers scoring WN images with different object diameters with eye-filter 6. e: residuals to the population fit. The error bars of both human and model d' represent 95% confidence intervals (CI) based on 10.000 bootstraps.

Table 1. Slope and r^2 for the eye filters and the different backgrounds

	CLB			WN		
	r^2	slope	offset	r^2	slope	offset
Filter 1	0.58	1.40	-0.80	0.28	0.84	0.12
Filter 2	0.32	1.79	-0.53	0.41	0.83	-0.22
Filter 3	0.48	2.02	-0.94	0.40	0.81	-0.13
Filter 4	0.60	1.37	-0.69	0.29	0.81	0.12
Filter 5	0.55	1.77	-1.02	0.32	0.82	0.03
Filter 6	0.45	2.67	0.04	0.42	0.75	-0.07
Filter 7	0.11	1.17	0.28	0.39	0.86	-0.31
No filter	0.56	7.18	-1.00	0.36	0.63	-0.22

Table 1 shows that on average the NPWE model observer has a better correlation with the human observer using CLB images (higher r^2). Furthermore, it is found that the slope is steeper for CLB images which means that the human observer read these images better. This might be caused by the fact that the human observer can, to some extent, prewhiten the structures of the noise. Moreover it is found that for most eye filters and both backgrounds the offset is close to or smaller than zero, meaning that the threshold SE at which d' starts increasing is smaller for model observers compared to human observers. This is desirable if d' predicted for human observer is estimated from the model observer d'.

For CLB images the NPWE model observer with eye filters 1 and 4 improves the relation between human and model performance in comparison with the NPW model observer (without eye filter). For WN images this was achieved with eye filters 2, 3, 6 and 7.

4   Discussion and Conclusions

The aim of this study was to evaluate different eye filters for the NPWE model observer in relation to human performance. In the literature several eye filters were reported with different behavior in the frequency domain. In this study it is shown that the eye filter has an impact on the response of the NPWE model observer. Furthermore it was found that some eye filters in combination with the NPWE model observer may improve the relation between model and human observers, especially for CLB images. For these backgrounds it was suggested that the dependency with diameter is reduced. This is in agreement with previous work of Burgess [4]. However, due to the different responses in the frequency domain the residuals might still show a dependence on diameter with some eye filters. For the evaluation of the eye filter we should therefore consider both r^2 and the residuals. In addition this study shows that the observer variability is substantial and therefore the eye filter which shows best agreement with humans might be observer dependent. However, for quality control procedures it is desirable to predict the impact to a population rather than an individual observer. Therefore we did not investigate the individual relations. Some eye filters need the mean display luminance as input, since the luminance has an impact on the shape of the human CSF. However, the models that include display luminance did not show a better performance. A possible explanation for this might be that the human CSF is determined for an ideal response and that the background variability needs to be taken into account as well.

For quality control procedures a methodology is needed which is sensitive to changes in image quality. Ideally the selected eye filter should match human and model performance for all diameters and be independent of the type of background. Since the NPWE model observer is a simple model observer that does not take into account noise correlations it is expected that this will never be achieved. Nevertheless, it is demonstrated that the NPWE model observer is capable of predicting human observer performance for a given task. In this study, only the impact of the selection of eye filters on the human model performance using two image backgrounds has been assessed. Since the eye filter that was most appropriate depended on the background, it is questionable whether a relation between human and model performance using the NPWE model observer would be valid if for example the color of the noise is changed. Further work regarding the implementation of model observers for quality control and their statistical validation is required to determine the impact of possible changes in image quality on the human model relation. In addition, the impact of background structures for the different tasks needs to be investigated.

References

1. Rolland, J.P., Barrett, H.H.: Effect of random background inhomogeneity on observer detection performance. J. Opt. Soc. Am. A 9(5), 58–649 (1992)
2. Burgess, A.E.: Statistically defined backgrounds: Performance of a modified nonprewhitening observer model. J. Opt. Soc. Am. A Opt. Image Sci. Vis. 11(4), 42–1237 (1994)
3. Castella, C., et al.: Mammographic texture synthesis: second-generation clustered lumpy backgrounds using a genetic algorithm. Optics Express 16(11), 7595–7607 (2008)
4. Burgess, A.E., Jacobson, F.L., Judy, P.F.: Human observer detection experiments with mammograms and power-law noise. Med. Phys. 28(4), 37–419 (2001)
5. Burgess, A.E., Li, X., Abbey, C.K.: Visual signal detectability with two noise components: Anomalous masking effects. J. Opt. Soc. Am. A Opt. Image Sci. Vis. 14(9), 42–2420 (1997)
6. Barten, P.G.J.: Evaluation of subjective image quality with the square-root integral method. Journal of the Optical Society of America a Optics Image Science and Vision 7(10), 2024–2031 (1990)
7. Bochud, F.O., Abbey, C.K., Eckstein, M.P.: Visual signal detection in structured backgrounds. III. Calculation of figures of merit for model observers in statistically non-stationary backgrounds. Journal of the Optical Society of America a Optics Image Science and Vision 17(2), 193–205 (2000)
8. Borasi, G., et al.: Contrast-detail analysis of three flat panel detectors for digital radiography (vol. 33, p. 1707, 2006). Medical Physics 33(9), 3580–3580 (2006)
9. Webster, M.A., Miyahara, E.: Contrast adaptation and the spatial structure of natural images. Journal of the Optical Society of America a Optics Image Science and Vision 14(9), 2355–2366 (1997)
10. Kelly, D.H.: Visual Contrast Sensitivity. Optica. Acta. 24(2), 107–129 (1977)
11. Barten, P.G.J.: Contrast sensitivity of the human eye and its effect on image quality, vol. PM72. SPIE Press book (1999)
12. Park, S., et al.: Incorporating Human Contrast Sensitivity in Model Observers for Detection Tasks. IEEE Transactions on Medical Imaging 28(3), 339–347 (2009)
13. Watson, A.B., Ahumada, A.J.: A standard model for foveal detection of spatial contrast. Journal of Vision 5(9), 717–740 (2005)
14. Kramer, M.: R2 statistics for mixed models. In: Proceedings of the Conference on Applied Statistics in Agriculture (2005)

It Is Hard to See a Needle in a Haystack: Modeling Contrast Masking Effect in a Numerical Observer

Ali R.N. Avanaki[1], Kathryn S. Espig[1], Albert Xthona[1],
Tom R.L. Kimpe[2], Predrag R. Bakic[3], and Andrew D.A. Maidment[3]

[1] Barco Healthcare, Beaverton, OR, USA
[2] BARCO N.V., Healthcare Division, Kortrijk, Belgium
[3] University of Pennsylvania, Department of Radiology, Philadelphia, PA, USA

Abstract. Within the framework of a virtual clinical trial for breast imaging, we aim to develop numerical observers that follow the same detection performance trends as those of a typical human observer. In our prior work, we showed that by including spatio-temporal contrast sensitivity function (stCSF) of human visual system (HVS) in a multi-slice channelized Hotelling observer (msCHO), we can correctly predict trends of a typical human observer performance with the viewing parameters of browsing speed, viewing distance and contrast. In this work we further improve our numerical observer by modeling contrast masking. After stCSF, contrast masking is the second most prominent property of HVS and it refers to the fact that the presence of one signal affects the visibility threshold for another signal. Our results indicate that the improved numerical observer better predicts changes in detection performance with background complexity.

Keywords: contrast masking effect, spatio-temporal contrast sensitivity function, channelized Hotelling observer, human visual system, virtual clinical trial, and psychometric function.

1 Purpose

Commonly used numerical observers cannot necessarily predict the behavior of a typical human observer in all observation scenarios. This is due to the fact that they are modeled after ideal observers (i.e., maximizing some detection performance metric) with some concessions for tractability (e.g., channelization). For example, a multi-slice channelized Hotelling observer (msCHO), without correct application of spatio-temporal contrast sensitivity function (stCSF), is unable to predict the fundamental effect of display contrast on detection of lesions in digital breast tomosynthesis (DBT) [1, 2].

Our goal is to enhance a numerical observer by making it perform more similarly to a human observer. Our approach towards this goal is to integrate important properties of the human visual system (HVS) as a pre-processing step to a commonly used numerical observer (msCHO). In other words, as the result of HVS modeling,

H. Fujita, T. Hara, and C. Muramatsu (Eds.): IWDM 2014, LNCS 8539, pp. 723–730, 2014.

"perceived" 3D image stacks are fed to msCHO. Previously we have reported on the benefits of integrating the HVS property of stCSF with msCHO [1, 2, 3].

In this work, we study the effect of modeling the contrast masking property of HVS in our numerical observer. Contrast masking refers to the phenomenon that the presence of a signal ("masker") makes detection of another signal ("maskee") more difficult.

1.1   Prior Work

Zhang *et al* channelized the input image in orientation and (spatial) frequency [4]. In the most sophisticated model used, an inhibitory component (denominator of Eq. 13 therein) is used to factor in the contrast masking effect.

Early channelization of the data in [4] is undesirable in our methodology. By postponing channelization to CHO (i.e., HVS simulation followed by a traditional numerical observer at the backend), one can replace msCHO by a more sophisticated observer to upgrade the pipeline. In other words, early channelization discards data that may be useful to the detection task to be performed at the backend. Also, the perception model in [4] is parametric and is unusable without a calibration to (psychophysical) experimental results.

Krupinski *et al* developed a perceptual numerical observer as follows [5]. Using a perceptual image quality metric, JNDmetrix, a lesion image (signal + background) is compared to the corresponding healthy image (background only). Lesion detectability is assumed to be correlated to the metric value which is an indication of the perceived difference between the two images. Contrast masking is one of the effects considered in the derivation of perceptual difference.

The perceptual observer proposed in [5] is double-ended. Our current pipeline is single-ended. This is an advantage in our application since unlike a double-ended observer, a single-ended observer does not require having both a version with and without lesion for every image stack.

Our current pipeline is designed for DBT (three dimensional, 2D space and 1D time; may be used for other 3D modalities, though not tested) and is able, for example, to show a peak in detection performance with slice browsing speed [2]. Numerical observers in above mentioned papers are spatial-only (2D).

2   Methods

2.1   Simulation Platforms and Preparation of Datasets

In this work, synthetic breast images were generated using the breast anatomy and imaging simulation pipeline developed at the University of Pennsylvania (UPenn). Normal breast anatomy is simulated by a recursive partitioning algorithm using octrees [10]. Phantom deformation due to clinical breast positioning and compression is simulated using a finite element model [11]. DBT image acquisition is simulated by ray tracing projections through the phantoms, assuming a polyenergetic x-ray beam without scatter, and an ideal detector model. Reconstructed breast images are obtained using the Real-Time Tomography image reconstruction and processing method [12].

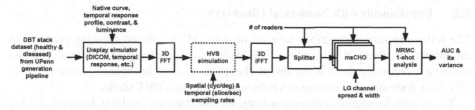

Fig. 1. Block diagram of the display and virtual observer simulation. The methods proposed in this paper are used in the dotted block.

The display and virtual observer simulation (Fig. 1) is implemented in MEVIC (Medical Virtual Imaging Chain) [13], an extensible C++ platform developed for medical image processing and visualization at Barco. DBT stack datasets (volumes of interest) with and without simulated lesions, generated using the UPenn pipeline, are input to the display and virtual observer simulation pipeline. For the experiments with numerical observer that are reported here, the "simple background" dataset (see next paragraph for details) consists of 3296 reconstructed 64x64x32 DBT image stacks, half with lesions and half without. Each stack is first decomposed into its spatiotemporal frequency components using a 3D fast Fourier transform (FFT). The stCSF [1, 2], contrast masking (Section 2.2), and psychometric function [1, 2] are modeled in the dotted block in Fig. 1 to determine the perceived amplitude of each frequency component. Then, an inverse 3D FFT is applied to the perceived amplitudes to transform the perceived stack into the space-time domain. Finally, the results are fed to a multi-slice channelized Hotelling observer (msCHO) developed by Platiša *et al* [14]. For further details of the simulation see [2].

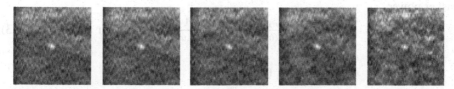

Fig. 2. From left to right: Slices #16 from the same image stack in datasets with background complexity level of 0 (simple background), 1, 2, 3, and 4. The insertion contrast for these images is increased to make the lesion (the bright spot in the center of each slice) visible for the purposes of publication.

To create datasets with varying background complexity, spatiotemporal low-pass Gaussian noise with four different levels of energy was added to the dataset from UPenn phantom. Slices #16 from a sample image stack in five datasets are shown in Fig. 2.

2.2   Experiments with Numerical Observers

The following section describes how we modeled HVS contrast masking property in the numerical observer. According to Winkler, we can disregard temporal contrast masking effect since there is no abrupt change in average luminance (Section 9.2 of [6]). This does assume a continuous browsing in viewing DBT stacks.

To account for spatial contrast masking, we use Barten's model (Chapter 6 of [7]), with the following considerations. Barten addressed the masking of a single spatial tone (single-frequency signal) by a band-pass noise. We assume each frequency component as masker for all other frequency components in a neighborhood determined by masker-maskee difference in frequency and orientation. This is done for every slice in the image stack and the result is used to adjust the CSF-only visibility threshold calculated for each spatio-temporal component of the image stack as follows (Eq. 2.50 in [7]):

$$m'_t = \sqrt{m_t^2 + k^2 m_n^2}, \tag{1}$$

where m'_t is the visibility threshold with masking, m_t is the CSF-only visibility threshold, m_n is the masker power, and k is Crozier coefficient. The rest of processing is the same as the CSF-only pipeline with psychometric non-linearity described in our prior work [1, 2].

To find $m_n(u, v)$, the masker power for a component with spatial frequency (u, v), we first approximate S, the spatial spectrum of the image stack, as follows.

$$S(u, v) = \sum_{\forall w} |I(u, v, w)|^2 \tag{2}$$

I is 3D DFT of the image stack. w denotes the temporal frequency. By generalizing Eq. 6.2 of [7] for 2D spatial frequencies, we derive the following formula for the masker power.

$$m_n(u, v) = \frac{\sum_{\forall (u', v')} w(u, v, u', v') S(u', v')}{S(0,0) \sum_{\forall (u', v')} w(u, v, u', v')}, \quad u \neq 0 \text{ or } v \neq 0, \tag{3}$$

$$and \ m_n(0,0) = 0.$$

The function $w(u, v, u', v')$ allows a higher weight for nearby components in (spatial) frequency and orientation and is given by

$$w(u, v, u', v') = \begin{cases} 0, & |\alpha| > 5° \\ e^{-2.2 \ln^2 \left(1 + \sqrt{\frac{(u-u')^2 + (v-v')^2}{u^2 + v^2}} \right)}, & |\alpha| \leq 5° \end{cases} \tag{4}$$

where α is the angle between (u', v') and (u, v). This weighting function above is derived by generalizing Eq. 6.4 of [7] for 2D spatial frequencies, and considering the fact that only excitations close in orientation mask one another (Eq. 5.18 in [8]).

Simulation parameters are the same as those used for human observer experiments (Section 2.3). For calculation of stCSF and the perceived amplitudes, see [2].

2.3 Experiments with Human Observers

The following section describes how we have established human observer detection performance in three levels of background complexity. From the same datasets used for experiments with numerical observer, 35 image stacks are randomly chosen for each of the six conditions. The set of conditions is the Cartesian product of {lesion, healthy} (i.e., lesion present or absent) and {0, 2, 4} level of background complexity (see Fig. 2), simulated by the image stacks without addition of noise, and the image stacks with medium and high energy noise added (the noise spectrum remained the same) respectively.

The total of 210 image stacks were presented to the human observer in a random order on a DICOM-calibrated BARCO MDMG-5221 medical display which is optimized and cleared by FDA for reading of DBT images and is equipped with Rapid-Frame temporal response compensation technology. Each image stack was displayed in cine mode at a constant browsing speed of 10 slice/sec twice. The recommended viewing distance from the display was about 40 cm (translates to a spatial sample rate of 18 pixel/degree) but was not strictly enforced for the observer's comfort. The maximum luminance of display (L_{max}) was set to 850 cd/m^2. In our viewing environment, the black point luminance of the display (i.e., the level of luminance associated with drive level of zero) was measured at $L_{min} = 1.75$ cd/m^2, using a Minolta CS-100A. Therefore, the effective contrast given by L_{max}/L_{min}, was 486.

The observer could repeat the presentation of an image stack (as described above) as many times as desired, or score the presence of a lesion in the spatiotemporal center of the stack. No temporal or spatial clue was provided for the location of lesion. That was because, given our presentation scenario, we found such clues unnecessary and even distracting from the lesion detection task in our pilot experiments. Scoring an image stack consisted of entering one number from the set {0, 1, 2, 3} meaning {certainly no lesion, probably no lesion, probably lesion, certainly lesion} respectively. When an image stack was scored, the process above was repeated for the next image stack. We considered the detection performance as the percentage of correctly identified (i.e., scored 2 or 3) lesion image stacks.

To have more stable results, the same set of image stacks that were randomly chosen for the first human observer was used for the experiments with other human observers as well.

The observers were required to have normal vision and pass a 10-minute training session to become familiar with the experiment and their task. The observers were not radiologist. This is justified considering the fact that the location of the lesion, if present, is always known (and constant), hence the detection task is simply reduced to recognizing a bright spot in a background with various levels of complexity.

3   Results and Discussion

The results of experiments with two human observers are given in Table 1. As expected, the detection performance for human observers falls with increasing background complexity. It is conceivable that with more experience, human observers who are aware of lesion prevalence rate (50% in our experiments) reach the chance performance (0.5) even in high background complexity.

Table 1. Percentage of correctly identified lesion stacks (of total) in three background complexity levels

Background Complexity	Low	Medium	High
Observer A	0. 9714	0. 7714	0. 2571
Observer B	0. 8000	0. 7143	0. 3429

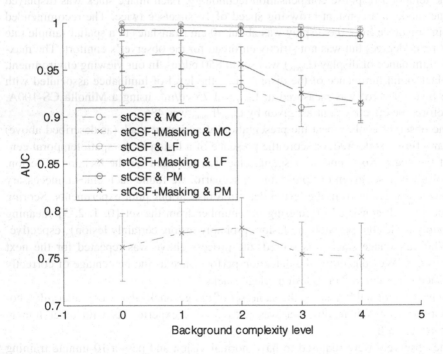

Fig. 3. Detection performance (in AUC) for datasets at various background complexity levels (Section 2.1)

Simulation results from modeling HVS with stCSF only, and stCSF plus contrast masking are compared in Fig. 3. In each case, three methods of calculating the perceived amplitudes using the visibility threshold are simulated: Monte Carlo (MC), probability map (PM), and linear filtering (LF). While both methods PM & MC use a nonlinear psychometric function, PM is deterministic and MC is not. For more information on calculation of the perceived amplitudes, see [2].

The inclusion of contrast masking makes the numerical observer more closely resemble the human observer performance, in the sense that it removes some of the over performance of numerical observer. Among the six graphs in Fig. 3, the one showing the results of modeling HVS with stCSF plus contrast masking using the PM method for perceived amplitude calculation demonstrates the most significant drop in detection performance with increasing background complexity. Even this graph, however, cannot match the fast drop of detection performance of human observers as listed in Table 1.

4   Conclusion

Our results indicate that by modeling the HVS contrast masking property, lesion detection becomes more difficult in a busier background, as expected from a typical human observer.

This is a work in progress. We plan to continue our work on this project in the following avenues. (i) Experiments are conducted with more human observers and the scores will be aggregated with one-shot multi-reader multi-case ROC analysis [9]. (ii) A more realistic model of background complexity including anatomical and quantum noise using our software phantom will be used to prepare the datasets. (iii) We will explore the extent of our claims for a variety of lesion sizes and types.

Acknowledgement. This work is supported by the US National Institutes of Health (grant 1R01CA154444). Ali Avanaki would like to thank Drs. Kyle Myers, Cédric Marchessoux, and Miguel Eckstein. Dr. Maidment is on the scientific advisory board of Real-Time Tomography, LLC.

References

1. Avanaki, A.N., Espig, K.S., Marchessoux, C., Krupinski, E.A., Bakic, P.R., Kimpe, T.R.L., Maidment, A.D.A.: On modeling the effects of display contrast and luminance in a spatio-temporal numerical observer. MIPS presentation, Washington DC (2013)
2. Avanaki, A.N., Espig, K.S., Maidment, A.D.A., Marchessoux, C., Bakic, P.R., Kimpe, T.R.L.: Development and evaluation of a 3D model observer with nonlinear spatiotemporal contrast sensitivity. To appear in Proc. of SPIE Medical Imaging (2014)
3. Avanaki, A.N., Espig, K.S., Marchessoux, C., Krupinski, E.A., Bakic, P.R., Kimpe, T.R.L., Maidment, A.D.A.: Integration of spatio-temporal contrast sensitivity with a multi-slice channelized Hotelling observer. In: Proc. SPIE Medical Imaging (2013)
4. Zhang, Y., Pham, B.T., Eckstein, M.P.: The Effect of Nonlinear Human Visual System Components on Performance of a Channelized Hotelling Observer Model in Structured Back-grounds. IEEE Trans. on Medical Imaging 25, 1348–1362 (2006)
5. Krupinski, E.A., Lubin, J., Roehrig, H., Johnson, J., Nafziger, J.: Using a human visual system model to optimize soft-copy mammography display: Influence of veiling glare. Acad. Radiol. 13, 289–295 (2006)

6. Winkler, S.: Issues in vision modeling for perceptual video quality assessment. Signal Processing 78, 231–252 (1999)
7. Barten, P.G.J.: Contrast sensitivity of the human eye and its effects on image quality. SPIE Optical Engineering Press, Bellingham (1999)
8. Barni, M., Bartolini, F.: Watermarking Systems Engineering: Enabling Digital Assets Security and Other Applications. CRC Press (2004)
9. Gallas, B.D.: One-shot estimate of MRMC variance: AUC. Acad. Radiol. 13, 353–362 (2006)
10. Pokrajac, D., Maidment, A.D.A., Bakic, P.R.: Optimized Generation of High Resolution Breast Anthropomorphic Software Phantoms. Medical Physics 39, 2290–2302 (2012)
11. Lago, M.A., Maidment, A.D.A., Bakic, P.R.: Modelling of mammographic compression of anthropomorphic software breast phantom using FEBio. In: Proc. Int'l Symposium on Computer Methods in Biomechanics and Biomedical Engineering (CMBBE). Salt Lake City, UT (2013)
12. Kuo, J., Ringer, P., Fallows, S.G., Ng, S., Bakic, P.R., Maidment, A.D.A.: Dynamic reconstruction and rendering of 3D tomosynthesis images. In: Proc. of SPIE, Medical Imaging (2011)
13. Marchessoux, C., Kimpe, T.R.L., Bert, T.: A virtual image chain for perceived and clinical image quality of medical display. J. of Display Technology 4, 356–368 (2008)
14. Platiša, L., Goossens, B., Vansteenkiste, E., Park, S., Gallas, B., Badano, A., Philips, W.: Channelized hotelling observers for the assessment of volumetric imaging data sets. J. of Optical Society of America A 28, 1145–1163 (2011)

Mammography: Radiologist and Image Characteristics That Determine the Accuracy of Breast Cancer Diagnosis

Mohammad A. Rawashdeh, Claudia Mello-Thoms, Roger Bourne, and Patrick C. Brennan

Medical Image Optimisation and Perception Group (MIOPeG), Medical Imaging & Radiation Sciences, Faculty Research Group, The Faculty of Health Sciences, The University of Sydney, Cumberland Campus, 75East Street, Lidcombe, NSW 2141, Australia
{mohammad.rawashdeh,claudia.mello-thoms, roger.bourne,patrick.brennan}@sydney.edu.au

Abstract. Variations in the performance of breast readers are well reported, but key lesion and reader parameters explaining such variations are not fully explored. This large study aims to: 1) measure diagnostic accuracy of breast radiologists, 2) identify parameters linked to higher levels of performance, and 3) establish the key morphological descriptors that impact detection of breast cancer. Methods: Sixty cases, 20 containing cancer, were shown to 129 radiologists. Each reader was asked to locate any malignancies and provide a confidence rating using a scale of 1-5. Details were obtained from each radiologist regarding experience and training and were correlated with jackknifing free response operating characteristic (JAFROC) figure of merit. Cancers were ranked according to the "detectability rating" that is, the number of readers who accurately detected and located the lesion divided by the total number of readers, and this was correlated with various mathematical lesion descriptors. Results: Higher reader performance was positively correlated with number of years reading mammograms (r=0.24, p=0.01), number of mammogram readings per year (r=0.28, p=0.001), and hours reading mammogram per week (r=0.19, p=0.04). For image features and lesion descriptors there was correlation between "detectability rating" and lesion size (r=0.65, p=0.005), breast density (r=-0.64, p=0.007), perimeter (r=0.66, p=0.0004), eccentricity (r= 0.49, p=0.02), and solidity (r=0.78, p< 0.0001). Radiologist experience and lesion morphology may contribute significantly to reduce cancer detection.

Keywords: Digital mammography, radiologist performance, lesion characteristics, lesion assessment, missed cancers.

1 Introduction

Early detection of breast cancer reduces the mortality rate, leads to more effective treatments [1] and is therefore a global health priority when developing national strategies for controlling breast cancer. Screening by mammography is currently the most effective method for the early detection of breast cancer, however, the sensitivity of

H. Fujita, T. Hara, and C. Muramatsu (Eds.): IWDM 2014, LNCS 8539, pp. 731–736, 2014.

mammography is in the 68–92% range [2-3]. The high incidence of breast cancer together with the rate of misdiagnosis highlights the need to direct efforts towards a better understanding of why lesions are being unreported.

Even though perception errors may be considered a principle reason for missing cancers in mammography [4], previous findings suggest that a comprehensive investigation of other features is required [5]. Bird et al. [5] found that missed cancers on mammograms commonly occur in denser breasts, were often present as developing densities, and were most likely to be located in the retroglandular regions. Other authors found that the missed cancers were significantly lower in density, were more often visible on only one of two views and were smaller in size [6]. It has been shown that masses, rather than calcifications, are more commonly undetected [6], which is of concern since a large number of lesions present as palpable, non-calcified tumors [7]. However, few data exist on the impact of other image and lesion appearances like shape and texture.

The accuracy of mammographic image reading among breast readers is highly variable and clinical experience and training can affect readers' performance [8]. Previous work, focused on mammograms, has investigated the effect of training and clinical experience on interpretive performance and have produced conflicting results, even when same populations of breast readers was compered [8,9]. This may be due to limited number of radiologists and mammographic cases along with the varying measures used to define characteristics such as clinical experience in the published studies. This highlights the need for a more detailed analysis of the impact of radiologists' experience and training on performance using a large number of expert readers.

If we are to understand why specific lesion types are being missed on screening mammograms and how detection can be improved, it is necessary to explore experience and training factors that can impact upon performance. In addition, accurate measurements of a number of lesion features are required along with an appreciation of how these features affect lesion detectability.

2   Methodology

Ethics review board approval was received from the participating institutions. A test set of mammograms was developed comprising of 60 digital cases, with each case consisting of four images: a caudal-cranial (CC) and medio-lateral oblique (MLO) projection for each breast. All images were collected by the State Radiologist, BreastScreen New South Wales. There were 20 abnormal cases, each having a biopsy proven malignant lesion. Examples of discrete masses (n=15), asymmetric density (n = 6), and architectural distortions (n = 3) were included and there were no microcalcifications because the focus of this study was mass lesion detection. To ensure that the cases were at least of reasonable difficulty, each malignant lesion had been missed previously by one reader in the course of a normal screen-read session (in Australia, regular clinical practice dictates that each mammogram is double read, with a third reader being used in case of disagreement). The other 40 cases were normal and confirmed by two independent normal screen reads, review of the cases by two expert readers and a follow-up negative screening mammogram two years later.

129 readers were asked to detect and localize the presence of cancer, and their levels of confidence were scored on a scale of 1-5 with 1 representing complete confidence that the case was normal and 5 representing complete confidence that a malignant lesion was present. For a controlled viewing environment, all readings took place in a specialized reading room with an ambient lighting within 12-20 lux at the position of the reader, measured with a calibrated photometer (Model Konica Minolta CL-200, Ramsey, NJ). All images were displayed using two Sectra and two Hologic workstations each driving 5MP reporting monitors. The Sectra workstation was linked to Barco MFGD 5621 monitors (8500 Kortrijk, Belgium) driven by a BarcoMed 5MP 2FH video card and the Hologic displayed images using Eizo Radiforce G51 (Ishikawa 924-8566 Japan) with a Matrox MED5MP-DVI video card. All monitors were calibrated to the Digital Imaging and Communication in Medicine Greyscale Standard Display Function (DICOM GSDF) using the Verilum software and luminance pod (IMAGE Smiths Inc., Germantown, Maryland) and the calibrated photometer described above. Details were obtained from each reader regarding reading experience, qualification, breast reading activities and demographic characteristics, and these were considered with jackknifing free response operating characteristic (JAFROC) figure of merit, location sensitivity and specificity using Spearman correlation.

A lesion was considered correctly detected when it received a confidence scores between 3 – 5 and the location was correctly marked by reader within 2 cm from the center of the lesion, as determined by an expert radiologist who did not participate as a reader in this study. In addition, each lesion was given a "detectability rating" that was calculated by dividing the number of observers who correctly detected and located the lesion by the total number of observers (n=129). Moreover, cancers were ranked according to the detection rate, and this was correlated with following quantities:

(1) Breast density: Each mammogram was categorized using the Breast Imaging Reporting and Data system BI-RADS [10] by a state radiologist (WL) with 20 years' experience reporting mammograms and was independently confirmed by other two expert readers

(2) Mean lesion size: Mean lesion sizes were calculated from three expert readers' measurements.

(3) Lesion shape: All lesions were manually segmented and a number of shape and texture features was then obtained and analyzed using Matlab (version 7.13 by math work). These shape and texture features are summarized here [11]:

- Perimeter: Circumferential distance around lesion boundary.
- Eccentricity: The ratio of the major axis to minor axis of the best fit ellipse which outlines the lesion.
- Solidity: The extent to which the external shape is smooth, calculated by the overall area divided by the convex area (an inverse indicator of the level of spiculation).

(4) Lesion Contrast: Represents the ratio of the signal intensity of the lesion to its background. Contrast was calculated for both local and global background areas as [12]:

- Local: (mean grey level value of lesion - mean grey level value of local background that compromised a region of 1 diameter immediately outside the lesion)/ $\sqrt{(\text{(standard deviation of the lesion)}^2 + \text{(standard deviation of the local background)}^2)}$.
- Global: (mean grey level value of lesion - mean grey level value of whole breast without pectoralis muscle)/ $\sqrt{(\text{(standard deviation of the lesion)}^2 + \text{(standard deviation of the global background)}^2)}$.

All data were analyzed using SPSS 21.0 for Windows (SPSS Inc, Chicago, IL, USA), and statistical significance was established at p<0.05.

3 Results

Median JAFROC figure of merit, location sensitivity and specificity scores across all 129 readers are shown in Table 1 along with 1st and lower 3rd quartile for median.

Table 1. Performance of readers

Score type	Median	1st quartile	3rd Quartile
JAFROC	0.81	0.72	0.87
Sensitivity	0.85	0.75	0.95
Loc sensitivity	0.61	0.58	0.83
Specificity	0.73	0.62	0.83

Table 2. Spearman correlation Analysis of the jack-knife free-response receiver operating characteristic (JAFROC), location sensitivity and specificity value with reader parameters. r values are shown in the table and p values are given in parentheses. Values shown in bold font are statistically significant.

| Parameters Investigated | Values measured | | |
	JAFROC	Location sensitivity	Specificity
Age	0.02 (0.73)	-0.1 (0.12)	0.06 (0.78)
Years of qualification	0.18 (0.05)	-0.16 (0.8)	0.08 (0.35)
Years of mammogram reading	**0.24 (0.01)**	0.6 (0.06)	0.09 (0.17)
Mammograms read per year	**0.28 (0.001)**	**0.25 (0.003)**	**0.18 (0.03)**
Hours reading mammograms per week	**0.19 (0.04)**	0.03 (0.6)	0.07 (0.4)

As might be expected, higher reader performance was positively correlated with number of years reading mammograms (r=0.24, p=0.01); number of mammogram readings per year (r=0.28, p=0.001); and hours reading mammogram per week (r= 0.19, p=0.04) (Table 2).

The "detectability rating" varied from 33% to 95% with mean 60%. For image features, there was a positive correlation between "detectability rating" with lesion size (r= 0.65; p= 0.005) and a negative correlation with breast density (r= -0.64, p= 0.007). In terms of lesion features, there was a significant positive correlation between the "detectability rating" and lesion perimeter (r= 0.66, p= 0.0004) lesion eccentricity (r= 0.49, p= 0.02) and lesion solidity (r= 0.78, p< 0.0001)(Table 3).

Table 3. Details on lesion features and the correlation between the "detectability rating" and the lesion features

Feature	Mean	Min	Max	r value	p value
Breast density	2.56	2	4	**-0.64**	**0.007**
Size (mm)	11.44	6	25	**0.65**	**0.005**
Perimeter	477.6	255	966	**0.66**	**0.0004**
Eccentricity	0.82	0.43	0.98	**0.49**	**0.02**
Solidity	0.67	0.41	0.98	**0.78**	**0.0001**
Local contrast	5.82	0.25	14.75	-0.29	0.18
Global contrast	0.87	0.07	3.69	-0.33	0.11

4   Discussion and Conclusions

Improved reader performance due to reader training and experience was found for years of experience reading mammogram, mammograms read per year and hours reading mammogram per week. In addition, the analyses performed here determined that breast density, lesion size and shape are the key image and lesion categories that affect detection accuracy. Breast density is well studied in the literature and once more highlights the obscuring potential of greater levels of fibroglandular tissue. Size is hardly a surprise but looking at the r and p values in Table 3, it is interesting to note that if a single descriptor of size is to be used, the widest diameter, simply defined by the radiologist using a basic post-processing tool is at least as effective as more procedurally or technically more challenging measures. With regard to shape, an array of key features were shown to improve detection, namely the level of perimeter, eccentricity and solidity. Overall these features imply that the more irregular the perimeter, the more likely radiologists are to miss the cancer.

In conclusion, the current work demonstrates key radiologist and lesion characteristics affecting diagnostic efficacy in mammography. The data should help the development of effective radiology training programmes and the design of future CAD algorithms.

References

1. Ferlay, J., Shin, H.-R., Bray, F., et al.: Estimates of worldwide burden of cancer in 2008: GLOBOCAN 2008. International Journal of Cancer 127(12), 917–2893 (2010)
2. Beam, C.A., Layde, P.M., Sullivan, D.C.: Variability in the Interpretation of Screening Mammograms by US Radiologists: Findings From a National Sample. Arch. Intern. Med. 156(2), 13–209 (1996)
3. Patel, M.R., Whitman, G.J.: Negative mammograms in symptomatic patients with breast cancer. Acad. Radiol. 5, 26–33 (1998)
4. Goergen, S.K., Evans, J., Cohen, G.P., MacMillan, J.: Characteristics of breast carcinomas missed by screening radiologists. Radiology. 204(1), 5–131 (1997)
5. Berlin, L.: Defending the "missed" radiographic diagnosis. AJR Am. J. Roentgenol. 176, 317–322 (2001)
6. Huynh, P.T., Jarolimek, A.M., Daye, S.: The false-negative mammogram. Radiographics 18(5), 54–1137 (1998)
7. Yankaskas, B.C., Schell, M.J., Bird, R.E., Desrochers, D.A.: Reassessment of breast cancers missed during routine screening mammography: A community-based study. AJR Am. J. Roentgenol. 177(3), 41–535 (2001)
8. Barlow, W.E., Chi, C., Carney, P.A., et al.: Accuracy of screening mammography interpretation by characteristics of radiologists. J. Natl. Cancer Inst. 96(24), 1840–1850 (2004)
9. Smith-Bindman, R., Chu, P.W., Miglioretti, D.L., et al.: Comparison of screening mammography in the United States and the United Kingdom. JAMA 290(16), 2129–2137 (2003)
10. American College of Radiology. Breast imaging reporting and data system, breast imaging atlas, 4th edn. American College of Radiology, Reston (2003)
11. Kallergi, M.: Computer-aided diagnosis of mammographic microcalcification clusters. Medical physics 31(2), 26–314 (2004)
12. Manning, D.J., Ethell, S.C., Donovan, T.: Detection or decision errors? Missed lung cancer from the posteroanterior chest radiograph. Br. J. Radiol. 77(915), 231 (2004)

Preliminary Study on Sub-Pixel Rendering for Mammography Medical Grade Color Displays

Katsuhiro Ichikawa and Hiroko Kawashima

Faculty of Health Sciences, Institute of Medical,
Pharmaceutical and Health Sciences, Kanazawa University
{ichikawa,hirokok}@mhs.mp.kanazawa-u.ac.jp

Abstract. The independent sub-pixel driving (ISD) technology, which utilizes sub-pixels included in each normal pixel for image rendering, had been developed for monochrome displays for mammography to improve their resolution and over–all noise properties, and displays with ISD technology has been used for the diagnostic reading on mammography in many institutions. The purpose of this preliminary study was to investigate a possibility of applying the ISD technology to medical color displays on mammography using quantitative resolution and noise evaluations and a visual comparison. A prototype 5 mega-pixel (MP) color display and a 5MP monochrome display were employed. To reduce the micro level color shifts caused by applying the existing ISD driver software to color displays, we implemented an additional low-pass filtering process to the driver software. The quantitative over-all resolution and noise properties for a magnification ratio of 0.4 which is routinely used in diagnostic initial reading of our hospital was measured for three conditions which included two conditions for the color display: Color with ISD (Color-ISD) and color without ISD (Color-normal) and one condition for the monochrome display: Monochrome-normal. Two radiologist visually compared Color-ISD with Monochrome-normal for resolution, noise and color shift using an ACR156 phantom image. Both over-all resolution and noise properties of ISD-color were superior to those of the others. In the visual comparison, Color ISD presented the similar resolution and superior noise properties as compared with Monochrome-normal. The color shift was visually ignorable in the phantom image displaying.

Keywords: color display, Independent sub-pixel driving (ISD), resolution.

1   Introduction

Color displays are increasingly used for diagnostic image readings, and recently some medical color displays for mammography with higher resolutions and maximum luminance have been commercially available and passed the Food and Drug Administration (FDA) clearances. On the other hand, for conventional 5 mega-pixel monochrome displays for mammography, a resolution enhancement technology by the Independent Sub-pixel Driving (ISD) has been developed, and several papers have demonstrated its performances of resolution enhancement and over-all noise reduction [1-5]. The ISD

H. Fujita, T. Hara, and C. Muramatsu (Eds.): IWDM 2014, LNCS 8539, pp. 737–743, 2014.

technology for monochrome displays enables rendering high resolution images by allocating an original image data to sub-pixels according to the sub-pixel pitch which is one third of the normal pixel pitch. By utilizing the sub-pixels for image rendering, an enhanced resolution with tripled Nyquist frequency is achieved in the sub-pixel direction [1]. Moreover, in shrunk (reduced) image displaying, the overall noise property is improved while maintaining the resolution because the aliasing noise contamination is reduce by the finer sampling pitch of the sub-pixel [3,5,6].

The purpose of this preliminary study was to investigate a possibility of applying the ISD technology to medical color displays for mammography using quantitative resolution and noise evaluations and a visual comparison.

2   Methods and Materials

2.1   Sub-pixel Rendering for Color Displays

When the driver software is applied to a color display, micro level color shifts were appeared, and the color shifts impair the quality of displayed image, while maintaining the original macro level white balance of the display. To reduce the color shifts, we implemented an additional low-pass filtering (LPF) by a three-point weighted average in the sub-pixel direction before the original sub-pixel rendering step in the ISD driver software. In the adjustment of the strength of LPF, we visually inspected displayed clinical mammography images of 20 cases with micro calcifications, and determined a strength by which the micro level color shifts became negligible and resolution degradation by LPF became minimal. The use of clinical mammography data was approved by the institutional ethics committees.

2.2   Displays and Measurements

A 5 mega-pixel (MP) monochrome display, MS51i2 (Totoku, Japan) and a 5MP prototype medical color display provided by Totoku both calibrated at a maximum luminance of 500 cd/m^2 were employed. We compared three display conditions which consisted of two conditions for the color display: color with ISD (Color-ISD) and color without ISD (Color-normal), and one condition for the monochrome display: Monochrome without ISD (Monochrome-normal). The bi-linear interpolation, one of the popular resampling technique for image displaying (image shrinking and maginification), was used in the image rendering for three conditions.

A bar-pattern test image which consisted of five bar-patterns with bar widths of 1, 2, 3, 4, and 6 pixels (Fig. 1a) was displayed with each condition for the resolution measurement. The magnification ratio was set to 0.4 (pixel by pixel: 1.0) which is routinely used in the diagnostic mammography reading of our university hospital. The displayed bar-pattern images were acquired with a high-resolution digital camera (D90, Nikon, Japan), and then the raw image data was analyzed using a dedicated software based on a previously published method for the modulation transfer function (MTF) of displays [7].

To measure overall noise properties, an X-ray image of an ACR156 mammography phantom, which was acquired by a full-field mammography system (Micro Dose Mammography L30, Sectra, Sweden), was used. The averaged glandular dose (AGD) of the image was 0.8 mGy. The phantom image was displayed with each condition with the magnification ration of 0.4. A flat area without any simulated objects in each displayed phantom image was acquired with D90 as shown in Fig. 1b, and then analyzed using a dedicated software based on a previously published method for the noise power spectrum (NPS) for displays [8].

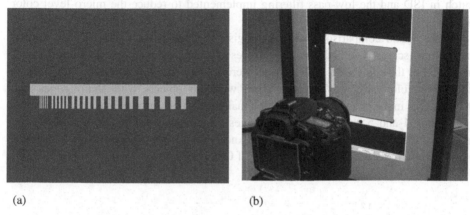

(a)   (b)

Fig. 1. (a) Bar-pattern test image for resolution measurement. (b)   experimental setup for overall noise measurement.

2.3   Visual Comparison

Two radiologists who had 18 and 33 years experiences visually compared the resolution and noise of the ACR156 phantom images displayed on the color display with Color-ISD and on the monochrome display with Monochrome-normal. The displays were placed side-by-side, and the observers evaluated Color-ISD compared with Monochrome-normal using a five-point scale (+2 = very good, +1 = good, 0 = fair, -1 = poor, +2 = very poor). Magnification ratios on both displays were 0.4. In addition, the observer evaluated the color shift in the displayed image of Color ISD using another five-point scale (1: no change, 2: negligible, 3: acceptable, 4: partly unacceptable, 5: unacceptable).

3   Results

Figure 2 shows MTF results in the sub-pixel direction for three conditions we examined. Color ISD presented a significantly higher MTF than those of the other conditions. Though the higher MTF was indicated by the sub-pixel rendering of ISD, conspicuous micro level color shifts occurred at edges of the bars was problematic. MTF of Color-normal was a little higher than that of Monochrome normal. This was caused by the sharp (triangle like) profile of each pixel, which was formed by the arrangement of red, green and blue sub-pixels in which the green has the highest luminance.

Figure 3 shows NPS results for three conditions. Color ISD indicated lower NPS values compared to the others in the frequency region less than 8.0 cycles/mm. This was due to the aliasing noise reduction caused by the oversampling with the sub-pixel pitch in ISD and the low-pass filtering implemented to reduce the micro level color shift.

In the visual comparison, both radiologists evaluated that ColorISD had similar resolution (scores = 0) and less noise (sores = +1) as compared with Monochrome-normal. For the color shift, both answers were 2 (negligible). It was suspected that the ignorable color shift was because there were no objects with sharp edges like bar-patterns in the phantom image, which make the color shifts visible.

Figures 4 and 5 shows displayed images of simulated micro calcifications with a size of 0.5 mm and a mass with a thickness of 2.0 mm, respectively. Noise was significantly reduced in displayed images of Color-ISD.

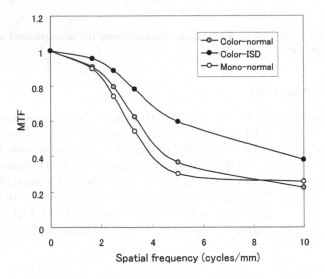

Fig. 2. MTF results of Color-ISD, Color-normal and Monochrome-normal in sub-pixel direction. Color ISD presented a significantly higher MTF than those of the other conditions, while conspicuous micro level color shifts occurred at edges of the bars in the bar-pattern test image.

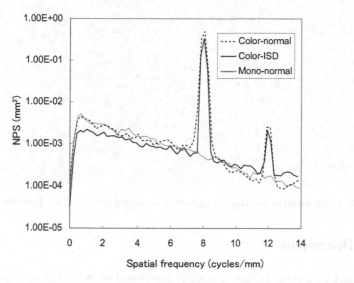

Fig. 3. NPS results of Color-ISD, Color-normal and Monochrome-normal in sub-pixel direction. Color ISD indicated lower NPS values compared to the others in the frequency region less than 8.0 cycles/mm.

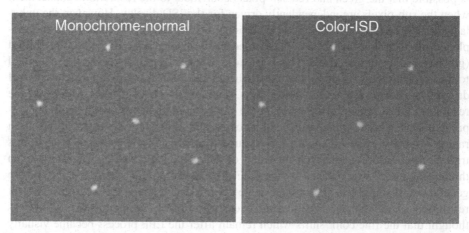

Fig. 4. Comparison of displayed images of simulated micro calcifications with a size of 0.5 mm

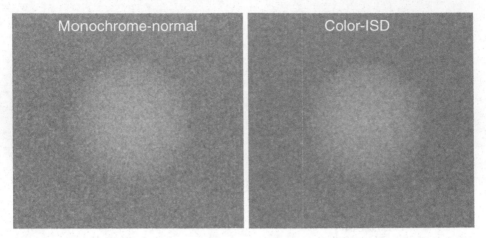

Fig. 5. Comparison of displayed images of a simulated mass with the thickness of 2.0 mm

4   Discussion

Each pixel on a color display is actually composed of individual red, green, and blue sub-pixels. Between them, the green sub-pixel has the highest luminance, followed by the red and blue sub-pixels. The luminance of blue sub-pixel is one sixth and one third of those of green and red sub-pixels in monochrome image displaying, respectively. Thus, the green and red sub-pixels are dominant for resolution rendering, and it is possible that the green and red sub-pixels contribute to the resolution enhancement when the sub-pixels are independently driven for the ISD display. However, the unbalanced sub-pixel drive levels cause a chromaticity change of the pixel, and the displayed monochrome image is contaminated by unnatural patterns with color-shifted (green or red weighted) pixels. This is because the ISD technique has not been applied to the color displays. In this study, we applied a LPF process to data for the sub-pixel driving, aiming to reduce the color shifts. Though this LPF of course reduced the resolution enhancement effect of ISD, the image contamination was effectively improved. This is because the visual evaluation results of resolution were "fair" for both radiologists. By using ISD, since the Nyquist frequency in the sub-pixel direction is tripled, the resolution enhancement effect of ISD is remarkable [1]. Therefore, even though the effect was reduced by the LPF process, some of the effect remained. In general, RGB sub-pixels appear as a single color to the human eye due to insufficient resolution of the human eye to resolve each sub-pixel. From this reason, it was thought that the fine color shifts which remain after the LPF process became visually negligible and simultaneously the remained resolution enhancement effect could not also be recognized.

Another preferable feature of ISD is overall noise (aliasing noise) reduction effect due to over sampling with the fine sub-pixel pitch [3,5,6]. The effect was fortunately enhanced by the LPF process, the overall noise property, when the phantom image was displayed, was significantly improved as shown in Fig. 4 and 5, and obtained evaluation scores of "good" from both radiologists. Since most of mammography images include noise depending on their radiation doses, it was suspected that this overall noise reduction would contribute the image quality improvement. In regards to question "Which display is preferable for mammography reading between these monochrome and color 5MP displays?", both radiologists answered "Color display" with additional comments that admired the lower black level of the color display. Though only the reduced display condition (magnification ratio = 0.4) was examined in this study, the ISD process did not cause any resolution change and color shifts for pixel by pixel or magnification conditions.

5   Conclusion

By applying the modified ISD driver software to the prototype 5MP color display, the resolution and the overall noise properties were improved as compared with the monochrome 5MP display for the reduced display condition which is routinely used for the initial display in diagnostic reading. Though the micro level color shift caused by the sub-pixel rendering was problematic for the test pattern image displaying, it was visually negligible in the phantom image displaying. Further investigations using clinical images would be needed to evaluate the effectiveness of ISD for color displays.

References

1. Ichikawa, K., Hasegawa, M., Kimura, N., Kodera, Y.: A new resolution enhancement technology using the independent sub-pixel driving for the medical liquid crystal displays. IEEE/OSA Journal of Display Technology 4(4), 377–382 (2008)
2. Ichikawa, K., Kawashima, H., Kimura, N., Hasegawa, M.: Clinical Usefulness of Super High-Resolution Liquid Crystal Displays Using Independent Sub-pixel Driving Technology. In: Krupinski, E.A. (ed.) IWDM 2008. LNCS, vol. 5116, pp. 84–90. Springer, Heidelberg (2008)
3. Ichikawa, K., Nishi, Y., Hayashi, S., Hasegawa, M., Kodera, Y.: Noise Reduction Effect in Super-high Resolution LCDs using Independent Sub-pixel Driving Technology. In: Proc. SPIE, 6917, 69171F:1-8 (2008)
4. Nishimura, A., Ichikawa, K., Mochiya, Y., Morishita, A., Kawashima, H., Yamamoto, T., Hasegawa, M., Kimura, N., Sanada, S.: Preliminary investigation of the clinical usefulness of super-high-resolution LCDs with 9 and 15 mega-sub-pixels: Observation studies with phantoms. Radiol. Phys. Technol. 3, 70–77 (2010)
5. Yamazaki, A., Ichikawa, K., Funahashi, M.: Theoretical demonstration of image characteristics and image formation process depending on image displaying conditions on liquid crystal display. In: Proc. SPIE 8318, 83181R:1-8 (2012)
6. Yamazaki, A., Ichikawa, K., Kodera, Y., Funahashi, M.: Overall noise characteristics of reduced images on liquid crystal display and advantages of independent subpixel driving technology. Med. Phys. 40(2), 021901 (2013) (in press)
7. Ichikawa, K., Kodera, Y., Fujita, H.: MTF measurement method for medical displays by using a barpattern Image. Journal of SID 14(10), 831–837 (2006)
8. Ichikawa, K., Hasegawa, M., Kimura, N., Kodera, Y., Takemura, A., Matsubara, K., Nishimura, A.: Analysis method of noise power spectrum for medical monochrome liquid crystal displays. Radiol. Phys. Technol. 1(2), 201–207 (2008)

Impact of Color Calibration on Breast Biopsy Whole Slide Image Interpretation Accuracy and Efficiency

Elizabeth A. Krupinski[1], Louis D. Silverstein[2], Syed F. Hashmi[1],
Anna R. Graham[3], Ronald S. Weinstein[3], and Hans Roehrig[1]

[1] Department of Medical Imaging, University of Arizona, Tucson, AZ USA
krupinski@radiology.arizona.edu
[2] VCD Sciences, Inc. 9695 E Yucca St. Scottsdale, AZ USA
[3] Department of Pathology, University of Arizona, Tucson, AZ USA

Abstract. Color LCD use is increasing in medical imaging especially in applications like telepathology. Standardized methods for calibrating, characterizing and profiling color displays have not been created. We used a validated calibration, characterization and profiling protocol for color medical imaging applications to determine if it impacts performance accuracy and interpretation time. 250 breast biopsy whole slide image (WSI) areas (half malignant, half benign) were displayed to 6 pathologists. In one condition the calibration protocol was used and in the other the same display was un-calibrated. Receiver Operating Characteristic area under the curve (Az) with the calibrated display was 0.8570 and with the un-calibrated one was 0.8488 (p = 0.4112). For interpretation time, the mean with the calibrated display was 4.895 sec and with the un-calibrated display was 6.304 sec (p = 0.0460). There is an advantage diagnostically using a properly calibrated and color-managed display and a significant advantage for potentially improving workflow via reduced viewing times.

Keywords: Color displays, diagnostic accuracy, color calibration, color management, pathology.

1   Introduction

There has been a lot of research on how to calibrate medical-grade and non-medical grade displays for radiology, but for the most part radiology uses monochrome displays and grayscale images, so the methods are not applicable to color. Color displays are needed in other diagnostic imaging applications such as pathology, ophthalmology and telemedicine, but the available displays and images vary in size, contrast, resolution, luminance, color primaries, color gamut, and white point.

Some standards exist for image acquisition [1-2], but guidance on display calibration lacks consensus [3-6]. There is no single validated color display calibration protocol in place for medical color image applications. A key barrier in adoption of whole slide imaging (WSI) in pathology is the display. To address this, we developed a calibration, characterization and profiling protocol for color-critical medical imaging applications [7].

H. Fujita, T. Hara, and C. Muramatsu (Eds.): IWDM 2014, LNCS 8539, pp. 744–748, 2014.
© Springer International Publishing Switzerland 2014

2   Methods and Materials

The color calibration protocol details are in [7], with a complete description of the black-level correction methodology compatible with the color profile structure specified by the International Color Consortium (ICC) methods for color management.

In sum, the process is a multi-step one that begins with calibrating a display using the manufacturer's software, internal LUTs and a standard luminance monitor. Ambient illumination is set at 35 lux. The X,Y,Z of the white point and R,G,B primaries are measured; then the values are normalized to Y (luminance) of the white point. The tone reproduction curves (TRCs) are then measured and a Chromatic Adaptation Matrix (Chad) is computed and applied.

In the next step, the TRCs are interpolated to 256 levels via cubic spline interpolation and the TRC values are normalized between 0 and 1. A black level correction is then applied. The ICC profile (V2/V4) is then generated and finally a color reproduction accuracy analysis is carried out.

Measuring and accounting for the display black level is important for color reproduction since the liquid crystal panel serves as an array of filtered light valves that modulate illumination from a backlight module that constantly emits light (i.e., there is always some light leakage even in the pixel off state). Physical characterization of displays calibrated with and without the protocol demonstrates that high color reproduction accuracy can be achieved.

Regions of interest from WSI stained breast biopsy specimens were selected from a set of 93 uncompressed WSIs (see Figure 1) as being those that contain diagnostic information. They were acquired with the DMetrix ultra-rapid WSI scanner that uses an array microscope for imaging and produces 1.5 x 1.5-cm virtual slides in less than 1 minute (0.47 μm per pixel resolution). Diagnoses were verified by the original report and a second confirmatory review by a Board Certified pathologist not participating in the study.

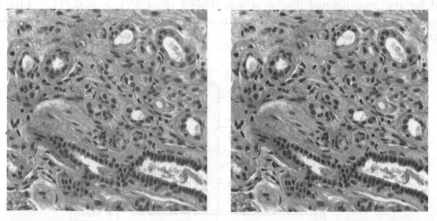

Fig. 1. Typical ROI from a case on a calibrated (left) and un-calibrated (right) display

Regions (512 x 512) were selected as those containing relevant diagnostic information for deciding if a case was benign or malignant. The ROIs were chosen to have good quality in terms of no blurring due to the scanning process, and no excess tissue material irrelevant to the task (e.g., blood cells). A total of 250 ROIs (half benign, half malignant) were selected.

Six pathologists participated in two sessions (counterbalanced and separated by a few weeks to promote forgetting of the cases). There were 2 Board certified pathologists, one senior Fellow, and 3 senior level pathology residents in the study. All of them had some experience with WSI.

One of the sessions used a calibrated/color managed NEC 2690 LCD (1920 x 1200; Lmax = 320 cd/m^2; contrast ratio = 1000:1; wide gamut) and the other session used a matched, non-medical grade, un-calibrated NEC 2690 LCD without color management. Images were shown at full resolution using a dedicated interface we developed for this study. They were not allowed to zoom/pan or adjust any of the viewing parameters (so as not to confound the main aspect of the study – the color rendering).

The pathologists were instructed to determine for each WSI if the tissue was benign or malignant and report their decision confidence using a 6-point scale (1 = benign, definite; 6 = malignant definite). Decision times were also recorded as a measure of diagnostic efficiency. Three of the subjects viewed the images on the color managed/calibrated display first then about 3 weeks later on the un-calibrated display; while the other three viewed the images in the opposite order. The room lights were set to 25 lux. Each subject was given Ishihara's Test for Color Deficiency (Kanehara Trading, Inc. Tokyo, Japan) and all passed.

3   Results

Multi-Reader Multi-Case Receiver Operating Characteristic (MRMC ROC) was used to generate Az (area under the curve) values [8]. Analysis of Variance (ANOVA) was used to test for significant differences. ROC Az for the calibrated display was 0.8570; and for the un-calibrated display it was 0.8488 (F = 0.71, p = 0.4112). Five of six readers had higher performance with the calibrated than un-calibrated display (see Figure 2).

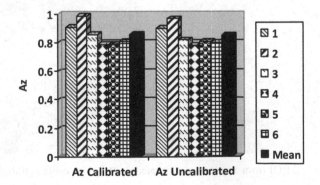

Fig. 2. Individual and mean ROC Az values for un-calibrated vs calibrated displays

For interpretation speed (see Table 1), the mean calibrated total viewing time was 4.90 sec; and the mean total viewing time for the un-calibrated display was 6.30 sec which was statistically significant (p = 0.0460).

Table 1. Viewing times for calibrated and un-calibrated displays

Reader	Calibrated (sec)	Un-calibrated (sec)
1	7.1	11.9
2	4.0	4.1
3	5.8	4.2
4	2.8	7.0
5	3.1	8.0
6	2.0	1.7
Mean	4.90	6.30

4   Discussion

This work represents one of the first studies to assess whether calibrating color displays for breast biopsy WSI impacts observer accuracy and efficiency and may have significant implications for how pathologists carry out quality control measures in digital reading rooms.

We did not observe a significant impact on accuracy with the color managed/calibrated display but there was a trend for performance being better with the calibrated display. We did observe a significant impact on efficiency. Times to view the WSI with the un-calibrated display were about 1 sec longer than with the calibrated display.

Recall that the images we used were small ROIs and not the whole version. If the whole images were used, the difference would likely increase and cumulatively could lead to significantly longer viewing times when viewing large numbers of cases over an extended period of time. There are other variables that impact viewing time, but if proper calibration of a display (which is a fairly simple thing to do) could reduce just this one factor it could increase overall efficiency and possible even greater use and acceptance of WSI.

With respect to why there was no significant difference in diagnostic accuracy, it may be that although color is important there are many other diagnostic features pathologists use when interpreting cases. Sophisticated color rendering and calibration just may not be as important as you would think. Features like the configuration of cells and cell structures are very important as well when determining whether a specimen is benign or malignant or what stage for example a cancer may be at. Color might help the pathologist visualize structures, but it may be that the physical configuration and relationship between the structures is more informative and important for diagnoses.

It also may be that un-calibrated non-medical grade displays are already really good in accurately reproducing and rendering color information. The improvements seen in physical characterizations with more sophisticated calibration methods may be dramatic but are only marginally important visually. It also may be that other types of pathology images with different stains, different diagnostic features etc. may require accurate color rending while breast biopsy specimens with the H&E stain may not.

Finally, the images we used may not be that dependent on the color information for their interpretation as another set might have been. There are often very distinct and significant differences in the appearance of different specimen samples depending on the organ, the disease, and the type of staining. Maybe breast biopsy specimens are not dependent on color information but other specimens may be. We need to conduct more research in this area and include other types of specimens and staining techniques.

5   Conclusions

We observed a marginal impact on diagnostic accuracy for breast biopsy WSI interpretation as a function of using a formally color managed/calibrated display - there was a trend for performance being better with the calibrated display. There was a significant impact on interpretation speed with the calibrated display yielding shorter viewing times. Further study is warranted since we only used one display and one specimen type.

Using eye-position recording might also reveal some interesting findings in terms of why search and thus viewing times are shorter with calibrated displays. For example, does it take less time to find relevant cells to view and make a decision? Further research is needed.

Acknowledgement. This work was supported in part by NIH/ARRA Grant 1R01EB007311-01A2.

References

1. Krupinski, E.A., Burdick, A., Pak, H., et al.: American Telemedicine Association's Practice Guidelines for Teledermatology. Telemed. J. eHealth 14, 289–302 (2008)
2. Cavalcanti, P.G., Scharcanski, J., Lopes, C.B.O.: Shading attenuation in human skin color. In: Bebis, G., et al. (eds.) ISVC 2010, Part I. LNCS, vol. 6453, pp. 190–198. Springer, Heidelberg (2010)
3. Li, H.K., Esquivel, A., Techavipoo, U., et al.: Teleophthalmology computer display calibration. Invest. Ophthalmol. Vis. Sci. 46, E-abstract 4580 (2005)
4. Li, H.K., Esquivel, A., et al.: Mosaics versus early treatment diabetic retinopathy seven standard fields for evaluation of diabetic retinopathy. Retina 31, 1553–1563 (2011)
5. Ricur, G., Zaldivar, R., Batiz, M.G.: Cataract and refractive surgery post-operative care: Teleophthalmology's challenge in Argentina. In: Yogesan, K., Kumar, S., Goldschmidt, L. (eds.) Teleophthalmology, pp. 213–226. Springer, Berlin (2006)
6. Van Poucke, S., Haeghen, Y.V., Vissers, K., et al.: Automatic colorimetric calibration of human wounds. BMC. Med. Imag. 10, 7 (2010)
7. Silverstein, L.D., Hashmi, S.F., Lang, K., Krupinski, E.A.: Paradigm for achieving color reproduction accuracy in LCDs for medical imaging. J. Soc. Info. Disp. 20, 53–62 (2012)
8. Dorfman, D.D., Berbaum, K.S., Metz, C.E.: Receiver operating characteristic rating analysis: Generalization to the population of readers and patients with the jackknife method. Invest. Radiol. 27, 723–731 (1992)

Author Index